Nursing
AND
Cancer

Nancy Burns, R.N., Ph.D.

ASSISTANT PROFESSOR
SCHOOL OF NURSING
UNIVERSITY OF TEXAS AT ARLINGTON
ARLINGTON, TEXAS

1982

W. B. Saunders Company

Philadelphia   London   Toronto   Mexico City   Rio de Janeiro   Sydney   Tokyo

W. B. Saunders Company: West Washington Square
Philadelphia, PA   19105

1 St. Anne's Road
Eastbourne, East Sussex BN21 3UN, England

1 Goldthorne Avenue
Toronto, Ontario M8Z 5T9, Canada

Apartado 26370 — Cedro 512
Mexico 4, D.F., Mexico

Rua Coronel Cabrita, 8
Sao Cristovao Caixa Postal 21176
Rio de Janeiro, Brazil

9 Waltham Street
Artarmon, N.S.W. 2064, Australia

Ichibancho, Central Bldg., 22-1 Ichibancho
Chiyoda-Ku, Tokyo 102, Japan

Library of Congress Cataloging in Publication Data

Burns, Nancy, Ph.D.

Nursing and cancer.

1. Cancer — Nursing.   I. Title. [DNLM: 1. Neoplasms —
  Nursing. WY 156 B967n]

RC266.B87	610.73′698	81–48467
ISBN 0–7216–2184–8		AACR2

Nursing and Cancer   ISBN 0-7216-2184-8

Last digit is the print number: 9   8   7   6   5   4   3   2   1

To Cancer Patients and Their Families

PREFACE

I remember as a new masters graduate how frustrated I was with the existing literature on cancer nursing. Little was available and that which was seemed to me to be very simplistic, examining only a small fragment of nursing care of the hospitalized patient. I remember visiting a publishing booth at a nursing convention. The person at the booth showed me one of the current books on cancer nursing. I told her how poor I thought the book was. The author happened to be in the booth. I was introduced to her, and she patiently sat and listened as I told her all of the things I thought were wrong with her book. I will always appreciate her tolerance, for from this exchange came the drive I needed to go beyond what was currently available — to search for greater knowledge, earn a doctorate, and write a book.

My original desire in writing this book was to make it perfect, to demonstrate a high level of knowledge in all areas of cancer nursing and thus contribute significantly to the quality of cancer nursing care. Eventually I realized that even 20 or 30 years of research and experience would not be enough to result in the perfect book. Therefore, after devoting much time and hard work to writing, I come to you with a book that reflects very much the present state of my knowledge. It is my hope that both students and those already in clinical practice will be able to use this book — the result of what I have experienced and learned thus far — in their care of patients who have cancer.

Nursing and Cancer is an unusual aggregate of theoretical orientations that can be useful in cancer nursing and practical down-to-earth strategies for providing care. The book examines the care that is now commonly given, the care that could be given, and the arena within which care occurs. The purpose of the book is to present a comprehensive examination of the newly emerging field of cancer nursing and to develop a framework of nursing practice within which this knowledge can be organized. I believe strongly that nursing practice must be broadly based on knowledge from many fields of study, including pathophysiology, psychology, and sociology. However, knowledge from these fields must be integrated carefully with nursing knowledge before it can be useful in nursing practice. A theoretical framework of nursing practice is not very useful unless it can be effectively applied in the many settings within which nursing occurs. I have tried throughout the book to tie theory to the realities of nursing practice.

The book is organized into four major sections: I, The Cancer Picture; II, The Medical Management of Cancer and the Nurse's Role; III, The Nursing Management of Cancer; and IV, Cancer Nursing Beyond the Hospital Walls. The first section consists of five chapters examining common beliefs about cancer that have a profound effect on society and health care, in addition to discussion of the physical development of cancer, the major theories of the etiology of cancer, physical assessment in the diagnosis of cancer, and the ethical implications of nursing practice involving cancer. The second section contains five chapters that describe in detail the medical management of the cancer patient and nursing responsibilities related to the medical care. Topics addressed in this section are the current state of the art of cancer nursing practice in the hospital, cancer surgery, radiotherapy, chemotherapy, and the very new field of immunotherapy. The third section includes four chapters, in which the most common nursing problems of cancer care are identified and discussed within the framework of the nursing process. Subjects considered are physiologic problems, psychosocial problems, situations unique to the child with cancer, and care of the dying patient. The fourth section examines cancer nursing within the realm of community health nursing, which includes rehabilitation of the cancer patient, support groups, home care, and the impact of cancer nursing on larger social and political systems.

So many people have influenced my knowledge in this field of study that the list could easily go on for pages. I would particularly like to thank Rhett Fredric, M.D., who helped me develop my skills in physical assessment of the cancer patient and who pushed me to seek knowledge of oncology far beyond where I thought I could go; Peggy Chinn, R.N., Ph.D., who helped me explore beliefs about cancer; Barbara Carper, R.N., Ed.D.; who guided me into the world of ethics and theories; Bernard Rubal, Ph.D., who helped me search through the field of pathophysiology; and Pat Mahon, R.N., Ph.D., who helped me explore the world of the inner self. My friends in clinical practice have been an invaluable source of information and support. They are, after all, the real "experts" in this field. They have been kind enough to review my writing and often provided helpful suggestions. I am also grateful to Donald Fernbach, M.D., for reviewing Chapter 13, "The Child with Cancer."

Support while writing is essential, for it can be a very lonely experience sometimes. I received encouragement from so many sources: The Dean and Faculty of the University at Texas at Arlington School of Nursing; all of my friends in the American Cancer Society, Texas Division; and most of all, from my family — Jerry, Robin, Melody, and Brady — who endured four years of the tremendous impact on family functioning that must occur with wife and mother completing a doctorate and writing a book at the same time.

CONTENTS

PART I
THE CANCER PICTURE 1

1 Cancer Beliefs, Social Expectations, and Health Care 3

2 The Nature of Cancer 19

3 The Etiology of Cancer: Current Theories 39

4 The Diagnosis of Cancer 62

5 Values, Ethics, and Ethical Dilemmas in Cancer
Nursing 77

PART II
THE MEDICAL MANAGEMENT OF CANCER AND THE
NURSE'S ROLE 87

6 Hospital Nursing Care for the Cancer Patient:
What It Is and What It Can Be 89

7 Surgery 102

8 Radiotherapy 122

9 Chemotherapy 146

10 Immunotherapy 191

PART III
THE NURSING MANAGEMENT OF CANCER 207

11 Nursing Care Related to Physiologic Conditions 209

vii

12 Psychosocial Aspects of Nursing Care 261

13 The Child with Cancer 288

14 Care of the Dying Patient.. 298

PART IV
CANCER NURSING BEYOND THE HOSPITAL WALLS 329

15 Rehabilitation and Cancer.. 331

16 Cancer Support Groups... 340

17 Home Care of the Cancer Patient 352

18 The Nursing Impact: Cancer and the Social and
    Political Systems.. 363

Index 383

1

The Cancer Picture

1

Cancer Beliefs, Social Expectations, and Health Care

INTRODUCTION

Cancer is a word that elicits an immediate emotional response, a response that seems to have no relationship to rational thinking, depth of knowledge of the individual, or the individual's role in society. The same response seems to occur in physicians, nurses, college professors, researchers, politicians, and unskilled laborers alike. It occurs in patients, families, friends of those who have cancer, people who think they may have cancer, or people who take the view that cancer is something that will happen to other people. In all of these groups, the feelings and mental images stirred up by the mention or thought of the word cancer seem to be practically identical.

CANCER BELIEFS

The Connotations of Cancer

The feelings and mental images aroused by the word cancer make up a complex of ideas that are tied together to form our concept of what cancer means. These ideas are all present to some degree and include an association of cancer with:

1. Death[44, 51, 84]
2. Feelings of hopelessness, helplessness, worthlessness, and shame[44, 51, 84]
3. Development of severe chronic intractable pain[14, 44, 51, 84]
4. Contagion[14]
5. Uncontrolled growth eating away inside the body[10, 26]
6. Social isolation[44, 84]
7. Rejection[44, 51, 84]
8. Not belonging[84]
9. Not being wanted and loved[84]
10. Feelings of dirtiness[51]
11. Foul smells[51]
12. Withering away of life's essential elements[51]
13. Chronic debility[51]
14. Costly medical care[44]
15. Punishment[3]
16. Mutilation[14, 44, 84]
17. Sudden, overwhelming life changes[84]
18. Uncertain future[44]

Because these ideas are very frightening and the incidence of cancer is high, people frequently think about and talk about cancer.[46] Cancer is associated uppermost with impending death, to the point that the two words are almost considered synonymous. Thinking about cancer increases our awareness that we are mortal and that we will die, possibly as a result of cancer. We feel that cancer is completely outside our control; that it is useless to try to do anything to prevent it, to slow it down, or to treat it; and that regardless of what is done, the ultimate result will be death.[46]

Social Consequences

Many people consider cancer to be the leprosy of our time. The social stigma asso-

3

ciated with it is devastating to both patient and family.[95] Many people feel that the person who has cancer does not deserve to receive treatment. They feel that these patients should not take up the valuable time of health care givers or use family resources to pay for the care or treatment they need. Because of the shame associated with cancer, the diagnosis is sometimes communicated to other people in whispers. Those who die of it are often said in their obituaries to have died of an "extended illness."

Sometimes the patient and family attempt to prevent the diagnosis of cancer from becoming known, often because of fear of the social isolation that they expect to occur when cancer is diagnosed. Friends and even family may begin to react differently to the person with cancer. There may be less touching, less eye contact. Conversations may be held standing at greater distances from the person.[15] Persons with cancer are often gradually left out of the social circles within which they normally operate. Sometimes they are even abandoned by their spouse.

Expressions in the Literature

Many articles and books on cancer refer to the emotional responses that cancer evokes. Some of the more vivid descriptions are included here as direct quotations to retain the precise wording and original emotional impact.

In the first place, cancer is the most feared of all diseases. People continue to think of cancer as a killer, and both patients and physicians use euphemisms to avoid the dreaded word. What is impressive is that the doctors themselves feel very much the same way.[2]

These phenomena of rejection, withdrawal and fear are further reflected in the stereotyped picture of cancer. People with cancer are expected to have a death-like look and to give off an odor of decaying flesh; cancer "consumes," causes persons to be eaten up by it! The course envisioned is that of rapid, downhill progression ending in painful and horrible death. Some patients reported that friends have made such statements as "You don't look — or smell — as though you have cancer!" As a result of such experiences, patients begin to realize that they are expected to be different and that they are perceived as different from others even though their cancer may not be visible.[26]

The diagnosis still tends to evoke irrational, emotional responses in both physician and patient — a legacy of terror centuries old. . . . Cancer as a chronic, progressive, often fatal disease evokes more terror and helplessness than other chronic, progressive, often fatal diseases. It is suggested that it is because the diagnosis is associated with fantasies of being devoured by a relentless, uncompromising, invidious process which is equated with death.[10]

Cancer is equated with more than death; it is equated with a manner of living and dying in chronic and endless debility accompanied by loss of muscular power and control. It is equated with a withering away of life's essential elements, and is associated with foul smells, feelings of dirtiness, hopeless irrevocability, severe and relentless pain and eventual death after weeks and months of this suffering. It is associated with fears of being a burden and fears of being abandoned.[51]

And when cancer itself is the leading actor in the prospective tragedy, all the usual emotions involved are magnified and generally new ones enter in. The word itself may very well be the most frightening one in our vocabulary and this is probably just as true for the doctor and his medical allies as it is for the layman. The big "C" is truly and literally the "fate worse than death" and the emotional stresses involved in dealing with its victims are augmented for the doctor in ways both real and imagined. Dedicated to preserving life, he faces the prospect of coping with his own feelings of helplessness, frustration and failure as his patient slips away. And no one is more acutely aware than he what an emotional upheaval the truth will precipitate for both victim and his family when they are told that Nemesis has struck, has recurred, or has metastasized.[21]

Loneliness and depression haunt cancer patients. Frequently they feel isolated by their new identity — "cancer patient." They often think of themselves as dying and they are related to as dying persons. Life changes, forced retirements, and limited social activities, all due to their cancer, contribute to their sense of loss and isolation.[73]

Fatalism and superstition sometimes cause people to believe that nothing can be done anyway, so why bother? They confuse the diagnosis of cancer with terminal illness, which is, of course, an incorrect assumption. However, prediagnostic pessimism often reflects a general attitude toward other problems: apathetic surrender, resistance is impossible, fate will have its way. There are also people who firmly believe that virtue is rewarded, and that being "good," i.e., abstemious, conscientious, prudent, and pious, will protect them. One man . . . was convinced that cancer is a dirty disease, not neat and clean, like a heart attack. Unfortunately, this is a common prejudice.[30]

Although the way in which disease mystifies is set against a backdrop of new expectations, the disease itself (once TB, cancer today) arouses thoroughly old-fashioned kinds of dread. Any disease that is treated as a mystery and acutely enough feared will be felt to be morally, if not literally, contagious. Thus, a surprisingly large number of people with cancer find themselves being shunned by relatives and friends and are the object of practices of decontamination by members of their household, as if cancer, like TB, were an infectious disease. Contact with someone afflicted with a disease regarded as a mysterious malevolency inevitably feels like a trespass; worse, like the violation of a taboo. The very names of such diseases are felt to have a magic power. . . . (Cancer patients are lied to, not just because the disease is (or is thought to be) a death sentence, but because it is felt to be obscene — in the original meaning of that word: ill-omened, abominable, repugnant to the senses.[85]

Research About Cancer Beliefs

Workers in nursing, medicine, and social work have all indicated interest in and concern about the connotations of the word cancer. Little research, however, has been done in this area. The American Cancer Society conducted national sample surveys in 1948, 1964, and 1979. The 1964 survey by Horn and Waingrow[45] indicated that 38 per cent of those interviewed felt that the patient is not likely to tell people that he or she has cancer; 12 per cent indicated that they would not be willing to work next to someone who had cancer; 12 per cent did not believe cancer was curable; and 6 per cent of those surveyed believed that cancer was contagious. The percentage of people who held these views had decreased since the 1948 survey.

The 1979 survey was conducted by Lieberman Research, Inc.[1] This study indicated that people continue to experience a considerable degree of fearfulness and anxiety about cancer. Forty-nine per cent agreed that the word cancer itself scared

them. Thirty-seven per cent believed that cancer was the worst thing that could happen to a person. Thirty-six per cent considered cancer to be a death sentence for most people. Twenty per cent skipped over news stories about cancer. Sixteen per cent did not believe that a cure for cancer would ever be found. Sixteen per cent stated that if they got cancer they would prefer not to know about it. Nine per cent would feel uncomfortable working next to someone who had cancer.

Other surveys have borne out the results of the American Cancer Society's findings. In 1965 public health nurses in England were surveyed to determine their opinions toward cancer. Twenty per cent of the nurses surveyed held the pessimistic attitude that hospital treatment for cancer was a waste of time.[27]

In 1968 Jenkins and Zyzanski conducted a carefully designed study comparing three diseases that had strong emotional connotations: poliomyelitis, cancer, and mental illness.[46] Of the three diseases studied, cancer was the most feared. The study indicated that those interviewed saw themselves as highly susceptible to cancer and they believed there was much public concern with this disease, with cancer being thought about and discussed frequently in groups. Pain and death were interrelated with feelings of high personal risk and community concern. Cancer had a social stigma and was associated with being dirty and disgraced. People associated cancer with helplessness and saw it as mysterious and impossible to prevent.

A survey of health care personnel at the City of Hope Medical Center in 1972 indicated that cancer was viewed by them as stronger, more cruel, more anxiety provoking, more unfair, less happy, and more worthless than even death.[68]

Effects on Health Care

The mental images and feelings that make up our concept of cancer influence our behavior as health care givers. The following groups of people have input on decisions concerning health care. All of these groups interact so that singularly or combined they have a major effect on cancer care.

The Physician. In seeking a cause for the patient's symptoms, the physician may block out cancer as a possibility — at least until all other reasonable causes have been ruled out. Informing the patient of the diagnosis of cancer is a much more difficult task than with other diseases and may be avoided, postponed, or presented in a vague manner. Decisions about future treatment, prognosis, depth of personal involvement, and time commitment are influenced by the physician's beliefs about cancer.

The Patient. The person who has symptoms that could be indicative of cancer may avoid going to a physician for diagnosis. When cancer is suspected, the period of testing prior to a definite diagnosis is a very emotion-laden time. According to research conducted by Volicer, "Thinking you might have cancer" was one of the two most stressful experiences for hospitalized patients.[91]

At the time of diagnosis, patients will often experience shock, disbelief, and a feeling of unreality that may make it impossible for them to continue hearing what the physician is saying. Even when the physician finds the courage to inform patients, the information may need to be repeated several times before they comprehend it. Compliance with treatment and beliefs about the effectiveness of treatment are influenced by common cancer beliefs. Self-esteem, the courage to fight the disease in the face of adversity, and the will to live will be influenced by these beliefs.

The Family. Family members have great influence on patient decisions such as seeking health care, compliance with treatment, and utilization of finances for health care. Emotional support of the patient comes primarily from family members. If the general consensus of the family revolves around negative cancer beliefs, the patient may not be supported during or after treatment.

Family members are also personally affected by the diagnosis and its consequences. The cancer stigma attaches itself to family as well as patient. The fear, grief, and family structure changes that often result can have serious implications for the future mental and physical health of all family members.

The Nurse. Nurses may react by avoiding caring for patients with cancer as well as by not reading professional literature on cancer or by not attending conferences or workshops on the disease. Often cancer patients are traded around so that the same nurse does not have to care for them daily. The nurse who works on a cancer unit or who specializes in cancer nursing may be considered somewhat strange and may experience some social isolation from other nursing professionals.

The nursing team may develop expected group behaviors and attitudes in relation to cancer care. A new nurse with a different approach to care of the cancer patient may meet with strong group resistance. For example, the nurse who spends time providing quality care (including emotional care) to the cancer patient may be told to spend time only with patients "who are going to live."

Nurses often find ways to avoid caring for the cancer patient. They can select clinical settings in which they are unlikely to encounter cancer. If cancer patients are present in the clinical setting, assignment to them can be avoided. If the nurses' clinical assignments include cancer patients, minimal physical care can be provided without having to deal with the cancer itself or its emotional impact.

For the most part, the nurse cares for cancer patients while they are in the hospital, and has little opportunity to know what happens to patients after they leave the hospital. The nurse sees only those who return to the hospital with advanced disease, and seldom see or hear of those who are cured.

Because they see only the dark side of cancer, nurses sometimes find it difficult to be optimistic or to recognize that there is another side. Providing treatments such as radical surgery, chemotherapy, and radiotherapy becomes much more reasonable viewed in the light of possible cure.

The Institution. Because of these negative cancer beliefs, institutions often place a low value on quality nursing care for the cancer patient. If a hospital has a cancer unit, it is often located in one of the oldest or least accessible parts of the hospital. Staffing patterns on nursing units with large numbers of cancer patients are frequently inadequate in number and quality of assigned personnel.

These institutions usually have a philosophy which encourages humanistic health care. Cancer beliefs are more primitive than intellectually espoused philosophies, and actions speak louder than words. Therefore, the beliefs actually in action in the institution may be the traditional cancer beliefs.

Conservative Philosophy of Cancer Treatment

The traditional approach to the treatment of metastatic cancer could be defined as conservative. In this approach, patients are seldom informed that they have cancer. It is believed by those who utilize this approach that people cannot cope with the knowledge that they have cancer. They think that if patients knew of the diagnosis, many might commit suicide or possibly give up hope and die early. If patients are not told of their diagnosis, they certainly will not be told of their prognosis.

Since the patient often does not know, decisions are made by the physician or by the physician and family together. The patient is a passive recipient of care and is not expected or allowed to participate actively in any way. The patient is expected to consider the physician the expert and let him or her "handle it."

In the conservative model of cancer therapy, early attempts to cure the cancer are primarily by surgery, although occasionally radiation or small amounts of chemotherapy will be used. If these attempts are not successful, no further treatment is advised.

Cancer is considered by these care givers to be a fatal disease. They believe the kindest thing to do is to allow patients to die quickly of their disease. Therefore supportive therapies such as antibiotics, blood transfusions, and IV therapy are used sparingly if at all. The patient is kept hospitalized, sometimes for many months.

Eventually the patient or family will be told that nothing more can be done. The physician may visit less and less frequently. Nurses are often forbidden to discuss their patients' illness with them. Family members keep conversation on a social level. Glaser and Strauss describe this as "pretense awareness."[32] Virtually total social isolation is established, with a solid wall of communication barriers placed around the patient.

As the patients near death, they are kept heavily sedated. Care givers who operate from this frame of reference believe that people cannot cope with dying and that therefore the best approach is to keep them so heavily sedated that they are not aware of dying. The heavy sedation serves another purpose: heavily sedated people do not interact with those around them. Therefore the physician, the nurses, and the family do not have to confront their feelings or those of the patients. The patients at this point may be treated as objects, not persons.

Occasionally the situation will progress to a state that Hinton calls "premortem burial."[42] In this case, the sedated patient is kept in a darkened room with the door shut and the window curtains closed. Conversations between family members are carried on in hushed whispers. Family members and nurses will stand across the bed from each other and talk across the patient. Occasionally family members will sit in the room and plan the patient's funeral. This behavior is similar to the social behavior that occurs in the "slumber room" of a funeral home as the family views the body in the casket.

MOVING TO A NEW SET OF BELIEFS

The Changing Impact of Cancer

As medical research has progressed, the expected trajectory for many kinds of cancer has changed. There is now much more reason for hope and extended and higher quality life. Unfortunately, changes in beliefs do not always occur at the same rate as medical research. Physicians, nurses, and patients continue to hold to old perceptions and make decisions based on old beliefs.

The association of cancer with death was a reasonable one in the past because the only hope for cure was surgery. If that failed, death was inevitable. This is no longer true. Radiotherapy or chemotherapy can and does cure cancer. We are accustomed now to the fact that people with some skin cancers, early cervical cancer, early breast cancer, and early laryngeal cancer have a high cure rate. Early Hodgkin's disease is often cured by either radiotherapy or chemotherapy. The cure of late Hodgkin's disease is possible if the patient responds well to chemotherapy. Radiotherapy is also curative in some cases of seminomas and head and neck cancers.

Chemotherapy has made a major difference in the cure rates of some cancers. In earlier years, a common sight on a pediatric ward was a child dying of leukemia. Now this is a much more infrequent occurrence. Today 95 per cent of children with acute lymphatic leukemia (ALL) can go into remission with chemotherapy. Ten years later 50 per cent of these children will still be in remission.

Patients with a number of other kinds of cancer respond well to chemotherapy, which slows the growth of the malignancy. Cures do occur among these people, even though they are less frequent. Adjuvant therapy is now common, combining early treatment by surgery, radiotherapy, chemotherapy, and sometimes immunotherapy. Combination treatment has greatly increased cure rates for many cancers.

Physicians use the word cured with great caution in relation to a specific person because in many cases the risk of dormant cancer cells is high for many years after all evidence of cancer is gone. It is safer under such circumstances to consider the person to be in remission rather than cured.

Aggressive Philosophy of Cancer Treatment

The aggressive approach is a much newer way to deal with cancer. In it there is much more openness and willingness of health care givers to deal with feelings, both their own and those of others.

In the aggressive approach, the patients are kept well informed. They are told the diagnosis, the possibilities of cure, and sometimes the prognosis. Decisions are made jointly by the health care givers and patients. Patients are made aware of alternative acceptable methods of treatment and their consequences, allowed to make choices, and made to feel that they and the health care givers will fight the disease together.

Early aggressive attempts, such as radical surgery, are made to cure the disease. These are followed by immediate additional therapies, such as radiotherapy or chemotherapy, to prevent possible recurrence. If these are unsuccessful and the disease does recur, it is aggressively treated in further attempts to achieve a cure or to induce a remission. If a cure is not possible, treatment is directed toward controlling the growth of the malignant cells.

Within this philosophy, cancer is considered a chronic disease with the focus on control of the disease and its symptoms. Palliative measures are used aggressively to control symptoms and maintain a high quality of life. These may include aggressive fighting of infections, transfusions, prompt treatment of obstructions, and frequent screening by laboratory or x-ray tests.

Long hospitalizations are avoided since it is believed they lower the quality of life. Patients are treated at home whenever possible and often continue to work. If patients are receiving chemotherapy, arrangements are made to schedule sessions for minimal interruption of job responsibilities.

Cancer is openly discussed. Patients openly express and explore their feelings with health care givers and talk freely among themselves about their illness and treatment. Family participation is encouraged by the health care team.

If cure becomes unlikely, the focus is switched from cure care to comfort care. Rigorous attempts continue to control symptoms. At no time is the patient abandoned. Pain is controlled in such a way that the patient can maintain conscious awareness and continue to interact with significant others. Families are allowed to remain with the patient during the dying process and receive support in their grief from health care givers.

Obviously, not all cancer care fits neatly into the conservative or aggressive philosophies described. These descriptions are given in order to differentiate clearly between the two philosophies. Some conservative care givers may be more open than those described. Some aggressive care givers may be aggressive to the extreme, continuing attempts to cure even until the death of the patient.

There is, however, a definite distinction between the two philosophies. They are based on a different set of assumptions and different beliefs about the nature of man. The aggressive approach seems to promote better mental health, a higher quality of care, and a higher quality of life for the patient. It allows patients to continue to behave in a mature and responsible way, feeling needed, useful, and loved.

SOCIAL ROLES AND CANCER

In recent years social scientists have begun to examine social roles in relation to illness. It is becoming apparent that social role expectations have a great impact on a patient's response to illness, the ability to cope with the situation, the quality of life, and possible chances of recovery or prolongation of life. These expectations have an impact not only on the patient but on everyone affected by the illness.

It is important for the nurse to assess messages of social role expectations that the client and family experience and also those social role expectations that the client and family have previously internalized. Nurses also need to recognize their expectations of the client and family and the expectations of other health care personnel. The expectations of health care givers will be communicated in one form or another, usually implicitly, and can influence client and family behavior, sometimes in a very negative way.

Before exploring sick roles, it would be helpful to examine the social expectations of the well person in relation to health. This would provide a standard by which to compare changes in expectations that have occurred as a result of taking on one of the sick roles. Unfortunately, there seems to be no wellness role, or health role defined as such, described in the literature. In 1969, Lipman and Sterne described the role of the independent person.[53] There seems to be much similarity between their description of independence and what would be expected of the healthy person.

The Independence Role

The expected performance of the independent person includes attitudinal, emotional, economic, and physical components. The independent person is expected to be economically self-supporting and behaviorally autonomous and is expected to deal effectively with his or her environment, including its personal, social, and cultural conditions and to fulfill reciprocal social obligations. The independent person is expected not to lean "unduly on others for emotional support."[53] In sum, the person "is expected to have and to attempt to maintain sufficient physical and mental health to allow himself to fulfill all of the foregoing behavioral and attitudinal patterns."[53]

This description leaves some important questions unanswered. Does society expect people to take actions to improve their health or is a minimum of health acceptable if social roles are fulfilled? Is the person who strives toward greater health deviant? Is deviance always bad or socially undesirable? What is the expected behavior of a person who is "at risk" of illness but who presently fulfills expected social roles? These questions have some relevance to cancer prevention, screening, self-examination for cancer, getting medical checkups, and controlling exposure to carcinogens.

Entrance into Sick Roles

Movement of a person from a healthy role to a sick role is socially controlled.[16] Supposedly the purpose of this control is to limit the number of people who are "officially sick" in order to decrease the impact of sickness on society. The question then arises: How does a person become "officially sick"? For a very brief sickness, such as a cold or influenza, people may be allowed simply to inform others that they have personally determined that they are sick. However, even this may vary depending on the status of the individual, with a person of low status often being required to bring a note from a higher status person verifying the illness.

The Gatekeeper Role. The gatekeeper is a person who has been authorized by society to officially declare that a person is sick. Parents perform this role with their children. School nurses and occupational health nurses may also function in this capacity. Most commonly in our society, however, this role is performed by the physician.[16]

Sanctions. Some role theorists say that sanctions are placed on those who are admitted to sick roles. A sanction is a form of punishment imposed by society. Sanctions may be such things as blaming, social isolation, loss of support systems, loss of economic support, or loss of other social roles.[16] The sanctions are imposed because of the debilitating effect that illness has on society, since people who are officially assigned to sick roles are nonproductive and released from social obligations. The sanctions differ depending on the social evaluation of how the illness should be classed:

either (1) illness over which the victim has no control or (2) illness that is a result of misconduct. The former has less social stigma and thus fewer sanctions.

From this point of view, some of the negative beliefs about cancer are a result of social sanctions imposed by society as a consequence of the diagnosis of cancer. These sanctions signify the imposition of a social stigma.

Acute Sick Role

In 1951 sociologist Talcott Parsons wrote a book entitled *The Social System*, which contained the first description of the sick role — the specific social expectations of the person who had been labeled sick.[70] Parsons believed that the state of illness is not the sick person's own fault and that the patient should be regarded as a victim of forces beyond his or her control. The patient should claim exemption from ordinary daily obligations and expectations. If the illness is sufficiently severe, Parsons stated, the patient should seek help from some kind of institutionalized health service agency. This seeking of help further includes the admission by the patient that being sick is undesirable (or deviant) and that measures should be taken to maximize the chances to facilitate recovery.[70]

Much controversy has arisen over Parsons' sick role.[31] Many have disagreed with the definition of sickness as deviant behavior.[59] Some believe that Parsons' description came at a time when physicians operated on a strict authoritarian basis, placing the patient in a completely dependent position, and that the role no longer fits our society today.[39] Another group believes that the sick role as defined by Parsons is too simplistic because he does not show how role expectations are dependent upon socioeconomic status, beliefs and values of referent groups, sex, type of illness, ethnic group, age, culture, and other social roles.[12, 17, 18, 28, 48, 82]

Concern has been expressed over the fact that the sick role as Parsons describes it does not adequately define all types of illnesses. Parsons' sick role seems to fit acute illness situations more adequately than illnesses such as cancer. Some theorists propose that the sick role be subdivided. The divisions suggested vary but usually include a chronic illness role and a terminally ill role.

Chronic Illness Role

Persons with chronic illnesses are expected to get treatment and to take personal responsibility for following through with medical instructions. If they do not follow medical directions, they are labeled as noncompliant. They are expected to fight against the onslaught of their illness, not give in to it.

Chronically ill persons are expected to continue participating in and contributing to society to the extent that their illness allows. This means that they should continue to work, maintain their roles within the family, and participate in social groups. A person with a chronic illness who withdraws and gives up is considered "bad" or "weak" by society.

Strauss and Glaser delineate the responsibilities of the person with a chronic illness.[87]

1. Prevent medical crises and manage them when they occur.

2. Control symptoms.

3. Carry out prescribed regimens and manage problems attendant upon carrying out the regimens.

4. Prevent or live with the social isolation caused by lessened contact with others.

5. Adjust to changes in the course of the disease, whether it moves downward or has remissions.

6. Normalize both interactions with others and style of life.

7. Find the necessary money to pay for treatments or to survive despite partial or complete loss of employment.

A comparison of the chronic illness role with Parsons' sick role indicates that a person with an acute sickness is expected to move toward resumption of social responsibilities whereas the chronically ill person must accept the fact that he or she will never fully resume previous social roles. The acutely ill person must overcome a temporary illness. The chronically ill person must adjust to a permanent condition. The person with an acute illness temporarily gives up autonomy and then regains it. Chronically ill persons focus on retaining what autonomy they have rather than losing more autonomy. Thus, in chronic illness, the person is concerned with maintaining autonomy and denying illness, whereas the person with acute illness must be willing to temporarily give up autonomy and accept the reality of illness. The chronically ill person views dependency as a real threat, whereas the person with an acute illness may use the opportunity to enjoy secondary gains.[48]

The situation of the person with cancer seems to more realistically fit into a chronic illness role rather than an acute sick role. Even if a cure is possible, the period of illness usually goes beyond that of acute illness. Of course, there are those fortunate situations of very early localized cancer that fit easily into Parsons' sick role. Even these people, however, may find it difficult to move back to a health role. They may be labeled by society as sick and a patient for long periods of time after successful treatment has been completed. The social stigma attached to a diagnosis of cancer can last a lifetime.

The Responsor Role

A person with a chronic illness requires help from other members of society. The responsor is a person or persons who have expected social responsibilities in caring for a person with a chronic illness and cooperating with health care providers.[35] Usually a person close to the chronically ill person fills the major role of providing needed care. Fulfilling the activities of this role requires courage, determination, will-to-cope, optimism, and commitment. The person in the responsor role usually has had a preexisting relationship with the patient. Taking on the role requires that the person acquire a set of duties and responsibilities that may be completely new. In order to take on this role, the person may have to give up previous activities and contacts that were important.

There are serious disadvantages shouldered by the person taking on this role. The person is not considered a part of the health care team, is not trained for the job, and may have little choice about doing the job and yet may have to work long hard hours. Responsors bear a heavy emotional load with little support. Their own needs constantly compete with the work requirements of the role. Often persons in the responsor role are limited in performing this role because of their own ailments.[35]

The responsibilities of this role include communicating with the health care team; administering drugs properly; and regulating diet, fluid ingestion, exercise, and habits such as smoking. Special exercises, use of equipment, and administering treatments may have to be learned. The responsor may have to perform very personal care such as bathing, dressing, toilet care, feeding, turning, and ambulating. Some chronically ill persons require constant supervision.[35]

The responsor role fills both a social need and the unique needs of a chronically ill individual. Major difficulties can occur when no one is available to fulfill the responsor role. Even if someone is available, inadequate response to this role may occur as a result of personal prejudices, personal problems, disinterest, or fear. Often the personal needs of the responsor are considered subordinate to societal needs and the needs of the chronically ill person. Thus responsors may be expected to sacrifice their own personal health and well-being in order to fulfill the needs of others.[35]

Members of communities, neighborhoods, and community agencies also have a responsibility for chronically ill persons. They are also fulfilling the responsor role. Community members may provide assistance to allow disabled persons to carry out their responsibilities. Members may also need to learn to watch for symptoms of illness or noncompliance to regimen. If these community efforts are to be effective, they must be coordinated. Coordination requires support systems, trust, interactional skills, and financial, medical, and family resources.[87] Unfortunately, in many cancer situations these community supports are lacking, leaving the family with total responsibility for the responsor role. Because of the heavy demands of this role, there is a serious threat to the physical and mental health of the family. This will be discussed further in Chapter 12.

Terminal Illness Role

The criteria used by society to classify an illness as terminal are not based on logic. People who have congestive heart failure, which is controlled by digitalis, are not considered terminally ill. People who have advanced diabetes, which is controlled by insulin, are not considered terminally ill. But patients with metastatic cancer, which is controlled by chemotherapy, are considered terminally ill. In fact, a cancer patient is often considered terminally ill from the time of diagnosis.

The impact of this label is great. A person who is thought to have a terminal illness may no longer be considered a contributing member of society. In this case, his or her social worth decreases greatly. A person with low social worth is not usually expected to make demands, either of society, family members, or health care givers. It is usually considered unreasonable for a person of low social worth to request or expect treatments or care that requires large expenditures of money or time from family members or health care givers.

For example, the patient may feel very guilty about receiving costly treatment and, feeling undeserving, may refuse to take it. Even after losing 60 to 80 pounds, patients may not be willing to buy new clothing or have false teeth relined because they feel that they are "going to die anyway," and that other family members have more right to the money. For the same reason, eyeglasses may not be changed in spite of vision changes.

When the patient is hospitalized there is often much reluctance to request care. The patient feels that the health care givers should take care of patients who are going to get well, not someone who is dying. Physicians are often excused by the patient for not making daily visits, or the patient might apologize for calling nurses or taking up their time. For this reason, poor nursing care may be accepted unchallenged.

Patients who are terminally ill are often expected to avoid exposing others to the fact that they are dying, since this makes everyone aware of the inevitability of death. Thus, it is not socially acceptable for patients to discuss the fact that they are dying or to express feelings about dying. Because the patient's mere presence makes others uncomfortable, the patient is often discouraged from attending social functions or working at a job. This is often couched in other terms, such as "you shouldn't tax yourself by coming" or some similarly disguised message.

The patient's function within the family also changes markedly. Dying people seem to be expected to become dependent family members. They may not be expected or even allowed to function as contributing family members. If they attempt to, they might get negative responses or reprimands from either family members or social groups.

Other family members may take over decision-making roles so that the patient no longer has the right to decide how the money is spent or how the children are disciplined. If the patient has been the breadwinner and chief authority in the family, this may be changed so that the patient no longer has authority. Sometimes patients even lose the right to make decisions about their personal belongings, which are sometimes discarded or given away without the patient's permission or even awareness.

The expected role behavior of the dying person has been discussed by a number of authors.[7, 49, 61, 84] The imposition of this role has very serious implications, particularly if the person attempts to function within the role for a long period of time, which often occurs after a diagnosis of cancer. As previously mentioned, people with cancer are often labeled by society as terminally ill at the time of diagnosis. The terminally ill role meets the needs of society to the detriment of the needs of the dying person. One could easily question whether it really meets the needs of society or simply supports our culture's denial of death.

There are many social values inherent in these role expectations: the denial of death is good, the dying person has little worth, and the needs of the health care givers are more important than those of the dying person. The following is a list of negative terminal illness role expectations. Most people confronted with this list would probably become angry and deny that these are socially expected behaviors. Observing and listening on the average hospital unit, however, may be sufficient to verify the validity of the list.

Social Role Expectations of the Dying Person. The patient should:

1. Maintain relative composure and cheerfulness.[7]

2. Face death with dignity.[7]

3. Not become isolated from the world.[7]

4. Continue to be a good family member.[7]

5. Be nice to other patients.[7]

6. Participate in the ward social life.[7]

7. Cooperate with the staff members.[7]

8. Avoid distressing or embarrassing staff members.[7]

9. Not shop around for impossible cures.[7]

10. Not make excessive demands.[7]

11. Not become noisy or hysterical.[7]

12. Not refuse to cooperate.[61]

13. Not become apathetic, hostile, or reproachful.[61]

14. Die with courage and grace.[61]

15. Not act to bring about his own death.[61]

16. Make health care providers comfortable.[61]

17. Avoid taking up health care givers' time.[61]

18. Conform to hospital organization.[61]

19. Not talk about death or related matters.[61]

20. Die well.[61]

21. Keep thoughts and feelings to self.[49]

Once a patient has indicated his awareness of dying, he becomes responsible for his acts as a *dying* person. He knows now that he is not merely sick but dying. He must face that fact. Sociologically, facing an impending death means that the patient will be judged, and will judge himself, according to certain standards or proper conduct concerning his behavior during his final days and hours.[84]

Family Responsibilities in Terminal Illness

The family of the dying person has all of the responsibilities as described under chronic illness. In addition, Benoliel describes two others:[8]

1. Facing the problem of maintaining some investment in the future while at the same time preparing for the patient's death through anticipatory mourning.

2. Facing the difficult problem of maintaining a sense of mastery and control while at the same time coming to terms with the terminal nature of the illness itself.

The Primary Caretaker Role

As in the chronic illness framework, there is usually a primary caretaker or responsor for a person who is dying. Kalish describes the role of this person.[47]

The role of the primary caretaker of the dying person has received little attention. In some families, one individual assumes — or has thrust upon her or him — the major responsibility for care. According to the British study, the average period of time for this task was 5 months. However, the duration of the task is highly variable. Not infrequently the primary caretaker becomes physically and psychologically exhausted during this period. Other family members are often relieved that the caretaking is being handled, and they may offer to help out either personally or financially to provide the primary caretaker with respite. There are forms of compensation for the job, nonetheless. The primary caretaker controls the information, the physical space, and the emotional contacts with the dying person. He or she (usually latter) can decide who visits and when, who is privy to what knowledge, and what messages are carried. The primary caretaker may also anticipate some financial reward (and can become bitter if it is not forthcoming), although this is probably rarely a major motive; he or she will also expect to receive proper recognition from other family members of the important task being conducted (and again may become bitter if it is not forthcoming). After the death, this person may find adjustment the most difficult in terms of reestablishing social activities, work career, or organizational involvement, but will probably have the least guilt and the fewest feelings of having unfinished business of anyone in the family.[47]

Dying in an Institution — Expected Behavior

When the person near death is brought to the hospital, certain behaviors are expected of the health care givers, the patient, and the family. When these have been accomplished, the death is considered satisfactory.

1. The successful death is quiet and uneventful. The death skips by with as little notice as possible; nobody is disturbed.

2. Few people are on the scene. There is, in effect, no scene. Staff is not required to adjust to the presence of family and other visitors who might have their own needs that upset the self-routined equilibrium.

3. Leave-taking behavior is at a minimum.

4. The physician does not have to be involved intimately in terminal care, especially as the end approaches.

5. The staff makes few technical errors throughout the terminal care.

6. Strong emphasis is given to the body during the care-giving process. Little effort is wasted on the personality of the terminally ill individual.

7. The person dies at the right time; that is, after the full range of medical interventions has been tried but before the onset of an interminable period of lingering on.

8. The patient expresses gratitude for the excellent care received.

9. After the patient's death, the family expresses gratitude for the excellent care received.

10. The staff is able to conclude that "we did everything we could for this patient."

11. The physical remains of the patient are made available to the hospital for clinical, research, or administrative purposes (via autopsy permission or organ gifts).

12. A memorial (financial) gift is made to the hospital in the name of the deceased.

13. The total cost of the terminal care process is determined to have been low or moderate: money was not wasted on a person whose life was beyond saving.[49]

Behavior and Social Roles

People may choose to behave according to specific social roles or they may have social pressures placed on them to take on those roles. In the latter case, the roles are imposed upon them. People can also resist or reject the taking on of particular roles. This may result in social sanctions, but in some instances the rejection of a role may be the most healthy thing to do. For example, patients may reject the sick role, or they may reject the terminally ill role in favor of the chronically ill role.

CANCER NURSING AND SOCIAL ROLES

The Cancer Patient Role

Cancer patients have taken on or have had imposed upon themselves two roles: patient and cancer patient. In taking on the role as patient they have had to accept some degree of dependence in order to seek help; they have had a loss of control and may have had to give up other desirable life roles.

In assuming the role of cancer patient, they take on a stigma and a decrease in social status or worth.[33] In addition, they may also have the terminally ill role imposed upon them. Because of the beliefs related to cancer, the role of cancer patient differs from that of other patients. Cancer patients are expected to tolerate more pain, endure suffering without complaint, be passive and submit to whatever the health care givers choose to impose upon them, make few demands upon others, ask no questions, and keep socially distant from others.

The Cancer Nursing Role

How nurses perceive the role of cancer nurse will depend to some extent on how they define nursing and what nursing theory they use as a base for their practice. For example, Orem's approach of promoting self-care, with the nurse becoming involved only in areas in which patients are unable to meet their own needs, would certainly revolutionize typical institutional care for cancer patients.[66a] Roy's approach of using adaptation could also maximize the quality of life possible for the cancer patient.[78a]

The cancer nurse can choose to function primarily on the technical level: administering medications, performing procedures, assessing the patient's physical condition, and moving rapidly from one task to another. A high level of technical competence is necessary to practice cancer nursing, but it is not sufficient.

Taking the risk of becoming involved with the patient on a personal basis is necessary. Communicating, caring, listening, supporting, encouraging, and functioning as a patient advocate are necessary, but even this is not sufficient. The cancer nurse must also be an analytical problem solver, a creative seeker of new ways of achieving high quality life for the cancer patient. This will require advanced knowledge in physiology, sociology, psychology, and nursing. Blended together in a way unique to nursing, these disciplines must be used in ever evolving ways to find solutions to problems that presently are seldom identified.

Nursing is a unique discipline, completely separate and different from medicine. A physician does not have the knowledge or skills necessary to practice nursing any more than a nurse has the knowledge and skills necessary to practice medicine. The nurse-patient relationship is just as important as and not subordinate to the physician-patient relationship.

Nurses and physicians, however, should not be rivals; they should function interdependently. Very little in health care can be done by a single person or a single discipline. Communication, mutual respect, and cooperation are necessary if quality patient care is to be provided. The cancer patient is the one who experiences the greatest loss if this relationship does not exist.

When Is a Cancer Patient No Longer a Cancer Patient?

People can be cured of cancer and live 30 or 40 years. But sometimes for the rest of their lives they are labeled a cancer patient. People often live with cancer for 15 years with treatment before they die of the disease. They can be in complete remission for long periods, but they are always seen and treated socially as cancer patients.

Is harm done to the person by the constant label of cancer patient? What are the consequences of using this label over a lifetime? Since the role of cancer patient is one with a stigma, and the social expectations of a sick role are inconsistent with independent or well role behavior, the cancer patient who attempts to move toward wellness behavior, even in remission or possible cure, is often rebuked by health care givers, family, and social support groups.[79] Could these blocked moves toward wellness affect the course of the disease, the state of mental health, or the development of other diseases?

It seems healthier to provide mechanisms for the patient to move out of the cancer patient role. Health care givers will have to provide the impetus for the social change necessary for cancer patients to be able to move toward wellness.

Is the Cancer Nurse's Responsibility Only to the Cancer Patient?

The life of the cancer patient is always inextricably intertwined with family members, social support groups, and significant others. It is impossible to provide effective nursing care for the cancer patient and exclude those with whom the patient's life is intertwined. The stresses confronting those persons in responsor or primary caretaker roles are overwhelming and can lead to future illnesses. An orientation to preventive health care requires concentrated nursing intervention with these families. Inability of family members or significant others to cope will also deter effective coping of the cancer patient. Limiting nursing care to the cancer patient alone will result in ineffective and limited nursing interventions.

BIBLIOGRAPHY

1. *A Basic Study of Public Attitudes toward Cancer and Cancer Tests.* Unpublished research report conducted for the American Cancer Society by Lieberman Research Inc., May 1979.
2. Abrams, R. D.: The patient with cancer — His changing patterns of communication. *New England Journal of Medicine.* 274:327–332, 1966.
3. Bahnson, C. B.: Psychologic and emotional issues in cancer: The psychotherapeutic care of the cancer patient. *Seminars in Oncology.* 2:293–309, 1975.
4. Baider, L.: The silent message: Communication in a family with a dying patient. *Journal of Marriage and Family Counseling.* 3:23–28, 1977.
5. Barkley, V.: The crises in cancer. *American Journal of Nursing.* 67:278–280, 1967.
6. Becker, M. H.: *The Health Belief Model and Personal Health Behavior.* Charles B. Slack, Inc., Thorofare, N.J., 1974.
7. Beilin, R. L.: *Managing Relations in Terminality: The Social Intelligibility of Denial of Death.* Paper presented at the meeting of the American Sociological Association, 1977.
8. Benoliel, J. Q.: Care, communication, and human dignity. In *Psychosocial Care of the Dying Patient,* ed. by C. A. Garfield. McGraw-Hill Book Co., New York, 1978.

9. Bouchard, R., and N. F. Owens: *Nursing Care of the Cancer Patient.* C. V. Mosby Co., St. Louis, 1972, p. 1.
10. Brauer, P. H.: When cancer is diagnosed. *Medical Insight.* 21:20–25, 1970.
11. Brennan, M.: The cancer gestalt. *Geriatrics.* 25:96–101, 1970.
12. Brown, J. S., and M. E. Rawlinson: Sex differences in sick role rejection and in work performance following cardiac surgery. *Journal of Health and Social Behavior.* 18:276–292, 1977.
13. Buehler, J. C.: What contributes to hope in the cancer patient? *American Journal of Nursing.* 75:1353–1356, 1975.
14. Burkhalter, P. K.: Sociocultural aspects of cancer. In *Dynamics of Oncology Nursing,* ed. by P. K. Burkhalter and D. L. Donley. McGraw-Hill Book Co., New York, 1978.
15. Burns, N.: *Nurse-Patient Communications with the Advanced Cancer Patient.* Unpublished Masters' thesis, Texas Women's University, 1974.
16. Calloway, J. C., and J. A. Baruch: Illness and social control. *Review of Social Theory.* 2:71–83, 1973.
17. Campbell, J. D.: Attribution of illness: Another double standard. *Journal of Health and Social Behavior. 21:114*–126, 1975.
18. Campbell, J. D.: The child in the sick role: Contributions of age, sex, parental status and parental values. *Journal of Health and Social Behavior.* 19:35–51, 1978.
19. Cancer: Bogey word to patient. *Australasian Nurses Journal.* 3:11, 1978.
20. Clapp, M. J.: Psychosocial reactions of children with cancer. *Nursing Clinics of North America.* 1:73–82, 1976.
21. Coping with the crisis of cancer. *Emergency Medicine.* 6:225–226, 1974.
22. Crane, D.: Decisions to treat critically ill patients: A comparison of social versus medical considerations. *Milbank Memorial Fund Quarterly.* 53:1–33, 1975.
23. Crane, D.: The social potential of the patient: An alternative to the sick role. *Journal of Communication.* 25:131–139, 1975.
24. Crary, W. G., and G. C. Gra: Emotional crisis and cancer. *CA — A Cancer Journal for Clinicians.* 24:36–39, 1974.
25. Creech, R. H.: The psychologic support of the cancer patient: A medical oncologist's viewpoint. *Seminars in Oncology.* 2:285–292, 1975.
26. Davis, M. Z.: Patients in limbo. *American Journal of Nursing.* 66:746–748, 1966.
27. Davison, R. L.: Opinion of nurses on cancer, its treatment and curability. *British Journal of Preventive and Social Medicine.* 19:24–29, 1965.
28. Eisenberg, L.: Disease and illness: Distinctions between professional and popular ideas of sickness. *Culture, Medicine and Psychiatry.* 1:9–23, 1977.
29. Francis, G. M.: Cancer, the emotional component. *American Journal of Nursing.* 69:1677–1681, 1969.
30. George, M. McG.: Long-term care of the patient with cancer. *Nursing Clinics of North America.* 8:623–631, 1973.
31. Gerson, E. M.: The social character of illness: Deviance or politics? *Social Science and Medicine.* 10:219–224, 1976.
32. Glaser, B. G., and A. L. Strauss: *Awareness of Dying.* Aldine Publishing Co., Chicago, 1966.
33. Goffman, E.: *Stigma.* Prentice-Hall, Inc., Englewood Cliffs, N. J., 1963.
34. Goleman, D.: We are breaking the silence about death. *Psychology Today.* 10:44–60, 1976.
35. Golodetz, A., et al.: The care of chronic illness: The "responsor role." *Medical Care.* 7:385–394, 1969.
36. Gottheil, E., W. C. McGurn, and O. Pollak: Truth and/or hope for the dying patient. *Nursing Digest.* 4:12–14, 1976.
37. Greene, R.: Physicians, pain, and cancer patients. *Hospital Physician.* 14:36–37, 1978.
38. Hackett, T. P., and A. D. Weisman: Denial as a factor in patients with heart disease and cancer. *Annals New York Academy of Science.* 164:802–817, 1969.
39. Hardy, M. E., and M. E. Conway: *Role Theory: Perspectives for Health Professionals.* Appleton-Century-Crofts, New York, 1978.
40. Harker, B. L.: Cancer and communication problems: A personal experience. *Psychiatry in Medicine.* 3:163–171, 1972.
41. Heimlich, H. J., and A. H. Kutscher: The family's reaction to terminal illness. In *Loss and Grief: Psychological Management in Medical Practice,* ed. by B. Schoenbert, et al. Columbia University Press, New York, 1970.
42. Hinton, J. M.: The physical and mental distress of the dying. *Quarterly Journal of Medicine.* 32:1–21, 1963.
43. Hobbs, P.: Changing attitudes to cancer. *Nursing Mirror.* 116:v+, 1963.
44. Holland, J. C. B.: Coping with cancer: A challenge to the behavioral sciences. In *Cancer: The Behavioral Dimensions,* ed. by J. W. Cullen et al. Raven Press, New York, 1976.
45. Horn, D., and S. Waingrow: What changes are occurring in public opinion survey. *American Journal of Public Health.* 54:431–440, 1964.
46. Jenkins, C. D., and S. J. Zyzanski: Dimensions of belief and feeling concerning three diseases, poliomyelitis, cancer and mental illness: A factor analytic study. *Behavioral Science.* 13:372–381, 1968.
47. Kalish, R. A.: Dying and preparing for death: A view of families. In *New Meanings of Death,* ed. by H. Feifel. McGraw-Hill Book Co., New York, 1977.
48. Kassebaum, G. G., and B. O. Baumann: Dimensions of the sick role in chronic illness. *Journal of Health and Human Behavior.* 6:16–17, 1965.
49. Kastenbaum, R. J.: *Death, Society and Human Experience.* C. V. Mosby Co., St. Louis, 1977.
50. Klagsbrun, S.: Cancer, nurses and emotions. *R.N.* 33:46–51, 1970.
51. Krant, M. J.: Problems of the physician in presenting his patient with the diagnosis. In *Cancer: The Behavioral Dimensions,* ed. by

Cullen, J., et al. Raven Press, New York, 1976, p. 270.

52. Kubler-Ross, E.: Coping with the reality of terminal illness in the family. In *Death: Current Perspectives*, ed. by E. S. Schneidman. Mayfield Publishing Company, Palo Alto, 1976.
53. Lipman, A., and R. S. Sterne: Aging in the United States: Ascription of a terminal sick role. *Sociology and Social Research*. 53:194–203, 1969.
54. Lord, E. A.: My crisis with cancer. *American Journal of Nursing*. 74:647–649, 1974.
55. Marcus, M. G.: The shaky link between cancer and character. *Psychology Today*. 10:52–54, 1976.
56. Marino, L. B.: Cancer patients: Your special role. *Nursing 76*, 1976, pp. 26–29.
57. Martini, C. J., and I. McDowell: Health status: Patient and physician judgments. *Health Services Research*. 11:508–515, 1976.
58. Mastrovito, R. C.: Cancer: awareness and denial. *Clinical Bulletin*. 4:142–146, 1974.
59. Meile, R. L.: Comment on Brown and Rawlinson's sick role rejection. *Journal of Health and Social Behavior*. 19:121–122, 1978.
60. Meinhart, N. T.: The cancer patient: Living in the here and now. *Nursing Outlook*. 16:64–69, 1968.
61. Mervyn, F.: The plight of dying patients in hospitals. *American Journal of Nursing*. 71:1988–1990, 1971.
62. Miller, C. L., P. R. Denner, and V. E. Richardson: Assisting the psychosocial problems of cancer patients: A review of current research. *International Journal of Nursing Studies*. 13:161–166, 1976.
63. Miller, R. N.: Psychosocial problems in rehabilitation. *Seventh National Cancer Conference Proceedings*. J. B. Lippincott, Philadelphia, 1973, p. 855.
64. Milton, G. W.: Thoughts in mind of a person with cancer. *British Medical Journal*. 4:221–223, 1973.
65. Oakes, T. W.: Primary group relations in sick role behavior — Perceived family and friends' expectations in patient compliance. *Dissertation Abstracts*. 31A:1916, 1970.
66. Olson, K. B.: Cancer and the patient. *Annals of Internal Medicine*. 81:696, 1974.
66a. Orem, D. E.: *Nursing: Concepts of Practice*. McGraw-Hill Book Company, New York, 1980.
67. Oster, M. W., M. Visel, and L. R. Turgeon: Pain of terminal cancer patients. *Archives of Internal Medicine*. 138:1801–1802, 1978.
68. Padilla, G.: *Second Quarterly Project Report to the American Cancer Society, California Division*. January, 1972.
69. Parkes, C. M.: The emotional impact of cancer on patients and their families. *Journal of Laryngology and Otology*. 89:271–279, 1975.
70. Parsons, T.: *The Social System*. The Free Press, New York, 1951.
71. Parsons, T.: The sick role and the role of the physician reconsidered. *Milbank Memorial Fund Quarterly*. 53:257–278, 1975.
72. Paulen, A., and S. Sylvester: Caring for the patient who's 'well'. *R.N.* 41:56–58, 1978.
73. Peebler, D.: How patients help each other. *American Journal of Nursing*. 75:1354, 1975.
74. Peterson, B. H., and C. J. Kellogg: *Current Practice in Oncology Nursing*. C. V. Mosby Co., St. Louis, 1976.
75. Priyadharsini, J.: Emotional reactions of adult patients with the diagnosis of cancer. *Nursing Journal of India*. 64:312, 1973.
76. Quint, J. C.: Obstacles to helping the dying. *American Journal of Nursing*. 66:1568–1571, 1966.
77. Rickel, L.: Human values and the quality of survival. *Journal of the Arkansas Medical Society*. 70:210–213, 1973.
78. Robbins, G. F., M. C. McDonald, and G. T. Pack: Delay in the diagnosis and treatment of physicians with cancer. *Cancer*. 6:624–626, 1953.
78a. Roy, C.: Adaptation: a basis for nursing practice. *Nursing Outlook*. 19:254–257, 1971.
79. Sanders J. B., and C. J. Karkinal: Adaptive coping mechanisms in adult acute leukemia patients in remission. *Journal of the American Medical Association*. 238:952–954, 1977.
80. Schoenberg, B., and R. A. Senescu: The patient's reaction to fatal illness. In *Loss and Grief: Psychological Management in Medical Practice*, ed. by Bernard Schoenberg et al., Columbia University Press, New York, 1970.
81. Schutt, B.: Penetrating the cancer patient's world. *American Journal of Nursing*. 66:745, 1966.
82. Segall, A.: Sociocultural variation in sick role behavioral expectations. *Social Science and Medicine*. 10:47–51, 1976.
83. Simonton, O. C., S. Matthews-Simonton, and J. Creighton: *Getting Well Again*. J. P. Tarcher, Inc., Los Angeles, 1978.
84. Smith, E. A.: *Psychosocial Aspects of Cancer Patient Care*. McGraw-Hill Book Co., New York, 1976, p. 42.
85. Sontag, S.: *Illness as Metaphor*. Vintage Books, New York, 1978, pp. 5–6.
86. Strauss, A. L., and B. G. Glaser: Awareness of dying. In *Loss and Grief: Psychological Management in Medical Practice*, ed. by B. Schoenberg et al. Columbia University Press, New York, 1970.
87. Strauss, A. L., and B. G. Glaser: *Chronic Illness and the Quality of Life*. C. V. Mosby Co., St. Louis, 1975.
88. Suchman, E.: Social patterns of illness and medical care. *Journal of Health and Human Behavior*. 6:2–27, 1965.
89. Sudnow, D.: *Passing On*. Prentice-Hall, Inc., Englewood Cliffs, N. J., 1967.
90. Veronesi, U., and G. Martino: Can life be the same after cancer treatment? *Tumori*, 64:345–351, 1978.
91. Volicer, B.: A hospital stress rating scale. *Nursing Research*. 24:352–359, 1975.
92. Wan, T. T. H.: Predicting self-assessed health status: A multivariate approach. *Health Services Research*. 11:464–477, 1976.
93. Weisman, A. D.: *On Dying and Denying: A Psychiatric Study of Terminality*. Behavioral Publications, Inc., New York, 1972.
94. Weisman, A. D.: *Coping with Cancer*. McGraw-Hill Book Co., New York, 1979, p. 16.
95. Winder, A. E., and J. R. Elam: Therapist for the cancer patient's family: A new role for the nurse. *Journal of Psychiatric Nursing and Mental Health Services*. 16:22–27, 1978.

2

The Nature of Cancer

NORMAL CELL BIOLOGY

For many years the cell has been labeled the basic structural unit of the body, and yet much remains to be known about the structures within the cell and how they function. Advanced technology has provided mechanisms for delving deeper into the mysteries of the cell and much research time and money have been spent in this search. This knowledge is necessary before the cancer cell can be probed in detail, as it is difficult to clearly define the abnormal unless the normal is known.

In cancer, the normal cell and the malignant cell reside side-by-side. Both are affected by normal processes, malignant processes, and treatment processes. Intelligent nursing intervention and prediction of nursing outcomes require knowledge of both the normal and the malignant cell.

Cell Structure and Function

Cell Membrane

The cell membrane is an important functioning part of the cell. It does a great deal more than encase the cell: it is a gate-keeper, a controller, and a communicator. Until very recently, little was understood about how the membrane was constructed, the mechanisms used to perform its functions, or even what all of its functions were. At present, much careful and detailed research is being conducted to learn more about the cell membrane.[35]

The cell membrane is complex in both organizational structure and function. There is some evidence that it may have as much influence on control of cell functions as does the nucleus. Until recently, the cell membrane was thought to be a very simple structure that controlled which substances entered the cell and which did not. A flurry of excitement occurred when active transport systems, including the carefully controlled sodium pump, were discovered.

Membrane receptors have been the subject of much study. These receptors are used as identifying markers for hormones, enzymes, and other chemicals. These markers maintain chemical communication with the rest of the body. As a result of this chemical communication, major changes in cell functioning can occur to meet body needs. If the cell membrane perceives a threat of attack by a foreign substance, the cell sends out chemical alarm signals, stimulating attack on the foreign substance from a variety of other sources within the body.[35]

The membrane receptors may sometimes function also as antigens. If other cells or body substances evaluate these antigens as foreign, an attack upon the cell will occur. This happens in autoimmune diseases, transfusion reactions, transplant rejection, and sometimes in cancer.

Electrical cell-to-cell communication is maintained by the cell membrane. In this way, groups of cells can act together as a body in their response to a situation. This communication takes place at small gap junctions or nexus junctions, which are small areas where cell membranes of adjacent cells come into close contact. These junctions allow for ion exchange between cells.[1]

Flow of fluids between cells is also controlled by the cell membrane. Tight junctions are regions of cell membrane that maintain intimate contact with adjacent cells. Ridges of one cell membrane fit into grooves of the adjacent cell membrane in such a way that a complete barrier to the passage of fluids is formed.[1]

The cell membrane controls cell movement. When cell membrane contact is made with another cell, movement of the cells stops. This is called contact inhibition. Many other intricate functions of the cell membrane are presently being identified and will add much to our understanding of the cell.

Cytoplasm

The cytoplasm is a viscous material found within the cell membrane and outside the nucleus. It is more dense near the cell membrane. The cytoplasm controls cell shape and transports substances within the cell. It contains many chemicals and proteins, transfer ribonucleic acid (RNA), and messenger RNA.

Organelles

Mitochondria are the powerhouses of the cell. They convert nutrients and oxygen to energy in a very complex chemical process involving the Krebs cycle. This is called aerobic metabolism. Energy is then stored in a compact high energy form called adenosine triphosphate (ATP). Anaerobic metabolism is utilized to a small extent in normal cells but results in the production of only very small amounts of ATP. Mitochondria have recently been found to contain deoxyribonucleic acid (DNA), but its function is not presently known.

Ribosomes are located both free in the cytoplasm and attached to the outside surface of endoplasmic reticulum. Ribosomes are composed of ribosomal RNA and function in the production of proteins. These proteins may be enzymes, hormones, or cell structural elements. Free ribosomes synthesize primarily soluble proteins. Ribosomes attached to endoplasmic reticulum manufacture membrane proteins and proteins to be secreted by the cell.[35]

Ribosomes manufacture proteins in coordination with messenger and transfer RNA. Messenger RNA attaches to the ribosome and is coded so that each amino acid

needed for the protein is indicated in sequence on the RNA. This sequence is called a codon. As each codon of the messenger RNA moves along the ribosome, transfer RNA carries that amino acid to the ribosome. The amino acid is connected by the ribosome to an increasing chain of amino acids to produce the protein programmed by the messenger RNA. These proteins are extremely long, and one amino acid out of place will alter the entire protein.[35]

Endoplasmic reticulum is a network of tubules and vesicles. There are two types: smooth and granular. One difference between the two is that granular reticulum has ribosomes attached to the exterior surface. Granular reticulum is involved in the process of producing proteins for secretion.[35] Smooth endoplasmic reticulum participates in lipid synthesis, glycogenolysis, drug detoxification, and conjugation of bile pigment.[25] Endoplasmic reticulum also has a very important role in the development of new cell membrane.[35]

The *Golgi complex* appears to be a specialized type of endoplasmic reticulum. These complexes gather substances to be secreted and transport them to the exterior of the cell. Golgi complexes assist in the production of glycoproteins. These complexes are also involved in lysosome formation. Cell membrane products manufactured in the endoplasmic reticulum must be routed through the Golgi complex before being transported to the cell membrane.[35]

Lysosomes are vesicles filled with hydrolytic enzymes. These enzymes are used to digest and remove foreign substances, such as bacteria, and damaged tissue.

Two pairs of *centrioles* are found in the cytoplasm of each cell. They are located near the nucleus and are active in cell division. During the process of cell division, they move apart and form the mitotic spindle.

The *nucleus* is responsible for the coordination and control of all cellular activities. Within the nucleus are long strands of DNA divided into sections called genes. The entire length of genes is called a chromosome.

It has been possible for a number of years

to identify the different chromosomes within the nucleus. All but the sex chromosomes are identified by number. The recognition of specific genes within a chromosome has been more difficult because of their very small size and the lack of appropriate technology. Recently, banding techniques have helped identify specific genes. It is now possible in some instances to identify the specific gene that controls a particular area of cellular function.[54]

Another structure within the nucleus is the nucleolus, which is made of RNA. The nucleolus is responsible for the production of ribosomal RNA, messenger RNA, and transfer RNA.

A double nuclear membrane encases the nucleus, controlling which substances are allowed to move into and out of the nucleus. The functions of this membrane are also complex and not fully understood.

The Cell Cycle

The cell cycle is an important process to understand in cancer nursing. This process will be referred to again in discussing both radiotherapy and chemotherapy. See Figure 2–1 for illustration of the cell cycle.

The cell cycle has two major divisions: interphase and mitosis. Interphase is the period between cell divisions. During interphase, cellular growth, protein production, and replication of DNA and RNA occur. Mitosis is the very brief period in which actual cell division occurs. Normal cell division occurs in order to replace cells that are lost as a result of cell aging or cell damage. When the number of lost cells has been replaced, cell division stops.

Interphase has been separated into three stages: G_1, S, and G_2. The length of each stage varies with the type of tissue; however, the usual or most common length of time for each stage has been identified.

G_1 lasts an average of 18 hours but is the most variable of the three stages. It is a period of cell growth that occurs immediately after cell division. Processes involving protein synthesis are active.

The S stage lasts 12 to 36 hours and is a period of DNA synthesis. During this stage, two sets of DNA are formed, doubling the usual amount of DNA in the nucleus.

G_2 lasts 3 hours and is a second period of cell growth that occurs after DNA synthesis is complete. During this period the cell doubles in size. RNA is synthesized and protein synthesis is active and rapid. When the cell reaches a "critical mass," mitosis will occur.

Mitosis requires about 1 hour to complete. The stages of mitosis have been broken down in a variety of ways. The sim-

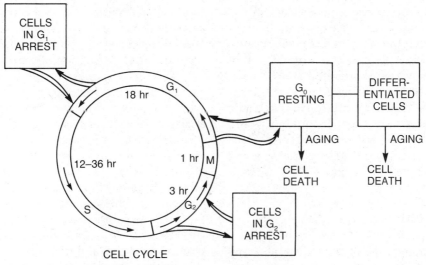

Figure 2–1. Diagram of the cell cycle.

plest and most common of these is the division into four stages: prophase, metaphase, anaphase, and telophase.[18, 23, 31]

Resting Cells

Only about 10 per cent of most types of cells are in the cell cycle at a given time, although some types of cells may have as much as 95 per cent of cells in the cell cycle. Many cells are in the resting state. These cells are capable of cell division, but are not involved in replication at that moment. G_0 has been used as the classification for the quiescent cells. Cells may also be blocked or arrested in G_1 or G_2 so that the cell cycle is not completed and mitosis does not occur. These cells are also considered resting cells.[18]

Resting cells require a stimulus in order to move back into the cell cycle. The longer they have been out of the cell cycle, the longer the period of time required and the greater the stimulus required before mitosis will occur. As people age, more of their cells are in the resting stage and greater stimulus is required to move normal cells into the cell cycle.[18]

Differentiated Cells

Some cells become highly differentiated as they mature. This allows those cells to function in a highly specialized manner without carrying on all of the normal cellular functions. One of the functions that these cells relinquish is replication. Therefore, highly differentiated cells will never be in the cell cycle. Dedifferentiation would have to occur for them to enter the cell cycle. This does occur normally in some instances; for example, in some types of white blood cells.

THE IMMUNE SYSTEM

The immune system is very complex and many of its processes are not well identified or understood. Much of the material presented in this section consists of hypotheses developed as a result of animal experimentation and cellular responses in test tubes. Within the human body the process is so complicated that it seems impossible to examine one segment of immune response in isolation from other segments of the immune system.

The immune system is roughly divided into two sections: humoral immunity and cell-mediated immunity. These two types of immunity often function together or duplicate the same function.

Humoral Immunity

Humoral immunity is involved in the production of antibodies. There are three phases in the production of antibody:

1. *Inductive phase* — The time between the first contact with an antigen and the first appearance of circulating antibody. The phagocyte handles the initial processing of the antigen. When antigen enters tissue with antibody-forming potential, it makes its first contact with phagocytic cells. These cells may be monocytes or tissue macrophages. The monocyte is located in peripheral blood. Tissue macrophages are found in lymph nodes, bone marrow, spleen, lung alveoli, adrenals, serous cavities, and skin. (Kupffer's cells of the liver are similar to tissue macrophages in function.) The phagocyte then passes the antigen or information about the antigen to a small lymphocyte. This lymphocyte undergoes differentiation and division, which results in the production of antibody.

2. *Productive phase* — The antibody rapidly increases in concentration.

3. *Stationary phase* — The amount of antibody remains constant.[22]

The antibodies produced are in the form of immunoglobulins of which there are five: IgA, IgM, IgG, IgE, and IgD. IgA is commonly found in the mucosa of the nose, bronchi, and tonsils. IgM is important in humoral immune reaction to gram-negative bacteria. IgG antibodies attack gram-positive bacteria and viruses. IgE is associated with allergies. The function of IgD is not yet understood.[22]

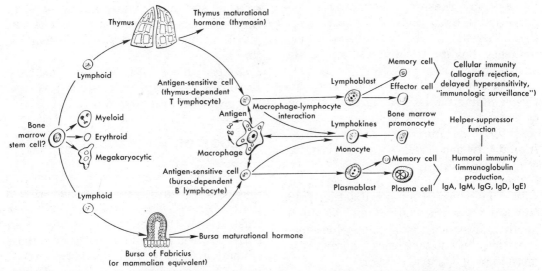

Figure 2–2. Schematic representation of the cellular events involved in adaptive immunity. (From Harris, J. E., and Sinkovics, J. G.: *The Immunology of Malignant Disease.* The C. V. Mosby Company, St. Louis, 1976. Used by permission.)

Cell-Mediated Immunity

Cell-mediated immunity is an important host defense against fungi, viruses, protozoa, and mycobacteria. Allograft rejection is also a cell-mediated process. The principal cell involved in cell-mediated immunity is a mononuclear cell. The events that result in the cellular immune response are not well understood. The process appears to be very complex and involves transformation of several types of lymphocytes. (See Figure 2–2.)

Newborns do not seem to have cell-mediated immunity; this function develops between 3 and 12 months of age. Cell-mediated immunity is gradually impaired as a person ages. Older people have a definite decrease in total circulating lymphocytes. T lymphocytes are decreased and sometimes there is a decrease in IgM and IgG. The thymus decreases in size. All of these changes could impair cell-mediated immunity.[22]

Thymus

The thymus is necessary for the maintenance of normal immune response, even in adults. However, the thymus' function in immunity is not clearly understood. The thymus seems to produce some lymphocytes and some chemical substances. Animal research studies have shown that one of these, thymosin, speeds up regeneration of lymphatic tissues, increases the number of antibody-forming cells, and increases immunocompetence. Thymosin seems to be primarily effective in stimulating cell-mediated immune responses; it appears to have no effect on humoral immunity. More recent studies indicate that thymosin may consist of more than one active ingredient.[22]

Other active substances found in the thymus are thymopoietin I and II, which cause bone marrow cells to develop T lymphocytes, and UBIP (ubiquitin), which induces T lymphocyte differentiation and affects B lymphocyte maturation.[22]

Lymphokines

Multiple factors are released by T lymphocytes and possibly by B lymphocytes when stimulated by antigens. The following is a list of those factors that have been identified. Whether all T lymphocytes release all factors or whether some factors are specific to particular lymphocytes is not known.[9]

Migration inhibitory factor (MIF) —

Released by sensitized lymphocytes apparently after reaction with a specific antigen. The MIF inhibits movement of macrophages, holding them at the site of the antigen reaction.[9]

Lymphotoxin — Destroys cells with antigens that stimulate sensitized lymphocytes.[9]

Proliferation inhibitory factor (PIF) — Inhibits division of cells with antigens that stimulate sensitized lymphocytes.[9]

Transfer factor (TF) — Active agent involved in transferring sensitization from one cell to another, from one person to another, or even across species. This sensitivity may last up to 2 years. There may be more than one transfer factor.[9]

Interferon — Produced by human lymphocytes after antigenic stimulation. Interferon is involved in the following activities:

1. Antiviral activity
2. Inhibiting cell division
3. Enhancing phagocytosis by macrophages
4. Enhancing cytotoxicity by sensitized lymphocytes
5. Inhibiting activity of colony stimulating factor[9]

Prostaglandins — A group of chemicals that have been identified only recently. Originally, the prostate gland was thought to produce them. Stimulation of lymphocytes has now been found to lead to the formation and release of prostaglandins. Their functions seem to be varied and are still being identified. In high doses, prostaglandins inhibit the cytotoxic activity of lymphocytes. They may act locally to control immunologic and inflammatory reactions.[9]

Colony stimulating factor — Stimulates the production of granulocytes and monocytes.[9]

Complement — Lymphocytes may synthesize some of the components of complement.[9] Complement is a system of factors found in normal serum, which are activated by antigen-antibody reaction. The system is very complex and involved in multiple plasma enzyme activities, such as the facilitation of phagocytosis and the blood-clotting system. Complement is involved in the lysis of antibody-coated cells and plays an important role in the inflammatory process.[31a]

Lymph node permeability factor — Produces capillary vasodilation, edema, and granulocyte infiltration.[9]

BIOLOGY OF THE CANCER CELL

For years attempts have been made to specifically identify the characteristics of the cancer cell. These attempts have been frustrated by the great variety of differences between cells of one tumor and those of another tumor — and even between cells within the same tumor. In spite of these differences, commonalities can be found. Even these vary in order of occurrence and do not always occur in every malignancy.[28, 55]

A vast amount of information has been gathered which describes *what* the cancer cell does and — to a lesser extent — *how* it does it. But the *why* evades us. We have been unable to define the malignant cell, save in broad terms by comparing it to its normal counterpart. The major problem appears to be that the malignant cell does so much. It is a chimera, mystifyingly composed of normal activities and structures, of phenotypic schizophrenia with embryonic, fetal and adult characteristics and occasionally a hint of unclassifiable capacity unique to malignant cells.[3]

Structure and Function

Cell Membrane

Multiple and varied changes occur in the cancer cell membrane. Decreased contact inhibition is one of the most striking.[1] Cancer cells continue movement when another cell is touched. Cell-to-cell communication is markedly decreased. There is a decrease in the number of small gap junctions and tight junctions. The cancer cell becomes autonomous, rather than maintaining physical contact with other cells. The cancer cell membrane also has a high negative surface charge that may repel other cells. Cell membrane antigens may be altered in cancer, thus changing communication with the rest of the body.[7]

Ryser[48] believes that cancer may be a membrane disease with loss of growth control as a result of membrane changes. Although the sequence of changes and the type of changes occurring may differ, the result — loss of growth control — may be the same.

Organelles

Mitochondria — Mutational changes may affect the functioning of the mitochondria in cancer. The mitochondria sometimes appear swollen. There are multiple alterations in metabolic functions. Metabolism is channeled into a simple pattern that requires less integration of genetic control.[7] Glucose utilization is higher than normal; however, the cell can adjust to lower levels of glucose. The cancer cell is able to utilize only about 50 per cent of available oxygen and utilizes anaerobic pathways of metabolism more frequently.[19] About 35 per cent of available glucose is converted to lactate.[19]

Ribosomes — There are more free ribosomes in the cancer cell. Protein production is oriented more toward structural proteins to support cell division. Enzyme products produced by the specialized normal cell decrease. Proteins normally produced only during fetal development may begin to be produced.[7]

Endoplasmic reticulum — Since it is a membrane, the endoplasmic reticulum may be altered by mutational changes. All membranes within the cell seem to undergo changes as the cell becomes more malignant.[7]

The *nucleus* — The nucleus may contain an abnormal distribution of chromosomes. Multiple mutations may have occurred. These changes do not necessarily affect the cell's ability to proliferate. The nucleus is much larger than normal, sometimes occupying most of the space of the cell. There is an increased production of DNA.[7] In many cases chromosome changes occur late in the evolution of the tumor; however, in some instances the tumor may develop as a result of chromosome changes.[56]

Cell Kinetics

Cell kinetics is a field of study that explores how cells grow. The growth process of cells is complex, dynamic, and frequently changing. Examining this process gives a much clearer picture of cell functioning than is possible by examining cell structure alone. Cell kinetics adds an invaluable dimension to our understanding of the neoplastic process.[31]

Terms used in the field of cell kinetics are not as familiar to nurses as those of histology, but they are very important for a broader knowledge of the process of cancer. Some of the terms used are growth curve, doubling time, growth fraction, cell cycle phases, cell loss, and growth coefficient. In the following discussion, these terms will be used and defined. Some of the findings of this complex and fascinating field of study will be described.

The Cell Cycle

Cancer cells have immortality in a way that normal cells do not. Normal cells age even though they are replicating and remain in the resting state longer as aging progresses, which ultimately results in cell death. Cancer cells can continue to replicate without aging and may not enter the resting state at all.

The chief function of the cancer cell is replication.[28] Cancer cells may move through the cell cycle more rapidly but are not necessarily dividing more frequently than normal cells.[31] The difference is that only 50 per cent of cancer cells differentiate, leaving 50 per cent of cells to continue replication (compared with 10 per cent of normal cells). The per cent of replicating cells is called the growth fraction. Malignancies have an increased number of cells that arrest in G_1 and G_2. Tumor cells may lose the capacity to move into the quiescent state of G_0.

Dedifferentiation

In dedifferentiation the cancer cell changes from the highly differentiated normal cell to a very primitive, undifferentiated cell called an anaplastic cell. Anaplastic cells replicate at a much more rapid rate.

Prehn and Prehn[45] identify five basic characteristics of the anaplastic cell:

1. *Neoplastic progression* — Cancer cells that are best able to replicate and those least able to differentiate outgrow the rest of the cells so that the cancer cell population with time tends to become more and more anaplastic.

2. *Convergence* — Almost all of the cells are undifferentiated and actively dividing. It is not possible to identify the tissue of origin, either chemically or structurally.

3. *Biochemical inflexibility* — Enzyme systems in the cell are unable to adapt to changes in the environment. A particular enzyme will be produced at a given level regardless of environmental changes.

4. *Aberrant differentiation* — Cell differentiation does occur but it is in bizarre and unexpected ways. Abnormal or unusual enzymes or hormones may be produced in large amounts.

5. *Neoantigenicity* — Cell membranes have new forms of antigens not found in normal cells.

TRANSFORMATION

Transformation is the process by which a normal cell changes into a malignant cell. Knowing how a cell transforms is very important in providing effective treatment and in planning approaches to prevent cancer. Because of the limits of our knowledge of molecular biology, many of the specific changes involved in this process are not known. In piecing together what is known, theories have been developed in attempts to describe the entire process.

Theory I

The original exposure of the cell to a carcinogenic agent changes the cell permanently to a malignant cell. After this event the malignant cell remains dormant for a long period of time. Emergence of the malignant cell from dormancy is a consequence of exposure to promoting agents that stimulate proliferation of the dormant but malignant cell.

This theory proposes that all people have malignant cells that may be developing regularly. The body's immune surveillance system rejects and destroys these cells. Therefore, a decrease in immunocompetence can allow the malignant cell to begin proliferating.

Theory II

The initial exposure to a carcinogenic agent causes a change in the cell. This cell, although changed, is not at this point malignant. Over a period of time, many more abnormal changes occur as the cell divides and is exposed to other carcinogenic substances. The ultimate result of all of these changes is the malignant cell. In effect, there is a progressive cellular evolution that stops only with the death of the person. This theory would explain easily why malignancies happen more frequently as aging occurs.[4]

Is Transformation an Irreversible Process?

Research scientists have conflicting answers to this question. Some scientists believe that the initial cell change makes a permanent alteration in the cell and that the process as it progresses from that point is irreversible. Other scientists believe that the first changes that occur in the cell are reversible but that past a certain point in the transformation process changes are irreversible.

Still other scientists believe that the entire malignant process is reversible. They believe that all of the changes occurring in the cell are epigenetic rather than genetic and that the movement of the cell toward dedifferentiation can be reversed. Genetic changes alter the DNA in the nucleus, implying mutation and irreversibility. Epigenetic changes are changes in the expression of existing genes, an example of which would be cell membrane alterations that change cell structure and function but do not alter DNA. Such changes would be reversible.[1]

If cancer cells are a result of abnormal dedifferentiation that causes epigenetic changes in cell functioning, anything that could reverse the process and cause the cells to differentiate would cure the cancer. The differentiated cells would move out of the cell cycle and overgrowth of cells would stop. Some scientists believe this will be the treatment of the future.[32]

CLONE FORMATION

After a cell has completed the transformation process, it must proliferate in order to form a clone of cells. The success of this process depends to a great extent on the interaction between the malignant cell and the host. This interaction involves substances produced by the malignant cell and substances produced by the host.

In essence, a battle begins, with both parties bringing out all their weapons and tactical maneuvers. If the host wins, the malignant cell is destroyed. If the malignant cell wins, a clone forms and develops into a tumor.

The Immune System

Much of the attack launched by the host is dependent on factors within the immune system.

Antibodies. Many cancer cells have altered antigens on the cell membrane surface. These altered antigens may be identified by the immune system as foreign. If this occurs, the complete antigen-antibody-complement process may take place, possibly resulting in the destruction of the cancer cells. Not all of the cancer cells within a tumor are alike, however. Those with strong antigens may be destroyed, leaving those with few or no antigens to continue growing.[9]

"Armed" Macrophages. Macrophages may be made to destroy specific cancer cells by the release of a factor produced by specifically sensitized T lymphocytes. The factor has not been definitely identified.[9] On the other hand, macrophages can have a protective effect on cancer cells that are sensitized with antibody and thus prevent cancer cell damage by antibody and complement or by cell-killing lymphocytes.[9]

Cellular Immunity. The cellular immune response seems to be very involved in the body's defense against cancer. Changes may occur in cellular immune responses as a result of the development of cancer.[9]

Thymus. Changes have been found in the thymus of patients with malignant disease. In research animals, the thymus is important in enhancing resistance to the growth of virus-induced cancer. The cause of the changes in the thymus and the effect of those changes on cell-mediated immunity are not known.[9]

Lymphokines. If cell-mediated immunity is in full operation, many of the lymphokines will be utilized in the battle against the cancer cell. However, since these are released only by sensitized lymphocytes, the cancer cells would have to be structured in such a way that sensitization would occur in order for lymphokines to be released.[9]

Immunologic Tolerance. Immunologic tolerance is a situation in which the immune system does not react to an antigen that ordinarily would cause a response. In order to induce tolerance, an antigen must be continually present in the body. It is more effective if the cells containing the antigen continue to replicate, providing a continuous source of antigen. If the antigen disappears, the host's ability to form antibody returns.

Tolerance may be induced by overwhelming the immune system with large amounts of antigen. In some cases, however, immunologic tolerance occurs when antigens are continually present at levels low enough that immune response is not stimulated. The process by which immune tolerance occurs is not known.[9]

Immune Escape Mechanisms. Obviously, a very complex immune reaction involving lymphocytes, macrophages, and soluble factors released by these cells is involved in the attack against cancer. Certainly there are host responses, whether or not an immune surveillance system as such exists. The question then arises — is it necessary for the immune system to malfunction in order for cancer to develop?

Several mechanisms have been proposed that would allow antigenic tumor cells to escape the attack by the intact immune system:

1. *Sneaking   through* — Cancer that begins as a single cell may not stimulate immunologic recognition during early growth. By the time the immune system recognizes it, the mass may be too large for effective attack by the body.

2. *Antigenic modulation* — The cancer cells mask or lose antigen when confronted by immunologic attack.

3. *Antigenic blindfolding* — Some tumors flood the body with tumor antigens. These antigens bind to the antibodies or receptors on lymphocytes, which prevents them from recognizing and destroying the tumor cells.

4. *Oncogenic viruses* — These viruses can infect the body at birth and remain unrecognized as foreign antigens.[43]

Blocking Factor

Blocking factors prevent the destruction of cells identified as foreign by lymphocytes. This process occurs normally in pregnancy. It also appears to be necessary in order to prevent autoimmune diseases. Blocking factors are related to the process of self-tolerance. These blocking factors are part of the immune system, but in cancer they can actually result in immunologic enhancement of tumor growth. Antigens, antibodies, and cytotoxic lymphocytes are involved in the blocking process.[9]

The process that seems to occur involves the shedding of antigens from cancer cell membranes into the blood stream. These excess antigens combine with all available antibodies to form antigen-antibody complexes, which inactivate T lymphocytes. This effectively immobilizes the immune system attack against the cancer cells (antigenic blindfolding), leaving them safe from attack and free to replicate. High blood levels of blocking factor are associated with rapid tumor growth. If a large bulk of tumor is removed, the level of blocking factor markedly decreases.[9]

Recognition Factor

Recognition factor is a substance produced by the immune system that combines with tumor cells before they can be attacked by macrophages. Healthy people and those with diseases other than cancer have high blood levels of recognition factor. People with cancer have lower levels of recognition factor. As the cancer progresses, the level of recognition factor decreases.[9]

Angiogenesis Factor

A good supply of blood is essential if the malignant cell is to develop into a clone. Some malignant cells secrete a substance called angiogenesis factor, which attracts capillaries to the cell. These capillaries then branch out, thus increasing the cell's blood supply. Without adequate vascularization, the clone will not grow beyond 3 to 4 mm in diameter.[23]

Chalones

A chalone is a mitotic inhibitor, a substance that prevents cell division. There is a different chalone for each type of tissue. Recognition of the existence of chalones is recent; therefore, understanding of the process by which they function is incomplete. Chalones are produced by the cells within a tissue. If a large part of the tissue is damaged or destroyed, there is also loss of chalone in the tissue, which stimulates an increase in cell division. As new cells, all containing chalone, are formed, a high level of the substance is reestablished and cell division stops.[6, 24]

It is believed that in cancer the malignant cells produce an adequate amount of chalone but fail to hold it within the cells. The chalone is apparently lost in the circulation.[24] It appears that the cell's loss of chalone is the result of a cell membrane abnormality.[6]

Experimental studies indicate that malignant cells will respond to artificially supplied chalones, although tumor cells are less sensitive to chalones.[24] Further research may reveal that chalones can be used as a treatment method.

Hormones

Hormones can either stimulate or interfere with the growth of cancer cells. The hormones' influence is dependent to some extent on receptors located on the cell membrane. As the cell dedifferentiates, hormones cease to affect cell growth, perhaps as a result of changes in cell membrane receptors.

Other Factors

Other substances are being considered in the search to understand the growth of malignant cells. The field of study is so new and complex that many substances are suspected of being present but have not been specifically identified. Some substances that are being mentioned in the literature are colony stimulating factor, diffusible granulopoietin stimulator, antichalones, leukocytosis inducing factor, and growth stimulating factor.[34]

The Growth Control System

The control of growth is a very complex system, with all of its components interrelated. The system seems to be very versatile. Much remains to be known about identifying components and mechanisms of control. From what is known, it appears that the host produces substances that tend to prevent abnormal or uncontrolled growth. The malignant cell produces substances that counter the effects of host defenses. The most effective defense prevails.

TUMOR STEMLINES

As the clone begins to develop into a tumor, additional cell changes occur. Further mutations, chromosomal changes, and cell membrane changes take place. The changes are not consistent from cell to cell. These cells, which differ from each other, begin to replicate, forming subpopulations of tumor cells called stemlines. Some of these stemlines have a selected advantage over others and predominate within the tumor.

As dedifferentiation occurs, these stemlines may be replaced by others, which are more primitive, less controllable, and more successful in replication. Solid tumors contain sectors of cells from the same stemline that are different from other stemline cells in other sectors of the tumor.[23]

Stem Cells

Not all of the cells in a tumor are in active cell division. Not all of the cells in the tumor are malignant; some are normal. Stem cells are those cells from the tumor stemlines, which have the capacity to divide rapidly and continuously. Stem cells make up about 10 per cent of a tumor. These cells are most active during the continuous replication that leads to the death of the host. Some of the other malignant cells may be in the resting state or may have differentiated in some bizarre way and therefore are no longer replicating.[23]

Doubling Time

The growth rate in a tumor is frequently expressed as doubling time. The doubling time may be measured in terms of volume, weight, or number of cells. The doubling time for human cancers ranges from 1 week to more than 1 year, with the median being 60 days.[23]

Factors Affecting Tumor Growth

Cell cycle time — The length of time required for cell division is dependent upon nutrients, including oxygen. Cells that are not near capillaries have a longer cell cycle time than those near capillaries. Tumor cells that produce angiogenesis factor have a distinct advantage, since this factor increases blood availability.

Growth fraction — The proportion of cells in the tumor that are actively dividing influences the rate of tumor growth. Tumors with a small growth fraction will grow slowly. The percentage of cells actively replicating varies from tumor to tumor, ranging from 10 to 70 per cent.[23]

Cell loss — Cells are lost in tumors as a result of a variety of processes. Cell death may occur as a result of cell aging and differentiation, nutrient deficiency, or destruction by host defense mechanisms. Cells also leave the tumor by means of exfoliation and metastasis. Cell loss in human tumors ranges from 60 to 90 per cent.[23]

STRUCTURE OF A SOLID TUMOR

In recent years, detailed research has been conducted on the makeup and function of solid tumors.

Necrotic Centers

Many solid tumors have necrotic centers. These necrotic centers contain dead tissue, which is digested in the interstitial spaces by macrophages and lytic enzymes. Originally this necrosis was believed to be caused by decreased blood circulation in the center of the tumor. Some scientists now believe the necrosis is not the result of decrease in circulation, since these regions have been found to contain large numbers of viable cells.[19]

Vascular Network

The blood vessels within a tumor are unlike those in the rest of the body. Capillaries in a tumor have a large diameter, and the endothelial lining and basement membrane are irregular and discontinuous. Sometimes the blood vessels are only irregular channels lined by tumor cells.[8, 19]

Blood vessels are abnormally connected: arteries and veins may be directly connected, and there may be complexes of vessels and unusual vessel growth patterns. These abnormal structures make up a very complex network of blood vessels. The vessels are more prevalent and best preserved at the edges of the tumor.[8]

Blood Flow

Blood flow in the tumor is equal to or higher than the flow in the tissue of origin. Vascular volume is 16 per cent of tumor size, which is greater than normal tissue.[19] The circulation patterns of blood within the tumors are different. Regurgitation and periods of blood stasis are common. When blood flow resumes, it may flow in an opposite direction. This may be caused by tissue pressures resulting from increased cell proliferation. When cell division is arrested or when many tumor cells are destroyed by treatment, vascular transport within the tumor improves.

Tumor Interstitial Fluid

The amount of interstitial fluid in a tumor is much greater than in normal tissue, making up 30 to 60 per cent of the tumor water.[19] Tumor tissue fluid content differs from normal tissue fluid by being higher in glucose, lactate, cholesterol, lipid phosphorus, and amino acids. Protein concentration is lower; the hydrogen concentration is twice that of arterial fluid; and bicarbonate ions are 20 per cent lower. This results in a state of acidosis within the tumor interstitial fluid.[19]

Cell Proliferation

Cell proliferation is more rapid on the surface of the tumor where the circulation is better. Cells near the center of the tumor grow much more slowly. Cell proliferation can be stimulated by many substances: steroids and other hormones, erythropoietin, colony stimulating factor, antichalones, leukocytosis inducing factor, growth stimulating factor, nerve growth factor, and epithelial growth factor. These factors apparently interact to influence cell growth. The mechanisms that control secretion of these substances are not completely understood.[34] Changes in the balance of these substances could alter proliferation rates.

Local Tumor Extension

The rate of tumor growth will determine its ability to spread. Malignant tumors spread by infiltration or erosion. This may involve necrosis, ulceration, or fibrous replacement of normal tissue. Infection or hemorrhage may occur in this damaged tissue.

Local extension and metastasis seem to be very complex processes with several influencing links. The growing tumor causes tissue damage, which results in inflammation. Inflammation causes multiple reactions including an increase in cell proliferation and damage to the blood vessel endothelium. Chemicals released to promote rapid division of normal cells also stimulate rapid division of cancer cells and increased cell motility. Because of the damage to blood vessels and inflammatory changes in nearby normal cells, these malignant cells can easily move into adjacent normal tissues or into the lumen of blood vessels.[34]

The growing tumor is not the only cause of tissue inflammation surrounding a tumor. Other causative factors are radiation, surgery, and mechanical injury. Any one of these factors will increase the probability of local spread.[34] Radiation damage also causes an increase in a chemical called growth stimulating substance (GSS). This chemical diffuses from the site of radiation out to surrounding normal tissues. GSS increases the rate of cell division of both normal cells and any malignant cells that have entered the area.[34]

The cancer cells advance along spaces where they meet the least resistance: this may be in interstitial spaces, along blood vessels, or along nerve pathways. Fibrous tissue is a barrier to tumor cell growth; thus, artery walls, organ capsules, and fibrous sheets will block growth except at points where they are penetrated by nerves or blood vessels.

Local spread occurs before metastasis. The increased bulk of the growing tumor will force cells to extend from the body of the tumor. Cell membrane changes that result in lack of contact inhibition and increase in cell movement also promote this process.[15]

METASTASIS

Separation

Cells separate from the primary lesion because of decreased or absent cell cohesion that results from cell membrane changes. The separation may occur as single cells or as clumps of cells. Since cancer cells have increased locomotion, movement away from the primary tumor and toward blood and lymphatic drainage systems is easily accomplished. Some scientists believe that detached cancer cells may be actively moving away from areas with inadequate nutrients and oxygen toward sites with higher nutrient levels.[51]

Distributive Systems

The two primary systems that distribute cancer cells to other parts of the body are the blood and lymphatic systems. Cancer cells are also transported by gravity from one part of a body cavity to another part of the same cavity; this is called seeding. Cerebrospinal fluid pathways may also serve as a transport mechanism.

The Lymph Route. The lymphatic system is the usual pathway for local metastasis. By mechanisms which are not understood, the regional nodes that drain a tumor are changed structurally before metastasis occurs. This is called premetastatic reactive hyperplasia. It is thought that this hyperplasia may be a body defense mechanism attempt to form a barrier to the tumor. These nodes produce immune cells that, although they are unable to protect the node from malignant invasion, may play an important role in the body's attempt to form an immune defense against the cancer. Because of this possibility, some scientists are questioning the wisdom of removing the lymphatic drainage system at the time of surgery.[8]

Cancer cells are usually caught in a lymph node by mechanical trapping, since the structure of a lymph node is somewhat like that of a maze. Once they enter the node, three things may occur: the cancer cells may die; the cancer cells may remain dormant within the node; or the cancer cells may proliferate and cause a metastatic lesion. Lymph node involvement is thought to occur early, possibly before the tumor has reached 1 mm in size.[8]

Cancer cells may travel through the lymph channels without being trapped in a node and be released into the blood stream, or they may become detached from metastatic nodes and travel through the lymph channels to the blood.

The Blood Route. There are several mechanisms through which cancer cells can enter the blood stream. As previously mentioned, blood vessels within a tumor are poorly constructed. Cells can simply break loose from the tumor and become a part of the blood stream. The tumor may actually invade the blood vessel by local extension and then cells could break away into the blood stream. Because of the increased locomotion of cancer cells and their ability to change shape, it is possible for them to squeeze through the lining of a vein (intravasation).[8] This is most likely to occur when pressure from the tumor becomes greater than the pressure within the blood vessel. Most distant metastases result from blood transport.

Survival in the Blood Stream

The majority of cancer cells that enter the blood stream apparently die.[8] Whether this is due to mechanical destruction, metabolic processes, or attack by elements in the blood is not known. There is no relationship between the number of cancer cells in the blood stream and the incidence of metastasis.[8]

If a cell survives, it must still succeed in implanting in a site suitable for growth to occur. It was once thought that the cancer cell implanted when it reached a place where the vessel was too small for the cell to continue. This has been found to be incorrect. The cancer cell can change shape and travel within small capillaries. It was also believed that the cancer cell attached and survived only in areas of rich blood supply. This also is not true. Certain types of cancers have affinity for specific types of tissue, and implantations at this site are most likely to result in the development of a metastatic lesion.[8] Inflammation in a tissue will increase the risk of metastasis. The administration of anti-inflammatory drugs, such as corticosteroids, has been found experimentally to reduce the number of lung metastases.[34]

Attachment

A complex process occurs when the cancer cell adheres to endothelial lining. In the blood stream, the cancer cell membrane becomes very sticky. Platelets then attach to the membrane. The cancer cell in turn sticks to the endothelial lining. The platelets may break open, releasing thromboplastin. Tumor cells also seem to be able to produce and release thromboplastin.[8, 34]

This causes the formation of a fibrin lattice, which surrounds the cell.[34] This process of fibrin formation around a cancer cell is called nidation. Experimentally, this process can be interfered with by administering heparin.[8]

Within 3 to 6 hours the cells break through the endothelium and begin to develop a vascular supply.[8] This is accomplished by the release of angiogenesis factor by the cancer cell. More thromboplastin is released and a fibrin framework is formed again around the cancer cell. This process occurs more readily in inflamed tissues and in the normal tissue surrounding a region that is being radiated.[34]

Growing

What happens to the cell at this point depends on host-tumor interactions.[8] The immune response is complex and involves specific antitumor antibodies that counteract the blocking antibodies.[8] Immune responses are apparently most effective in preventing the start of metastatic growth. Once that growth is established the immune defenses are relatively ineffective.[8]

If growth is established, several things can occur: the tumor cells may begin to grow and then regress "spontaneously"; the cells may remain dormant for as long as 20 years or more and then begin to grow (little is understood about how dormancy is maintained); or the cells may begin to replicate and form a metastatic lesion.[8]

Neoplastic Progression

After metastasis is established, the tumor cells begin to change. Stem cells, which proliferate more rapidly, predominate. With the rapid proliferation come additional abnormal cell changes. The cells become less and less like the normal cells from which they originated. These malignant cells also become more and more different from the malignant cells in the primary tumor. They are then defined as anaplastic. At this point, dissemination of malignant cells throughout the body occurs very rapidly.[34]

PRODUCTS PRODUCED BY TUMORS

As they differentiate, tumors produce unusual hormones, enzymes, and other chemicals as a result of alterations in gene expression. The number of abnormal chemicals increases as the tumor grows.[21] Normally, enzyme levels are regulated by diet, hormones, or metabolic controls. The enzymes produced by cancer cells are slightly different chemically and do not respond to any controls.[21] These products may cause major alterations in body functioning or they may have no known impact on the body.[42] Some of these substances are useful in diagnosing or determining the growth rate of tumors.

One group of substances produced are fetal antigens. These are thought to be the result of derepression of genes that normally function only during the embryonic period or during cell differentiation.[55] These antigens are usually located on the cell membrane and sometimes stimulate host immune responses to the cancer cell.

Carcinoembryonic Antigen

Carcinoembryonic antigen (CEA) was the first fetal antigen detected. When it was first discovered, CEA was thought to be produced only by gastrointestinal cancers and there were high hopes that it could be used to diagnose cancer in the gastrointestinal (GI) tract. Unfortunately, CEA was also found to be present in small amounts in people with cirrhosis of the liver, uremia, alcoholism, emphysema, inflammatory bowel disease, and peptic ulcer, in heavy smokers, and in some normal people. The amounts (≤ 10 ng/ml) were never as high as the levels present in malignancy (≥ 10 ng/ml) but CEA caused too high an incidence of false positive results to allow its use as a screening device.

Fewer than half of early curable cancers have elevated CEA, thus causing false negative results.

As the disease progresses, however, the CEA level becomes increasingly elevated. Because of this elevation, measurement of CEA is used to determine the effectiveness of cancer treatment. If the CEA decreases, the treatment has been effective. Patients with known disease who seem to be in clinical remission can be monitored by measuring their CEA level. If the level begins to rise, it is an indication of regrowth of tumor occurring before clinical signs appear.

CEA is frequently present in the following cancers: colon, stomach, pancreas, lung, and breast tumors; and sarcomas, leukemias, and lymphomas.[38, 55]

Alpha-fetoprotein

Alpha-fetoprotein (AFP) is found in patients with cancer of the liver, testis, or ovary. Bronchogenic carcinoma and gastric and pancreatic cancer may also produce AFP. No relationship has been found between the level of AFP and the prognosis.[55]

Other Fetal Antigens

In recent years other fetal antigens have been found in malignant tissues. Studies to determine the types of cancer in which they are found and their levels in the blood are not complete.

Paraneoplastic Syndromes

Some of the substances produced by cancer cells cause the development of paraneoplastic syndromes. These are disorders that can occur together with a malignancy. The number of syndromes that can occur is extensive. They cause hormone disorders, connective tissue and skin disorders, neuromuscular disorders, and vascular, gastro-intestinal, immunologic, and hematologic difficulties. These syndromes may appear before the malignancy is diagnosed.[14]

SYSTEMIC EFFECTS OF TUMOR GROWTH

Some of the effects of growing tumors are local and a direct result of increasing occupation of space by the tumor. Other effects are systemic and the processes that cause them to occur are not well understood. These systemic effects may occur weeks, months, or even years before clinical signs of cancer appear.[42]

Pressure

Tumors cause pressure because they are taking over space usually occupied by body organs. They also cause pressure because of rapid cell division. Pressure within the tumor is greater than pressure of adjoining body structures. One consequence of this pressure is the obstruction of tubular structures such as the esophagus, ureters, bronchi, bowel, ducts, blood vessels, and lymphatic channels. Another consequence is a decrease in blood supply to the region. Decreased blood supply may also occur because available blood is directed into the tumor.

As a result of inadequate blood supply, normal tissue may become necrotic and then ulcerate. As ulcerated areas erode deeper into normal tissue, hemorrhages occur. Small hemorrhages increase the risk of infection in the area.[25]

Anemia

Many patients with cancer are anemic; the cause of this is not well understood. It is possible that chemicals produced by the tumor interfere with the production of red blood cells. The metabolites usually used to manufacture red blood cells could be used instead by the tumor. Iron, for example, has been shown to be taken into the tumor rather than deposited normally into the liver. Therefore, anemia may be a result of iron being lost to the tumor. Alteration of iron deposition alone is not the basic problem, because administration of iron will not reverse the anemia. Further studies will need to be done before there is a clear understanding of the mechanisms involved.[25]

Decreased Immunocompetence

Persons with cancer have decreased immunocompetence, which becomes more severe as the disease progresses. Length of survival is related to the level of immunocompetence. People who have a better functioning immune system are usually long-term survivors of their illness, regardless of the treatment used. People with very low immune functioning will die quickly, regardless of the treatment. The cause of decreased immunocompetence is not well understood.

Increased Incidence of Clotting

Cancer patients have a high risk of blood clotting, even very early in the disease. There is a high incidence of thrombophlebitis. The primary cause of pulmonary embolus is cancer. The cause of the change in the clotting mechanism is not known.

Change in Sense of Taste

A change in taste occurs in cancer patients often before clinical signs of the disease appear. The specific changes are not consistent from patient to patient. Most commonly, beef and pork begin to taste bitter and will usually be rejected by the patient. Some patients experience a decreased ability to taste sweet foods, requiring that foods be very sweet in order to taste sweet; other patients cannot tolerate sweet tastes at all. Salty and sour foods are usu-

ally better tolerated. Again, the cause of these changes is not known.

Altered Food Intake

There seem to be two separate mechanisms for controlling food intake: (1) receptors in the portal-hepatic area that send post-absorptive signals controlling the duration of feeding and (2) central receptors that respond to the depletion of energy reserves and control the efficiency of feeding. In cancer both of these mechanisms malfunction, the former early in the disease and the latter during progressive disease.[37]

Metabolic Changes

Multiple metabolic changes occur in cancer. Some of these changes develop early, before clinical diagnosis of the disease is possible. If the changes are severe, they may cause the patient to seek medical care, resulting in the diagnosis of cancer. These changes — along with some of the other systemic changes occurring in cancer — result in the development of cachexia, a metabolic disease characterized by weakness and emaciation.

Protein Metabolism. Protein depletion seems to be a generalized phenomenon in cancer, varying with different tumors. Cancer patients have a low serum albumin level. As the cancer progresses, the hypoalbuminemia becomes more severe. There seems to be a decrease in the synthesis of albumin by the host. Since amino acids are utilized to synthesize albumin, many researchers turned to extensive study of the metabolism of amino acids in cancer. Theologides[52] proposed that as the tumor grows larger, amino acids are released from muscle tissue into plasma and are extracted from plasma by the tumor. Even when the host is adequately fed, normal cells may not benefit from the increased intake of nutrients. The tumor utilizes all the nitrogen from the dietary intake and takes the building materials from normal tissues. The tumor's need for growth somehow supersedes the requirements of the host. The nitrogen in the tumor becomes trapped and is not available to normal tissue.[52] For this reason, the tumor is often labeled a "one-way nitrogen trap." A negative nitrogen balance is reported in a large percentage of advanced cancer patients. However, the patient may be in calorie deficit and show a positive nitrogen balance because most of the nitrogen is being retained by the tumor.[52] More recently Busch[7] has shown that uptake of proteins by cancerous and normal cells is the same. What is different is the way that the amino acids are utilized: tumor cells incorporate amino acids into the nuclear protein, whereas normal cells incorporate them into the cytoplasmic structures.

Lipid Metabolism. In cancer patients there is a progressive decrease of body fats to as little as 10 per cent of that normally found. Lipid loss is not due entirely to inadequate food intake because force-feeding does not prevent the loss. Marked hyperlipidemia may be present. Increased metabolic rate and greater caloric expenditure seem to be the cause of the mobilization of stored fats.

Other changes also occur in cancer patients that affect the storing of body fat. Normally, excess glucose or acetate is stored in adipose tissue. Even in starvation, acetate continues to be deposited into adipose tissue. However, in cancer, neither glucose nor acetate is deposited in adipose tissue, even if they are provided in excess of body needs. There may be a decreased ability to synthesize fat.

With 80 per cent of fat lost, it is possible that the structural lipids in the cells are almost destroyed, with irreversible consequences for vital cellular function. This fat loss is also a significant factor in the development of cachexia, a metabolic disease prevalent in cancer.[13] Much remains to be understood about the complex changes that occur in lipid metabolism during cancer.

Carbohydrate Metabolism. Tumors seem to flourish optimally in the presence of an adequate supply of insulin. A relationship based on both clinical and biochemical data has been established between neoplasms and impaired carbohydrate metabolism.

As the tumor grows, it consumes ever-increasing amounts of glucose at the expense of the host's energy reserves. Low liver glycogen levels are frequently present in the host.

Although most cancer cells have enzyme systems for oxidative metabolism, experimental evidence suggests that the majority of the glucose and the products of gluconeogenesis are metabolized via the anaerobic glycogenic cycle — an inefficient, low energy-yielding system that liberates the lactic acid that often must be resynthesized into glucose before being utilized.[11]

There is some evidence that glycolysis may be inhibited by an acid pH. Tumor cells that metabolize large quantities of glucose by way of the glycolytic cycle liberate lactic acid, which lowers the pH. When large amounts of glucose are provided by intravenous hyperalimentation, the blood and urine sugar levels remain normal, indicating that the glucose is being taken into cells and metabolized. As a result, the host gains weight and increased energy. The tumor does not increase in bulk even though more glucose is available for metabolism. There is possibly a limit to the rate at which the tumor can metabolize large amounts of glucose.[11]

Water. In cancer patients, total body water content increases to 10 per cent above normal.[12] This might account for the failure to observe significant weight changes even though there are major losses of adipose and muscle tissue.

Sodium. Sodium is retained by the cancer patient, with 120 per cent of the sodium found in the healthy individual being found in the cancer patient. It is possible that as a result of the decrease in available energy there is a breakdown in the sodium pump within the cells.[12] There is an increase in the body's total sodium as the tumor grows larger and a transfer of sodium from the host to the tumor. The amount of sodium in the tumor accounts for almost all of the dietary sodium retained.[12]

Since most of the sodium is retained within the tumor, the host is actually sodium poor. In sodium depletion in otherwise normal subjects, there is decreased palatability and appeal of food.

Increased Metabolic Rate. In cancer there is an increased energy expenditure and an inability to adjust the metabolic rate in spite of malnutrition. There are two possible reasons for this. First, the growth of neoplasm continues throughout the entire day rather than the diurnal pattern of the metabolic activity of normal tissues, in which there is periodic decrease of caloric expenditure. Second, selective removal of nutrients by the tumor causes changes in the intermediate metabolic pathways of the host, requiring the host to utilize more expensive pathways in terms of energy and nitrogen metabolism. Some biochemical reactions previously available to the host may not be possible because the involved metabolites have been utilized by the tumor.[53]

BIBLIOGRAPHY

1. Ambrose, E. J.: Surface properties of tumor cells. In *Biology of Cancer,* ed. by E. J. Ambrose and F. J. C. Roe. John Wiley & Sons, Inc., New York, 1975.
2. Baserga, R. L.: Cell cycle dependency of transformation. In *Neoplastic Transformation: Mechanisms and Consequences,* ed. by H. Koprowski. Abakon Verlagsgesellschaft, Berlin, 1977.
3. Becker, F. F.: *Cancer: A Comprehensive Treatise, Vol. 3: Biology of Tumors: Cellular Biology and Growth.* Plenum Press, New York, 1975, p. V.
4. Berenblum, I.: Established principles and unresolved problems in carcinogenesis. *Journal of the National Cancer Institute.* 60:723–726, 1978.
5. Braun, A. C.: Differentiation and dedifferentiation. In *Cancer: A Comprehensive Treatise, Vol. 3: Biology of Tumors: Cellular Biology and Growth,* ed. by F. F. Becker. Plenum Press, New York, 1975.
6. Bullough, W. S.: Chalones and cancer. In *Growth Kinetics and Biochemical Regulation of Normal and Malignant Cells,* ed. by B. Drewinko and R. M. Humphrey. Williams and Wilkins, Baltimore, 1977.
7. Busch, H.: *The Molecular Biology of Cancer.* Academic Press, Inc., New York, 1974.
8. Carter, R. L.: Metastasis. In *Biology of Cancer,* ed. by E. J. Ambrose and F. J. C. Roe. John Wiley & Sons, Inc., New York, 1975.
9. Castro, J. C.: *Immunological Aspects of Cancer.* University Park Press, Baltimore, 1978.
10. Clifton, K. H., and B. Sridharan: Endocrine factors and tumor growth. In *Cancer: A Comprehensive Treatise, Vol. 3: Biology of Tumors: Cellular Biology and Growth.,* ed. by F. F. Becker. Plenum Press, New York, 1975.
11. Copeland, E. M., et al.: Intravenous hyperalimentation as an adjunct to cancer chemotherapy. *American Journal of Surgery.* 129:167–173, 1975.
12. Costa, G.: Cachexia, the metabolic component of neoplastic disease. *Progress in Experimental Tumor Research.* 3:321–369, 1963.
13. Costa, G., and A. P. Weathers: Cancer and the nutrition of the host. *Journal of the American Dietetic Association.* 44:15–17, 1964.
14. Davies, J. N. P.: Spread and behavior of cancer and staging. In *Clinical Oncology,* ed. by J. Horton and G. J. Hill. W. B. Saunders Co., Philadelphia, 1977.
15. Easty, G. C.: Invasion by cancer cells. In *Biology of Cancer,* ed. by E. J. Ambrose and F. J. C. Roe. John Wiley & Sons, Inc., New York, 1975.
16. Farber, E.: Carcinogenesis — cellular evolution as a unifying thread: Presidential address. *Cancer Research.* 33:2537–2550, 1973.
17. Folkman, J.: Tumor angiogenesis. In *Cancer: A Comprehensive Treatise, Vol. 3: Biology of Tumors: Cellular Biology and Growth,* ed. by F. F. Becker. Plenum Press, New York, 1975.
18. Gelfant, S.: A new concept of tissue and tumor cell proliferation. *Cancer Research.* 37:3845–3862, 1977.
19. Gullino, P. M.: Extracellular compartments of solid tumors. In *Cancer: A Comprehensive Treatise, Vol. 3: Biology of Tumors: Cellular Biology and Growth,* ed. by F. F. Becker. Plenum Press, New York, 1975.
20. Guyton, A. C.: *Textbook of Medical Physiology.* Philadelphia, W. B. Saunders Co., 1981.
21. Harrap, K. R.: Deviant metabolic patterns in malignant disease. In *Biology of Cancer,* ed. by E. J. Ambrose and F. J. C. Roe. John Wiley & Sons, Inc., New York, 1975.
22. Harris, J. E., and J. G. Sinkovics: *The Immunology of Malignant Disease.* C. V. Mosby Co., St. Louis, 1976.
23. Hill, H. Z., and H.-S. Lin: Carcinogenesis and tumor growth. In *Clinical Oncology,* ed. by J. Horton and G. J. Hill. W. B. Saunders Co., Philadelphia, 1977.
24. Houck, J. C., and A. M. Attallah: Chalones (specific and endogenous mitotic inhibitors) and cancer. In *Cancer: A Comprehensive Treatise, Vol. 3: Biology of Tumors: Cellular Biology and Growth,* ed. by F. F. Becker. Plenum Press, New York, 1975.
25. Hubbard, S. M.: Neoplastic processes. In *Medical Surgical Nursing,* ed. by D. A. Jones, C. F. Dunbar, and M. M. Jerover. McGraw-Hill Book Co., New York, 1978.
26. Jansson, B.: Cell ecology: Deductive and dynamic

models for proliferation, differentiation and competition of tumor cell populations. *Theoretical Biology.* 68:43–51, 1977.

27. Kent, S.: Cell regeneration, the aging process, and cancer control. *Geriatrics.* January 1978, pp. 112–116.

28. Koller, P. C.: Chromosomes: The genetic component of the tumor cell. In *Biology of Cancer,* ed. by E. J. Ambrose and F. J. C. Roe. John Wiley & Sons, Inc., New York, 1975.

29. Koprowski, H.: *Neoplastic Transformation: Mechanisms and Consequences.* Abakon Verlagsgesellschaft, Berlin, 1977.

30. Lewinsky, B. S., and D. G. Baker: The genetic control of immunity and its relationship to carcinogenesis. *Oncology.* 26:481–494, 1972.

31. Lightdale, C., and M. Lipkin: Cell division and tumor growth. In *Cancer: A Comprehensive Treatise, Vol. 3: Biology of Tumors: Cellular Biology and Growth,* ed. by F. F. Becker. Plenum Press, New York, 1975.

31a. Likhite, V. V.: On the frontiers of immunology. In *The Handbook of Cancer Immunology,* ed. by H. Waters. Garland Publishing, Inc., New York, 1978.

32. Lipkin, G., M. Rosenberg, and M. Knecht: Factors affecting growth of normal and malignant cells. *Vitro Biochemical Pharmacology.* 25:1333–1337, 1976.

33. Little, N., and R. A. Cooper, Jr.: Overview of cancer pathology. *Physical Therapy.* 56:914–918, 1976.

34. LoBue, J., and M. Potmesil: Stimulation. In *Cancer: A Comprehensive Treatise, Vol. 3: Biology of Tumors: Cellular Biology and Growth,* ed. by F. F. Becker. Plenum Press, New York, 1975.

35. Lodish, H. F., and J. E. Rothman: The assembly of cell membranes. *Scientific American.* 240:48–63, 1979.

36. Medina, D.: Tumor progression. In *Cancer: A Comprehensive Treatise, Vol. 3: Biology of Tumors: Cellular Biology and Growth,* ed. by F. F. Becker. Plenum Press, New York, 1975.

37. Morrison, S. D.: Generation and compensation of the cancer cachectic process by spontaneous modification of feeding behavior. *Cancer Research.* 36:228–233, 1976.

38. Nathanson, L.: Remote effects of cancer on the host. In *Clinical Oncology,* ed. by J. Horton and G. J. Hill. W. B. Saunders Co., Philadelphia, 1977.

39. Neville, A. M., and T. Symington: Systemic factors produced by human neoplasms. In *Biology of Cancer,* ed. by E. J. Ambrose and F. J. C. Roe. John Wiley & Sons, Inc., New York, 1975.

40. Nicolson, G. L., and G. Poste: The cancer cell: Dynamic aspects and modifications in cell–surface organization. Part I. *New England Journal of Medicine.* 295:197–203, 1976.

41. Nicholson, G. L., and G. Poste: The cancer cell: Dynamic aspects and modifications in cell–surface organization. Part II. *New England Journal of Medicine.* 295:253–258, 1976.

42. Odell, W. D., and A. Wolfsen: Ectopic hormone secretion by tumors. In *Cancer: A Comprehensive Treatise, Vol. 3: Biology of Tumors: Cellular Biology and Growth,* ed. by F. F. Becker. Plenum Press, New York, 1975.

43. Old, L. J.: Cancer immunology. *Scientific American.* 236:62, 1977.

44. Pitot, H. C.: The stability of events in the natural history of neoplasia. *American Journal of Pathology.* 89:703–716, 1977.

45. Prehn, R. T., and L. M. Prehn: Pathobiology of neoplasia. *American Journal of Pathology.* 80:529–550, 1975.

46. Roesel, C. E.: *Immunology: A Self-Instructional Approach.* McGraw-Hill Book Co., New York, 1978.

47. Roitt, I. M.: Essential immunology. *Blackwell Scientific Publications,* London, 1977.

48. Ryser, H. J-P.: Special Report: Chemical Carcinogenesis. *Ca — A Cancer Journal for Clinicians.* 24:351–360, 1974.

49. Schwind, J. V.: Cancer: Regressive evolution? *Oncology.* 29:172–180, 1974.

50. Silagi, S.: Reversible suppression of malignancy and differentiation of melanoma cells. *American Journal of Pathology.* 89:671–684, 1977.

51. Strauli, P.: The spread of cancer in the organism: Facts and problems. *Naturwissen Schaften.* 64:403–409, 1977.

52. Theologides, A.: Pathogenesis of cachexia in cancer: A review and a hypothesis. *Cancer* 29:484–488, 1972.

53. Theologides, A.: Generalized perturbations in host physiology caused by localized tumors. The anorexia-cachexia syndrome: A new hypothesis. *Annals of the New York Academy of Science.* 230:14–22, 1974.

54. Thompson, J. S., and M. W. Thompson: *Genetics in Medicine.* W. B. Saunders Co., Philadelphia, 1980.

55. Uriel, J.: Fetal characteristics of cancer. In *Cancer: A Comprehensive Treatise, Vol. 3: Biology of Tumors: Cellular Biology and Growth,* ed. by F. F. Becker. Plenum Press, New York, 1975.

56. Wolman, S. R., and A. A. Horland: Genetics of tumor cells. In *Cancer: A Comprehensive Treatise, Vol. 3: Biology of Tumors: Cellular Biology and Growth,* ed. by F. F. Becker. Plenum Press, New York, 1975.

3

The Etiology of Cancer: Current Theories

THE SEARCH FOR THE CAUSE

For many years, there has been a search for *THE CAUSE* of cancer. This search has taken place primarily as a result of the expectations and demands of the American public. The search has been heavily funded by grants from the federal government and by private contributions from the public, chiefly through the American Cancer Society.

Causality

The contemporary concept of causality began in the early nineteenth century when research scientists began to discover pathogenic organisms. They focused on an intense search for germs, to the exclusion of considering other environmental factors. This led to a very simple sequential model of causality:

$$A \longrightarrow B$$

This tunnel vision led to the thought that each illness had a single cause, and medical research was designed with that idea in mind. The ideal way to demonstrate the cause of a disease was to identify a suspected factor and expose a group of subjects to it. If, in a carefully controlled experiment, 100 per cent of the subjects exposed to that factor developed the disease whereas subjects not exposed to the factor never developed the disease, the causality of the disease had been identified. Unfortunately, the cause of most human illness is not that simple.

More recent studies in epidemiology, animal, and clinical research have indicated that illnesses have multiple causes. More aspects are now examined in relation to a disease. The social and cultural environment; effects of the physical environment including pollution, radiation, and climate; and emotional stress are being considered as determinants.

By focusing on multiple causality, we get a much more logical picture of the etiology of cancer. A number of causes of cancer have been identified, and attempts are now being made to explain the relationship of these causes to the disease.

Assumptions

Large expenditures of time and money on cancer research were based on five major assumptions that have been more implied than expressed:

1. Cancer is a single disease.
2. There is a single cause for cancer.
3. With enough money and scientists focused on searching for a cause, the cause will be found.
4. Increasing the amount of money available for research on the cause of cancer will lessen the time required to find the cause.
5. Once a cause for cancer is found, it will be a very brief time until a cure for cancer is developed.

Although these assumptions have not all proved to be accurate, the research has been fruitful in understanding and dealing with the cancer situation.

Research Approaches

Epidemiology

Many of the current theories on the etiology of cancer are based on epidemiologic studies. Epidemiology is a method of demonstrating relationships between identified factors and an illness. Epidemiologists attempt to determine patterns in the incidence of a particular illness. They collect information on factors such as sex, age, geography, economic status, ethnic background, employment history, family history, and life patterns. Epidemiologists are searching, probing detectives who gather clues and logically relate those clues in order to make correct inferences.

MacMahon defines epidemiology as "the study of the distribution and determinants of disease prevalence in man."[41] According to Susser, a determinant can be "any factor, whether event, characteristic, or other definable entity, so long as it brings about change, for better or worse in a health condition."[73]

Epidemiologic Techniques. Rather than examining each case of a disease as it occurs, epidemiologists study patterns of a disease as it occurs in a population. Epidemiologic studies generally follow this sequence:

1. Study pattern of disease in the population.

2. Conduct statistical studies to evaluate data.

3. Make inferences (educated guesses) about patterns of disease.

4. Identify determinants.

5. Make inferences about relationships of determinants.

A relationship may be very simple, such as

$$A \xrightarrow{\text{(Causes)}} B \xrightarrow{\text{(Causes)}} C$$

or it may be much more complex, such as

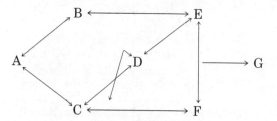

The science of epidemiology requires critical thinking and analysis. Difficulties may occur that may cause incorrect conclusions. Faulty reasoning can result in misinterpreting the relationships that are found. The presence of a factor can be circumstantial and have nothing to do with the etiology of the illness. It is also possible to completely overlook determinants when defining the relationships between factors and illness.

Types of Studies. Two types of studies are conducted in epidemiology: descriptive and prospective. Descriptive studies attempt to identify determinants. Prospective studies select a sample of people who are associated with the identified determinants of an illness but do not have the illness. These people are followed over a period of years. The development of illness in this group is then compared with the development of illness in people who do not have those determinants.

The biggest epidemiologic study of cancer in the United States was conducted by the American Cancer Society beginning in 1959. Entitled "The Cancer Prevention Study," the prospective investigation followed one million people over the age of 30 in 25 states. The subjects filled out detailed questionnaires and were tracked for approximately 20 years. This study generated a great deal of information about cancer and our environment.

Animal Research

Reasons for Animal Research. After determinants have been identified by epidemiologic studies, laboratory studies are conducted in an attempt to demonstrate the role of those determinants in the etiology of cancer. Since this type of experimentation cannot be conducted using humans, biologically similar animals are used. If the determinant causes cancer in animals, there is a high probability that it may cause cancer in humans. Some known exceptions do occur, however. Arsenic is known to cause cancer in humans, whereas animals in laboratory studies do not develop cancer after exposure to the substance.[32] Viruses, which commonly cause cancer in a variety of animals, have not been proved to cause cancer in humans; however, viruses are strongly suspected of causing several human cancers.

Research Design. Research studies that demonstrate chemical carcinogenesis in animals are frequently misunderstood and criticized by the general public. This is often because the reason for the research design is not fully understood.

To test one chemical capable of causing 20,000 human cancers, 30,000 mice or rats are needed. Thousands of chemicals need to be tested in this manner to determine the carcinogenic hazards now being released into the environment. To study each chemical costs about $70,000 and requires more than 3 years to complete.[13]

The dosage of the chemical given to animals is usually much higher than that to which humans are commonly exposed. There are several reasons for the higher dosage. There is normally a latent period between exposure to the chemical and the appearance of cancer. If this period is long, it may exceed the lifespan of the animal and no tumors will be observed. The higher dosage increases the number of tumors that will appear in a given number of animals and shortens the latent period so that if tumors develop, they will appear sooner.[29] Higher doses will *not* cause the development of tumors if the chemical is not a carcinogen. "There is no basis for the contention that all chemicals are carcinogenic when tested at high doses."[19]

Sometimes animals are exposed to the chemical in a different way than exposure occurs in humans. For example, the chemical may be applied to the skin rather than ingested. The purpose is to document that the chemical *is* a carcinogen, not to exactly reproduce the way that the chemical causes cancer in humans. This may not be possible in animals, whose metabolic pathways may be different.

Animal research studies are not sufficient evidence to prove carcinogenicity in humans, and the findings must be combined with epidemiologic studies before conclusions are reached. However, it is often unwise to wait for conclusions when the health and lives of large numbers of people are involved. Action must be taken on the basis of the evidence available.

Clinical Case Studies

Clinical researchers often collect case histories of patients with a particular type of cancer in order to identify commonalities. These case studies are useful as the basis for thorough epidemiologic studies but are not sufficient to demonstrate determinants. The key disadvantage to the clinical case studies approach is that there is no control group and, therefore, no way to show that a randomly selected group of people without cancer would not have the same commonalities. These case histories are often reported in the literature, and it is easy for the unwary reader to mistake the findings for facts concerning causes of cancer.

Cancer Registries

Cancer registries are set up to collect information and statistics about diagnosed cases of cancer. Data from these registries can be used in epidemiologic studies. They can be very valuable resources in cancer research. However, there are problems with registries: an inadequate number of registries exist; there are multiple deficiencies in existing registries; histologic data on reported cases are usually not available; physician reporting is slow; all cases may not be reported; reports submitted by the registry may be inadequate to meet the needs of the researchers; and the population included in the registry may not be representative.[62]

Molecular Biology Research

A primary interest of cancer etiologists is cellular physiology and biochemical pathways. It is believed that increased knowledge in this area will paint a much clearer picture of the origins of cancer. This knowledge is needed to understand the situation and how time factors are involved. Virologists enter into this picture by studying the interactions of human cells and viruses. Geneticists search for increased knowledge of human genes and chromosomes and how they interact with cellular components. All of these sciences must converge in putting together the pieces of the cancer puzzle.

IDENTIFIED DETERMINANTS OF CANCER

The following are the major factors that have been identified as determinants of cancer:

1. Genetic factors
2. Chemical carcinogens
3. Radiation
4. Viruses
5. Immune system failure
6. Rapid tissue proliferation
7. Hormone changes
8. Diet
9. Emotional factors

There are multiple theories about the etiology of cancer. Scientists often believe strongly in one particular theory and base their findings on it. Those working in genetics are convinced that genetic mutations are the primary factor in cancer etiology, whereas virologists are convinced that viruses are the real etiologic agent and that genetic changes occur only after the viral invasion.

In the following discussion an attempt will be made to reflect the major theories and the most significant differences of opinion of current scientists in the field of cancer etiology.

Genetic Factors

The relationship of genetics to cancer can be examined from several perspectives. By whatever means the relationship is examined, more questions will be found than answers and more theories than known facts.

Much research is being conducted in the area of genetics and molecular biology. Before the development of cancer can be thoroughly understood, much more needs

to be known about which factors affect genetic functioning, the location and role of specific genes, and why genes begin to function or cease functioning.

Theories

Two-Hit Theory. The two-hit theory was developed by Knudson.[37] A "hit" in this instance means a genetic mutation. Knudson developed his theory while studying retinoblastoma. He found that children who developed retinoblastoma could be separated into two groups. The children in one group develop the disease early and are inclined to have multiple tumors. The children in the other group are older when the tumor develops and have only one tumor.

Knudson believes that in the first group, the initial "hit" occurs in the parent's germinal cells; therefore, the retinoblastoma is inherited. The second "hit" is a somatic mutation. A somatic mutation occurs in a normal body cell at the time of cell division. The reason that the mutations occur is not presently understood.

In the second group, both "hits" are thought to be somatic mutations. In other words, two mutations occur at different times in the same cell in the retina; therefore, the retinoblastoma in the second group is not inherited.

Wilms' tumor, neuroblastoma, and pheochromocytoma all fit the two-hit pattern. Knudson believes that the theory applies to all childhood cancers. This information is very important to know in providing genetic counseling to parents. It is possible that all cancer fits the two-hit pattern, with hereditary cancers occurring earlier in life and occurring more often in multiple sites.[30]

Derepression. Proponents of the derepression theory believe that genes involved in early embryo development remain in genetic material throughout the individual's life.[12] These genes are repressed after development of the embryo is complete. The repression is maintained by inhibiting genes, which produce chemicals designed to maintain repression of the first gene. If the inhibiting gene is lost or ceases to function, derepression will occur, causing the development of a malignant cell. The malignant cells then dedifferentiate to primitive cells similar to those existing during the embryonic period.[12]

Genetic Changes

Multiple chromosomal mutations are apparent in the cancer cell. These changes seem to be the result rather than the cause of cancer. The mutations vary markedly from cell to cell.

Some people may have genetic abnormalities that are inherited and cause them to be more susceptible to cancer than the average person. Attempts are being made to specifically identify these abnormalities so that people who have them can be carefully screened for cancer. Identifying these abnormalities would also assist scientists in understanding the process of cancer development.

Genetic abnormalities can be the result of chromosomal changes, alterations in a single gene, or polygenic changes. Chromosomal abnormalities are associated both with congenital defects and with being cancer prone.[30, 48] See Table 3–1 for a list of genetic defects that are associated with a high risk of cancer. Persons with each of these genetic defects are at high risk of developing a specific cancer. In addition, even if they are cured of that cancer, they are still in danger of developing other malignancies.

In animals, abnormal genes associated with development of a specific cancer may be single or multiple. For example, a single gene is associated with susceptibility to mouse mammary tumor virus.[30] At least four genes are involved in the inheritance of lung tumors in animals. Murine leukemia virus in animals involves at least ten genes.

Table 3–1. Genetic Conditions Predisposing Toward Cancer*

Condition	Mode of Inheritance	Type of Cancer
Cancer as the primary manifestation:		
Retinoblastoma	Dominant	Ocular – childhood
Neuroblastoma	Dominant	Thoracic and abdominal
Pheochromocytoma	Dominant	Catecholamine production
Wilms' tumor	Dominant	Embryonal renal cancer
Sipple's syndrome	Dominant	Parathyroid adenoma, medullary thyroid cancer, pheochromocytoma
Basal cell nevus syndrome	Dominant	Basal cell epithelioma
Cancer in association with inherited condition:		
Tylosis	Dominant	Esophageal
Familial polyposis of colon	Dominant	Squamous carcinoma
Gardner's syndrome	Dominant	Gastrointestinal – colon
Fanconi's anemia	Recessive	Lymphoreticular
Bloom's syndrome	Recessive	Lymphoreticular
Xeroderma pigmentosum	Recessive	Squamous carcinoma
Inherited disease of immune system in association with:		
Wiskott-Aldrich syndrome	Dominant	Lymphoreticular
Ataxia-telangiectasia	Recessive	Lymphoreticular
Agammaglobulinemia	X-linked, recessive	Lymphoreticular
Cancer in association with chromosomal aberrations:		
Down's syndrome (trisomy 21)		Leukemia, lymphoma
Bloom's syndrome		Lymphoreticular
Fanconi's anemia		Lymphoreticular
Klinefelter's syndrome (XXY)		Breast
Turner's syndrome (XO)		Gonadal

*From Hill, H. Z., and Lin, H. S.: Carcinogenesis and tumor growth. In *Clinical Oncology,* edited by Horton, J. and Hill, G. H. II. Philadelphia: W. B. Saunders Co., 1977. Used by permission.

Philadelphia Chromosome

The Philadelphia chromosome is the only chromosomal abnormality that has been consistently associated with a malignant disorder. From 70 to 90 per cent of patients with chronic myelocytic leukemia have the Philadelphia chromosome in their blood cells. Therefore, the presence of this chromosome is of important diagnostic significance. In chronic myelocytic leukemia, the long arms of chromosome 22 are translocated to the long arms of chromosome 9. It is possible that small portions of chromosomes 9 or 22 may be lost in the translocation process.[48] This chromosomal abnormality is not present in individuals before they develop leukemia. It is very likely a result rather than a cause of cancer.

Heredity and Cancer

Some cancers occur more frequently within families.[3, 30] These cancers may be limited to a specific site, or there may be a high incidence of all types of cancer.[30] It is not clear whether the increased risk is a result of genetic factors, environmental influences, or both.

Significant increases in risk have been found for persons whose family members had cancer of the stomach, breast, large intestine, uterus, or lung; childhood brain tumors; or sarcomas. These persons are at high risk of developing the same type of cancer as their family members. Melanomas, leukemias, and lymphoreticular cancers sometimes have familial tendencies.

Lung Cancer.   First degree relatives of lung cancer patients have a fourfold risk of developing lung cancer if they do not smoke. If there is no family history of lung cancer, the person who smokes has a five times greater risk of developing lung cancer than the nonsmoker. The combined effect of smoking and a family history of lung cancer results in a fourteenfold increase in lung cancer deaths.[3] It would be interesting to see if there is an increased risk for those who have a family history of lung cancer and who are heavily exposed to secondhand smoke (the air contaminated by cigarette smoke of other smokers).

Breast Cancer.   First degree relatives of breast cancer patients have two to three times the risk of breast cancer that the general population has. If the patient has bilateral breast cancer, the risk for relatives is five times that of controls. If the patient is premenopausal and has bilateral breast cancer, the risk for relatives is nine times that of controls. This seems to indicate that breast cancer that is premenopausal and bilateral (as in Knudson's model) is more likely to be genetically determined.[4]

Genetic Susceptibility.   Some people seem to have an increased susceptibility, which may be inherited, to developing any type of cancer. The susceptibility alone may cause very few cancers, but if this susceptibility is combined with exposure to environmental factors that cause cancer, the increased risk may be very great.[48]

Chemical Carcinogens

What Are They?

"Chemical carcinogens are nonviral and nonradioactive substances which, under appropriate circumstances, cause malignant tumors to develop in multicellular organisms in significantly greater incidences than would occur spontaneously."[45]

Where Are They?

Chemical carcinogens were first identified in epidemiologic studies. The first identified cancer-causing agent was soot, which was found to cause scrotal cancer among chimney sweepers. As our society became more complex, the number of chemicals utilized increased rapidly. Scientists began to recognize the need for more rapid and more sophisticated techniques for identifying chemical carcinogens.

Methods were developed to detect carcinogens by animal studies.

Each year, more and more chemicals, most of which were never tested for carcinogenicity, were dumped into our environment. If epidemiologic studies showed a possibility that a chemical was a carcinogen, animal studies were conducted. These studies usually were conducted many years after the chemical was introduced into the environment, allowing large numbers of people to be exposed to the chemical before measures were taken to control it.

How Do They Act?

Recently it has been demonstrated that all carcinogens are mutagens, apparently causing cancer by inducing cell mutation. Tests have been developed using bacteria to demonstrate this ability. If the chemical causes the bacterial genes to mutate, it may cause human genes to mutate, resulting in cancer. More recently, human cells in culture are being used to detect chemicals that cause cell mutation. The chemical can then be classed as a potential carcinogen, and animal studies can be conducted. In the meantime, use of the chemical in the environment can be controlled.

Classification

Chemical carcinogens are now being classified into groups. These classifications are not yet distinct and separate, but the terms are being commonly used.

A *precarcinogen* is a substance that can be converted to a carcinogen by chemical reaction with other substances. This may occur metabolically within the body.

A *cocarcinogen* is a substance that will cause cancer only in the presence of another specific chemical.

An *ultimate carcinogen* is a chemical that directly causes the cell to become malignant.

A *tumor promoter* is a chemical that shortens the latent period and increases the possibility of tumor production. Some of these chemicals promote cell division.[60]

A *weak carcinogen* is a chemical with cancer-causing effects that cannot be easily detected by current testing methods. Epidemiologic studies are not likely to show a clear relationship between it and cancer. As a result, these carcinogens may be more hazardous than more potent carcinogens. Examples of weak carcinogens are pesticides, food additives, and air pollutants.[18]

A *potent carcinogen* is a substance that can be identified readily with current testing methods and is easily related to the development of cancer in humans.

The National Cancer Institute has stated that 80 to 90 per cent of cancer is the result of environmental factors and that about 60 per cent is the result of chemicals.[55] Two or more chemical carcinogens may have additive or multiplicative effects on carcinogenesis.[65] This means that the risk of developing cancer increases as an individual is exposed to greater numbers of carcinogens.

The Biology of Chemical Carcinogenesis

How susceptible a person is to chemical carcinogens seems to be genetically predetermined. Chemicals apparently cause cancer by inducing genetic mutations; however, changes in molecular biologic processes not detectable by present scientific methods could be caused by chemicals. Whatever changes do occur as a result of chemicals seem to be irreversible and transmittable to daughter cells. This change in the cell may result in cancer after exposure to a second or third chemical carcinogen.

Cancer can result from a single dose of a carcinogen; however, it is usually caused by multiple exposures and is dose dependent, which means the greater the dosage, the more powerful the effect. At present, there is *no* way to determine if there is a threshold dosage below which a chemical carcinogen is harmless.[60]

A period of latency lasting from several months to 50 or more years follows the initial exposure to a chemical carcinogen. This period can be shortened by tumor promoters.

Many chemical carcinogens that are ingested have to be metabolically converted to an ultimate carcinogen. Metabolism of one precarcinogen can give rise to several ultimate carcinogens. Carcinogens can also be metabolically inactivated so that they can no longer cause cancer. Speeding up metabolic inactivation may decrease the cancer-causing effect of some chemicals.[60]

Carcinogens may act at several sites in the body:

1. Site of initial contact
2. Site of selective organ
3. Site of accumulation of the chemical within the body
4. Site of metabolism
5. Site of excretion

Some carcinogens act at only one site; others may act at multiple sites.[19]

Carcinogens in Our Environment

Industry. In industry there are approximately 2000 chemicals that are known or suspected carcinogens. Numerous other chemicals used in industry have never been tested for carcinogenicity. Since present indications show that about 20 per cent of cancer is job related, industrial carcinogens can be considered to have a major impact on health.

Industrial carcinogens can affect the health of various groups of people: employees; families of employees who are exposed to the carcinogen by clothing worn home from work; those who live in the vicinity of the industrial plant; and consumers of the industrial product.

Since most cancer develops 10 to 25 years after initial exposure, it is difficult to relate the disease to the chemical. Seldom do researchers taking patient health histories go back further than 25 years. Even if they do, they may not be aware of the specific chemicals with which the patient was working, and the patient may not even know this information.

In order to detect which chemicals in industry may be carcinogens, researchers are investigating the health records of industrial employees and are attempting to trace employees who have left jobs to determine their health record after leaving. This is a tedious, time-consuming procedure. When adequate information is gathered, the incidence of cancer in those employees is compared with that of the general population. If an increased incidence is found, animal research studies are conducted on the chemicals used in the industry.

Pattern of Industrial Carcinogens. The typical pattern of chemical carcinogens in our environment can be demonstrated by the history of the industrial use of vinyl chloride. Vinyl chloride is a gas used in producing polyvinyl chloride, the base for most of our plastics. The industrial manufacture of plastics in large volume began about 30 years ago. At that time, a very rare type of cancer called angiosarcoma of the liver occurred only infrequently in the United States. In recent years, epidemiologists began to notice an increase in the number of people who developed the disease. Each year an increasing number of people developed this rare type of cancer for which there is no known successful treatment. Careful questioning of the patients and/or their families demonstrated that most patients were employed in industries in which plastics were manufactured. Studies were done on employees working in plastics plants. A number of employees were found with liver damage that could not be explained by alcoholism, hepatitis, or other factors. Vinyl chloride was identified as a causative agent of angiosarcoma of the liver. Because there was no prior reason to suspect that the chemical was dangerous, no attempt had been made by the plastics industry to control exposure of employees to this substance.

Today the use of this chemical in industry is carefully controlled: instruments measure the presence of vinyl chloride gas in the air; employees use protective clothing and masks; and all employees are frequently checked for changes in liver function. However, the development of cancer in those who have been exposed — including people living near the industrial plants — cannot be controlled as easily. The length of time between exposure and the development of this cancer can be 10 to 25 years.[65]

Asbestos. Asbestos is an unusual carcinogen. It is not known whether it causes cancer by directly changing the cell, by functioning as a chronic irritant, or by allowing other carcinogens to adhere to its outer surface. Asbestos enters the body in long needle-like slivers that embed in tissue and remain there for the rest of the person's life. Any chemicals adhering to the outer surface of the asbestos fibers would likewise be carried into the tissue.

Asbestos acts as a causal agent in a number of types of cancer, including lung cancer, gastrointestinal cancer, and pleural and peritoneal mesothelioma.[65] Exposure to asbestos alone does not seem to increase the risk of lung cancer. However, the smoker who has been exposed to airborne asbestos has a 92 times greater risk of developing lung cancer than the nonsmoker who does not work with asbestos.[65] The risk of combining these two carcinogens is so great that if a nonsmoker is exposed to airborne asbestos and frequently breathes secondhand smoke, the risk of developing lung cancer is 40 times that of the nonsmoker who does not work with asbestos. Other types of cancer caused by asbestos do not seem to be associated with smoking.

Searching for persons who have been or who are being exposed to asbestos has become an enormous task. Asbestos has been used in a multitude of industries including shipbuilding, housing and construction, insulation, and asbestos factories. Family members of workers using asbestos are at high risk because the workers' clothing contains asbestos. People working or living in buildings that have been insulated with asbestos are at risk. Many children attend schools that have asbestos insulation.

Asbestos has been found in several public water supplies. Pipes carrying water to homes are sometimes made of materials containing asbestos. Whether the asbestos from these pipes is or can be released into the water is unknown.

Asbestos is used to filter wine, beer, and soft drinks and is used in a variety of processes in the production of alcoholic beverages. Although doses may be very small, total accumulated body doses from drinking water, food, and industry must be considered, since this substance is permanently retained by the body.

Water. Chemicals are constantly being deposited into rivers and lakes, which are sources of our drinking water. In 1974 studies were conducted to determine the presence of chemical carcinogens in the drinking water in New Orleans. The results of the studies set off a heated controversy. Sixty-six chemicals were present in the New Orleans water supply. Most of the chemicals were present only in trace amounts, but several known carcinogens were found, including chloroform, carbon tetrachloride, and dieldrin.

The majority of the chemicals found had never been tested for carcinogenicity. Some of the chemicals detected in the water supply, including carbon tetrachloride, were found in the blood plasma of residents. However, it cannot be proved that the chemicals in the blood plasma were there as a result of the drinking water. New Orleans does have a higher incidence of cancer than the national average, but it is not possible to attribute this directly to the drinking water.

Since these studies, other water supplies have been tested and some have been found to contain carcinogens. Tests to detect possible carcinogens in water supplies are difficult to carry out, expensive, and infrequently done. Current public health laws are designed to prevent communicable disease transmission by water supplies; they are not designed to control toxic or carcinogenic chemicals. Moves are being made to require carbon-filtering systems in public water supplies. The carbon will filter out many of the dangerous chemicals, but in order for the carbon to function effectively, it must be changed frequently and this is very costly. Therefore, there is strong resistance to these measures.

Chemicals enter the water supply from two sources. Point pollution is the deposit of substances into water from a specific place, usually an industry. Nonpoint pollution is the deposit of chemicals into the water from such sources as pesticides and herbicides sprayed on crops, lawns, and gardens, and the tire marks on the streets. Rainwater washes these chemicals into the nearest river or lake.

Attempts are being made to control both point and nonpoint sources of water pollution. The problems involved in doing this are multiple. Dumping waste into water supplies is a cheap and easy method of waste disposal and will be difficult to monitor. Controlling nonpoint pollution will require banning the use of some chemicals and might alter the lifestyle of the general public.

Air. The air we breathe has been heavily polluted with a variety of chemicals from industrial by-products, automobile exhausts, and cigarette smoke. Some of these chemicals are known or potential carcinogens. The main class of carcinogens in air are polycyclic aromatic hydrocarbons, the primary sources of which are coal furnaces, refuse burning, coke production, and automobile and truck emissions. Epidemiologic studies have indicated a definite correlation between air pollution and the incidence of cancer.

Recent studies show a very high incidence of nasopharyngeal cancer in regions that have a large number of oil refineries. People who smoke cigarettes and live in an area of high air pollution have a greater risk of cancer of the lung than those who smoke and live in areas with low levels of air pollution.

Trace amounts (25 mg.) of extracts (of air pollution) from some cities, particularly those with predominant usage of solid fuel, produced a high incidence of tumors of the liver, lymphatic system (lymphomas), and lung (multiple adenomas) in animal studies. Such amounts would be inhaled in about three to four months by a man living in one of the cities considered.[53]

Skin Contact. Our skin comes in contact daily with a variety of chemicals. We once believed that substances applied to intact skin were not absorbed systemically. Recent studies show that chemicals contained in materials with which our skin has had contact can be found in varying amounts in blood and urine. Thus, chemicals contained in cosmetics, shampoos, hair conditioners, soaps, lotions, hair dyes, deodorants, and the many other potions alluringly hawked by enterprising businesses to make us appear young, beautiful, soft skinned, and nice smelling may very well be absorbed through our skin and react biochemically within our bodies. Most of these chemicals have not been tested for carcinogenicity. Until recently, the chemicals contained in these substances were carefully guarded secrets.

Recent studies have shown that the majority of semipermanent hair dyes are mutagens.[23] Hair dyes are aniline dyes made of polycyclic hydrocarbons from coal tar. These dyes are known to be absorbed through the skin. Preliminary epidemiologic studies indicate a higher incidence of lung cancer in beauticians. Research reported in 1976 indicates that women with breast cancer have an abnormally high use of hair dye and hair bleach. Another report found that 86 per cent of the authors' patients with cancer of the uterus bleached their hair.[66]

Other chemicals are incorporated in the material of the clothing we wear. Detergents, softeners, and chemicals used to make clothing crease resistant or permanently pressed, and fillers added to the fabric by the manufacturer to give the fabric more body until the first washing, can sometimes be absorbed through the skin.

Chemicals used in lawn care, gardening, farming, house maintenance, and industry may also be absorbed through the skin. This could occur from direct skin contact or as a result of inhalation of airborne droplets or powders. Recently it has been discovered that farmers have a higher incidence of cancer than the general public.

Tobacco

Smoking Statistics. Forty per cent of all cancer in men is caused by smoking. As the number of women who smoke increases, the percentage of female cancer caused by smoking also increases.[49] In addition, the cigarette is responsible for about 75,000 deaths a year from lung cancer. When the smoker is also a heavy drinker, he or she is 15 times more likely to develop oral cancer than either the nonsmoker or the drinker. Smoking is also a cause of throat, stomach, bladder, and esophageal cancer.

Cigarette smoking as a cause of cancer is one of the best documented facts in cancer research. Not only has it been definitely proved that smoking causes cancer, it has been possible to demonstrate that the risk of developing lung cancer increases with the length of time a person has smoked and with the number of cigarettes smoked each day. Levels of tar and nicotine are also associated with the incidence of lung cancer. Death rates increase with the depth of inhalation of smoke and are much higher in those who start smoking in their early teens.[24]

Carcinogens in Cigarette Smoke. A number of tumor promoters, initiators, and accelerators have been identified in cigarette smoke. Among these are polynuclear aromatic hydrocarbons (very potent carcinogens), chlorostilbenes and catechols (accelerators), phenol and substitute phenols (promoters), nitrosonornicotine (potent carcinogen), and hydrazide (potent carcinogen).[78]

Other forms of tobacco usage such as cigars, pipes, chewing tobacco, and snuff have less incidence of lung cancer than cigarette smoking. Lung cancer from cigar and pipe smoking is less prevalent because of decreased inhalation. Cigarette smokers who switch to cigars or pipes continue to inhale and continue to have a high risk of lung cancer. Chewing tobacco and snuff are strongly related to oral cancers.

Secondhand Smoke. Research studies have indicated that the nonsmoker who inhales secondhand smoke has increased blood levels of several chemicals absorbed from the cigarette smoke. Considering the number of cancer-related chemicals in cigarette smoke, it seems reasonable to assume that an increased risk of cancer could occur from secondhand smoke.

Advertising and Smoking. In spite of these facts, many of which have been known for years, advertisements continue to tempt the nonsmoker to take up the habit. Advertisements use role models who are young, beautiful, successful, rich, and appealing to the opposite sex. Implied is the idea that by smoking, the person will become like the role model. Although the total number of people smoking in the United States has decreased, there has been a marked increase in smoking by the adolescent female. Children are beginning to smoke at a much earlier age; it is not unusual to find fourth and fifth grade children who smoke. Although the number of physicians who smoke has decreased, the number of nurses who smoke has increased.

Alcohol. People who consume large amounts of alcohol have a high incidence of cancer of the mouth, throat, larynx, esophagus, liver, and gastrointestinal tract. It is not known how alcohol functions in carcinogenesis. It may function as a chronic irritant, it may be a direct carcinogen, it may be a cocarcinogen, it may promote the action of other carcinogens, or it may diminish the body's own internal defenses in such a way that a malignancy can easily grow. Some researchers think that contaminants in the alcohol rather than the alcohol itself are the true carcinogens.[59]

Drugs. In recent years, a number of drugs have been identified as carcinogenic. Most of these drugs were used to treat cancer. Originally, there was little concern about this because patients treated with these drugs seldom lived long enough to develop a second cancer. Now, some patients taking chemotherapy are long-term survivors, and the development of a second cancer is a serious concern. The possibility of long-term survival is now taken into consideration in selecting drugs for treatment. However, if the drug that is carcinogenic is the only effective treatment for a certain type of cancer, it will be used, since the patient would die without the treatment.

Although drugs have been carefully tested for short-term toxic effects, very few studies have been conducted to determine

Table 3–2.   Cancers Related to Drug Exposures in Man*

Drug	Related Cancer
Radioisotopes	
Phosphorus (P^{32})	Acute leukemia
Radium, mesothorium	Osteosarcoma, sinus carcinoma
Thorotrast	Hemangioendothelioma of liver
Immunosuppressive drugs (for renal transplantation)	
Antilymphocyte serum	Reticulum cell sarcoma
Antimetabolites	Soft tissue sarcoma, other cancers (skin, liver)
Cytotoxic drugs	
Chlornaphazine	Bladder cancer
Melphalan, cyclophosphamide	Acute myelomonocytic leukemia
Hormones	
Synthetic estrogens	
Prenatal	Vaginal and cervical adenocarcinoma (clear-cell type)
Postnatal	Endometrial carcinoma (adenosquamous type)
Androgenic-anabolic steroids (for aplastic anemia)	Hepatocellular carcinoma
Others	
Arsenic	Skin cancer
Phenacetin-containing drugs	Renal pelvis carcinoma
Coal-tar ointments	Skin cancer
Phenytoin?	Lymphoma
Chloramphenicol?	Leukemia
Amphetamines?	Hodgkin's disease
Reserpine?	Breast cancer

*From Hoover, R. and Fraumeni, J. F. Jr.: Drugs. In *Persons at High Risk of Cancer,* edited by Fraumeni, J. F. Jr. New York: Academic Press, Inc., 1975. Used by permission.

long-term chronic effects such as cancer. Therefore, the carcinogenic potential of most drugs is unknown. For a list of drugs classified as carcinogenic, see Table 3–2.[32]

Radiation

Causality in humans has definitely been established between certain types of cancer and both ionizing and nonionizing radiation. Ionizing radiations include photons (gamma rays and x-rays), uncharged particles (neutrons), and charged particles (electrons, beta particles, and alpha particles). The nonionizing radiations are primarily ultraviolet radiations, which have been associated with skin cancers. Nonionizing radiation has a low penetrating ability but is highly damaging to deoxyribonucleic acid (DNA).

When Does Radiation Cause Cancer?

Both epidemiologic and animal studies have linked increased risk of cancer with increased exposure to x-rays. Higher rates of leukemia are found in radiologists and people treated by long-term x-ray therapy, for example, in treatment of ankylosing spondylitis. Exposing the pregnant mother to abdominal x-rays seems to increase the incidence of cancer in the child. Exposure to atomic explosion fallout increases the risk of leukemia. Exposure to x-rays for diagnosis or treatment during the first 2 years of life is associated with the development of cancer later in life. Children under 10 years old are more sensitive to radiation-induced cancer than adults. Long-term low level radiation may also be related to the development of cancer. See Table 3–3 for groups of people studied epidemiologically who were exposed to radiation and the types of cancers associated with them.

How Does Radiation Cause Cancer?

The process by which radiation causes cancer is not completely understood. Even after exposure to large doses of radiation, the probability of the patient's developing cancer is very small.[34] The latent period extends to at least 30 years.

Tumor induction from radiation — as from other determinants — is a complex process that is dependent upon the tissue, hormonal state, and age of the patient as well as other factors.

Radiation damages DNA and causes mutation and chromosome breaks and rearrangements. In one animal study, radiation carcinogenesis was found to result

Table 3–3. Cancers Related to Radiation

Group Studied Epidemiologically	Types of Cancers Occurring
Children exposed to atomic bomb explosion	Leukemia Thyroid Brain Salivary gland Gastrointestinal (GI) tract
Adults exposed to atomic bomb explosion	Leukemia Respiratory tract Breast GI tract Lymphosarcoma Thyroid
Ankylosing spondylitis patients treated with long-term x-ray therapy	Leukemia Pharynx Pancreas Bronchus Lymphatic Hematopoietic Gastric
Children irradiated for supposedly enlarged thymus glands	Leukemia Thyroid Salivary gland
Women treated with x-ray therapy for postpartum mastitis Patients undergoing multiple fluoroscopies during treatment of tuberculosis Persons exposed to atomic bomb radiation	Breast
Women treated with x-ray therapy for cancer of cervix	Uterine corpus
Radium dial painters	Bone sarcoma Carcinoma of paranasal sinuses and mastoid
Patients given thorotrast as contrast medium for x-rays	Liver Leukemia
Miners exposed to high atmospheric levels of radon	Lung
Children treated with radium-224 for bone tuberculosis	Bone sarcoma
Prenatal irradiation	Leukemia
Patients given ^{32}P to treat polycythemia vera	Leukemia

from the interaction of radiation with an oncogenic virus. The mice harbored an oncogenic virus in a latent form that was released following exposure to radiation.[30]

Dose-Response Relationship

An unsolved issue is whether there is a dose-response relationship in the development of radiation-caused cancer. Dose is the amount of radiation to which a person is exposed; response is the development of a malignancy. In studying dose-response relationships epidemiologically, three factors have to be considered:

1. Number of individuals exposed
2. Number of individuals with tumors
3. Dosage of radiation[46]

If there is a dose-response relationship, the number of individuals with tumors within an exposed group would increase as the dosage increased.

"Safe" Levels

Another interest in this area is the concern about "safe" levels of radiation. Is there a threshold below which there are no harmful effects? In order to determine this, a control group with no prior radiation exposure would be required. This is impossible since small amounts of radiation are emitted from the earth and the sun. "The most prudent policy would be to assume that there is no threshold for radiation carcinogenesis and that every exposure is potentially carcinogenic."[30]

Viruses

The Virus Search

One of the most elusive quests in the search for the etiology of cancer has been in the field of virology. For years viruses have been known to cause animal cancers. This has led scientists to strongly suspect that viruses are involved in the etiology of some types of human cancers.

Proving this is a difficult task. Demonstrating the presence of a virus in tumor tissue does not mean that the virus caused the cancer. The virus may simply be taking advantage of an already abnormal situation that provides a convenient and supportive environment for its growth. Even in animal cancers known to be caused by viruses, the virus itself is not usually in the tumor.

The Process of Viral Oncogenesis

An intensive search for the process by which viruses cause animal cancers has been conducted in the last few years. Bits and pieces of information have emerged gradually, resulting in several theories.

Cells can be classified according to how they respond to an oncogenic virus:

1. *No interaction* — the cells do not interact at all with the virus.
2. *Permissive* — the cells support the reproduction of the viruses to create more viruses (infection).
3. *Nonpermissive* — the cells do not permit reproduction of the viruses but can be transformed by them into malignant cells.[30]

Viruses have been categorized as ribonucleic acid (RNA) viruses or DNA viruses. Both types of virus cause cancer in animals. RNA viruses in animals have been associated with leukemia, sarcoma, and breast cancer.

Since in the process of causing animal cancers the genetic material of the virus combines with the DNA of the cell, researchers have sought evidence for this viral genetic material in human cancers. DNA sequences not contained in normal human cells have been found in human leukemias, lymphomas, sarcomas, breast cancer cells, Hodgkin's disease, and Burkitt's lymphoma.[30]

Herpesviruses

Herpesviruses are a type of DNA virus that is the most likely to cause cancer in humans. Epstein-Barr virus is a herpes-like virus that can almost always be found in Burkitt's lymphoma. This virus is believed to be the cause of infectious mononucleosis. Antibodies to this virus are commonly found among the African children in whom almost all Burkitt's lymphoma occurs. Epstein-Barr virus may also be a causal factor in a nasopharyngeal cancer that occurs in China.[28] It is possible that the Epstein-Barr virus infections may be the *result* of defective immune response rather than the *cause* of cancer. If these are a cause of cancer, other factors must be involved as well.[26]

Herpes simplex type 2 (HSV-2) antibodies are frequently present in women with cervical cancer. Eighty per cent or more of women with cervical cancer, in situ carcinoma of the cervix, or cervical dysplasia have antibodies to HSV-2. Only 30 per cent of women in control groups have these antibodies.[44]

Herpes simplex type 1 (HSV-1), which causes fever blisters, has been associated with head and neck cancers[26] and with squamous cell carcinoma at the site of recurrent fever blisters.[30, 56]

Oncogene Theory

A great debate has centered around when the invasion of the oncogenic virus occurs. Proponents of the oncogene theory believe that the genetic material of oncogenic viruses is present in the normal gene pool of all vertebrates and is transmitted genetically from one generation to the next. This oncogene is normally repressed but is derepressed under certain conditions such as radiation, chemical carcinogens, or aging.[1, 30, 33] The oncogene theory sounds very much like the derepression theory, but it is not the same. In the derepression theory, the gene that is derepressed is one that has the important function of influencing embryo development, and the gene is repressed when this task is complete.

The oncogene is considered alien to the normal cell, a segment of viral DNA that has invaded the cell and does not contribute to its useful function. This gene is always repressed in the normal cell.

One group of researchers studied identical twins, one of whom in each pair had cancer. The children with cancer had extra genetic material that was not present in the cells of their identical twins.[70] This would be evidence against the oncogene theory, but not evidence against viral causality.[30]

Transmission Theories

Vertical transmission is the passing of the virus from the parent to the child either through the parent's germinal cells or congenitally in the uterus, through paternal virus in semen,[22] or by perinatal exposure through breast milk.

Horizontal transmission is the passing of the virus from one individual to another.

After transmission, the virus genes merge with the cellular genes and remain latent for long periods of time. Radiation or chemical carcinogens could activate these virus genes, causing their transformation from nonmalignant to malignant cells.

Viral Etiology and Human Cancers

The human cancers that have a possible viral etiology include leukemia, Hodgkin's disease, Burkitt's lymphoma, sarcomas, breast cancer, head and neck cancer, and nasopharyngeal carcinoma. Borden[9] believes that the evidence of a viral origin is sufficient enough that breast-feeding should be discouraged by mothers with first degree relatives who have breast cancer or by mothers whose husband has first degree relatives with a history of breast cancer. In some families, adult patients with breast cancer have a positive history of having been breast-fed as infants.[30]

An intense study of viruses and cancer is continuing. If there is a viral cause of cancer, it probably acts with many other factors. Viruses may simply accelerate or trigger already existing malignant processes.[26] Serious consideration is being given to the development of vaccines to prevent invasion of oncogenic viruses or to block the oncogenic process after cellular invasion.[31]

Immune System Failure

The role of the immune system in the etiology of cancer is very controversial. One reason for the controversy is the inadequate knowledge we have about the complex workings of the immune system. We know that the immune system definitely affects cancer in many ways. But is it directly involved in the etiology of cancer, or is it involved in providing a milieu that is either favorable or unfavorable to the growth of a cancer cell that has already developed?

An immune system that is deficient because of inherited disorders or drug immunosuppression for organ transplants results in an increase in cancers of the lymphatic system, but not in other types of cancer.[30, 35, 52] These lymphoid cancers could be caused by genetic mutations, increased activity of oncogenic viruses, or the immune surveillance system's decreased ability to recognize and destroy malignant lymphoid cells.[4]

Cancer patients frequently have abnormalities in both humoral and cell-mediated immunity. The severity of the immunodepression progresses as the disease advances and may be a result of the cancer. It will be necessary to do prospective studies to determine whether or not the immune defect was present before the cancer developed. This will be difficult since at this point it is not possible to determine when cancer begins. Some researchers believe that cancer may exist in a subclinical state for 10 to 15 years before diagnosis. Could small undetectable groups of cells alter the immune response?

Some oncogenic viruses are immunosuppressive. Chemical carcinogens can also be immunosuppressive. Could these substances alter the immunocompetence of an individual sufficiently enough to promote tumorigenesis? Is it necessary for the immune system to be suppressed in order for malignancy to begin?

Rapid Tissue Proliferation

A number of seemingly miscellaneous factors have been associated with the etiology of cancer. These factors include pipe smoking (with cancer of the lip), ill-fitting dentures or broken teeth (with oral cancer), burn scars, chronic wounds,[72] and occasionally the site of an acute trauma.[47] All of these conditions cause rapid proliferation of tissue, and any situation that increases cell proliferation increases the risk of cancer.[60]

In animal experiments tissue trauma alone will not cause tumors, but if a chemical carcinogen is placed on the animal's skin and at a later date the tissue is traumatized, a tumor will develop.[30] What relation this has, if any, to the development of human cancers is not known.

Hormones

Epidemiologic studies have found similarities in the known risk factors in cancer of the breast, uterus, and ovary. See Table 3–4 for risk factors in breast cancer.[27] The risk factors are interrelated. When these risk factors are carefully examined, they seem to center around ovarian or pituitary function. Because of this, research has focused on searching for an abnormality in ovarian function. The findings of this research have indicated that cancer of the breast may be a result of an underlying abnormality of hormone secretion. Breast cancer is associated with elevated levels of estradiol and estrone (two fractions of the hormone estrogen). Increased secretion of specific pituitary hormones may also be associated with the tumor. These may not be the only hormonal changes involved in the etiology of breast cancer, and all breast cancer may not have the same etiology.

Women who have cancer of the breast

Table 3–4. Known Risk Factors in Female Breast Cancer*

Category	Risk Factors
Demographic	Old age Higher socioeconomic status Caucasian
Menstrual	Earlier age at menarche Later age at menopause Decreased frequency of artificial menopause
Reproductive	Never married Increased age at first full-term delivery Fewer pregnancies
Hormonal	Increased use of exogenous estrogens (oral contraceptives, hormones at menopause)?
Other	History of benign breast disease Family history of breast cancer Increased total body size

*From Henderson, B. E., Gerkins, V. R., and Pike, M. C.: Sexual factors and pregnancy. In *Persons at High Risk of Cancer*, edited by Fraumeni, J. F. Jr. New York: Academic Press, Inc., 1975. Used by permission.

have twice the risk of developing cancer of the ovary, and vice versa. Cancer of the ovary is associated with fertility problems and thus seems to be a result of a defect in pituitary or ovarian functioning.

Women with endometrial cancer have a higher frequency of diabetes and hypertension and twice the risk of developing cancer of the ovary or breast. Also associated with this disease are infertility, irregular menses, late menopause, obesity, excessive menstrual bleeding, and premenstrual breast swelling.

Further research needs to be done on the endocrine profile of women with these cancers. The long-term effects of ingestion of hormonal preparations need to be more closely examined. Long-term use of estrogens doubles the risk of breast cancer and greatly increases the risk of uterine cancer. Vaginal cancer has been associated with maternal intake of diethylstilbestrol (DES) to prevent abortion. Long-term effects of birth control pills will not become evident for several years.

More studies need to be conducted on hormonal relationships in cancer of the cervix, gallbladder, prostate, and testis. Studies also need to be conducted on the effect of diet on hormone levels.

Diet

In recent years much interest has developed in the possibility of diet as a cause of cancer. Diet has been associated with cancers of the large bowel, prostate, breast, endometrium, and ovary.[8] This idea originated from epidemiologic studies showing significant increases in numbers of colon cancers in groups of people who moved from a country with a low frequency of colon cancer to a country with a higher frequency.

There are two aspects of diet that have been associated with the development of cancer:

1. Foods making up the diet
2. Chemicals added to foods for various purposes

Types of Food

Several dietary determinants have been related to a high incidence of cancer. The determinants identified in epidemiologic and animal studies are:

1. Low fiber diet
2. High fat diet
3. High cholesterol level in bowel
4. Different population of intestinal flora
5. Increased protein intake
6. Increased intake of refined carbohydrates (particularly sugar)
7. Slow bowel transit time
8. Decreased physical activity
9. Increase in bile acids and sterols in bowel
10. Ingestion of chemical carcinogens[57, 75, 76]

Low Fiber Diet. A low fiber diet is believed to slow the bowel transit time. Studies have also indicated that low amounts of fiber promote increased breakdown of bile salts into bile acids and sterols, which are considered tumor promoters or cocarcinogens. Decreased feces bulk means bile acids will be more concentrated.

High Fat Diet. The high fat diet has a variety of effects. Increased fats promote the breakdown of bile salts into bile acids and sterols. The high fat diet is associated with a change in normal bacterial flora. With a high fat diet, increased amounts of cholesterol are present in the bowel. Bile acids form mixed micelles during fat digestion. Liquid-soluble carcinogens could be incorporated into these micelles and transported through the small bowel to the large bowel.[58]

Cholesterol. Cholesterol is considered by some researchers to be a cocarcinogen. Therefore, its presence would promote carcinogenesis.

Intestinal Flora. An intestinal flora containing such anaerobic bacteria as *Clostridium paraputrificum* and *bactercides* is present in people with colon cancer and people who eat a low fiber, high carbohydrate, high fat diet. This bacterial flora is able to retoxify chemicals that have been metabolically inactivated in the liver.[58] Thus, chemicals could be changed back to ultimate carcinogens by this bacterial flora and absorbed by the blood stream.

High Protein Diet. The relationship of increased protein intake to colon-rectal cancer is recognized but its role is not understood. The only explainable factor is that a high protein diet increases the amount of fat in the diet.

Refined Carbohydrates. Increased intake of refined carbohydrates — particularly sugar — is associated with alterations in bacterial flora. Also, diets high in these substances are usually low in fiber.

Slow Bowel Transit Time. Slower bowel transit time is thought by some researchers to allow an increased exposure of the bowel wall to carcinogens or increased systemic absorption of carcinogens. Decreased physical activity is associated with slow bowel transit time.

Some researchers believe that these dietary processes alone can result in carcinogenesis in susceptible individuals without exogenous carcinogens. Others believe that carcinogens found in food and water allow this dietary process to cause the development of an ultimate carcinogen, resulting in carcinogenesis. (See Fig. 3–1.)

Chemicals in Food

Aflatoxins. Aflatoxins occur naturally and are produced by *Aspergillus flavus*, a fungus that grows in high humidity conditions. In rats, aflatoxins are highly potent carcinogens. This mold grows on peanuts, corn, barley, peas, rice, soybeans, fruit, and some meats, milk, and cheddar cheese.[60] Growth of aflatoxins is dependent upon food storage methods, and in some parts of the world the fungus is thought to be a major cause of some types of cancer. Its growth on stored food is carefully monitored in the United States. Small amounts can be found in peanut butter, milk, and cheese.

Nitroso Compounds. Nitrosamines are very powerful carcinogens in animal studies; they can cause cancer in very low concentrations. Nitrosamines and their precursors (nitrates and nitrites) are found frequently in foods. Nitrite is used as a preservative in human and in animal food. Ham, bacon, and canned meat are preserved with nitrite. Nitrate fertilizer raises the nitrate content of vegetables; spinach, celery, and other green vegetables are rich in nitrates. Nitrates are readily reduced in the body to nitrites.[40]

Nitrites alone have been found to be carcinogenic in animal studies. Nitrites also easily combine with available amines to form nitrosamine. This chemical formation can occur in the soil, during food storage, during food preparation (such as the frying of bacon), or in the body. Intestinal bacterial flora can convert nitrate to nitrite or act as a catalyst in the combination of nitrites and amines. Vitamin C blocks the formation of nitrosamines from nitrites and amines.[7]

Polycyclic Aromatic Hydrocarbons. Benzpyrene is the most common of the

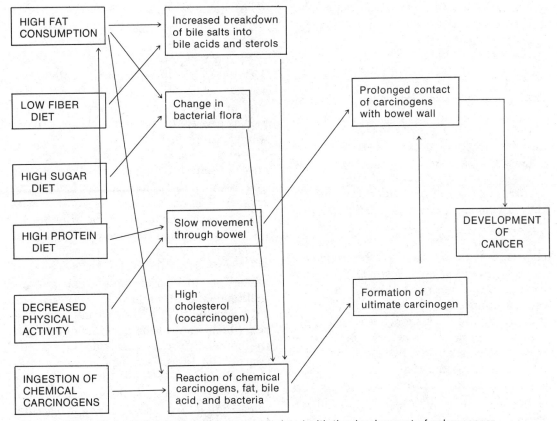

Figure 3–1. Relationships of factors associated with the development of colon cancer.

polycyclic aromatic hydrocarbons occurring in foods, and is found in smoked fish, ham, barbecued beef, cooking oil, and coffee. It is classified as a very potent carcinogen.

Talc. Talc particles are sometimes found in gastrointestinal tumors. This does not prove that talc causes cancer but its presence is a source of concern. Talc is used in a variety of ways related to food. Rice is polished by talc and some remains on the rice. Talc is used in salami, peanuts, and chewing gum.[8]

Saccharin. Saccharin is an artificial sweetener that has recently been identified as a weak carcinogen and a tumor promoter. Since a large market has been developed using saccharin in low caloric food products, this discovery has led to a heated controversy over whether to remove it from the market or not. Some people believe that sugar causes greater harm than saccharin.

Vinyl Chloride. Although vinyl chloride is not an ingredient of foods, much food packaging and wrapping is plastic. Foods are often heated in boiling water in plastic bags. With the advent of microwave ovens, food is heated in plastic dishes. Baby bottles are made of plastic, and the baby's milk is heated in a plastic bottle. We eat from plastic dishes and sometimes use plastic tableware.

Heating plastic to high temperatures is known to cause sufficient release of vinyl chloride to pollute the surrounding air. Is it possible that heating plastic to a lower temperature could release trace amounts of vinyl chloride into food?[60, 67]

Other Carcinogens Related to Diet. Many chemicals are added to foods for preserving, increasing flavor, adding color, artificially sweetening, and other purposes. Not all of these substances have been tested for carcinogenicity. Some of them are thought to be precarcinogens, cocarcinogens, or weak carcinogens. They can be converted to ultimate carcinogens during the digestive process, in the liver, or during metabolic processes.

Vitamins and Trace Elements

Deficiencies and excesses of vitamins and trace minerals have been associated experimentally, and in some cases in humans, with the etiology of cancer.[8]

Increasing vitamin A intake decreases the carcinogenic effect of chemicals, perhaps by altering the metabolic pathways. Deficiency in vitamin A has been implicated as a contributing factor in the etiology of some types of cancer.[8] Research has been conducted to examine the analogs or retinoids of vitamin A. The naturally occurring analogs of vitamin A are too toxic to give to humans in large doses and do not disperse well through the body. Synthetic retinoids are being developed that hold the promise of stopping or reversing the process of chemical carcinogenesis during the latent phase.[71]

Emotional Factors

Since the late 1800s it has been suspected that there is a psychosocial component to the etiology of cancer. Multiple research studies have been conducted in attempts to identify emotional factors associated with cancer. Some of the characteristics that have been identified are:

1. Masochistic character structure[6]
2. Inhibited sexuality[6,12]
3. Inhibited motherhood[6]
4. Inability to discharge or deal with anger[6,39]
5. Aggressiveness or hostility and unresolved hostile conflicts with the mother[6]
6. Delay in securing treatment[6]
7. Loss of an important relationship[36,39]
8. Unresolved grief[39]
9. Poor outlets for emotional discharges[36]
10. Adverse life events[36]
11. Despair, depression, and hopelessness[36,61]
12. Poor handling of stress[36]

One of the more interesting studies was conducted by Schmale and Iker.[61] They administered a psychologic test designed to measure despair and hopelessness in 68 women who were admitted to the hospital for cervical conization to diagnose cancer after a positive Papanicolaou (Pap) smear. The tests were administered before the surgery. The researchers were able to predict 73.6 per cent of the time whether or not the women had cancer by indications of hopelessness on a psychologic test.

The research studies that have been conducted in this area have some serious methodologic problems. The studies are conducted on people who already have cancer, which leads to the question of whether the personality characteristics caused the cancer, the cancer caused the personality characteristics, or neither. Many times control groups have not been used or were selected inappropriately. Attempting to develop a rigorous research design to study this topic is extremely difficult. Prospective studies need to be developed using larger sample sizes.

Emotional factors are probably related to functioning of the immune system.[69] If this is true, any type of counseling that improved coping mechanisms, raised self-esteem, and encouraged assertiveness, thus making one feel better about one's self, would influence the immune system and the body's response to cancer.

If poor mental health interferes with the functioning of the immune system, and if an ineffective immune system is a causal factor in cancer, it can be said that emotional factors are involved in the etiology of cancer.

SUMMARY

The etiology of cancer is a complex process that is not completely understood at the present time. Many factors interact, apparently in many ways, to influence the development of cancer. Intensive research is being conducted in epidemiology, in animal research, in molecular biology, and in virology to unravel the cancer puzzle.

It is commonly believed by the general public that scientists will one day make a miraculous discovery of the cause of cancer and find a miraculous way to cure it. However, we cannot wait for this miraculous discovery before taking action. We must take the information we have now and use it in efforts to prevent cancer.

It seems likely that the prevention of cancer will come from major economic, political, and lifestyle changes that will have a marked effect on the functioning of our society as a whole. In essence, the control of cancer will require a national commitment.[51]

Our industry, our government, and we ourselves are crisis-oriented. It is difficult to establish an urgency about something that *may* cause cancer 25 years from now. In order to influence important changes in our society, nurses need to place high values on both individual and public health and take actions — however unpopular — that will support those values.

Nurses need to become more active in patient health teaching, public actions to support and improve public health, and political work to support legislation influencing public health.

Needed Changes in our Society

Before carcinogenic factors can be eliminated or controlled, it seems that several things need to occur:

1. The public needs to become aware of the seriousness of the threat to its present and future health.

2. The public has to be willing to accept changes in its lifestyle in order to decrease the risk of development of cancer.

3. Legislative bodies have to accept responsibility for establishing effective control of carcinogenic factors presently in our environment and carcinogenic factors that could be introduced into our environment at a future date.

4. Industries have to accept the responsibility for or be forced to make alterations in the method of disposal of waste and chemicals used in production of their products and in the exposure of their employees to dangerous chemicals, with the intent in mind of decreasing the incidence of cancer.

BIBLIOGRAPHY

1. Allen, D., and P. Cole: Viruses and human cancer. *New England Journal of Medicine.* 286:70–82, 1972.
2. American Cancer Society, Inc.: *1980 Cancer Facts and Figures.* 1979.
3. Anderson, D.: Familial susceptibility. In *Persons at High Risk of Cancer,* ed. by J. F. Fraumeni, Jr. Academic Press, Inc., New York, 1975.
4. Anderson, D. E.: A genetic study of human breast cancer. *Journal of the National Cancer Institute.* 48:1029–1034, 1972.
5. Ashley, D. J. B.: The two 'hit' and multiple 'hit' theories of carcinogenesis. *British Journal of Cancer.* 23:313, 1969.
6. Bacon, C. L., R. Renneker, and M. Cutler: A psychosomatic survey of cancer of the breast. *Psychosomatic Medicine.* 14:453, 1952.
7. Benyesh-Melnick, M., and J. S. Butel: Oncogenic viruses. In *The Molecular Biology of Cancer,* ed. by H. Busch. Academic Press, Inc., New York, 1974.
8. Berg, J. W.: Diet. In *Persons at High Risk of Cancer,* ed. by J. F. Fraumeni, Jr. Academic Press, Inc., New York, 1975.
9. Borden, E. C.: Viruses and breast cancer. *Johns Hopkins Medical Journal.* 134:66, 1974.
10. Busch, H.: *The Molecular Biology of Cancer.* Academic Press, Inc., New York, 1974, p. 377.
11. Clark, J.: Preventing cancer in the environment. *Cancer News.* 32:11–13, 1978.
12. Comings, D. E.: A general theory of carcinogenesis. *Proceedings of the National Academy of Sciences.* 70:3324–3328, 1973.
13. Commoner, B.: Cancer as an environmental disease. *Hospital Practice.* 10:83–84, 1975.
14. Croce, C. M., and H. Koprowski: The genetics of human cancer. *Scientific American.* 239:117–125, 1978.
15. Deinhardt, F.: Introduction to virus-caused cancer: Type C virus. *Cancer.* 34:1363–1366, 1974.
16. DeRouen, T. A., and J. E. Diem: The New Orleans drinking water controversy. *American Journal of Public Health.* 65:1060–1062, 1975.
17. Donovan, P. J., and J. A. DiPaolo: Caffeine enhancement of chemical carcinogen induced transformation of cultured Syrian hamster cells. *Cancer Research.* 34:2720, 1974.
18. Epstein, S. S.: Chemical hazards in the human environment. *CA — A Cancer Journal for Clinicians.* 19:276–281, 1969.
19. Epstein, S. S.: Environmental determinants of human cancer. *Cancer Research.* 34:2425–2435, 1974.

20. Failkow, P. H.: The origin and development of human tumors studied with cell markers. *New England Journal of Medicine.* 291:26–35, 1974.

21. Farber, E.: Carcinogenesis — Cellular evolution as a unifying thread. *Cancer Research.* 33:2537, 1973.

22. Hadden, J. W.: Possible involvement of semen in cancer. *Clinical Bulletin.* 5:161–163, 1975.

23. Hair dyes and cancer. *Lancet.* 2(7927):218, 1975.

24. Hammond, E. C.: Tobacco. In *Persons at High Risk of Cancer,* ed. by J. F. Fraumeni, Jr. Academic Press, Inc., New York, 1975.

25. Haney, C. A.: Illness behavior and psychosocial correlates of cancer. *Social Science and Medicine.* 11:223–228, 1977.

26. Heath, C. W. Jr., G. G. Caldwell, and P. C. Feorino: Viruses and other microbes. In *Persons at High Risk of Cancer,* ed. by J. F. Fraumeni, Jr. Academic Press, Inc., New York, 1975.

27. Henderson, B. E., V. R. Gerkins, and M. C. Pike: Sexual factors and pregnancy. In *Persons at High Risk of Cancer,* ed. by J. F. Fraumeni, Jr. Academic Press, Inc., New York, 1975.

28. Henle, W., and G. Henle: Epstein-Barr virus and human malignancies. *Cancer.* 34:1368, 1974.

29. Higginson, J.: Cancer etiology and prevention. In *Persons at High Risk of Cancer,* ed. by J. F. Fraumeni, Jr. Academic Press, Inc., New York, 1975.

30. Hill, H. Z., and H.-S. Linn: Carcinogenesis and tumor growth. In *Clinical Oncology,* ed. by J. Horton and G. H. Hill, II. W. B. Saunders Co., Philadelphia, 1977.

31. Hilleman, M. R.: Human cancer virus vaccines and the pursuit of the practical. *Cancer.* 34:1439–1445, 1974.

32. Hoover, R., and J. F. Fraumeni, Jr.: Drugs. In *Persons at High Risk of Cancer,* ed. by J. F. Fraumeni, Jr. Academic Press, Inc., New York, 1975.

33. Huebner, R. J., and G. J. Rodaro: Oncogenes of RNA tumor viruses as determinants of cancer. *Proceedings of the National Academy of Sciences.* 64:1087, 1969.

34. Jablon, S.: Radiation. In *Persons at High Risk of Cancer,* ed. by J. F. Fraumeni, Jr. Academic Press, Inc., New York, 1975.

35. Kersey, J. H., and B. P. Spector: Immune deficiency diseases. In *Persons at High Risk of Cancer,* ed. by J. F. Fraumeni, Jr. Academic Press, Inc., New York, 1975.

36. Kissen, D. M.: Psychological factors, personality and lung cancer in men aged 55–64. *British Journal of Medical Psychology.* 40:29, 1967.

37. Knudson, A. G., Jr.: Mutation and cancer: Statistical study of retinoblastoma. *Proceedings of the National Academy of Sciences.* 68:820–823, 1971.

38. LeShan, L.: Psychological status as factors in the development of malignant disease: A critical review. *Journal of the National Cancer Institute.* 22:1, 1959.

39. LeShan, L., and R. E. Worthington: Some psychological correlates of neoplastic disease: A preliminary report. *Journal of Clinical Experimental Psychopathology.* 16:281, 1955.

40. Low, H.: Nitroso compounds. *Archives of Environmental Health.* 29:256–260, 1974.

41. MacMahon, B.: *Epidemiology: Principles and Methods.* Little, Brown & Co., Boston, 1970.

42. Marcus, M. G.: The shaky link between cancer and character. *Psychology Today.* 10:52–54, 1976.

43. Marx, J. L.: Drinking water: Another source of carcinogens. *Science.* 186:809, 1974.

44. Melnick, J. L., E. Adam, and W. E. Rawles: The causative role of herpes virus type 2 in cervical cancer. *Cancer.* 34:1375–1384, 1974.

45. Miller, E. C., and J. A. Miller: Biochemical mechanisms of chemical carcinogenesis. In *The Molecular Biology of Cancer,* ed. by H. Busch. Academic Press, Inc., New York, 1974.

46. Mole, R. H.: The dose-response relationship in radiation carcinogenesis. *British Medical Bulletin.* 14:184, 1958.

47. Monkman, G. R., G. Orwall, and J. C. Ivims: Trauma and oncogenesis. *Mayo Clinic Proceedings.* 49:157–163, 1974.

48. Mulvihill, J. J.: Congenital and genetic diseases. In *Persons at High Risk of Cancer,* ed. by J. F. Fraumeni, Jr. Academic Press, Inc., New York, 1975.

49. Newell, G. (Acting Director of the National Cancer Program, National Cancer Institute): *Statement Before the Intergovernmental Relations and Human Resources Subcommittee.* September 30, 1977.

50. Old, L. J.: Cancer immunology. *Scientific American.* 236:62, 1977.

51. Pelfrene, A. F.: Prevention of cancer: A luxury or an indispensability? *Biomedicine.* 24:2–3, 1976.

52. Penn, I.: Chemical immunosuppression and human cancer. *Cancer.* 34:1474–1479, 1974.

53. Pike, M. C., and P. G. Smith: Clustering of cases of Hodgkin's disease and leukemia. *Cancer.* 34:1390–1394, 1974.

54. Pike, M. C., et al.: Air pollution. In *Persons at High Risk of Cancer,* ed. by J. F. Fraumeni, Jr. Academic Press, Inc., New York, 1975.

55. Rademacher, P., and H.-G. Gilde: Chemical carcinogens. *Journal of Chemical Education.* 53:757–761, 1976.

56. Rapp, F., and R. Duff: Oncogenic conversion of normal cells by inactivated herpes simplex viruses. *Cancer.* 34:1353–1362, 1974.

57. Reddy, B., T. Narisawa, and J. H. Weisburger: Effects of a diet with high levels of protein and fat on colon carcinogenesis in F344 rats treated with 1,2-dimethylhydrazine. *Journal of the National Cancer Institute.* 57:567–569, 1976.

58. Renwick, A. G., and B. S. Drasar: Environmental carcinogens and large bowel cancer. *Nature.* 263:234–235, 1976.

59. Rothman, K. J.: Alcohol. In *Persons at High Risk of Cancer,* ed. by J. F. Fraumeni, Jr. Academic Press, Inc., New York, 1975.

60. Ryser, H. J. P.: Special report: Chemical carcinogenesis. *CA — A Cancer Journal for Clinicians.* 24:351–360, 1974.

61. Schmale, A. H., and H. P. Iker: The affect of hopelessness and the development of cancer. *Psychosomatic Medicine.* 28:714, 1966.

62. Schneiderman, M. A.: Sources, resources, and

tsouris. In *Persons at High Risk of Cancer,* ed. by J. F. Fraumeni, Jr. Academic Press, Inc., New York, 1975.

63. Schwind, J. V.: Cancer: Regressive evolution? *Oncology.* 29:172–180, 1974.

64. Segelman, A. B., et al.: Sassafras and herb tea, potential health hazards. *Journal of the American Medical Association.* 236:477, 1976.

65. Selikoff, I. J., and E. C. Hammond: Multiple risk factors in environmental cancer. In *Persons at High Risk of Cancer,* ed. by J. F. Fraumeni, Jr. Academic Press, Inc., New York, 1975.

66. Shafer, N., and R. W. Shafer: Potential carcinogenic effects of hair dyes. *New York State Journal of Medicine.* 76:394–396, 1976.

67. Shubik, P.: Potential carcinogenicity of food additives and contaminants. *Cancer Research.* 35: 3475–3480, 1975.

68. Simonton, O. C., and S. S. Simonton: Belief systems and management of the emotional aspects of malignancy. *Journal of Transpersonal Psychology.* 7:29–47, 1975.

69. Solomon, G.: Emotions, stress, the central nervous system, and immunity. *Annals of the New York Academy of Sciences.* 164:335–343, 1969.

70. Speigelman, A., et al.: Human cancer and animal viral oncology. *Cancer.* 34:1406, 1974.

71. Sporn, M. B., et al.: Prevention of chemical carcinogenesis by vitamin A and its synthetic analogs (retinoids). *Federation Proceedings.* 35:1332–1338, 1976.

72. Stephenson, J. R., and W. J. Grace: Life stress and cancer of the cervix. *Psychosomatic Medicine.* 16:287, 1954.

73. Susser, M.: *Casual Thinking in the Health Sciences.* Oxford University Press, New York, 1973.

74. Temin, H. M.: Introduction to virus-caused cancers. *Cancer.* 34:1347–1352, 1974.

75. Walker, A. R. P.: Colon cancer and diet, with special reference to intakes of fat and fiber. *American Journal of Clinical Nutrition.* 29:1417–1426, 1976.

76. Walker, A. R. P., and D. P. Burkitt: Colonic cancer, hypothesis of causation, dietary prophylaxis and future research. *American Journal of Digestive Diseases.* 21:910–917, 1976.

77. Wein, A. J., W. Graham, and H. P. Royster: The malignant change in chronic wounds. *Industrial Medicine.* 41:12–14, 1972.

78. Wynder, E. L., et al.: Interdisciplinary and experimental approaches: metabolic epidemiology. In *Persons at High Risk of Cancer,* ed. by J. F. Fraumeni, Jr. Academic Press, Inc., New York, 1975.

4

The Diagnosis of Cancer

THE MAGNITUDE OF THE CANCER PROBLEM

Cancer is the second leading cause of death in the United States. Twenty-five per cent of the population will develop some type of cancer and 20 per cent will die of cancer.[4] In the 1970s there were an estimated 3.5 million cancer deaths, 6.5 million new cancer cases, and more than 10 million people under medical care for cancer. Over 54 million Americans now living will eventually have cancer. About 690,000 new cases of the disease are diagnosed yearly. Each year about 385,000 people die of cancer —1055 people a day or one person every 1½ minutes. Cancer does not discriminate; it strikes all age groups. It kills more children ages 3 to 14 years than any other disease.[1] (See Figs. 4–1 to 4–6 and Tables 4–1 and 4–2, pp. 63–68.)

THE DETECTION OF CANCER

A disease with such a powerful impact on both individuals and society as a whole demands major attempts to prevent or limit its devastating toll. The most effective way to approach this disease is with an orientation toward prevention. The theories and strategies associated with prevention will be discussed in detail in Chapter 18.

The focus of this chapter is on the detection of cancer, whether early or late in the disease process. In some instances, early detection of cancer greatly increases the chance of cure. Early detection can often provide both prolongation and a higher quality of life. In some situations, detection may be a matter of identifying cancer as the causative factor for the presenting symptoms, when the symptoms could be due to a variety of other disorders.

Feelings — Their Impact on Diagnosis

Cancer is a difficult disease to detect. Symptoms usually appear late in the disease process and often are common to many other disease entities. Patients may minimize or completely fail to mention symptoms that they have. Sometimes the patient is aware of a symptom and has already decided that the symptom is due to a specific cause; for example, bright red lower bowel bleeding may be thought to be an indication of hemorrhoids. It is very easy for the examiner to simply accept the patient's diagnosis without considering other possible explanations.

The fear of cancer may be so great in some individuals that they may attempt to relay information in such a way that cancer will not be considered as the diagnosis. Other people feel that the examiner is the expert and should be able to detect problems with little or no information about their symptoms.[9]

Examiners themselves may block out thoughts of the possibility of cancer because of negative personal beliefs about the disease. They may take an approach equivalent to an ostrich sticking its head in the sand — if cancer is not found, it is not there. Often all other diagnoses are ruled out before cancer is considered; this can cause a long delay in beginning treatment. The examiner may not wish to be the one to bestow upon an individual the label of having cancer and may avoid the responsibility by referring the person to someone else. The consequence of this action may be repeated delays in diagnosis and in the institution of treatment.

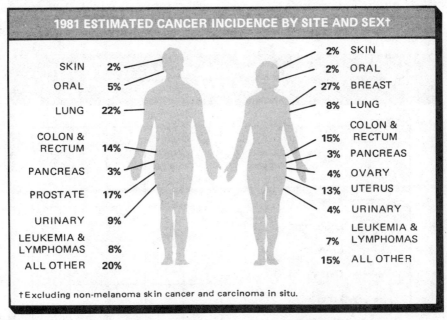

Figure 4–1. Estimated cancer incidence by site and sex for 1981. (From SEER Program: Cancer Statistics, 1981. *CA — A Cancer Journal for Clinicians.* 31:13, 1981. Used by permission.)

The Diagnostic Process

It would be impossible in a book of this nature to describe the entire process of performing a history and physical examination on a patient. This process cannot be learned entirely from a textbook, since it requires both guidance from a person experienced in the technique as well as the opportunity to practice the skills. Therefore, the material will be presented in this book under the assumption that the reader has the basic knowledge and skills required to perform these activities.

Text continued on page 68

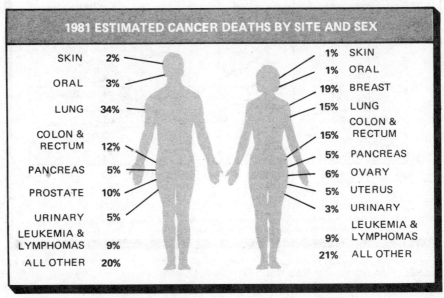

Figure 4–2. Estimated cancer deaths by site and sex for 1981. (From SEER Program: Cancer Statistics, 1981. *CA — A Cancer Journal for Clinicians.* 31:13, 1981. Used by permission.)

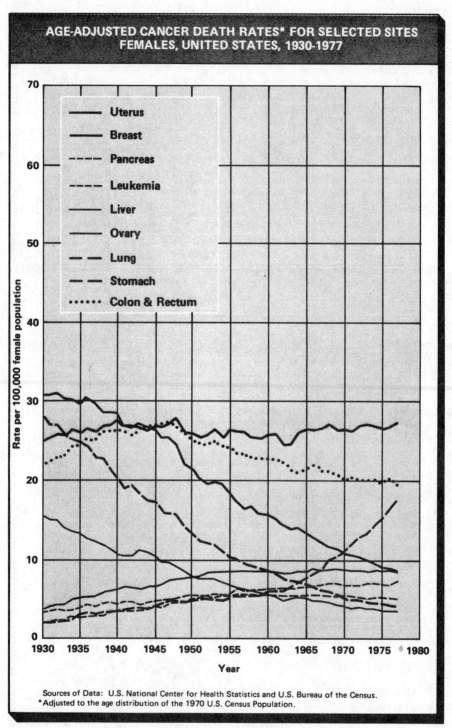

Figure 4–3. Age-adjusted cancer death rates for selected sites for females in the United States from 1930 to 1977. (From SEER Program: Cancer Statistics, 1981. *CA — A Cancer Journal for Clinicians.* 31:18, 1981. Used by permission.)

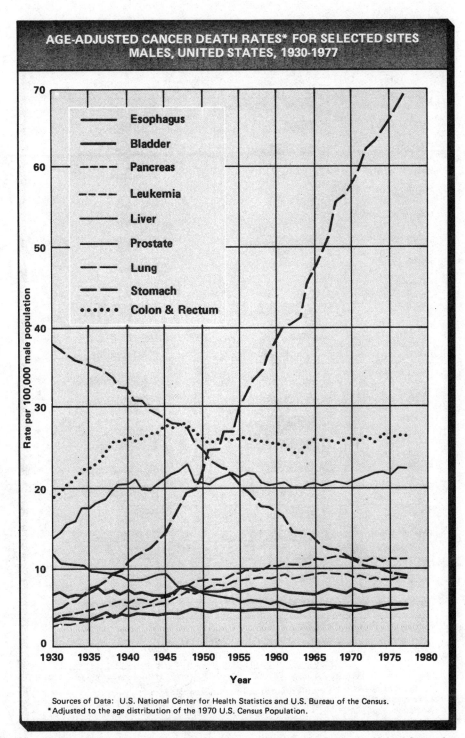

Figure 4–4. Age-adjusted cancer death rates for selected sites for males in the United States from 1930 to 1977. (From SEER Program: Cancer Statistics, 1981. *CA — A Cancer Journal for Clinicians.* 31:19, 1981. Used by permission.)

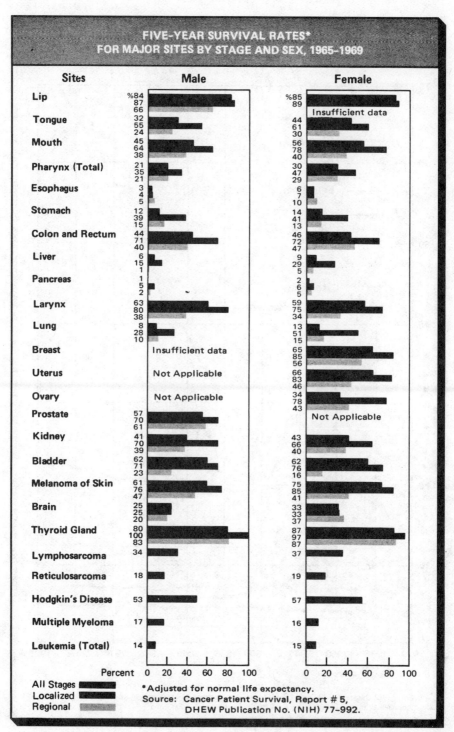

Figure 4–5. Five-year survival rates for major cancer sites by stage and sex, 1965 to 1969. (From SEER Program: Cancer Statistics, 1981. *CA — A Cancer Journal for Clinicians,* 31:26, 1981. Used by permission.)

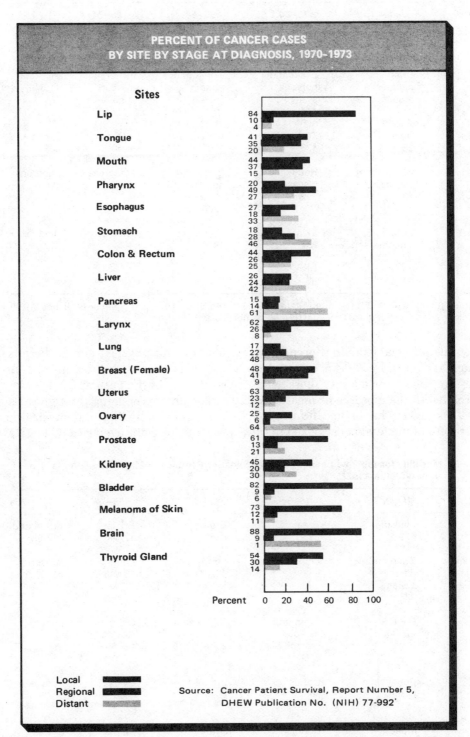

**PERCENT OF CANCER CASES
BY SITE BY STAGE AT DIAGNOSIS, 1970-1973**

Sites

Site	Local	Regional	Distant
Lip	84	10	4
Tongue	41	35	20
Mouth	44	37	15
Pharynx	20	49	27
Esophagus	27	18	33
Stomach	18	28	46
Colon & Rectum	44	26	25
Liver	26	24	42
Pancreas	15	14	61
Larynx	62	26	8
Lung	17	22	48
Breast (Female)	48	41	9
Uterus	63	23	12
Ovary	25	6	64
Prostate	61	13	21
Kidney	45	20	30
Bladder	82	9	6
Melanoma of Skin	73	12	11
Brain	88	9	1
Thyroid Gland	54	30	14

Percent 0 20 40 60 80 100

Local
Regional
Distant

Source: Cancer Patient Survival, Report Number 5,
DHEW Publication No. (NIH) 77-992`

Figure 4–6. Percentage of cancer cases by site by stage at diagnosis, 1970 to 1973. (From SEER Program: Cancer Statistics, 1981. *CA — A Cancer Journal for Clinicians*, 31:27, 1981. Used by permission.)

Table 4–1.   Mortality for the Five Leading Cancer Sites for Males in Major Age Groups, United States – 1977*

All Ages	Under 15	15–34	35–54	55–74	75+
Lung 68,481	Leukemia 633	Leukemia 755	Lung 10,110	Lung 44,112	Lung, 14,060
Colon and rectum 24,984	Brain and nervous system 414	Brain and nervous system 474	Colon and rectum 2434	Colon and rectum 13,504	Prostate 11,645
Prostate 20,790	Bone 58	Testis 423	Pancreas 1307	Prostate 8851	Colon and rectum 8811
Pancreas 10,938	Connective tissues 50	Hodgkin's disease 352	Brain and nervous system 1200	Pancreas 6378	Pancreas 3205
Stomach 8688	Lympho-sarcoma and reticulosar-coma 49	Skin 254	Leukemia 1046	Stomach 4652	Bladder 3121

*Source: Vital Statistics of the United States, 1977. (From SEER Program: Cancer Statistics, 1981. CA — A Cancer Journal for Clinicians. 31:15, 1981. Used by permission.)

A routine physical examination must be thorough and should not focus on a search for only one disease or for only those symptoms related to the diseases or disorders a patient is known to have. Significant problems are often completely overlooked in the history and physical simply because they are not directly related to the primary complaint of the patient.

The process of going through the steps of performing a history and physical is fairly routine, perhaps even ritualistic. However,

Table 4–2.   Mortality for the Five Leading Cancer Sites for Females in Major Age Groups, United States – 1977*

All Ages	Under 15	15–34	35–54	55–74	75+
Breast 34,481	Leukemia 422	Breast 623	Breast 8348	Breast 17,341	Colon and rectum 11,953
Colon and rectum 26,608	Brain and nervous system 302	Leukemia 553	Lung 4528	Lung 13,045	Breast 8166
Lung 22,029	Bone 47	Brain and nervous system 316	Colon and rectum 2283	Colon and rectum 12,190	Lung 4341
Uterus 10,842	Connective tissues 46	Uterus 303	Uterus 2093	Ovary 6000	Pancreas 3778
Ovary 10,653	Kidney 35	Hodgkin's disease 235	Ovary 2063	Uterus 5573	Uterus 2970

*Source: Vital Statistics of the United States, 1977. (From SEER Program: Cancer Statistics, 1981. CA — A Cancer Journal for Clinicians. 31:15, 1981. Used by permission.)

the previous experience, knowledge, attitudes, and value system of the examiner may influence how the examiner interprets what the patient says; what physical findings are noted; and the importance placed on these findings. When the orientation of the examiner is medical and disease-related, importance may be placed on those findings that logically tie in with a known disease, and a further search may be made for additional signs related to the same disorder or disease. If the examiner is a nurse, the patient's sociologic and cultural background will more often be tied together with psychologic and physical findings in an attempt to view the patient's current problems as a part of a whole. There must be an awareness that multiple problems may be present, some totally unrelated to others from a point of view of disease states.

NURSING HISTORY

The Establishment of Trust. The establishment of trust in a therapeutic relationship is essential if the patient is to feel safe in revealing symptoms and intimate feelings. Part of this trust develops from signals from the nurse that indicate a willingness to listen to and an acceptance of the patient as he or she is. It is important that nurses do not discount the information a patient provides by considering it unimportant or by being inattentive. It is also important that nurses not make premature judgments without sufficient data. Nurses should seek the patients' physical and emotional strengths as well as weaknesses, their areas of health as well as areas of disorders.[9]

Approach. One effective approach to the history is to allow patients to begin by describing their present state of health and how they view themselves and their lives. The reasons for the present examination can be explored. Many fears and imaginings of the patient may not be verbally expressed. Skills in perceiving nonverbal communication and in verbal reflective techniques can be useful in eliciting a maximum amount of information from the patient. The verbal reflective technique involves repeating a word or phrase used by the patient, with a pause afterward to encourage elaboration. The examiner can also reflect a patient's nonverbal communication by describing observed behavior; for example, "You seemed tense when you were telling me about _____ . Do you have some concerns about that?" The advantage of the reflective technique is that it provides information from the patient that has not been influenced by the examiner's value system. One disadvantage of the technique is that an extremely verbose patient may take a long time to provide the needed information.[9]

Cancer Symptoms. A variety of symptoms can be indicative of cancer. The seven warning signals listed by the American Cancer Society are important to keep in mind. These include a change in bowel or bladder habits, a sore that does not heal, unusual bleeding or discharge, a thickening or lump in the breast or elsewhere, indigestion or difficulty in swallowing, an obvious change in a wart or mole, and a nagging cough or hoarseness.[5] Some types of cancer have no symptoms until very late in the course of the disease. Asymptomatic tumors are usually smaller and more easily cured than those with symptoms.[13]

General symptoms that may be present are: rapid and unexplained weight loss, anorexia, nausea and vomiting, fatigue, weakness, confusion, fever, dyspnea, edema, effusions, frequent infections, and pain. Symptoms that have been described by the patient should be explored in detail by inquiring about their location, characteristics, intensity, time of onset, pattern of development since onset, circumstances surrounding the occurrence of the symptoms, aggravating and alleviating factors, and associated symptoms. At this point the temptation to jump to conclusions about the cause of the symptoms and to direct all further questions toward that end should be avoided.

Past Health History. It is important to explore the patients' past health history. Many physicians call this a health history, when in fact their approach to it could better be termed a disease history. In order to get a broad nursing perspective, the patients' previous and present attitudes toward health and health care should be examined. Actions taken by the patients to improve their level of health should be noted. Patterns in diet, weight control, exercise, smoking, and alcohol use should be identified. Questions should be oriented toward determining if the patients are in a high risk group for cancer, using the criteria provided in Chapter 3 of this book. When exploring the patients' past health history, it is important to note their occupations for the past 25 years in order to determine possible exposure to chemical carcinogens. If the patient smokes, the examiner should find out the age at which the individual started smoking and how many cigarettes a day are smoked. It is important to remember that a person who presently has or has previously had cancer is more likely to develop a second cancer.[6] Symptoms caused by a second primary tumor are often mistakenly attributed to anxiety or to complications of previous cancer treatment.

Family History.   The family history of the patient should be explored. A pedigree should be developed that indicates the cause of death and age at death of all known family members and the present state of health of living family members. Any diagnosis of cancer that has occurred in family members should be listed. This pedigree should extend as far as possible beyond the immediate family to include relatives such as cousins, aunts, uncles, great-aunts, and -uncles. If 10 per cent of the family members have a history of diagnosed cancer, the family is labeled a "cancer family," and the patient has a much higher risk of developing cancer. In some families, the type of cancer that occurs is similar; for example, one family may have a pattern of cancer within the gastrointestinal tract. Other families may exhibit no clear pattern of cancer type.

Personal and Social History.   The personal and social history should include the patient's current and past relationships with others, family members in particular. Inability to establish intimate relationships, unresolved grief, or presence of a feeling of despair may indicate an increased risk of cancer for the patient. The examiner should try to determine the patient's usual coping mechanisms and their effectiveness. One way to get this information is to inquire about previous crisis situations in the patient's life and how they were resolved.

Systems Review.   The last section of the history is the systems review, which can be very effective in detecting symptoms and problems that have failed to surface in previous sections of the interview. Since cancer is a multisystem disease, this section of the history may be very significant. A helpful source for improving the technique of history-taking is Morgan and Engel's book *The Clinical Approach to the Patient.*[9]

PHYSICAL EXAMINATION

The following is a description of some of the more common findings that could be indicative of cancer. A complete discussion of this topic would require a book in itself.

General Overview.   An accurate weight determination is important, since cachexia is occasionally the presenting symptom of cancer.

Skin.   The skin should be visually examined in totality for abnormal-appearing moles or growths and palpated for unusual lumps.

Head.   Scalp lesions, which are concealed by hair, may be present. The skull should be palpated. Some malignancies invade the skull bone and cause softened areas within the skull.

Eyes.   Eyes are examined for equality in size and shape. Malignant lesions in the retinal area are sometimes easily observed by simple visual examination, but may require use of the grid on the ophthalmoscope to detect variations in the contour.

Mouth.   The lips and interior surface of the mouth should be visually inspected.

However, most malignancies in the mouth cannot be detected by visual examination and require the use of palpation. This is most effectively done with a gloved hand. The roof of the mouth should be palpated, and the cheek walls should be examined by palpating both internal and external cheeks simultaneously. The tongue should be palpated for masses. Bimanual palpation should be used to thoroughly examine the floor of the mouth and the tongue. For some reason, the examination of the mouth seems offensive and is not usually included as part of the regular physical examination. Few dentists conduct this type of examination for a malignancy. Thus, cancer in the mouth may go undetected for years.

Neck. Cervical nodes should be examined carefully. Nodes that are malignant are inclined to be firm, nontender, and fixed in position and at times are attached to underlying structures. Nonmalignant nodes are soft, movable, and frequently tender. However, this does not always hold true and it is somewhat dangerous to make this assumption. Nodes that are not enlarged may also prove to be malignant on microscopic examination. The trachea should be examined to determine deviation from the midline, which can indicate a malignancy within the bronchial tree. The thyroid should also be palpated for masses.

Chest. Abnormal breath sounds can be indicative of a malignancy, as can absence of breath sounds from a particular area of the lung field. Regions where changes in lung sounds are heard may also be dull to percussion. Pleural effusions from cancer may also alter normal breath sounds.

Breast and Axilla. The breasts are examined in a circular motion beginning with the nipple and working outward. Breast tissue extends upward to the clavicle and is also located on the chest wall under the arm. The largest number of malignant breast lesions are found in the upper outer quadrant of the breast. Visual inspection of the breast should be made with the patient sitting with arms at the side, with arms elevated above the head, and with hands pressed on the hips. Each breast should be carefully inspected for drainage from the nipple; for changes in size or shape; for nipple inversion; and for symmetry with the other. The pectoral, subscapular, lateral axillary, and supraclavicular nodes should be examined. The supraclavicular nodes can more easily be palpated by standing behind the patient, pressing inward and down slightly behind the clavicles, and requesting that the patient cough. With the cough, enlarged nodes will pop up behind the clavicle. Because of the location of these nodes in relation to the thoracic duct, enlargement of these nodes may be the first indication of a malignancy elsewhere in the body.

Abdomen. The abdomen should be inspected for changes in contour that can occur as a result of ascites or abdominal masses. Auscultation may indicate the site of partial obstruction due to abdominal tumors. Percussion may reveal the presence of solid masses and may also be used to determine increased size of the liver and spleen. Light and deep palpation can be used to detect abdominal masses.

Genitalia in Men. Both inspection and palpation should be used to examine the penis and scrotal area for the presence of skin lesions or masses. Skin lesions on the penis may be malignant. Palpate the testes carefully for small nodules, which may be the only sign of testicular cancer in young men. Early testicular cancer is now a very treatable disease.

Genitalia in Women. Examine the external genitalia, using inspection and palpation. A vaginal examination should be done with careful inspection of both cervix and cervical os, looking for signs of inflammation, ulceration, nodules, masses, discharge, or bleeding. A three-slide Papanicolaou (Pap) smear should be done. First, an endocervical swab should be taken by inserting a moistened cotton applicator into the os of the cervix. The second slide should be made from a cervical scraping. The third slide should be made from material obtained from a cotton applicator rolled on the floor of the vagina below the cervix. The purpose of the third slide is to pick up cells that may have shed from the endometrial lining. For some unfortunate reason, many physicians do not include the third slide as part of the Pap smear. Endometrial cancer is much more difficult to detect than cervical cancer, and results in a later diagnosis and a poorer prognosis. The risk of endometrial cancer increases markedly after menopause.

The vaginal wall should also be examined for masses, ulceration, inflammation, or discharge. A bimanual examination should be done to palpate the vaginal wall, the cervix, the uterus, and the ovaries. Pelvic masses that may be present can also be detected during this examination. Cancer often causes tissue to feel hard, inflexible, rigid, and, when in an advanced state, to feel very different from normal tissue.

Anus and Rectum. A large percentage of cancers of the large intestine are near enough to the anal sphincter to be detected by digital examination. Unfortunately, digital examination of the rectum is seldom conducted except during complete examination and sometimes not even then. Perhaps some of the reasons for this are the negative social connotations associated with rectal examination. Since most colon cancers are adenocarcinomas and metastasize when they reach one centimeter in size, early detection may literally mean the difference between life and death. Lesions just above the reach of the finger tip can occasionally be felt by asking the patient to strain down. In the male, the prostate is examined during the rectal examination. The prostate can be felt through the interior wall of the rectum and should have two clearly defined lobes with a median sulcus between them. Notation should be made of size, shape, nodularity, and tenderness. Cancer does not always cause the prostate to enlarge, so it is unwise to make the assumption that if the prostate is within normal size and shape, cancer is not present. As cancer develops in the prostate, the consistency of the gland changes from soft to firm.

A test for occult blood should be administered on the feces adhering to the gloved finger after it is removed from the rectum. The American Cancer Society has recently made available material to test feces for occult blood and this material is now being used as a screening test for cancer.[5] There are obviously many causes for the presence of occult blood in the stool. However, since adenocarcinoma of the colon is vascular, the tumor bleeds easily, and often bleeding occurs early in the course of the disease. Therefore a test for occult blood is very useful as a screening device for colon cancer.

Extremities. Extremities should be examined for masses and for lymphedema. Since many tumors obstruct lymphatic flow as they grow, varying degrees of lymphedema may be present. Lymphedema as a result of cancer is often attributed to other causes such as varicosities.

Neurologic Examination. A thorough examination of neurologic functioning can be useful in detecting brain tumors, tumors of the spinal cord, and tumors that are interfering with the function of the peripheral nervous system. Abnormalities found will vary greatly, depending on the location of the tumor.

PATIENT TEACHING

The physical examination presents a good opportunity for patient teaching. Women can be encouraged to do monthly breast examinations and can be taught adequate procedures for examination of the breast. Health habits and their relationship to the risk of development of cancer can be discussed with the patient. The importance of routine physical examinations can be discussed. It is also important to make sure that the patient understands that a physical examination does not guarantee that cancer is not present, since many types of cancer are not detectable by examination.

DIAGNOSTIC TESTS

Radiographic Examinations. A variety of diagnostic tests may be used in an attempt to detect or rule out the presence of cancer. X-ray examinations are the most frequently used and include such procedures as upper gastrointestinal (GI) studies, barium enemas, and intravenous pyelograms. Routine chest x-rays are not usually a very effective means of detecting early cancer. Chest tomograms are much more accurate in indicating the presence and location of tumors in the lung.

Mammography is utilized for the detection of breast cancer, particularly in patients at high risk of this disease. Mammography can detect breast cancers that are not yet detectable by manual palpation. Some question has arisen over the possibility that increased radiation exposure to the breast from mammography causes an increase in the risk of cancer. Thus, mammography is being used only for postmenopausal women who are at high risk of breast cancer.

Contrast angiography is now being used both to detect the presence of cancer and to determine the vascular supply of known malignancies, in order to more intelligently plan treatment approaches.

Radioactive isotopes are being used very frequently for scans in order to detect the presence of cancer. The most common scans now in use are brain, bone, liver and spleen, and thyroid scans, and lymphangiograms.[6]

Blood Tests. For many years, it has been hoped that a blood test could be developed that would indicate the presence of cancer somewhere in the body. Many research studies have been conducted with the aim of developing such a test. No blood test has yet been developed to accomplish this purpose. Blood tests that show variation from the normal values of chemicals within the body have been useful in diagnosing specific types of cancer; for example, carcinoid syndrome and choriocarcinoma. M protein is present in patients with myeloma, and high copper levels are detectable in patients with Hodgkin's disease. Acid phosphatase, serum glutamic-oxaloacetic transaminase (SGOT), and SGPT are elevated in patients who have metastatic disease; however, these changes are the result of cell destruction and are certainly not specific to cancer. As the size of the tumor increases, amounts of both carcinoembryonic antigen (CEA) and alpha-fetoprotein (AFP) increase in the blood. However, the accuracy of these tests is not sufficient to make them useful in diagnosing cancer.

Pap Smears. Papanicolaou (Pap) tests can be used to detect cancer in many body sites. The most familiar site for the Pap test, of course, is the cervix; however, the same test can be used for detecting cancers in the mouth or bronchial tree, or by fluid aspiration from the chest or abdominal cavities.

Endoscopic Examinations. Endoscopic examinations may be used to visualize lesions and to obtain biopsy material. Endoscopic examinations are utilized in examining the bronchial tree, the esophagus, the stomach, and the small bowel; proctoscopic examinations are used in examining the lower colon; and flexible fiberoptic instruments are useful in examining the entire colon. The development of flexible fiberoptic endoscopes has made possible the examination of areas that were previously inaccessible except by surgical exploration.

When to Use Diagnostic Tests. The difficult problems come when deciding which of these examinations to use in attempts to detect cancer. This decision is usually made by the physician. The cost of conducting all of these procedures yearly on a healthy individual would be prohibitive, and the resulting number of cancer cases found would not be sufficient enough to justify their use. Therefore, some discretion is necessary in making decisions about when to use these tests. Persons at high risk of developing a particular type of cancer should be screened frequently for that type of cancer. Persons who have symptoms that could be indicative of a cancer in a specific site should have all of the screening procedures necessary in order to detect the presence of cancer in that area. These tests are also used to determine sites of metastases in a patient who has already been diagnosed as having cancer, since the results may influence the decision as to which type of treatment is appropriate. The tests may also be used to determine the effectiveness of treatment already implemented. In patients with breast cancer, brain scans, bone scans, and tomograms may be done before breast surgery is performed, since if cancer is present in any of these areas, the results may influence the type of surgery done.

Biopsies. The only method of obtaining a definite diagnosis of cancer is from cytologic examination of tissue obtained from biopsy or exfoliative cytology. There are three types of biopsy in common use: excisional, incisional, and needle biopsy.

Excisional Biopsy. Excisional biopsy is performed by removing an entire palpable mass. The mass is then cut into very thin slices that are entered under the microscope. This type of biopsy is commonly used in detection of early breast cancer and in examination of lymph nodes.

One very important factor in the accuracy of the results from an excisional biopsy is the attention to detail shown by the pathologist performing the microscopic examination. Some pathologists take only three or four sliced sections from the biopsy specimen to examine for malignant cells. However, unless the cancer is very advanced, cancer cells can be randomly scattered throughout a mass in which a high percentage of normal cells are present. By examining only three or four sections, it is very possible for the pathologist to completely miss any cancer cells that might be present. In order to detect those cancer cells, it is necessary to examine 25 to 50 sections of a small node. If lymph nodes are being examined, it is very possible for some of the nodes within a chain to contain malignant cells and for other nodes to be completely normal. Enlarged nodes are not always the ones that contain malignant cells. If several nodes are enlarged in a particular area, the surgeon will very frequently remove the largest node possible for pathologic examination. These nodes are very often necrotic in the center and of little use in pathologic diagnosis.

Many times the first biopsy proves to be negative. The patient continues to experience symptoms, and two or three other biopsies may be required over a period of several months before a diagnosis is made. This is a loss of very valuable time when effective treatment could be implemented to cure or control the growth of the cancer.

Incisional Biopsy. Incisional biopsies are performed on tumors too large to remove or those located in an area where complete removal is not feasible. The accuracy of diagnosis from these biopsies is again dependent on the careful attention to detail exhibited by the pathologist performing the cytologic study.

Needle Biopsy. Needle biopsies are performed in areas where surgical removal of a portion of the mass is not feasible either because of location or because of the physical condition of the patient. One common site of needle biopsy is the liver. Because of the vascularity of the liver, there is a risk of hemorrhage after the biopsy, and the patient should be very closely watched for signs of internal bleeding. Needle biopsies are the least accurate type of biopsy because there is no direct visual examination of the area being biopsied and because only a very small portion of a large mass of tissue is removed. It is possible to completely miss scattered islands of malignancy within the organ.

Bone Marrow Aspiration. Bone marrow aspiration may be conducted in order to diagnose leukemia, lymphomas, and other cancers that may have invaded bone marrow tissue. The sternum and the iliac crest are the two most common sites of bone marrow aspiration.

Biopsy and cytologic study are the only means for definitive diagnosis of cancer, and — except in rare cases such as brain tumors — most responsible physicians will not institute treatment for cancer without this diagnosis.

WAYS OF CATEGORIZING CANCER

In addition to determining the presence or absence of malignant cells within the tissue examined, it is the responsibility of the pathologist to describe the cells in detail and to categorize them into class, grade, or stage.

Class

Papanicolaou tests are categorized into classes:

Class 1 — Absence of atypical or abnormal cells.

Class 2 — Atypical cytology but no evidence of malignancy.

Class 3 — Cytology suggestive of, but not conclusive for, malignancy.

Class 4 — Cytology strongly suggestive of malignancy.

Class 5 — Cytology conclusive for malignancy.

Grading

Grading is a process done by the pathologist and consists of categorizing the number of malignant cells in relation to the number of normal cells in a tissue sample seen under a microscope. In grade one, most of the cells are normal, with scattered malignant cells present. Progressive degrees of malignancy are seen in grades two, three, and four. Grade four shows mostly malignant cells with very few normal cells present.

Another factor considered in this process is the degree of malignancy of the cell seen under the microscope. Some malignant cells have an appearance very similar to that of normal cells. More and more changes appear in cell structure as malignancy progresses. In early cancer cells, it is very easy for the pathologist to identify whether the cells are from breast tissue, lung tissue, or gastrointestinal tissue. In extreme stages of malignancy, the cancer cell is classified as anaplastic, or dedifferentiated. Cells that are anaplastic cannot be identified as to site of origin. The nucleus is extremely large and takes up most of the cell space. The cells are very grotesque in appearance and vary markedly in shape and size from one cell to another. Most commonly, cells from early states of cancer are grade one or two and cells from very advanced malignancy tend to be grade four. However, this is not always true. With grade four cells, there is a much greater risk of metastasis since these cells have lost contact inhibition.

Staging

Staging and grading are very often confused in the mind of the health care provider. The purpose of staging is to identify the extent of the malignancy's spread. Cancers seldom have a specific sequence in which they spread from one location to another within the patient's body. However, some significance can be placed on whether the malignancy is confined to the primary site, has spread locally through the lymphatic system, or has metastasized to distant sites. Staging methods have been developed for many different kinds of cancer, with each type having its own staging system. Staging systems have been developed for breast cancer, for Hodgkin's disease, for non-Hodgkin's lymphomas and for many other malignancies. The first staging systems that were developed varied from one country to another and even from one researcher to another. This made it difficult to compare results of research studies.

Staging systems were developed for several reasons: to make communications between researchers more meaningful; to aid in the selection of treatment techniques for a particular cancer and a particular degree of progression; to allow the physician to determine probable prognosis; to compare research findings; and to evaluate the effectiveness of various treatment techniques. In 1959 an attempt was made to standardize the staging of all kinds of cancer. A system called the TNM system was developed, with the capital T representing the primary tumor and subscripts indicating increases in size of the tumor or involvement by direct extension. The capital N indicated lymph node involvement, with subscripts further breaking down categories of nodal involvement. The capital M indicated distant metastases.

Staging procedures require involved diagnostic tests to determine all possible identifiable sites of metastasis. These may include x-ray examinations, scans, fiberoptic examinations, or exploratory laparotomy with extensive node dissection. It is sometimes difficult for nurses and physicians to understand the rationale for performing an exploratory laparotomy on a patient who has just had a nodal biopsy in the neck and been told that he or she has Hodgkin's disease. Because the rationale behind the staging process is not always clearly understood or accepted, the family physician may often discourage the patient from allowing these procedures to be done. If treatment is to be intelligently planned with the greatest chance of survival for the patient, staging is absolutely essential. For example, if radiation to the chest region is ordered for a patient with Hodgkin's disease who has not had prior staging, it is very possible for the disease to have progressed to the spleen, liver, and periaortic nodes with no evidence of symptoms. If this is the case, malignancies in the abdominal area will continue to grow uncontrolled while the radiation is being administered to the chest area. The patient's chances of long-term survival will be markedly diminished.

CANCER CLASSIFICATION

Cancer is not a single disease but many diseases, each of them unique. For many years, attempts have been made to classify these diseases by some type of logical system. Most of these classifications have become obsolete as our knowledge of cancers

Table 4–3. Classification of Very Common Types of Cancer

Tissue	Cancer
Epithelial	Carcinoma Squamous cell Adenocarcinoma
Nonhematopoietic Mesenchymal	Sarcoma
Hematopoietic and lymphoid	Leukemia Lymphoma Myeloma
Neural	Glioma
Miscellaneous	Melanoma Embryonic tumor

has increased. No single classification system is presently being used. The system most commonly used classifies cancers according to the tissue of origin. However, the classification does give health care givers and researchers a point of reference. See Table 4–3 for the classification of very common types of cancer. Only the most common types are listed, as it would take many pages, or perhaps an entire book, to list all the identified cancers.

BIBLIOGRAPHY

1. American Cancer Society, Inc.: 1980 Cancer Facts and Figures, 1979.
2. Bates, B.: *A Guide to Physical Examination.* J. B. Lippincott Co., Philadelphia, 1979.
3. Burns, K. R., and J. Johnson: *Health Assessment in Clinical Practice.* Prentice-Hall, Inc., Englewood Cliffs, N.J., 1980.
4. Epstein, S. S.: *The Politics of Cancer.* Anchor Press/Doubleday Publishing Co., Garden City, N.Y., 1978.
5. Holleb, A. I.: Self-examination in the asymptomatic patient. In *Cancer Medicine,* ed. by J. F. Holland and E. Frie, III. Lea and Febiger, Philadelphia, 1974.
6. Horton, J., and D. Daut: Detection and recognition of cancer. In *Cancer Oncology,* ed. by J. Horton and G. J. Hill, II. W. B. Saunders Co., Philadelphia, 1977.
7. Macleod, J., E. B. French, and J. F. Munor: *Introduction to Clinical Examination.* Churchill Livingstone Inc., New York, 1977.
8. McCray, N. D.: Oncology patient assessment tool. *Oncology Nursing Forum.* 6:15–18, 1979.
9. Morgan, W. L., and G. L. Engel: *The Clinical Approach to the Patient.* W. B. Saunders Co., Philadelphia, 1969.
10. Moritz, D. A.: Nursing histories — A guide, yes. A form, no! *Oncology Nursing Forum,* 6:18–19, 1979.
11. Prior, J., and J. S. Silberstein: *Physical Diagnosis: The History and Examination of the Patient.* C. V. Mosby Co., St. Louis, 1973.
12. Schottenfeld, D.: Patient risk factors and the detection of early cancer. In *Cancer: Pathophysiology, Etiology, and Management,* ed. by L. C. Krause, J. L. Reese, and L. K. Hart. C. V. Mosby Co., St. Louis, 1979.
13. Shimkin, M. B.: Introduction: cancer detection and prevention. In *Cancer Medicine,* ed. by J. F. Holland and E. Frie, III. Lea and Febiger, Philadelphia, 1974.
14. Smith, C. E.: *Cancer: Nursing Assessment and Care, a Self-learning Text.* McGraw-Hill Book Co., New York, 1980.
15. Thompson, J. M., and A. C. Bowers: *Clinical Manual of Health Assessment.* C. V. Mosby Co., St. Louis, 1980.

5

Values, Ethics, and Ethical Dilemmas in Cancer Nursing

There are three components that must be included in considering the impact of nursing on the cancer situation: feelings, factual knowledge, and ethics. These three are interrelated and must be integrated into a meaningful whole for the provision of quality nursing care. Chapter 1 focused on feelings and beliefs about cancer. Chapters 2, 3, and 4 were primarily concerned with the factual knowledge of cancer. This chapter will explore the third component, ethics.

VALUES

One of the key concepts in the area of ethics is that of moral value. A moral value is a belief about what ought to be.[13] Intertwined in our thinking about the meaning of value are words such as worth, desirability, excellence, usefulness, importance, significance, and ideals. Many of the values that we hold were first instilled in us in early childhood.[41] Both the acculturational process and the educational process involve the taking on of values. Taking on a moral value involves acting consistently in accordance with that value. The taking on of moral values is part of becoming a rational human being.[41] Unfortunately, for many people the taking on and "owning" of values never became a conscious process. Many people are unaware of the values they hold. Thus it is possible for their decisions and behavior to be based on unrecognized values.

For the taking on of moral values to become a conscious process, it is first necessary to recognize the need for a value, identify alternative values, and choose the preferred value. The person may first wish to consider the consequences of selecting each alternative value.

Identifying Values. Thoughts or statements that include words such as should, ought, good, bad, better, best, right, or wrong are value-laden. If any of these words is involved, a value is probably hidden somewhere in the thinking about that subject.

People may hold many different positions regarding a specific value. For example, they may believe that: (1) nurses should spend their time taking care of patients who are going to live; (2) nurses should spend time allowing dying patients to express their feelings about dying; (3) it is better to first provide nursing care to patients who are going to live and then to care for the cancer patients; (4) people have a right to health care; (5) patients should be told their diagnosis.

Many decisions require only the consideration of facts; they are called "clinical judgments"[9] since they are based to some degree on professional knowledge. In these cases, a decision-making process can be used that is effective in providing a consistent guide for weighing the factors in factual decisions. However, if the decision involves values, an ethical decision-making process is required. Many decisions require consideration of a combination of facts and values. Using only facts and disregarding values can never provide a final answer in these types of decisions.[9]

What Is the Difference Between Facts and Values? A fact tells us what is. A fact involves that which is considered true or real or known to exist. It becomes known by experience, observation, or research. Facts could be considered the body of knowledge that makes up a professional discipline. For example, if a patient with impaired mobility is left lying in one position for a long period of time, decubiti will probably develop. There are no differing opinions about this; it is a fact. The fact itself is not considered good or bad; it is considered true or false.

A moral value expresses a view of the world as the individual would like it to be. Values give us goals to work toward. They direct our behavior. Several alternative values can exist in a particular situation. Values cannot be true or false, they can be considered good or bad, or right or wrong.

Facts and Values in Science. For the last 100 years, science has been considered a completely factual area. In order to be scientific, a person had to put all values aside. Decisions were made based only on what were termed "the facts." Research was expected to be designed in such a way that biases or values were avoided. Medicine, as a science, reflected this orientation. Education, in both medicine and nursing, was supposedly based only on facts. Everything had to be rational and objective, rather than emotional and subjective. To be "value-neutral" or "value-free" was good; to be "value-laden" was bad.[42]

In more recent years, it has become apparent that although some provinces of science are indeed value-free, there are some basic scientific concepts that are value-laden. Anatomy is value-free, whereas clinical medicine is value-laden.[42]

As medical science has progressed, the consequences of medical decisions have become more apparent to the general public. A new field called bioethics has developed. Human subjects review committees and institutional review boards have appeared

on the scene. The ethical implications of who should receive renal dialysis and when a person should be considered dead have been debated publicly. A new focus on health has stirred further discussion about ethics.

Values in Nursing Education. Many of the values that are related to nursing are acquired during basic nursing education. Unfortunately, these values are seldom identified as such in the curriculum and discussed openly in the classroom. They are taught from what might be called a hidden curriculum. For example, nursing students hear the faculty evaluate nursing practice and discuss "good" nursing care. Examples of "bad" nursing care may be pointed out in the clinical area. But the values on which the labels "good" and "bad" are based are rarely identified or explored.

MAKING ETHICAL DECISIONS

The totality of a person's moral values is called a value system. If a person has consciously selected specific values and uses them consistently, he or she is said to have an ethical value system. In order to be logically consistent and rational, ethical value systems need to be based on a particular theory.

Ethical Theories

There are three basic theories of ethical reasoning that have relevance to health care situations: utilitarianism, formalism, and justice. Each of these provides a systematic way of making ethical decisions.

Utilitarianism. Utilitarianism holds that moral decisions must always be based on the greatest good for the greatest number of people or the greatest amount of pleasure over pain. This way of measuring right and wrong considers only the consequences of the action. The principal theorist of utilitarianism was John Stuart Mill,[28] a nineteenth century philosopher and economist. A question commonly asked is what would happen if everyone did that. This theory is the primary one to which hospitals hold and to which (as Murphy[4] believes) most nurses have been socialized by the hospital bureaucracy.

Utilitarianism has two main divisions: act-utilitarianism and rule-utilitarianism. Act-utilitarians hold the position that the greatest good for the greatest number must be the only consideration in ethical decisions. Rule-utilitarians take the position that there are recognized rules that are generally used to make ethical decisions. These rules were established in the belief that following the rules will always lead to the greatest good for the greatest number.[18]

Formalism. Formalist theories posit that ethical decisions must be based on general rules that have been established by society (or previous ethical theorists). These rules should be followed regardless of the consequences to oneself or others. If you take the position of "letting your conscience be your guide," this is probably your standard of ethics. The principal theorist was the eighteenth-century philosopher Immanuel Kant.[24] Kant identified absolute duties such as virtue, truth, and promise-keeping.

More recently, Ross has identified a priori rules or obligations or duties.[37] These are:

1. The obligation to keep promises.
2. The obligation to make restitution for harm done.
3. The obligation of "gratitude" to return benefits.
4. The obligation to distribute rewards and punishments in accordance with merit.
5. The obligation to do good to others.
6. The obligation to improve ourselves in respect of virtue and intelligence.
7. The obligation to abstain from injuring others.

Some other theorists in this area define absolute duties such as virtue, truth, and justice.

Justice. Another ethical position regards justice as fairness. The main proponent of this position is John Rawls.[34] Rawls believes that the least advantaged should share equally with others in the benefits of society. Ethical decisions and policies must be based on the benefit received by the least advantaged. Ethical principles must apply to everyone, not just to a few select people. The principles must be publicly recognized and have priority over the demands of law and custom.

Ethical Dilemmas

An ethical dilemma occurs when a person is faced with a conflict between two values in a situation in which the individual has the power to make a decision between courses of action. The values may be related to the action itself or the consequences of that action.[9] Ethical theories do not establish priorities of values. Therefore, when two values conflict, the individual must make a choice between them. For example, a nurse may believe that patients who are dying should be allowed to express their feelings about dying. The same nurse may believe that it is bad to allow a patient with impaired mobility to develop a decubitus.

This nurse would experience an ethical dilemma in the following situation: The unit is very busy. Nurse J has a heavy assignment including Patient A, who is dying, and Patient B, who has impaired mobility. Other nurses on the unit do not have time to help Nurse J. Nurse J enters the room of Patient A, who has hitherto been unwilling to talk about feelings. Patient A begins, with some fear and hesitation, to express those feelings. Nurse J is aware that it is past time to turn Patient B. Patient B already has reddened areas that appear close to skin breakdown. Nurse J is also aware that if an explanation is given to Patient A along with reassurance that Nurse J will return, Patient A will likely interpret that as rejection because of previous avoidance by nurses and will probably make no further attempts to express feelings.

If skin breakdown occurs in Patient B, Nurse J will be reprimanded. If Patient A does not express feelings and withdraws, Nurse J will not be held responsible. Both facts and values are involved in this situation. The facts are that: (1) remaining in one position for long periods causes decubiti; (2) further skin damage will occur if Patient B is not turned; (3) poor emotional coping with dying will speed up the physical deterioration of Patient A.

How would Nurse J decide what to do? How would Nurse J place differing weights on each factor? Nurses often act intuitively, relying on the feelings of the moment without evaluating what they are feeling or understanding of the implications of their actions. Sometimes nurses avoid making decisions or leave decisions to someone else. However, not making a decision *is* a decision. Leaving it to someone else is a decision to relinquish power to others. Nurse J has no one to leave the decision to, and if a decision is made on the basis of the facts alone, it will not be sufficient.

Who Should Make Ethical Decisions?

As a result of the team approach to health care, all health care givers are now involved in the process of making ethical decisions. At the present time, no one member of the health care team is more knowledgeable or competent in ethical decision-making than another. Conflicts, as a result of differing ethical stands, are becoming more common in health care today. The nurse and the patient are both more assertive and autonomous in their roles and each may claim the right to take an ethical stand on an issue and act according to it.

RIGHTS AND DUTIES

In recent years, rights in relation to health care have become a major issue. This is an area in which nurses need to exercise ethical decision-making. The increased awareness of rights seems to be very much linked with changes within our society.[12] Defining a right is difficult. Bandman and Bandman[5] define rights as justifications for action. They have identified three kinds of rights — option rights, welfare rights, and legislative rights.[5]

Option rights, which are associated with personal freedom, define our areas of autonomy. We can exercise an option right without interference from others. We can also choose not to exercise this right; for example, we have a right to overeat, or we can choose not to overeat.

Welfare rights are associated with well-being. They involve public provision of food, clothing, shelter, education, and health care to those in need. The existence of one person's welfare rights implies that other people have a duty to ensure that those rights are fulfilled. If duties are imposed on people, this limits their option rights and thus their freedom. One person's right can limit another person's right. For example, if a person has a right to health care, the medical profession has a duty to provide that care. This limits the freedom of those in the medical profession, prohibiting them from providing medical care only to patients whom they select.

Legislative rights are associated with justice. Some believe that without justice there are no rights. Legislative rights result from the development of rules or laws determining the extent and limits of welfare rights and option rights. If by law a patient has a right to informed consent, the freedom of the health care giver to withhold information from the patient is limited. The health care giver has a duty to inform the patient.

QUALITY OF LIFE

Quality of life is frequently talked and written about in nursing today. It is something that nurses seem to value greatly. Quality of life is one of those very important concepts that mean something highly significant, and yet its meaning cannot be fully defined. A high quality of life might mean one thing to one person and something very different to another.

In spite of its intangible nature, there are some definitions of quality of life with which most people would agree. Some kinds of life are better than others.[9] A high quality of life may be associated with productivity, high self-esteem, self-actualizing experiences, a high level of health, wholeness, opportunities for creativity, and opportunities to share intimacy and feelings with significant others and family.

Many experiences related to illness and the present methods of health care lower the quality of life. For most people, staying in a hospital means a lower quality of life than being at home. Being in pain decreases the quality of life. The quality of life may become so low that death may be preferable.

Other experiences not as dramatic and yet very significant to the patient are the depersonalization and loss of control that occur with hospitalization and illness. Institutional rules decrease the quality of life, for example, by limiting the patient's contact with significant others. Personal grooming and usual self-care measures that are associated with self-esteem may not be possible for the patient to perform and frequently are not provided by health care personnel. The lack of privacy in a hospital also diminishes the quality of life.

It is not possible in this book to consider all of the dimensions of quality of life; many others could be mentioned. The numerous dimensions give a clearer picture of the value placed on quality of life.

NURSING DECISIONS AND QUALITY OF LIFE

Nurses constantly make decisions in the process of their nursing practice. Most of these decisions are considered to be clinical judgments, but when they are examined more closely, values are almost always involved. Often, more than one value is present. This means that if the values conflict, the nurse is in an ethical dilemma. How do nurses weigh the importance of values in making a nursing decision? Let

us examine a few situations commonly found in cancer nursing.

Pain Relief

Many values are present in a nursing decision related to pain control. The following are some examples: (1) drug addiction is bad; (2) it is better to endure a little pain than to risk drug addiction; (3) people should be able to tolerate minimal amounts of pain without complaining or needing medication; (4) a nurse's time is valuable; (5) patients should not take up a nurse's time by complaining or asking for medication unless they have severe pain; (6) patients should understand that nurses have many responsibilities and should not expect pain medication to be brought to them immediately; (7) it is better to administer routine medications on time than to stop and give pain medications; (8) patients should know when the change of shift occurs and not ask for pain medication at that time; (9) patients should not be critical or complain about their nursing care; (10) patients who complain about inadequate pain relief or nursing care should not get their medication as quickly as those who do not; (11) patients who have cancer should learn to endure some pain; (12) postoperative patients should be given pain medication before cancer patients; (13) patients should be kept free from pain; (14) pain-free patients have a higher quality of life; (15) a high quality of life is good; (16) nurses should give medication for pain as soon as they are asked; (17) nurses should never claim that a patient is not experiencing pain; (18) good nurses find ways to relieve the patients' pain.

If the nurse is to make an ethical decision, as many as possible of the values influencing the decision must be identified. These values are then considered in making the decision. If you use the formalist approach to reasoning, the values will need to be categorized as rules, duties, or obligations and placed in order of priority. The decision will be based on the rule with the highest priority. If a utilitarian approach is used, the consequences of making a decision based on each value must be considered and the option with the best consequence chosen. Another consideration involves whether the values used to make the decision should be those of the nurse, the patient, the physician, the institution, the family, or others. Sometimes these values will conflict.

Consider this sample case and test your use of ethical decision-making. Mrs. W is 35 years old, married, and has three elementary school age children. Her husband is a public school teacher. Mrs. W has been previously diagnosed as having Hodgkin's disease, stage 4B, and is receiving chemotherapy. Recently it was discovered that she also has primary ovarian cancer. Mrs. W complains constantly about the low quality of nursing care. She also complains constantly of pain. She has a doctor's order for Demerol 100 mg and Phenergan 25 mg every 2 hours as needed. Her physician told her to let him know if she does not get medication when she asks for it. He frequently criticizes the nurses for not giving Mrs. W the pain medication.

Mrs. W keeps a record of medications she receives, noting in a little black notebook at what time the drug was given, what nurse administered it, and what the nurse said to her. She and her husband have twice sent written complaints to the hospital administrator. She keeps an alarm clock in her room and sets it so that it awakens her when medication is due, particularly at night when she is likely to sleep past the time.

The nurses do not feel that Mrs. W should receive the medication if she does not appear to be in pain. They are very angry about the use of the alarm clock at night, since they believe that if she is asleep, she is not in pain and should not receive medication. Mrs. W says that if she does not receive it, she awakens in severe pain later and cannot sleep the rest of the night.

Nurses are taking turns being assigned to care for Mrs. W. Most of the nurses intentionally spend as much time as possible at the end of the hall away from her room, so that they will not have to answer her light. They delay taking pain medication to her as long as possible after she requests it, using any excuse to postpone the trip to her room. It is their custom to automatically delegate Mrs. W to float nurses who are assigned to the floor. You are a float nurse assigned to their floor, and you are in charge of Mrs. W. The nurses tell you their story about her and ask you to follow their pattern of care.

What facts and values are involved in this situation? What is the ethical dilemma? Some facts that could be identified are: (1) Mrs. W is experiencing pain; (2) Mrs. W will eventually die of her illness; (3) Mrs. W is angry; (4) narcotics given over long periods cause addiction. Values involved could include: (1) patients should or should not endure a moderate amount of pain; (2) pain is good or pain is bad; (3) pain interferes with quality of life; (4) a high quality of life is good; (5) narcotic addiction is always bad; (6) heavy narcotic use lowers the quality of life.

There are several ethical dilemmas that can be identified in this situation. The dilemma that will be discussed is the conflict between the experiencing of pain and the administration of narcotics.

The nurses on the unit do not believe that Mrs. W has as much pain as she complains of. There are values inherent in this belief: (1) nurses cannot believe what patients say about their pain; (2) nurses are better judges of patients' pain than are patients; (3) tolerating pain is good; (4) suffering builds character; (5) nurses are the best people to decide what is good for patients; (6) patients should be submissive to what nurses decide is best for them. They may also believe that narcotic addiction is always bad and that overuse of narcotics lowers the quality of life.

Suppose the float nurse believes that Mrs. W experiences the amount of pain she claims to have. Perhaps the nurse believes that experiencing pain is bad and lowers the quality of life. This nurse probably has some other values that conflict with those of the nurses on the unit, such as: (1) patients give accurate information to nurses; (2) patients should be allowed to control their situation; (3) suffering lowers the quality of life and is bad; (4) patients are the best judges of what is good for them; (5) the patient and the nurse should plan together the care the patient will receive; (6) addiction in dying patients is not bad; (7) use of narcotics to relieve or prevent the development of pain is good; (8) pain should not be allowed to occur in the dying patient.

Mrs. W apparently believes that: (1) pain is bad and lowers the quality of life; (2) addiction is not bad in dying patients; (3) patients should demand things they need; (4) patients should control what happens to them in a hospital situation. Mrs. W's physician apparently also agrees with this position.

Who is right? Who should make the decision? There is no one correct answer. The answer depends on the ethical stand that you take.

Basic Patient Care

Basic care for the cancer patient is also heavily influenced by values. Some of the values you may find associated with basic patient care are as follows: (1) cancer patients are no longer useful to society and should be given a minimum amount of the nurse's valuable time; (2) cancer patients are responsible for their own illnesses and should not be pampered; (3) patients who will live should be cared for before cancer patients; (4) cancer patients will be in and out of the hospital over a long period of time and should learn to conform to the ward routine; (5) since cancer patients are familiar with the ward routine, they should understand and be more tolerant of delays in care than other patients; (6) cancer patients should be given extra attention since cancer is such a terrible disease; (7) basic patient care is very important to enhance the quality of life; (8) increasing the quality of life is important for the cancer patient.

Consider a sample case in basic patient care. Mrs. A is a 45-year-old widow and has one married son. Mrs. A has advanced ovarian cancer and weighs about 60 pounds. Because of severe intractable pain, a subcutaneous cordotomy was performed, which left Mrs. A partially paralyzed below the waist. She has developed severe decubiti. To treat the decubiti, Mrs. A was placed on a Circoelectric bed, which she hates. She is unable to lie in comfortable positions, and the narrowness of the bed disturbs her.

At 7 PM her physician writes an order for her to be transferred to a regular hospital bed, which has an alternating pressure mattress. Mrs. A is very excited about this. You are a young staff nurse who has been assigned to care for Mrs. A. Mrs. A talks of nothing else but looking forward to sleeping on a "real" bed that night.

When you go out to the nurses' station, the evening charge nurse has read the order and angrily tells you that if the physician wants something like that done, the physician should write the orders earlier in the day. The physician is disliked by the nursing staff. The nurse states that staff is not available to make the transfer and that it will have to wait until the following morning. You explain Mrs. A's excitement about the change. The charge nurse states that since Mrs. A has waited this long, she can wait one more day. You again attempt to explain the importance of the transfer for Mrs. A. Finally, the charge nurse impatiently says, "If you want it done, do it yourself. I will not help you." Your evaluation of the situation is that the charge nurse resents the physician frequently making rounds so late. There is an orderly on the unit who can assist you in the transfer. If you make the transfer, you risk incurring the wrath of the charge nurse, which later could have some unpleasant consequences for you.

What is the decision to be made? What facts and values are involved? The decision is whether or not to transfer Mrs. A from the Circoelectric bed. The ethical decision involves the importance of both promise-keeping and the quality of life. The facts involved in this decision include: (1) the nursing unit is short-handed; (2) the physician wrote the order late in the day; (3)

Mrs. A expects to be transferred; (4) Mrs. A's physician promised her that she would be transferred.

The values of the charge nurse are that: (1) the physician should write orders earlier in the day; (2) Mrs. A's satisfaction is not as important as ensuring care for the rest of the patients on the unit; (3) Mrs. A should be willing to wait one more day to be transferred; (4) getting all the work done is more important than meeting the needs of one patient.

The staff nurse could have the following values: (1) nurses should put the patient's needs before their own; (2) promises should be kept; (3) nurses should place a high value on quality of life; (4) nurses should care about their patients; (5) the patient's needs are more important than showing the doctor who is in control.

Again, there is no correct decision. Your ethical stand will determine this.

In conclusion, values and ethical dilemmas are important factors in nursing care. These will be discussed in relation to specific topics throughout the remainder of the book. The present chapter provides the orientation needed for later discussions.

BIBLIOGRAPHY

1. Alfidi, R. J.: Informed consent, a study of patient reaction. *Journal of the American Medical Association.* 216:1325–1329, 1971.
2. Annas, G. J.: The patient has rights: how can we protect them. *Hastings Center Reports.* Sept. 1973, pp. 8–9.
3. Aroskar, M. A.: Anatomy of an ethical dilemma: the theory. *American Journal of Nursing.* 80:658–660, 1980.
4. Bandman, E. L., and B. Bandman: *Bioethics and Human Rights.* Little, Brown & Co., Boston, 1978.
5. Bandman, E. L., and B. Bandman: The nurse's role in protecting the patient's right to live or die. *Advances in Nursing Science.* 1:21–36, 1979.
6. Barbus, A. J.: The dying person's bill of rights. *American Journal of Nursing.* 75:99, 1975.
7. Baumrind, D.: Principles of ethical conduct in the treatment of subjects. *American Psychologist.* 26:887–896, 1971.
8. Beauchamp, T. L.: The foundations of ethics and the foundations of science. In *Knowing and Valuing: The Search for Common Roots*, ed. by H. T. Engelhardt, Jr. and D. Callahan. The Hastings Center, New York, 1980.
9. Brody, H.: *Ethical Decisions in Medicine.* Little, Brown & Co., Boston, 1976.
10. Carper, B.: The ethics of caring. *Advances in Nursing Science.* 1:11–20, 1979.
11. Cassell, E.: Response to H. Tristran Englehardt, Jr. In *Knowing and Valuing: The Search for Common Roots*, ed. by H. T. Engelhardt, Jr. and D. Callahan. The Hastings Center, New York, 1980.
12. Davis, A. J., and M. A. Aroskar: *Ethical Dilemmas and Nursing Practice.* Appleton-Century-Crofts, New York, 1978.
13. Engelhardt, H. T. Jr.: Knowing and valuing: looking for common roots. In *Knowing and Valuing: The Search for Common Roots*, ed. by H. T. Engelhardt, Jr. and D. Callahan. The Hastings Center, New York, 1980.
14. Engelhardt, H. T. Jr.: Doctoring the disease, treating the complaint, helping the patient: some of the works of Hygeia and Panacea. In *Knowing and Valuing: The Search for Common Roots,* ed. by H. T. Engelhardt, Jr. and D. Callahan. The Hastings Center, New York, 1980.
15. Ewing, A. C.: *Ethics.* The Free Press, New York, 1953.
16. Flaherty, M. J.: The nurse and orders not to resuscitate. *Hastings Center Reports.* Aug. 1977, pp. 27–28.
17. Fletcher, J.: Ethics and euthanasia. *American Journal of Nursing.* 73:670, 672, 1973.
18. Frankena, W. K.: *Ethics.* Prentice-Hall, Inc., Englewood Cliffs, N.J., 1973.
19. Fried, C.: Rights and health care — beyond equity and efficiency. *New England Journal of Medicine.* 293:241–245, 1975.
20. Gorovitz, S., et al.: *Moral Problems in Medicine.* Prentice-Hall, Inc., Englewood Cliffs, N.J., 1976.
21. Griffin, J. J.: Family decision, a crucial factor in terminating life. *American Journal of Nursing.* 75:794–796, 1975.
22. Hollander, R.: Patient's rights still not established. *Hasting Center Reports.* Aug. 1976, pp. 10–11.
23. Hunt, R., and J. Arras: *Ethical Issues in Modern Medicine.* Mayfield Publishing Co., Palo Alto, 1977.
24. Kant, I.: From *Fundamental Principles of the Metaphysics of Morals.* In *Moral Problems in Medicine,* ed. by S. Gorovitch, et al. Prentice-Hall, Inc., Englewood Cliffs, N.J., 1976.
25. Kelly, L. Y.: The patient's right to know. *Nursing Outlook.* 24:27–32, 1976.
26. Macklin, R.: Moral concerns and appeals to rights and duties. *Hastings Center Reports.* Oct. 1976, pp. 31–38.
27. Milgram, S.: Some conditions of obedience and disobedience to authority. *Human Relations.* 18:57–76, 1965.
28. Mill, J. S.: From *Utilitarianism.* In *Ethics in Medicine: Historical Perspectives and Contemporary Concerns,* ed. by S. J. Reiser, A. J. Dyck, and W. J. Curran. The MIT Press, Cambridge, Mass., 1977.
29. Moser, D., and J. M. Cox: Perspectives: resolving an ethical dilemma. *Nursing 80.* 10:39–43, 1980.
30. Outka, G.: Social justice and equal access to health care. *Journal of Religious Ethics.* 2:11–32, 1974.

31. Pepper, S. C.: Values and value judgments. *Journal of Philosophy*. 46:429–434, 1959.
32. Ramsey, P.: *The Patient as Person*. Yale University Press, New Haven, 1970.
33. Ramsey, P.: *Ethics at the Edge of Life*. Yale University Press, New Haven, 1978.
34. Rawls, J.: Justice as fairness. In *Ethics in Medicine: Historical Perspectives and Contemporary Concerns*, ed. by S. J. Reiser, A. J. Dyck, and W. J. Curran. The MIT Press, Cambridge, Mass., 1977.
35. Reich, W.: The physician's 'duty' to preserve life. *Hastings Center Reports*. April 1975, pp. 14–15.
36. Reiser, S. J., A. J. Dyck, and W. J. Curran: *Ethics in Medicine: Historical Perspectives and Contemporary Concerns*. The MIT Press, Cambridge, Mass., 1977.
37. Ross, W. D.: From "What makes right acts right?" In *Ethics in Medicine: Historical Perspectives and Contemporary Concerns*, ed. by S. J. Reiser, A. J. Dyck, and W. J. Curran. The MIT Press, Cambridge, Mass., 1977.
38. Schorr, T. M.: The right to die. *American Journal of Nursing*. 76:53, 1976.
39. Sigman, P.: Ethical choice in nursing. *Advances in Nursing Science*. 1:37–52, 1979.
40. Simons, S. M.: The obligation to live vs. the option to die. *Southern Medical Journal*. 65:731, 757, 1972.
41. Stent, G. S.: Science and morality as paradoxical aspects of reason. In *Knowing and Valuing: The Search for Common Roots*, ed. by H. T. Engelhardt, Jr. and D. Callahan. The Hastings Center, New York, 1980.
42. Toulmin, S.: How can we reconnect the sciences with the foundations of ethics. In *Knowing and Valuing: The Search for Common Roots*, ed. by H. T. Engelhardt, Jr. and D. Callahan. The Hastings Center, New York, 1980.
43. Van den Berg, J. H.: *Medical Power and Medical Ethics*. W. W. Norton and Company, Inc., New York, 1978.
44. Veatch, R. M.: *Case Studies in Medical Ethics*. Harvard University Press, Cambridge, 1977.

II

The Medical Management of Cancer and the Nurse's Role

6

Hospital Nursing Care for the Cancer Patient: What It Is and What It Can Be

INTRODUCTION

Nursing care for the cancer patient is in a state of rapid change, which makes generalizations about it difficult, if not impossible. In some settings, patient care is still primarily guided by the conservative philosophy described in Chapter 1. In others, the nurse is seen as a technician, providing highly complex physical care, but with little time or encouragement to intervene at the psychosocial level. Some institutions consider psychosocial care to be the responsibility of the physician or social worker, and the nurse may be instructed to stay out of this arena of patient care. More progressive settings seek and facilitate the practice of using skilled oncology nurses to provide high quality comprehensive care to cancer patients and their families. In large institutions, oncology nurses may function as members of a multidisciplinary team in the provision of cancer care.

Cancer care occurs in a variety of settings, from the small rural hospital to the large urban research center. The temptation is to assume that the poorest care occurs in the small general hospital and the best care in the large research center. Whereas this may sometimes be the case, it is not always true.

Although the provision of high quality nursing care is certainly separate and distinct from the provision of high quality medical care, the two are complementary. Both must be present in order for comprehensive cancer care to occur. The provision of this care is a highly complex process requiring its practitioners to have a strong knowledge base within a holistic, humanistic framework.

There is an increasing trend toward the development of oncology units and outpatient clinics for cancer patients. In many instances, this occurs as a move from conservative care philosophy, and the attitudes of the institution do not necessarily change with the same speed as the change in clinical facilities. The oncology unit may exist, but inadequate staffing, unqualified nurses, lack of a support system, and restraints on nursing practice severely limit its effective functioning.

Oncology nursing is developing into a specialized area of nursing practice. The specialty has emerged so rapidly that nurses prepared to function in this area are scarce. Continuing education courses and formal course work in oncology nursing are available, but are not yet sufficient in number. The Oncology Nurses Society has grown rapidly in the past few years. Two professional nursing journals, *Cancer Nursing* and *Oncology Nursing Forum*, have developed to meet the growing need for information about this area.

Even though cancer care is changing, many problems exist in current hospital care. Oncology units and nurses prepared to practice oncology nursing are the exception, not the rule. The majority of cancer patients are cared for in general hospitals, not in specialized settings. And in some of these hospitals, the cancer patient receives poorer quality care than other patients. This is not planned; in most cases it is not even recognized. But it has a definite impact on the quality of life of the cancer patients and their families.

PROBLEMS IN CURRENT CARE

Feelings About Cancer Nursing

Providing nursing care for the cancer patient, particularly the advanced cancer patient, has never been a popular field of practice in nursing. The work is demanding, complicated, and sometimes unpleasant. Nurses, as well as other health professionals, may hold strongly negative beliefs about cancer. Also, there has not been the element of excitement, challenge, and drama that is often present in other areas of nursing practice. The merging of these factors has generally made cancer nursing an undesirable field of practice.

Staffing Problems

Medical units are frequently considered a low priority in planning the staffing for a hospital. If a staffing shortage exists, the medical units will usually be the ones that are shortchanged first. This is particularly true of medical units that have large numbers of cancer patients.

Since many nurses do not like cancer nursing, it is difficult to find nurses interested in working on these units. Nursing administration personnel may reward "good" nurses by assigning them to a more desirable area of the hospital. Conversely, nurses may be punished by being assigned to the cancer unit. Therefore, the nurses working on a medical unit that consists primarily of cancer patients will often be overworked and have a low self-esteem and a low group morale. Although some nurses working on these units will be highly motivated, productive, and interested in cancer nursing, others (more than on other nursing units) will have low motivation and work problems of some sort. Nurses in the latter group may have been assigned to the unit because of their problems. Others

may develop problems as a reaction to understaffing, low morale, frustration, or other experiences. Turnover rates on these units are high; management problems are great; and quality of care is usually poor.

Poor Quality Care

Cancer patients, particularly those who are hospitalized with advanced disease, often receive poorer quality care than other patients. This is not simply a result of inadequate staffing, because poor care may occur even when staffing is adequate. Insufficient care may stem from the beliefs, philosophy, and values discussed in Chapters 1 and 5.

Cancer patients are hospitalized more frequently, and often for longer periods of time, than other patients. Nurses often expect them to adjust to the hospital routine and not complain. They are expected to "understand" delays, short-staffing, and other inconveniences. Family members who complain about the quality of care are dismissed as overreacting to the patients' illness. Therefore, complaints to the physician, nursing administration, and the hospital administrator are often to no avail.

Vachon and colleagues' study of widows of cancer patients indicated that they had many more complaints about the nursing care that their spouses received than did widows of cardiovascular patients.[51] The memory of poor quality care seemed to have an impact on the widows' ability to move through the grieving process.

The widows of men who die of cancer are highly likely to express anger towards the medical care system. While the causes of this anger frequently lie within the woman as a projection of her guilt or a lashing out against the pain of her bereavement, the anger is often appropriate. Despite the best of intentions members of the health care team are often less sensitive and accessible than they should be. There are many reasons for this, including insufficient staff, inadequate training in the areas of coping with death and bereavement, and often our own need to deny death in ourselves and our patients, which may lead us to avoid contact with dying patients.

The three major areas our group of widows

singled out for complaint were: (a) quality of nursing care, (b) accessibility of physicians and (c) accuracy of information.

Nurses were often accused of neglecting cancer patients and giving them poor care. In some instances the women believed that such poor care hastened death. . . . The hospital system in general was resented even more bitterly. . . .

When we are told by so many widows that the stress of living with cancer as a terminal illness is far worse than the stress of widowhood, it behooves us to question how much we and our hospital system contribute to unnecessary suffering of these women and their families and to determine what we can do to alleviate such suffering.[51]*

Family members who are concerned about the quality of care being given are much more reluctant to leave the cancer patient alone. They spend long hours with the patient, sometimes attempting to give care themselves. This has a direct impact on the physical and mental health of the family members. Of course, allowing the family to assist in care is sometimes a very helpful thing, but it should not occur because the family members fear that their loved one will not receive adequate care if they do not help to provide it.

Personal Care

The fine art of nursing is often not applied to cancer patients. This can be seen in terms of the finishing touches to personal care that have a limited direct effect on matters of life and death, but a great impact on the quality of life.

The problems related to personal care are more apparent in the care given to advanced cancer patients. They may be among the last to receive their bath each morning. This may very well be because their bath requires more nursing time than other patients'. It may seem better to get all of the other patients' baths done earlier and thus make fewer patients unhappy. Cancer patients, however, are often hospitalized for long periods of time. It is difficult to look forward, for the rest of one's life, to half a day of disorder and discomfort. Mouth care is seldom adequate. Hair

is often left uncombed. Body positioning is disregarded or done in a sloppy, haphazard manner. (Frequently, the hospital does not provide adequate numbers of pillows to allow for proper positioning.)

Arrangement of the room for tidiness and placement of personal belongings within easy access of the patient are important parts of personal care. Providing fresh ice water, clean sheets, and a nurse call cord within easy reach are such simple measures that they are often overlooked in the flurry of "important" activities, but these touches are very meaningful to both the patients and their families.

The types of activities just described have been relegated to the "nice but not necessary" category in many institutions. They are done when time permits, but time has been permitted for these activities less and less often in recent years. In order to deal with the frustration of not having the time to do them, we have simply devalued them. Thus, even when time is available, these activities are still not done. Our memories of the satisfaction of a clean, fresh-smelling patient in a tidy room have somehow faded to the dim and distant past when things were more simple. Is it possible, given the scientific and technologic complexities of today's nursing practice, to merge these two worlds and achieve a depth of holistic, humanistic cancer care never before possible?

Food trays are often left in cancer patients' rooms long after mealtime. The reason why this occurs is not clear. It may be an avoidance behavior, or the nursing personnel may think that the longer the tray is left in the room, the more the patient will eat. Whatever the reason, it is often interpreted by the patients and their families as neglect and rejection.

Inadequate attention is paid to how much or what the patient eats. Too often patients' eating patterns and food preferences are disregarded in favor of hospital routine. Feeding patients who cannot feed themselves is usually done hurriedly. Somehow the nurturing that should accompany nourishment has been lost in the hustle and bustle of the modern nursing unit.

---

*Originally published in *Canadian Medical Association Journal* Vol. 117, November 19, 1977.

The constipation and diarrhea that are consistent problems of advanced cancer patients are not monitored as closely or dealt with as quickly as they should be, leaving the patient to experience unnecessary discomfort. If bowel movements were carefully recorded, which they would be if they were considered important, treatment measures could be used more quickly, improving the patient's appetite and general sense of well-being and lessening the possibility of serious complications.

Medication for the relief of pain and other symptoms is often delayed. The severity of symptoms — particularly pain — is often minimized by nursing personnel. Postoperative patients are medicated much more quickly than cancer patients. Patients and families frequently evaluate the quality of care given primarily in terms of the effectiveness of pain control. Certainly it is impossible to provide good pain control without sufficient orders from the physician; however, even when medical orders are adequate, nurses may not provide satisfactory pain control.

Rehabilitative measures designed to maximize the cancer patient's potential are often not utilized. Many nurses get caught up in the hopelessness associated with cancer. This leads to the feeling that nothing nurses do will make any difference anyway; all efforts seem futile. What the nurses see is continuous physical decline in spite of what they do. So why put all that time and effort into rehabilitative activities? Is it worthwhile to invest time and effort to help patients to function nearer their potential, even though — in spite of all that is done — they will continue to deteriorate physically and will eventually die?

The hopelessness that many nurses feel regarding cancer patients is reflected in their observation of and intervention in these patients' symptoms. All symptoms tend to be blamed on the disease in the assumption that nothing can be done. Nurses may also feel that minor problems are of little importance when viewed in the light of the overwhelming fact that the patient has advanced cancer.

On the contrary, minor symptoms such as a rash, a runny nose, a sore toe, or a sheet burn on the elbow are of major concern to patients. Care that diminishes or eliminates these problems will seem a minor miracle to them. They do not expect the nurse to cure their cancer. At this point, their concern is comfort.

Advanced cancer patients are at high risk of developing decubiti; and yet in many settings they are not turned and positioned frequently. The turning that is done is not carefully charted, so that there is little coordination between nurses or between shifts in this endeavor.

The careful charting of an activity is a good measure of how important that endeavor is considered. The physician's orders are meticulously charted and carefully monitored by institutional supervisors. Nursing care is often not adequately charted and is monitored less carefully in many settings.

Nursing care on a general medical unit does not usually lend itself to day-to-day communication and cooperation between shifts or even between nurses. The charting does not usually supply adequate information about previous care that has been provided, how it was provided, or the present condition of the patient.

Between-shift reports are usually limited to the medical condition and medical treatments given, not to the nursing care of the patient. There is often little agreement or discussion between nurses as to what care should be provided or how. Nurses consider the time when they are caring for the patient as their own domain. Attempts by other nurses or other shifts to influence or modify that care may be seen as an unacceptable invasion. There is little predictability to the care that is given. The philosophy of care differs according to each nurse.

This leaves the patients and their families in the position of having to "psych out" each nurse who cares for them and then determine how best to manipulate the nurse to get what they need. This is certainly not the most mature way to act, but when the cancer patient is confronted with the unpredictability, helplessness, depersonalization, and loss of control that are usually inherent in hospitalization, this is the most effective alternative left. Certainly, advanced cancer patients are going to need more meticulous attention to their personal care than other cancer patients who are more able to care for themselves. However, because of the psychologic impact of cancer, attention must be paid to the patient's personal care during all stages of cancer, even if it consists only of encouraging and supporting the patient in self-care measures. Decreased motivation for self-care frequently occurs in cancer patients as a result of emotional reactions to the illness and physiologic responses to treatment.

Good personal care is certainly not all there is to nursing practice, but it is the foundation on which all other nursing care must be based. If the personal care is of poor quality, the effectiveness of all other nursing care deteriorates. Professional nurses cannot, in every situation, directly provide all of the personal care; however, this does not diminish their accountability for overseeing and reinforcing this care. Other levels of nursing personnel that the professional nurse supervises may have different sets of beliefs and values influencing their decisions about nursing care in cancer. Their practice may be based on primitive beliefs and intuition rather than knowledge, adequate assessment, and rational decision-making.

Psychosocial Care

Psychosocial care is extremely important in cancer care; however, it is an area for which nurses are seldom held accountable. The evaluation systems in a hospital seldom include these areas for examination except in general happiness data. Happiness data are acquired from evaluation forms that ask very broad questions such as "How would you rate the nursing care you received?" Institutional reward systems rarely acknowledge nurses for providing good psychosocial care. In fact, for the most part, a nurse's superiors — and peers — may be totally unaware of the psychosocial interventions used by him or her. Nurses may have a general reputation for "being good with" patients who are emotionally upset or they may be criticized as "wasting time talking with patients" when they should be "getting their work done." A low value is generally placed on psychosocial interventions.

The beliefs and values associated with cancer have strongly influenced psychosocial interventions. Cancer is closely associated with death. If cancer patients have a type of cancer with a low probability of cure, they will be treated as though they are dying, even though death may be months or years away. This results in avoidance behavior by nurses.[52] The patient may be placed in a room at the end of the hall with the door kept shut, ostensibly to provide quiet for the patient. Nurses may go to the room less frequently. They may hold conversations standing farther away from the bed. There is less touching and less eye contact. Communication is kept at the social and factual levels. Expression of the patient's feelings is not encouraged. The nurse, not the patient, maintains control of topics discussed.[12]

Although the situation is more acute in the patient with metastatic disease, it also occurs at other times in the course of the disease, when effective psychosocial intervention, not avoidance, is called for. There are several periods of crisis possible in the cancer situation. The first occurs when cancer is suspected and diagnostic tests are being conducted. The second occurs when the diagnosis is made and the patient and family are informed. A third crisis occurs when metastasis is discovered. Another crisis is experienced when the patient and family are told that the present treatment is no longer controlling the growth of the cancer and that no further treatments are available to halt the malignant growth.

At each of these crisis times, nurses on general medical-surgical units often fail to provide effective psychosocial intervention. The patient is not avoided totally; in fact, more time may be spent in task-oriented activities with the patient. However, there is a marked change in the level of communication. Patients may first detect that a decision has been made, even before they are told, by changes in the nurses' nonverbal behavior. The amount of conversation may be increased, but kept at the social level. The patient's questions about the illness or treatment will not be answered directly. Feeling-level communication will be avoided.

In between these crises, communication may appear to be more normal. The cancer, and its portent for the future, can be put on the back seat and more attention focused on the tasks at hand. Also, the patient is likely to leave the hospital in between crises, thus seemingly absolving the nurses of any further responsibility for dealing with the situation.

Families are usually kept on the periphery, rather than being included in the patient care situation. The nurses may tend to see them as irritants, troublemakers, or hindrances, or they may simply disregard them. Family members may be discounted in many ways. They will usually be classified as "good" or "problems." "Good" family members do not express their feelings or seek emotional support; they are cheerful and accept the situation; they help with patient care and do not criticize or complain; and they encourage the patient to comply with the nurses' expectations. They are complimentary of nursing care, tolerant of problems caused by short staffing, and do not take up the nurses' time. They follow the rules, do not ask that exceptions be made, and are grateful if a rule is bent for them.

Many nurses have difficulty dealing with shock, anger and depression. Patients or family members experiencing these feelings are classified as "problems" and will be avoided. Nurses may not attempt to intervene therapeutically. Rather, they may react defensively and let the situation mushroom into almost impossible dimensions. Nurses are seldom provided with any outside support to help them cope with the situation. The family and patient often react by accusing nurses of incompetency, questioning the adequacy of the hospital, and making unreasonable demands of the hospital administration.

Nurses seem to like denial. It is so much easier to handle that they may actually promote its maintenance. There are some instances when denial may be a very useful coping strategy, but purposefully blocking the movement of a patient's attitude from denial to acceptance is not healthy.

Not providing effective psychosocial interventions has serious consequences, not only for the patient, but also for the nurse. Personal growth is often a two-way interactive process, with each person learning from the other. There is much that nurses can learn from patients with cancer and their families. If instead, nurses isolate themselves, they will have less to give to the next patient, and they will be moving in the direction of rigidity, entrenchment, security, and defensiveness rather than personal growth.

Fragmentation of Care

Fragmentation is a serious problem throughout the health care system. The cancer situation is no exception and, because of its complexity, the implications of fragmentation are very serious. Medical care, nursing care, and institutional care all are fragmented. Patients may see five or more physicians before the diagnosis of cancer is made. After diagnosis, patients may at various times be seen by oncologists, surgeons, radiotherapists, and family physicians. At times, they may not even know who their present physician is. For example, their family physician may have referred them to a surgeon for diagnosis and surgery. The surgeon has dismissed them and they have an appointment to see the oncologist in 3 weeks. There is great reluctance, at this point, to seek out any of these physicians for help.

Each physician whom patients see may treat them in a different health care institution, sometimes in different cities. It becomes difficult for patients to identify with an institution that operates as a base for their care. All of the people they deal with — social workers, counselors, financial and bookkeeping personnel, physical therapists, nutritionists, and personnel in volunteer agencies — may be affiliated with different institutions or may be functioning independently in the community. There may be little coordination or communication among these individuals.

Nursing care is also fragmented at many levels and stages. Each time patients are admitted, they are sent to a different unit of the hospital. Patients may be on a surgical unit for diagnosis and surgery and in later admissions be sent to various medical units. Upon each admission they will probably encounter nurses who know nothing about them or their illness. The nurse, knowing that the encounter with the patients is limited to the present hospital admission, feels little motivation to learn their social history or to plan long-term nursing interventions. The nurse feels no accountability to the patients beyond their present hospital stay.

Even if patients are readmitted to the same nursing unit, it is unlikely that they will be cared for by the same nurse, since assignments are decided primarily by chance. On the nursing unit, patient assignments are frequently rotated, so that the same nurses will not be continually caring for the same patients. This again diminishes the commitment of an individual nurse to continuity, coordination, or long-term planning. The nurse's focus will be primarily on accomplishing the tasks of the day. Or the nurse may be aware of the patients' problems and the nursing interventions that need to be implemented, but may feel helpless about having an impact on the present situation.

If patients are hospitalized for longer periods of time, they may become better known by the nurses. If they are "good" patients, their care may develop more of a sense of continuity. However, if they are "problem" patients or are labeled terminal by the nurses, arrangements may be made to rotate assignment of the patients' care. In this case, the float nurse will often be assigned to care for them. Thus, patients may see a new nurse each shift and each day.

After patients have been discharged, they often feel cut off from contact with nurses. Patients usually do not feel that they can call the nursing unit they left. The nurse who works with the patients' physician may or may not be accessible and helpful. Patients are reluctant to contact physicians about matters they feel might be considered trivial, even if the matter is important to them. Therefore, they feel very much alone to deal with whatever problems arise. They are in a state of limbo even more in matters requiring nursing care.

PROVIDING QUALITY HOSPITAL CARE FOR THE CANCER PATIENT

Quality nursing care must be defined more broadly than simply the exciting technical skills that burst on the horizon of nursing practice each day. Certainly these are important in assisting the physician to provide current comprehensive medical care. But nursing care is much more than this. Nursing deals more with the patients' response to their illness than the treatment of the illness itself. This response is so important that it can influence the quality of life and can alter the course of the illness.

There are general goals that must be attained if high quality care is to be provided. A positive philosophy of cancer care must be adopted by all health care providers. The health care system must be organized in such a way that a high level of personal and psychosocial nursing care can and will be given. The situation must be one that supports the provision of a high level of medical care. The professional nursing staff must have an adequate background in oncology nursing. The nursing staff must be free to practice nursing at a professional level. A support system must be provided for the nursing staff. Use of continuing education courses to increase knowledge of the practice of oncology nursing must be encouraged. Continuity of care for both patient and family must be a major goal.

Developing an Oncology Unit

One of the most logical ways to accomplish these goals is by an oncology nursing unit. The existence of this unit will not alone ensure that these goals will automatically be achieved. Changes in the institution's system of providing care and perhaps a change in philosophy will usually be necessary. Neither of these changes is easy to accomplish.

The level of care on an oncology unit is between that of a general medical-surgical unit and that of an intensive care unit. Length of time required for care and complexity of care are both greater than on general care units. Therefore, staffing patterns and salary levels may need to be adjusted.

On oncology units, the nurses are exposed to a high incidence of stress. They may experience the death of patients with whom they have developed long-term close relationships. This requires nurses with a high level of commitment and maturity, who have to some extent dealt with their own feelings about death. It certainly is no place for nurses with serious personal problems or those trying to work through their own grief. A person with work problems or relationship problems will not survive long on an oncology unit. Therefore, prospective nursing staff must be carefully screened.

If these measures and goals are adopted, the oncology unit will have a greater opportunity to operate effectively, with a highly motivated, highly cohesive group providing quality care. If these measures are not taken, there are serious risks in establishing an oncology unit. Nurse turnover will be rapid; recruitment of new staff will be difficult; internal conflicts among staff will be frequent; physicians will be unhappy with the situation; and patient satisfaction will be low.

Establishing a Philosophy of Care. In establishing a philosophy of care, it may be helpful to first determine the philosophy presently functioning in the institution. There may be a variety of philosophies in operation among various groups. Determine which ones have the greatest influence on decision-making. The written philosophy of the institution may not be the one utilized in actual practice. Look for the values and meanings given to human beings in general, patients, health, nurses, and nursing care. All of these values will influence the decisions made about the nursing care being provided.

Identify concepts or theories that might be helpful to you in establishing a framework from which an approach to nursing care can be developed. Some that might be helpful are humanism, holism, adaptation, self-care, and role theory.

Begin to establish some values that you will be using in making decisions about nursing care. Answering the following questions may be helpful in clarifying your values.

Human Beings in General — Should a person be used as a means to an end? Do people have worth only if they are contributing to society? What is the value of a day of life? Is the value of life a function of the quality of life? Are people rational, logical beings or are they irrational? Do people have some control over what happens in life or are they helpless victims of fate?

Patients — When does a person become a patient? Does a patient have the same worth as a human being? When does a patient cease to be a patient? Should patients have any control over their care? Should patients passively receive nursing care or should they be active participants?

Health — What is health? Is it possible for a person to have a high level of health during a serious illness? Can a dying person have a high level of health? Can people work to achieve higher levels of health or should they learn to accept (or adapt to) their present level of health? Is health the best possible goal or are other things sometimes more important?

Nurses — How should a nurse relate to a patient? What is the role of a nurse? When is a nurse responsible for providing nursing care? To whom is a nurse accountable for nursing care?

Nursing Care — What is the goal of nursing care? What constitutes nursing care? Is it a part of medical care, or is it different? Who should make decisions about nursing care — the nurse or the patient?

Developing Goals for Care. Many times goals are viewed as something taught in nursing school that have to be written on nursing care plans for teachers, but can be forgotten after graduation. It really is difficult to get somewhere, however, if you do not know where you are going. For much of nursing practice, the overriding goal is for the patient to get well and/or go home from the hospital in relatively good condition. This goal is not usually written, but it is the rule by which the effectiveness of nursing care is measured. What, then, is the goal if the patient has metastatic cancer and will gradually deteriorate physically and eventually die, perhaps not during this hospitalization, but in the foreseeable future? If the goal remains the same, nurses will consider themselves to be failures. One approach is to switch the focus from cure care to comfort care. Comfort is indeed a valuable contribution, but is it sufficient? And what is cure care? Are nurses ever really involved in cure? What is a cure? Can one person ever cure another? If so, one would have to use a strict, simplistic medical model to define illness. Is illness really that simple?[1] When patients are cured of a disease, are they often left with the same problems that caused the disease to develop? Is the nurse concerned with the disease, the illness, or the health deficit? Or are they the same thing?

If health was considered separate from illness and a nursing goal was to promote health, the nurse could aim toward helping patients maximize their health potential. This would include providing social relationship activities and comfort measures with attention given to physical care. It would be very possible to identify more specific, achievable goals. The question thus becomes, who identifies the goals: nurses, with their "superior" knowledge; nurses and patients jointly; or patients?

Designing a Plan of Care. Nursing care plans are required by accrediting bodies, dutifully written on by nurses, and scrupulously ignored in nursing practice. They can be effective tools if their focus is nursing care, not medical care. Nursing practice has become too complex for intuitive nursing to be effective, and without a plan of care, nursing is intuitive; the nurse reacts to the situation rather than acting to influence or alter it.

The nursing care on an oncology unit should be based on a carefully designed and individualized plan. The plan should be more comprehensive than those usually found on general hospital units, because the time period involved will be longer and the care more complex.

A plan of care should be based on a careful and thorough collection of baseline data. This baseline data should include information obtained from the nursing history and physical examination and a social history of the patient and family. The plan should include all nursing activities that require consistent nursing action across shifts and days. The nursing care plan is the design for achieving the goals of care.

Merely writing down activities on the care plan by no means ensures that they will be done. That is only one step. The nursing staff must be committed to a logical, rational, knowledge-based, decision-making, goal-oriented model of nursing care. They must value the continuity of care. They must have similar philosophies of nursing practice. Each nurse must feel very much a part of a team effort.

Cancer patients need to be active participants in their own care and should be equal partners in both planning and implementing the care plan. They should be involved in self-care as much as possible. The family also needs to be involved in the care plan. Leaving a copy of the plan at the patients' bedside is a very effective way of including the patients and their families. This also accomplishes several other things: it tends to make the nurses more directly accountable to the patients and conversely it increases the patients' responsibility for their own care.

Sharing the care plan with the patient is a change in the power situation between the nurse and the patient and is very threatening to some nurses. Withholding information is a very effective way of maintaining power. As long as something seems mysterious, unknown, and unpredictable, the person who knows it has considerable power over the person who does not.

Cancer patients who are active participants in their care survive longer and respond physiologically to their treatment more effectively. Therefore, it is critical that oncology units be designed to facilitate this patient response. The customary nursing care unit facilitates the passive, compliant patient. The oncology nursing unit must develop effective, perhaps novel, ways to encourage active patient involvement.

When the patient is discharged, the nursing care plan should be retained either as a part of the patient's record or in a file kept on the oncology unit. When the patient returns for another hospitalization, this valuable data will then be available. If an outpatient oncology clinic operates in the same institution, the nurses in the clinic can refer to the nursing care plan, thus further promoting continuity of care. Of course, the written form will be more useful if nurses from the two areas have the time and opportunity to discuss patient care.

Providing Personal Care. The importance of personal care has been stressed in a prior section of this chapter. Sometimes on oncology units, the administration of medications and technologic procedures requires almost all of the professional nurses' time. Personal care is given by other personnel. If the unit is to function optimally, personal care must be highly valued and at least closely supervised by professional nurses. Methods must be devised to reward nursing personnel who provide high quality personal care. Charting of care should be sufficiently detailed to supply information to other nurses and to promote continuity of care.

Providing Symptom Control. On an oncology unit, symptoms should be carefully searched for and considered important. A major aim of the unit should be symptom control. Particular attention should be given to control of pain, constipation, and decubiti. Thrombophlebitis and pulmonary embolus are common among cancer patients and should be monitored closely. Nurses should search for infections, which are also common among cancer patients. Medical treatments will cause specific complications that should be closely watched for.

The oncology unit not only cares for the patients who will eventually die, but also for those receiving treatment that will result in long years of life or possibly cure of their disease. The focus on symptom control and personal and psychosocial care, as well as medical treatment, is quite appropriate and ideally provides an arena in which medical treatment can have the maximum effect.

Providing Psychosocial Care. The oncology unit should provide an environment that will allow patients and their families to perceive it as a warm, familiar, caring, and helping place to come. Touching and eye contact should be used therapeutically. The focus should be on the patient as a person. Listening should be a skill utilized effectively by all nursing personnel on the unit. Expression of feelings should be encouraged. Care should be taken to avoid categorizing patients as problems, but rather as persons who have problems. A more detailed discussion of psychosocial care will be found in Chapter 12.

Providing Family Centered Care. Families must be an integral part of the focus of care on an oncology unit. They need to be included as members of the team and included in the care that is being provided.

Patients cannot be viewed as isolated beings, unaffected by the world around them. Patient-Family-Society make up a gestalt that cannot be dissected for treatment. Any factor that alters one part will affect the whole. Effective nursing interventions must include the entire gestalt.

The patient has traditionally been the

target of nursing interventions. If family members were included in nursing actions, they were treated as secondary to the patient. The entire gestalt should be viewed as the patient, with the nurse's focus changing as needed from one part to another, in order to move the entire gestalt toward a higher level of health.

The Oncology Outpatient Clinic

As medical treatment for cancer has progressed, it has been possible to provide much of cancer care on an outpatient basis. Outpatient clinics, when effectively designed, can facilitate the continuity of care and greatly increase the quality of life for the cancer patient. The clinics usually have a progressive philosophy and use interdisciplinary teams. Some clinics are small and primarily provide an arena for the administration of chemotherapy. Other clinics, often located in medical centers, are large and complex in the types of care they provide.

The clinics offer many opportunities for teaching, psychosocial interventions, and group discussions. Patients and families usually feel free to call the outpatient clinic when problems occur. Relationships are often developed between staff and clients, which allows for much more open communication.

Many oncology outpatient clinics are in hospitals that also have oncology units. In order for care to be coordinated, nursing communication between the unit and the clinic is necessary. The patient's data base, social history, disease history, and nursing care plan should be shifted from unit to clinic and back, as the patient's care shifts. Nurses from both units need opportunities to discuss the patient's care and common problems. These discussions can greatly enhance the continuity of care provided.

Home Health Care

Home health care agencies have provided a much needed service to the cancer patient. Although most care is provided to advanced cancer patients, postsurgical cancer patients also use these services. This type of health care makes it possible to care for patients at home, who otherwise would require some type of institutional care. The care provided is interdisciplinary in nature and can include such professionals as nurses, social workers, dietitians, and physical and occupational therapists. Nurse's aides may be available to give daily baths and other personal care. Housekeeping services may also be available.

Some hospitals are attempting to improve the continuity of care by providing an oncology unit, an outpatient clinic, and home care for the cancer patient. If services (including psychosocial care) are well coordinated, this arrangement could supply a level of care not previously available to cancer patients.

The Oncology Intensive Care Unit

Hospitals that have extensive programs of chemotherapy may also have an oncology intensive care unit. These units are necessary to treat the patient experiencing complications as a result of aggressive therapies. Facilities for reverse isolation (protective units for the patient with an extremely low white blood count) may often be part of the intensive care unit. These units may also treat patients with infections resulting from low white blood counts. Cancer patients are prone to thrombophlebitis, pulmonary embolus, and pneumonia, any of which may require intensive care.

The Comprehensive Community Cancer Center

A comprehensive community cancer center is a hospital with major focus on cancer care. To be classified as such, these hospitals must meet specific criteria, including regularly scheduled interdisciplinary tumor conferences and a tumor registry. These hospitals tend to be more progressive in their philosophy of cancer care and offer more innovative types of services to cancer patients.

The Comprehensive Cancer Research Center

Cancer research centers provide care for cancer patients from a large region. These centers are usually associated with medical schools and are heavily involved with experimental therapies and teaching. The center is usually part of a cooperative research group that conducts organized research on cancer care. Some of these centers also support nursing research.

BIBLIOGRAPHY

1. Antonovsky, A.: *Health, Stress, and Coping*. Jossey-Bass Publishers, San Francisco, 1979.
2. Arenth, L.: Administrative support for cancer nurses. *Proceedings — Fifth Annual Congress of the Oncology Nursing Society*. A94, p. 57, 1980.
3. Arenth, L.: Multidisciplinary discharge planning project. *Proceedings — Fifth Annual Congress of the Oncology Nursing Society*. A95, p. 57, 1980.
4. Armstrong, A. and K. M. Thaney: The efficacy of a separate inpatient oncology unit in a community hospital. *Proceedings — Fourth Annual Congress of the Oncology Nursing Society*. A78, p. 43, 1979.
5. Baird, S. B.: Nurses' perceptions of stressors in oncology nursing practice. *Proceedings — Fourth Annual Congress of the Oncology Nursing Society*. A181, p. 69, 1979.
6. Barrett, K. G. and N. L. Carr: Stress reducers for oncology nursing. *Abstracts — Third Annual Convention of the Oncology Nursing Society*. A49, 1978.
7. Beck, J. A.: Primary nursing and oncology: a program for patient care. *Abstracts — Third Annual Convention of the Oncology Nursing Society*. A30, 1978.
8. Bedell, C.: Development of primary care nursing on a cancer research unit. *Proceedings — Fifth Annual Congress of the Oncology Nursing Society*. A117, p. 63, 1980.
9. Belis, L., R. B. Weiss, and D. Trush: The oncology clinic: a primary care facility. *Cancer Nursing*. 3:47–52, 1980.
10. Bell, B. and K. G. Skelton: Advocating for yourselves and your patients: one approach to justify staffing needs. *Proceedings — Fifth Annual Congress of the Oncology Nursing Society*. A110, p. 61, 1980.
11. Boyer, M. and R. Selgas: A nursing care plan which is kept as part of the official record. *Proceedings — Fourth Annual Congress of the Oncology Nursing Society*. A41, p. 34, 1979.
12. Burns, N.: *Nurse-Patient Communication with the Advanced Cancer Patient*. Unpublished Master's Thesis. Texas Woman's University, 1974.
13. Carpenter, L. C.: Coordinating cancer nursing care in a community hospital without an oncology unit. *Proceedings — Fifth Annual Congress of the •Oncology Nursing Society*. A20, p. 38, 1980.
14. Carter, P. and C. Varriechie: Utilization of the Betty Neuman model in oncology nursing practice. *Proceedings — Fifth Annual Congress of the Oncology Nursing Society*. A103, p. 59, 1980.
15. Champagne, E.: Developing cancer nursing teams in community hospitals. *Abstracts — Third Annual Convention of the Oncology Nursing Society*. A8, 1978.
16. Corley, B. N.: Participative management on a cancer research unit. *Proceedings — Fourth Annual Congress of the Oncology Nursing Society*. A85, p. 45, 1979.
17. Cox, S. and R. Tiffany: A review of cancer nursing services in North America. *Nursing Mirror*. 141:66–68, 1975.
18. Craytor, J. K., J. K. Brown, and G. R. Morrow: Assessing learning needs of nurses who care for persons with cancer. *Cancer Nursing*. 1:211–220, 1978.
19. Dailey, K. S.: Quality cancer care in the community hospital. *Abstracts — Third Annual Convention of the Oncology Nursing Society*. A27, 1978.
20. Dunphy, J. E.: Annual discourse on caring for the patient with cancer. *New England Journal of Medicine*. 295:313–319, 1976.
21. Dunphy, J. E.: On caring for the patient with cancer. *CA — A Cancer Journal for Clinicians*. 27:109–118, 1977.
22. Early, A. J. and M. Boyer: Enriching life experience of the poor prognosis cancer patient. *Proceedings — Fifth Annual Congress of the Oncology Nursing Society*. A91, p. 56, 1980.
23. Eisenhauer, J. and M. L. Kaup: Development of a cancer care unit in a private hospital. *Abstracts — Third Annual Convention of the Oncology Nursing Society*. A20, 1978.
24. Elliott, C. St. J.: The application of individualized nursing standards and evaluation by a nursing audit to determine quality nursing care. *Abstracts — Third Annual Convention of the Oncology Nursing Society*. A17, 1978.
25. Fallon, G. A.: The multidisciplinary team approach. *Proceedings — Fifth Annual Congress of the Oncology Nursing Society*. A119, p. 63, 1980.
26. Fox, L., P. Amaral, and A. Nehemkis: Staff inservice and support: an integrated multidisciplinary approach. *Proceedings — Fifth Annual Congress of the Oncology Nursing Society*. A28, p. 40, 1980.
27. Habech, M. C. and F. E. McLaughlin: Health care professionals' role expectations and patient needs. *Nursing Research*. 26:288–298, 1977.
28. Hayes, D. M.: Perceptions of cancer care by pro-

fessionals and nonprofessionals. *Evaluation and the Health Professions.* 1:29–56, 1978.

29. Isler, C.: Delivering total care — everywhere. *RN.* 41:59–62, 1978.

30. Levitt, B. W.: Expanded role of community oncology nurse in a community based oncology project. *Proceedings — Fifth Annual Congress of the Oncology Nursing Society.* A51, p. 46, 1980.

31. Louis, J. and M. Havlovie: Life and living: the holistic concept in the care of the cancer patient (abst). *Proceedings of the American Society of Clinical Oncology.* 18:348, 1977.

32. Luel, J. K. and J. J. Dawson: Quality of life. *Seminars in Oncology.* 2:323–327, 1975.

33. Mayer, A.: Position statement on cancer patient care evaluation. *American College of Surgeons' Bulletin.* 61:18–19, 1976.

34. McCorkle, R.: A new beginning: the opening of a multidisciplinary cancer unit. *Cancer Nursing.* 2:269–278, 1979.

35. Mellette, S. J. and W. Regelson: Quantification of rehabilitation outcomes in a multiteam cancer rehabilitation program. *Proceedings of the American Society of Clinical Oncology.* 19:367, 1978.

36. Murphy, P. P.: The multidimensional role of the oncology nurse specialist in the community hospital. *Proceedings — Fourth Annual Congress of the Oncology Nursing Society.* A18, p. 29, 1979.

37. Newlin, N. J. and D. K. Wellisch: The oncology nurse: life on an emotional roller coaster. *Cancer Nursing.* 1:447–449, 1978.

38. Nightingale, F.: *Notes on nursing: what it is, and what it is not.* Harrison, London, 1859.

39. *Outcome Standards for Cancer Nursing Practice.* Oncology Nursing Society and American Nurses' Association Division on Medical-Surgical Nursing Practice, 1979.

40. Owen, W. L., P. S. Anderson, Jr., and W. L. Parry: Health services delivery to prostatic cancer patients. *Oklahoma State Medical Association Journal.* 70:436–442, 1977.

41. Plant, J.: Teaching hospital nurtures growth of community oncology clinics. *Hospitals.* 52:121, 1978.

42. Priest, P., B. Piper, and B. Bell: Oncology care units in community hospitals. *Proceedings — Fifth Annual Congress of the Oncology Nursing Society.* A111, p. 61, 1980.

43. Rickel, L.: Human values and the quality of survival. *Journal of the Arkansas Medical Society.* 70:210–212, 1973.

44. Robinson, J.: Against a subtle enemy: the dissenting voice of Jean Robinson. *Nursing Mirror.* 147:111, 1978.

45. Saunders, J. P.: The cancer center: its coordinating role. *Hospital Practice.* 13:11, 1978.

46. Shell, J.: How stress affects the coping mechanisms of the oncology nurse within the hospital setting. *Proceedings — Fifth Annual Congress of the Oncology Nursing Society.* A162, p. 74, 1980.

47. Silverman, D. C., A. D. Turnbull, P. L. Goldiner, and W. H. Howland: The value of the therapeutic intervention scoring system in a cancer center intensive care unit. *Clinical Bulletin.* 5:106–108, 1975.

48. Smith, M.: The development of an oncology care unit. *Abstracts — Third Annual Convention of the Oncology Nursing Society.* A3, 1978.

49. Strauss, A. L. and B. G. Glaser: *Chronic Illness and the Quality of Life.* C. V. Mosby Company, St. Louis, 1975.

50. Terrill, L. and B. Wagner: Work-study program in cancer nursing. *Proceedings — Fifth Annual Congress of the Oncology Nursing Society.* A19, p. 38, 1980.

51. Vachon, M. L., S. K. Freedman, A. Formo, J. Rogers, W. A. L. Lyall, and J. J. Freeman: The final illness in cancer: the widow's perspective. *Canadian Medical Association Journal.* 117:1151–1154, 1977.

52. Wegmann, J. A.: Avoidance behaviors of nurses as related to cancer diagnosis and/or terminality. *Oncology Nursing Forum.* 6:8–14, 1979.

53. Wegmann, J. A.: Methods of staff support in a new oncology unit. *Proceedings — Fifth Annual Congress of the Oncology Nursing Society.* A13, p. 37, 1980.

54. Wilkes, E.: Some problems in cancer management. *Practitioner.* 213:82–86, 1974.

55. Wilkes, E., A. G. O. Crowther, and C. W. K. H. Greaves: A different kind of day hospital for patients with preterminal cancer and chronic disease. *British Medical Journal.* 6144:1053–1056, 1978.

56. Yasko, J. and A. Butz: Holistic care of the patient with cancer — a nursing process data collection tool. *Proceedings — Fifth Annual Congress of the Oncology Nursing Society.* A101, p. 59, 1980.

7
Surgery

INTRODUCTION

Until very recently, surgery was considered the primary treatment modality for cancer and the only curative therapy. The big question was — and usually still is — "Did you get it all?" To "not get it all" was a sentence of death. Chemotherapy and radiotherapy are now considered to be effective treatment modalities for the cure and control of cancer. All three forms of modalities may be used at various stages in the treatment of a specific type of cancer. The surgeon was once considered the primary physician for cancer. Now, the medical oncologist is more likely to be the primary physician, with surgeons and radiotherapists providing care at specific stages of treatment. Surgery will probably remain the treatment of choice for early cancer; however, we are now coming to understand how seldom cancer is detected in early stages, when surgery is most effective.

THE CHANGING PHILOSOPHY OF SURGICAL TREATMENT FOR CANCER

In any discipline, the philosophy and strategies that predominate are based on the existing level of scientific knowledge and on the beliefs held by those in positions of power and influence within the profession. Sometimes their power is so great that alternative theories or approaches receive little consideration.[2] This has been true in cancer surgery. Even when advances in scientific knowledge have shown the rationale to be inaccurate, many surgeons have continued to hold steadfast to the old and familiar approaches.[13, 31, 41]

Nurses have been dependent on the physicians with whom they work for an understanding of the rationale behind therapy. They have been inclined to adopt physicians' beliefs with little understanding of the biologic basis for treatment. If nursing care is to have a rational, scientific base, nurses must acquire more knowledge of the rationale behind therapies. The provision of medical therapies is part of the nurse's job, but a knowledge of medical therapies and the biologic processes involved is necessary in order to provide intelligent and effective nursing care.

History of Cancer Surgery

The notion of curing cancer by cutting it out is a very primitive and compelling idea. Ancient man attempted to destroy some cancers — primarily of the skin, bone and breast — by surgery and cautery.[41] In the second century AD, Galen considered cancer to be a systemic disease associated with an excess of black bile. Because of this belief, cancer was not considered curable by surgery and surgery was seldom used before the eighteenth century.[13] Two centuries ago, the microscope was discovered and gradually the cellular nature of cancer was recognized. The neoplastic nature of cancer and the phenomenon of metastasis were recognized and studied.[41]

In the eighteenth century, surgeons began to develop a rationale for cancer surgery. Valsalva, in 1704, believed that cancer was a local lesion capable of cure by surgery. He believed that cancer spread by way of the lymphatics to regional lymph nodes and that it was inclined to recur. Le Dran (1757) and Morgagni (1769) continued to develop this thesis. From these scientists came the assumption that cancer is a local disease that is curable if found early.[13]

The principles on which present-day cancer surgery is based were developed a century ago. The most influential person in this development was William S. Halsted. His name is most closely associated with the radical mastectomy, but his precepts have served as the basis for all cancer surgery for nearly 100 years.[13]

Halsted placed little significance on the blood stream as a mechanism for metastases. He believed that cancer spread locally by contiguous growth from the original tumor, extending along the fascia and the walls of lymphatic vessels. In 1860, Virchow formulated the precept that lymph nodes served as a barrier to the passage of cancer cells. Another assumption, in keeping with Halsted's concept, also developed. It was believed that cancer remained localized for a long period of time; then, at some instant in time, spread to the regional lymph nodes; and then, after another interval of time, systemic dissemination occurred.[13]

Based on these assumptions, an anatomic basis developed for cancer surgery. "Effective" cancer surgery consisted of removal of the primary tumor along with regional lymphatics and lymph nodes. This was accomplished by an "en bloc" dissection, meaning that the tumor, the lymphatics and lymph nodes, and a surrounding region of normal tissue were removed in one large piece. Since the growth of cancer was believed to be contiguous, surgical failures were blamed on the surgeon for not being extensive enough in the dissection. It was thought that removing one more node or cutting out a little more tissue would have cured the patient.

Thus, the concept of radical surgery developed. As surgical techniques and postoperative care improved and antibiotics were developed, the surgery became more and more radical. Procedures such as extended radical mastectomy, hemipelvectomy, forequarter amputation, pelvic evisceration, and hemicorporectomy are based on the assumptions described above.[13]

When research studies began to be conducted on cancer treatment, it became increasingly obvious that, in spite of highly skilled and radical surgery, the length of patient survival and cure rates were scarcely different from those of patients who received no treatment. On the basis of these studies and new knowledge concerning tumor biology, cancer surgery is changing. As is true of any change, the process is slow. It is difficult to give up old ideas and practices.

New Assumptions About Cancer

Current knowledge of the biologic processes involved in cancer are discussed in detail in Chapter 2. Some of the discoveries most influential in the changes taking place in cancer surgery will be outlined here.

Cancer as a Systemic Disease. Cancer is now viewed as a systemic disease. Almost all patients with solid tumors have disseminated disease at the time of diagnosis. This position has been taken on the basis of studies of cell doubling times and treatment failures of patients surgically treated for "early" cancer.

Cell Doubling Time. (See Fig. 7–1.)

When cancer is first detectable it is a 1 cm mass. At this point it has already gone through two-thirds of its growth, usually about thirty doublings. A billion cancer cells are already present, and it is almost certain that since cell shedding increases with age and tumor bulk, many cells may have shed into lymph nodes and/or peripheral blood by the time of diagnosis. If metastases grow and the tumor is unchecked, in as little as five more doublings a tumor mass as large as one foot in diameter could be present; with five more doublings, sufficient tumor is present to kill the host. In a sense then, cancer is advanced at diagnosis. Even with apparent complete removal of tumor, up to 10^3 cells can be scattered throughout the body without recognition as cancer cells.[11]

There are several weaknesses in the concept of cell doubling time: (1) the assumption that the malignancy began from a single cell; (2) the assumption that all of the cells within the tumor will divide; and (3) the assumption that all of the cells will

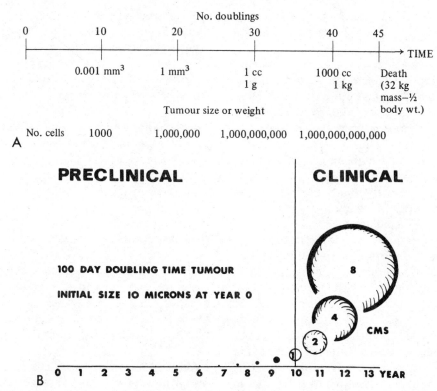

Figure 7–1. *A,* Number of doublings versus tumor size or weight. *B,* Growth of 100 day doubling time tumor. (From Walter, J.: *Cancer and Radiotherapy.* London: J. & A. Churchill, 1971. Used by permission.)

survive after cell division and will continue to replicate. In spite of these weaknesses, the concept can be helpful in understanding why metastases are so common, even in small tumors.

Treatment Failures. Another good indication of the systemic nature of cancer is the rate of recurrence of cancer that has been clinically judged to be early and curable. Ten years after a radical mastectomy was performed 50 per cent of the patients have had recurrence. Twenty-four per cent of those patients with no positive lymph nodes will have recurrence within 10 years. Treatment failure rates of other common cancers are: pancreas — 99 per cent, lung — 90 per cent, prostate — 70 per cent, bowel — 60 per cent.[13]

It does not necessarily follow that patients who do not have a recurrence had no residual tumor cells at the time of surgery. The tumor cells left may have been small enough in number for normal body defenses to destroy.[13, 41]

Impact of Removal of the Primary Tumor. As discussed in Chapter 2, the primary tumor has many effects on body functioning; this is true even when the tumor is very small. When the primary tumor is surgically removed, body functioning will be altered. In addition, removal of the primary tumor may alter the growth pattern of micrometastases. Fisher[13] has given an excellent review of the literature in this area.

Alteration of Immune Responses. After surgery, immune responses will change in several ways. There is a decrease in serum blocking activity, and cell-mediated immunity may improve. Circulating antitumor antibodies usually increase; however, two studies find loss of tumor immunity after removal of the primary tumor, followed by increased numbers of metastases.[13] Spontaneous regression of metastases has also been known to occur. There are mixed findings on the effect of surgery and anesthesia on the body's immune mechanisms. Some studies have revealed alterations in cell-mediated immunity. Lymphocyte transformation has been shown to be depressed. Antibody-producing cells have been found to be reduced in number in some circumstances and enhanced in others. Phagocytosis and depression of the reticuloendothelial system occur.[13]

Effect of Residual Metastases. If host immune responses do not destroy the metastases, the rate of metastatic growth may increase. The primary tumor seems to slow down growth at metastatic sites. When the primary tumor is removed, these sites (which often contain more anaplastic cells and have higher proportions of cells in the cell cycle) will begin more rapid growth. Surgery, if it is the only treatment used, may actually speed up the time of death. However, these rapidly growing cells may be very susceptible to destruction by chemotherapy or radiotherapy.[13]

The Role of Lymphatics and Lymph Nodes. Cancer cells that break away from the primary tumor may travel through the lymphatics to a lymph node or may bypass nodes, entering the blood stream through the thoracic duct. Not all nodes near a tumor will contain tumor cells, even when the tumor is widely metastasized. Regional lymph nodes appear to retain immunologic capacities, despite the presence of growing tumors. The presence or absence of positive nodes may simply be an indication of the immunocompetence of the host, rather than an indication of whether or not metastasis has occurred. This would explain the serious implications of finding positive nodes at the time of surgery.[13, 31]

Multicentric Cancers. All cancers do not develop from a single malignant cell. This has been found to be true for breast cancer in particular. If the primary tumor is removed and the breast tissue left intact, other clusters of malignant cells may begin to grow. Little is understood about the kinetics of tumor foci. Does the removal of the primary tumor affect their growth? Are they similar to distant metastases in their response? How responsive are they to chemotherapy? This information is needed for

surgeons to make intelligent decisions about surgical strategies for treatment of breast cancer.[13]

Current Surgical Strategy

Surgery is still the main curative modality available for cancer; however, the role of the surgeon in the treatment of cancer has changed. Cancer surgery is now seen as one stage in a much more comprehensive scheme of care. Surgery is often very effective in local control of cancer growth and at the least may give the patient added time or increased quality of life. Adjunct therapy with radiotherapy or chemotherapy may further lengthen life or greatly increase the possibility of cure. The surgeon must remain informed about the place of the surgery in the whole system of treatment. Otherwise the patient's chances for cure or lengthened life will be diminished.[16]

Some of the purposes for performing surgery have changed. In the past, the major purpose of surgery was to cure cancer. With current knowledge, we know that it is possible that surgery alone will not cure cancer. The cure may be more dependent on the patient's immune response.[13, 41]

If the sole purpose of the surgery is to remove the primary tumor, less radical surgery may be utilized. En bloc dissection may not be considered necessary. The surgery may also be conducted in such a way that reconstructive surgery is facilitated.

The state of the patient will be more closely considered in future decisions to perform surgery. In the past, it was commonly believed that since the patients had cancer, they had nothing to lose by having surgery and that the surgery might save them. However, if patients are at high risk, surgery may actually shorten their life.[16]

There is still a debate about the advantages of one-stage and two-stage surgical procedures for cancer, breast cancer in particular. In a one-stage procedure, a biopsy is done, the pathologist performs a frozen section, and, if the diagnosis is cancer, surgery is performed. In a two-stage procedure, a biopsy is done and the patient returns to the hospital room. If the pathology examination indicates the presence of cancer, the patient is told, alternative approaches are discussed with the patient, and physician and patient together decide on the surgical approach.

Those who favor the one-stage procedure believe that there is an additional risk of metastasis if the lump is removed for biopsy and more extensive surgery is performed later. Their beliefs are based on Halsted's approach to cancer surgery. These surgeons also object to the additional risks involved in administering two general anesthetics in so short a period of time. Some also criticize the two-stage procedure because it requires a hospital bed for a longer period of time and increases the cost of the procedure. Additionally, if the patient has already decided on the desired operative procedure in case of cancer, or if there are no options, there is no reason to postpone the surgery.

Proponents of the two-stage procedure believe the extra time allows the patient time to adjust more easily to the surgical procedure. Some surgeons are performing the biopsy under local anesthesia or sometimes as an outpatient procedure.

Removal of Tumor Mass. Surgery to remove a large mass of solid tumor is often performed in order to make chemotherapy or radiotherapy more effective. If lymph nodes are removed, it is usually for the purpose of diagnosing the extent of the disease, not for curing the patient. Some surgeons believe that all of the tissue from which the malignancy originated should be removed, since the tissue has already shown vulnerability to cancer and will likely give rise to more new tumors. Examples of this would be breast and stomach tissue.[16]

Staging. Surgery may be performed for the purpose of determining the extent of disease; this is called staging. In staging operations, samples of lymph nodes are removed and biopsies of various organs and structures are taken. In some cases, the spleen is removed. This type of surgery just to obtain a diagnosis may seem extreme, but an accurate determination of the extent of disease is essential for the provision of effective treatment. Radiotherapy may not be the treatment of choice if evidence of disease is found in distant sites. An example of this is Hodgkin's disease. Stage I or II may be effectively treated by either radiotherapy or chemotherapy, but stage III or IV must be treated only with chemotherapy. If properly staged, this disease has a high cure rate even in late stages. If the staging is done solely by physical examination the disease will often be defined as an earlier stage than it actually is, and the patient could die unnecessarily.

Diagnosis. As discussed earlier, surgery may be performed to determine if the patient has cancer. Often this entails obtaining a biopsy of some type. Diagnosis is also more demanding now. To merely detect cancer is not sufficient. Diagnosis also involves staging and determining the histology of the tumor, its differentiation and its pattern of growth. The state of the patient must also be carefully evaluated. The surgeon has a major role in this process. Information obtained from these procedures will be used in making decisions about appropriate therapy.

Palliation. Patients with metastatic disease have complications of their disease process that can sometimes be relieved surgically. Procedures have been developed to relieve pain. These may involve blocking or severing nerves, or they may involve removing a tumor mass that is causing pain due to pressure on a strategic area. Other procedures have been developed to relieve obstructions of hollow viscera — most commonly the bowel and the ureters. Although these procedures may not prolong the patient's life for long, they usually improve the quality of life.

Reconstruction. For many years, reconstructive surgery for cancer was frowned upon. If done, it was delayed for 2 or more years after the original surgery, in order to monitor for local recurrence. Now reconstructive surgery is becoming simply another phase of the treatment protocol for breast cancer and head and neck cancers, in particular. These procedures do much to improve quality of life after mutilating surgery.

COMMON SURGICAL PROCEDURES IN CANCER

Mastectomy

There has been more controversy about the appropriate treatment for breast cancer than any other malignancy. For the last century, the radical mastectomy has been considered the only effective treatment. The radical mastectomy involves removing the breast tissue, the lymph node chains under the arm, the pectoralis muscle, the lymph node chains over and under the pectoralis muscle, and most of the skin covering the breast. This surgery is accomplished with an en bloc approach, leaving the patient with an obvious chest deformity and decreased functioning of the shoulder. Research studies found, however, that the length of survival of patients after the radical mastectomy was little different from that of those who had no treatment. Other approaches began to be used. These approaches included the modified radical mastectomy and removal of only the breast mass, sometimes called a lumpectomy by those favoring more radical surgery.

Studies comparing the three types of surgery found little difference in cure and survival rates between the radical and the modified radical mastectomy. Results after removing only the breast mass are conflicting. Therefore, the current treatment of choice is usually the modified radical mastectomy. In this surgery, the pectoralis muscle is left intact, as are the lymph node chains under the muscle. Removal of skin over the breast is not as extreme. Breast reconstructive surgery is considered more acceptable and may be planned for at the time of the original surgery. Breast implants are often placed under the pectoralis muscle, resulting in much more natural-appearing breasts.

If any nodes are found to be malignant, chemotherapy is usually begun shortly after the original surgery. Some physicians still use radiotherapy after breast surgery if the disease is believed to be confined to the regional lymph nodes. Breast cancer is usually a slowly growing malignancy and seems to be able to lie dormant for many years after the original surgery. Metastasis can occur 10 to 25 years after the primary lesion is removed. The most common sites of metastasis are the lung, bone, brain, and liver.

Colostomy

A colostomy is the creation of an artificial anus — a new opening for the colon is made, usually on the abdominal wall. A colostomy is usually performed when a malignancy is found in the lower third of the descending colon. Unless the tumor is extensive, the anus and rectum may also be removed. If the tumor is higher in the colon, a colon resection is often possible. A colostomy may also be performed in the transverse or ascending colon. Construction of a permanent end colostomy begins by removing the section of colon containing the tumor and a surrounding region of normal tissue. Lymph nodes draining the region are also removed. The colon above the surgery is then attached to the abdominal wall and a stoma is created.

Patients with advanced cancer may have large abdominal masses obstructing the bowel. These patients are usually in poor physical condition and cannot tolerate extensive surgical procedures. In these patients, the bowel is opened and brought to the abdominal wall for the development of a stoma. The lower end of the colon is left intact. This is called a double barreled colostomy. It allows decompression of the bowel and passage of fecal material.

Colon cancer usually metastasizes by the time the tumor is 1 cm in size. The most common sites of metastasis are the regional lymph nodes and the liver. Chemotherapy may be utilized if nodes are positive; however, chemotherapy is not as effective with colon cancers as it is with other types of tumors. Control of growth is more possible than is cure.

Head and Neck Surgery

Head and neck cancers are usually basal or squamous cell in origin. They tend to spread locally rather than to distant parts of the body. They are frequently slow growing. Because of these factors, surgery is often utilized to cure or to slow down growth. The surgery is often mutilating; however, it must be considered that the uncontrolled malignancy will disfigure the patient even more. The exact nature of the surgery will vary with the location of the malignancy, but may involve removal of a facial or jaw bone, removal of an eye or an ear, removal of the tongue or a portion of it, a permanent tracheostomy, or a radical neck dissection that consists of excision of lymph node chains in the neck and removal of some of the anterior neck muscles.

These patients are frequently heavy smokers or alcoholics or both. They may be physically and nutritionally in poor condition for surgery. Infections are common after surgery, and wound healing is a frequent problem. These patients require complex postoperative care and may have to adjust to a permanent tracheostomy or tube feeding or both for the rest of their life.

Some of these tumors are very sensitive to radiotherapy, which may be utilized after surgery. Chemotherapy may also be utilized, but is not considered highly effective with head and neck tumors.

DETERMINING SURGICAL RISK

According to Luckmann and Sorensen:

The degree of surgical risk is based upon four factors: (1) the physical and mental condition of the patient, (2) the extent of the disease, (3) the magnitude of the required operation, and (4) the resources and preparation of the surgeon, nurses and hospital.[26]

Using these criteria, the cancer patient will usually be in a high risk category. Even when the patient's physical condition appears to be good, the malignant processes may have effects that are not easily visible. Even "early" tumors often cause metabolic changes that can have an effect on the patient's response to surgery. The patient may be in negative nitrogen balance. Utilization of sodium may be altered. There may be changes in metabolic pathways. Most of these changes have not yet been studied in relation to the cancer patient's response to surgery.

Because of the negative connotations of the diagnosis of cancer, the patients' psychologic state places them in a high risk category. The level of stress is usually higher for these patients than for the average surgical patient. The extent of disease may not be known at the time of surgery. The magnitude of the surgery is likely to be great, since most cancer surgery is radical in nature.

THE PHYSIOLOGY OF SURGICAL CONVALESCENCE

Recovery from surgery has not been thoroughly studied. Most of the studies that have been conducted examined convalescence from trauma. Since surgery is a type of trauma, these data have often been generalized to include surgery. The process of convalescence from surgery occurs over a much longer period of time than is generally expected. Six months to 1 year after surgery, some body processes are not back to their presurgical functioning state. There are numerous metabolic changes that continue for several months after surgery. The metabolic changes seem to be proportional to the extent of the injury or surgery.[14] Changes occurring with surgery are not usually as extensive as those resulting from trauma situations.

Metabolic responses to trauma include weight loss, fatigue, weakness, and some degree of starvation.[2] The factors causing these changes are complex and interrelated. (See Fig. 7–2.) The changes that occur have been divided into phases. In the initial phase, responses include: (1) depression of body activities; (2) stabilization of cardiopulmonary function; and (3) mobilization of tissue fuel supplies. In the catabolic phase, which lasts from days to

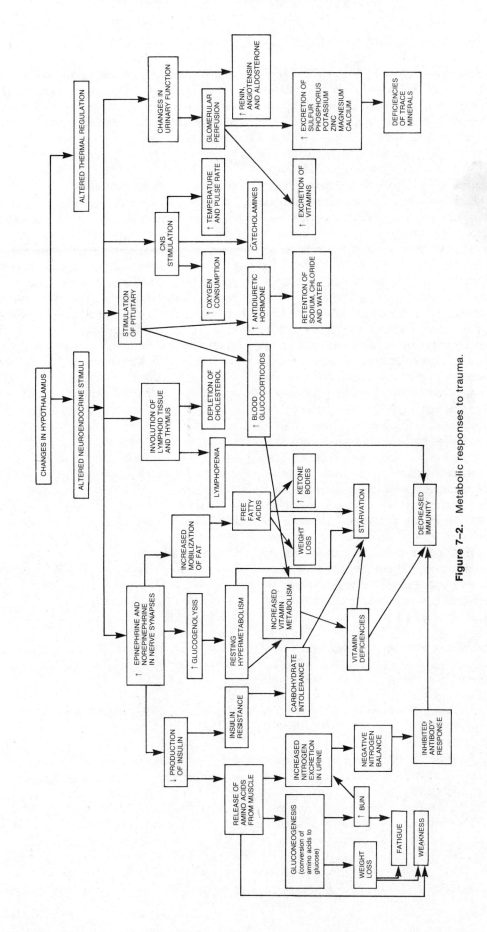

Figure 7-2. Metabolic responses to trauma.

weeks, changes include: (1) resting hypermetabolism; (2) increased nitrogen loss; (3) carbohydrate intolerance; and (4) increased fat mobilization. The anabolic phase, which lasts from weeks to months, is involved with: (1) wound healing; (2) replacement of muscle proteins; and (3) replacement of fat stores.[2, 20] These phases are not clearly distinguishable. Catabolic and anabolic processes occur simultaneously, but one or the other predominates.[25]

Resting Hypermetabolism

After injury or surgery, the patient continues to maintain a higher than normal metabolic rate, even when at rest. Normally, the metabolic rate decreases markedly when a person is at complete rest. The increased rate means that the patient continues to utilize oxygen and nutrients and produces heat at high rates even when at rest. A patient who underwent uncomplicated abdominal surgery will have a 10 per cent increase in metabolic rate. A person with a femoral fracture has an increase of 20 per cent. The person with a serious infection, such as peritonitis, has an increased rate of 20 to 40 per cent. An extensive third-degree burn will cause an increase of 50 to 100 per cent. Fever alone increases the metabolic rate 10 per cent for each degree centigrade above normal.[25]

Alterations in Protein Metabolism

Immediately after trauma, a rapid breakdown of skeletal muscle protein begins to occur. This process is most acute in young, heavily muscled men in previously good nutrition and is less intense in women, the elderly, and the poorly nourished.[20] Muscle protein is broken down into amino acids and then converted to glucose. This process is called gluconeogenesis. The high rate of gluconeogenesis is thought to be a result of imbalances in insulin, catecholamines, cortisol, and glucagon.[2] The result of this process is an elevated blood urea nitrogen (BUN) level,

increased nitrogen excretion in the urine, and a state of negative nitrogen balance. As a consequence, the patient will experience weight loss, fatigue, and muscle weakness.

Alterations in Carbohydrate Metabolism

The mechanisms of carbohydrate metabolism after injury are complex and not well understood. Research is discovering some of the processes, but many connecting links remain to be explained. During the initial phase of trauma, insulin secretion is suppressed. At the same time, blood glucose levels are rising rapidly. In the catabolic phase, there is an abnormally high insulin level but a peripheral insulin resistance resulting in carbohydrate intolerance. (Peripheral insulin resistance occurs when the cells will not permit the insulin to enter. Since the job of insulin is to transport glucose across the cell membrane into the cell, glucose remains in the blood and is not used by the cells.) Metabolic pathways for utilization of glucose are altered. Because of hypermetabolism and increased heat production, there is an increased need for energy production. All available glucose will be oxidized. Very little glucose will be converted to glycogen or stored in fat cells. In order for oxidation of glucose to occur in the Krebs cycle, amino acids must be converted to metabolic intermediates of the Krebs cycle. This allows rapid production of high energy adenosine triphosphate (ATP).[20]

Alterations in Fat Metabolism

The body's fat reserves make up 5 to 25 per cent of body weight. The energy reserves in this fat are much greater than those freely available from protein or carbohydrates. Mobilization of fat reserves involves the conversion of triglycerides to fatty acids and glycerol. This process is stimulated by norepinephrine, epinephrine, thyroxine, and glucagon. It is discouraged by insulin and prostaglandins.

Fatty acids are converted to carbon dioxide and water and energy. By-products of this process are ketone bodies. Therefore, ketosis may occur.

In addition to mobilization of stored fats, other substances (blood cholesterol, triglycerides, lipoproteins, and phospholipids) will also be metabolized for energy. Since these substances all have important body functions, this process carried to the extreme can be threatening to the patient's life. Another danger is that fatty acids accumulate more quickly than they can be metabolized to energy. These fatty acids collect in the liver, interfering with liver function, and can also cause fat embolism.[10]

Alterations in Vitamin Metabolism

All of the metabolites are interrelated; changes affecting one will cause changes in the others. Therefore, it is likely that metabolism of all of the vitamins is affected by injury. However, much of the research that has been conducted examines only the relationship between injury and vitamins C and A. Many of these studies have been conducted using animal models. Very few studies have examined human vitamin metabolism during illness or injury.

Vitamin C is vital to the production of collagen, which is essential to wound healing. Vitamin A is important for vision, reproduction, maintenance of epithelium, immune responses (particularly cellular immunity), and a number of other activities. The presence or absence of one vitamin affects the availability of other vitamins. For example, one of the first effects of vitamin A deficiency is depletion of vitamin C reserves. Vitamin E enhances the absorption, storage, and utilization of vitamin A.[25]

In the initial phase of injury, there is an abrupt and sustained drop in adrenal, urinary, and white and red blood cell levels of vitamin C.[25] Similar drops have been reported for thiamine and nicotinamide. The high levels of cortisone secreted by the body after injury speed up the depletion of vitamin A. Extra vitamin A is needed in the wound healing process.

If the intake of the vitamins was marginal before the injury, the problem is even more serious. For example, animals that were on a lowered intake of vitamin A before injury lost weight rapidly from relatively minor wounds, and half of them died. Less collagen was formed and incision strength was poor. Blood glucose levels were much lower in vitamin A deficient animals. Treatment with vitamin A caused an immediate response of weight gain and improvement of incision strength. Topical application of vitamin A to the wound also increased incision strength. Administration of cortisone to animals mildly deficient in vitamin A resulted in severe weight loss and impairment of wound healing. Extra vitamin A counteracted the adverse effects of cortisone on wound healing.[25]

Pretreatment of animals with vitamins greatly improves their response to injury. Animals pretreated with large doses of vitamin C before injury had increased survival rates. Administration of thiamine before injury increased both blood pressure and the rate of survival after injury.[25] Supplemental vitamin A before injury prevented the adrenal hypertrophy and the thymus atrophy that often occur after injury.

The increased need for vitamins seems to continue throughout the period of convalescence. For example, because they are healing, scars are metabolically more active than normal connective tissue for long periods after the injury. Higher vitamin C levels are needed to maintain this activity.

Imbalance of Trace Minerals

Little is known about the functioning of trace minerals after injury; however, these minerals do function on the metabolic pathways. Many of the trace minerals, including sulfur, phosphorus, potassium, zinc, magnesium, and calcium, are rapidly excreted in the urine after injury. The decreases in the average elective surgery patient are minimal and seem to cause no difficulties.[12]

Altered Thermal Regulation

Thermal regulation controls heat production and heat loss. As a result of changes in the hypothalamus following injury, there is an alteration in thermal regulation throughout the body. Marked increases in metabolism and heat production occur. Heat is more easily lost by the body. This may be a consequence of increased levels of catecholamines. Environmental temperature has a greater impact on body metabolism in the injured person than in the healthy person.

Consequences of Metabolic Changes

From the previous discussion, it is apparent that the body's reaction to injury involves most of the metabolic pathways. The reaction is dynamic, but it follows a predictable pattern. The pathogenesis of many of the changes is not yet understood. Many factors affect the metabolic response: the patient's age, sex, pretrauma nutritional status, injury severity, body temperature, and environmental temperature and humidity. The disturbances of metabolic pathways can have serious consequences for the surgical or injured patient.[25]

Weight Loss. The postoperative patient will usually lose 4 to 8 per cent of body weight as a consequence of increased catabolism. The losses will tend to be 13 per cent protein, 13 per cent fat, and 74 per cent water. The weight loss is usually complete 10 to 14 days after surgery. Weight loss can be serious because of its extent and its rapid rate of development. As weight loss increases, so does risk of death. Often, weight loss is not recognized in the postoperative patient because of extracellular water retention.[21]

Fatigue and Weakness. Postoperative fatigue is a consequence of several factors. Cells destroyed at the time of surgery are broken down and excreted. In-creased protein metabolism is occurring. Both of these processes cause elevations of uric acid and BUN levels that result in fatigue. Muscle weakness is a consequence of the breakdown of skeletal muscle protein. After surgery the last thing to revert to normal is the ability to work a complete day without fatigue. Returning to normal work capacity requires at least 2 to 3 months. Recovery is not complete until muscle mass, muscle function, and adipose tissue losses are restored.[21]

Starvation. Even though nutrients are being metabolized at a faster than normal rate, the body cells may be in a state of starvation because nutrients are unavailable to meet cell needs. If this progresses to a critical point, cells begin to die. This point is seldom reached in the average surgical patient because metabolism is not that greatly increased.

Decreased Immunity. Decreased immunity after surgery is a consequence of involution of the lymphoid tissues and thymus, lymphopenia, inhibited antibody response, and vitamin deficiency. This decrease in immunity increases the patient's susceptibility to infection. For the cancer patient, it can mean increased rate of growth of any remaining malignancy.

Effective Interventions for Metabolic Changes

Metabolic changes are so complex that intervening at one point changes many other factors in an unanticipated manner. This can be favorable or unfavorable. Some interventions can diminish metabolic changes or their consequences. Providing good nursing care can make the difference between life and death. Researchers have found that trauma patients cared for in an environment maintained at 30°C with a relative humidity of 35 to 45 per cent do not experience the resting hypermetabolism, increased protein catabolism, or increased oxygen consumption of those kept in an environment of 20°C. Wounds heal more rapidly at 30°C. The nutritional state of the patient is easier to maintain. There is also a decrease in nitrogen loss.[9, 14] One study indicated that 28°C was just as effective;[14] however, this temperature is above the comfort level of health care providers caring for the patient. Since the metabolic rate is not as elevated after surgery, it might be sufficient to allow the patients to select the room temperature most comfortable to them, keeping in mind that it may tend to be warmer than usual.[24]

Increasing the patient's nitrogen intake will improve the nitrogen balance, but will not decrease the rate of breakdown. However, nitrogen balance is the first step in restoring the body cell mass that is optimal for that patient. Infusion of glucose will not inhibit the gluconeogenesis that is occurring. High doses of intravenous glucose may simply increase the blood sugar level. Administration of vitamins prior to, during, and after surgery seems to be helpful in preventing problems related to increased vitamin metabolism.

Cancer Metabolism and Surgical Metabolism

Cancer metabolism (discussed in Chapter 2) often causes metabolic alterations early in the course of the disease. Since most patients facing cancer surgery are considered to have advanced cancer, it is very possible that some metabolic changes that could have an effect on surgical metabolism have previously occurred. This does not seem to be discussed in the literature.

Even if all tumor cells are removed, metabolic alterations that had occurred would require time to return to normal. If the patient has metastatic disease, the problem may be even more complex. Nutritional deficiencies may cause the patient to be at higher risk for surgery. Vitamin deficiencies may be greater. Cancer patients may already have cachexia at the time of surgery. What impact do these factors have on postsurgical metabolic changes in these patients? Are the changes different? Are they more serious?

Wound Healing After Cancer Surgery

The normal process of wound healing has been much more carefully studied than the process of surgical convalescence. Many health care providers think of the wound as healed when a strong scar has developed. This process occurs within about 14 days. Complete wound healing actually takes much longer. One year later, the wound region is still metabolically more active than normal tissue and can deteriorate as a result of nutritional deficiencies or radiation therapy.

The factor in both cancer and surgical metabolism that seems to have the greatest impact on primary wound healing is the nutritional state. If the cancer patient is in reasonably good nutritional condition, wound healing should progress normally. Wound infections occur with greater frequency in cancer patients. Both surgical and cancer metabolism diminish the effectiveness of immune responses.

NURSING CARE DURING SURGICAL INTERVENTION FOR CANCER

Preoperative Care

Discovery of a Mass

Nurses may encounter a cancer patient for the first time in many different settings. Many of these encounters occur in off duty hours. A woman who has found a lump in her breast will often seek out a nurse before she contacts a physician. This contact will usually be casual and informal. At this point, the nurse has to decide whether or not to intervene therapeutically with this person. Nurses cannot live their lives intervening therapeutically with every person with whom they interact 24 hours a day. The decision to function as a nurse in this situation is based on ethics and values. Nurses need to identify what they consider to be their responsibilities to society, to their family, and to themselves. The three are interrelated. If nurses do not take care of their own mental and physical health needs, they will be unable to meet their responsibilities to family or society.

If the nurse elects to function as a nurse with this person, an implicit contract is made between the two of them. The nurse then switches from social interaction to therapeutic intervention. The contract may be as brief as 5 minutes or it may span years in time. It is possible to relate to a person both as a friend and as a nurse. The style of interaction between them will change when they switch into a nurse-patient mode.

A woman who has found a breast lump and seeks out a nurse is often hoping to be told that it is nothing to worry about, it will go away, and she will not need to contact a physician. It is very easy for the nurse to accept the woman's denial and tell her what she wants to hear. When the woman is advised to see a physician or when the nurse examines the breast and verifies the presence of a lump, the woman will react to the threat to her health and to her feelings about cancer. She will need help in recognizing and expressing these feelings before she can decide to seek medical care.

At this point, the woman may move in one of two directions. She may attempt to see the physician immediately or she may minimize the urgency of the situation by postponing a doctor's appointment for several months. She may feel that she has to complete other life activities before seeing the physician, thus decreasing the impact of possible surgery on her world. This avoidance can continue indefinitely, since there is always another activity on the horizon that must be tended to before contacting the physician.

Nursing Care Before Hospitalization

The time between discovery of a mass anywhere in the body and a definite diagnosis of cancer is one of the most difficult. This time is lonely, frightening, and uncertain. The thought of cancer pervades all of a person's thinking. It is impossible to "put it out of your mind," and yet daily activities must go on. At this point the nurse can function in a supportive role. People who can explore the possible outcomes and picture in their minds how they could cope with those outcomes seem able to better accept the entire situation. They also need opportunities to express whatever they are feeling.

Family members also need help. If the nurse plans to continue a therapeutic relationship, this is an ideal time to assess the strengths and weaknesses of family dynamics, the health status of family members, and past and present coping patterns. Social support groups need to be identified. The financial resources of the family should also be assessed. Family members need to examine what the situation means to them, how they see it affecting their lives, and how they imagine themselves coping with the diagnosis of cancer. The family needs to consider changes that might occur in family roles if the diagnosis is cancer and how the family as a group will function. In order to accomplish this, the nurse will have to function in a nurse-client relationship with the symptomatic person, each family member, and the family as a group.

The nurse needs to assess the nutritional status of the symptomatic person and encourage good nutrition before hospitalization. Adequate nutrition, moderate physical exercise, adequate rest, avoidance of people with infections, and minimization of the stress level will facilitate an optimum state of health for surgery. Teaching relaxation strategies can be very helpful at this point.

Hospital Preoperative Care

In many instances, the nurse's first contact with the patient will be upon admission to the hospital. The admission may be for diagnostic tests and biopsies, or surgery may be scheduled. Upon admission to the hospital the patient and family are directly confronted with the awesome threat to their life and their world. Anxiety will be high, even if they maintain calm exteriors. Nursing interventions should be directed toward minimizing anxiety-producing situations resulting from the hospital environment.

On a busy surgical nursing unit, preoperative patients require the least amount of physical nursing care. Faced with the urgency of other responsibilities, it is difficult to take time to provide adequate nursing assessment and interventions to the preoperative patient. If the patient is having a biopsy, it is easy for the nurses to tell themselves that the biopsy will probably be negative. For example, only 15 per cent of the women admitted for breast biopsy will have cancer.

However, the preoperative care sets the stage for optimum recovery from the surgery and, in many instances, for optimum response to the illness. Establishment of a strong nurse-patient relationship at this point can greatly facilitate a positive patient response to the cooperative venture of the nurse and patient in postoperative care. A thorough nursing assessment is important at this point and should include a nursing history and baseline physical assessment. The nursing history should include nutritional patterns, weight changes, recent history of infections, level of stress, usual coping strategies, family relationships, support systems, knowledge of the illness and its treatment, and beliefs about cancer.

The care plan, both preoperative and postoperative, should begin at this point. This plan needs to be developed with the patient as an active participant in the process. This plan, along with the nursing history and physical examination, should accompany the patient throughout the hospitalization, to all nursing units involved in the patient's care. Of course, the plan will be modified as treatment progresses, but the basic plan provides a logical pattern of continuity to all of the care provided. As more information about the patient is acquired, it should be added to the nursing history and the care plan.

Most preoperative patients are eager to learn about the surgical procedure and postoperative period. Because the pending surgery is a crisis situation, there is an increased need for help and an openness to suggestions or teaching. Tasks that need to be accomplished by the patient postoperatively are best prepared for during this time. Teaching should include such activities as coughing, deep breathing, nutrition, and positioning, with the goal of moving the patient toward feeling good and experiencing a higher level of wellness.

Patients need to be prepared for experiences that they will have in surgery, the recovery room, and the first few postoperative days. This preparation should involve what the experience will be like and how it will feel, rather than an intellectual explanation of the reason why it is occurring. It is helpful to assist patients in imagining how they might cope with each experience. The nurse can suggest alternative ways of coping for the patient to consider. Postoperative nursing care measures and the reasons for them can be explained.

Health professionals who are cancer patients are often neglected in the area of preoperative teaching. It is assumed that they know about the care they will receive and why they are receiving it. This knowledge, however, is at an intellectual level and additionally is often incomplete or inaccurate. Since this may be their first experience as cancer patients, they need the same careful attention as others. Since health professionals and very bright people may tend to overintellectualize their feelings, more careful attention must be focused on describing reactions and experiences that they may have and strategies for coping with them.

Negative beliefs about cancer have a strong impact on the coping strategies that patients use, how they see themselves, and their recovery from surgery. Patients need opportunities to express their feelings in an accepting environment. Nursing interventions may include communicating acceptance and positive regard for the patient, communicating that a diagnosis of cancer will not alter that regard, providing accurate information, and proposing alternative beliefs for the patient's consideration. Some patients are not aware that other beliefs about cancer exist. Just telling the patients that they are wrong and giving them new information will do little to alter beliefs. This must be accomplished at an affective rather than an intellectual level and must be accomplished over a period of time. Nurses who have very negative beliefs about cancer will have difficulty helping the patients in this area.

Family members also need nursing care in the preoperative period. Nurses need to establish a primary nurse-client relationship with each significant family member with whom they come into contact. The nurse should assess each family member's level of health, coping strategies, and beliefs about cancer; the impact of the situation on the person's lifestyle and health; and the support systems available to that individual.

Planning and intervention involve providing opportunities for family members to ask questions and to express feelings and concerns. They need to explore the coping strategies that they plan to use. They need the same opportunities as the patient to become aware of and consider alternative beliefs about cancer. Intervening with family members in this manner is not easy. Perhaps this is why it is not usually done. There are occasions when the nurse will encounter conflicts between what patients want or need and what the family members want or need in order to maintain or improve the patients' physical and mental health. These situations sometimes place the nurse in an ethical dilemma.

The family as a group should also be a client of the nurse. It is possible to intervene effectively with a family even though direct contact is not made with every family member, since changes that are made by other family members will have an impact on those who are absent. The nurse needs to assess family relationships and dynamics, watching for changes in roles or dynamics brought about by the effects of illness or the diagnosis of cancer.

Families often need to be made aware of the choices they are making and the consequences of those choices for the future.

This may include changes in communication patterns so that the patient suddenly is not kept informed or changes in roles so that the patient is no longer allowed to make decisions. This will be discussed in more detail in later chapters.

The nurse will often have contact with people within the patient's social system, such as friends or neighbors. If the nurse interacts with the people to meet their personal needs, it is a nurse-client relationship. If the nurse interacts with them to intercede on the part of the patient, it is not a nurse-client relationship.

In a sense, all nurse-client relationships occur within a health situation. The situation being explored in this book is cancer. Contacts may include the patient, individual family members, the family as a group, and individuals in the social system, all of whom are being affected by the same situation. The nurses' focus changes as they provide nursing care, first to one member and then to another. They move (at least psychologically) in closeness and perceptual point of view from one member to another, helping each to respond to the situation in the healthiest way possible for that individual at that time.

The interventions described above begin in the preoperative period and continue for the duration of the nurse-client relationship. The goal for the preoperative period is to facilitate movement of the patient, the family, and members of the patient's social system toward an optimum state of physical and mental health, in order to promote the optimum response to surgical intervention and the recovery from surgery to a higher level of health.

Operative Care

The goal of nursing care in the operating room is to help maintain the patients' optimum physical and mental health so that the patients can respond healthily to the trauma of surgery. This can be accomplished most effectively by continuing to interact with the patients as persons, not as objects, whether they are awake or anesthetized. This more likely occurs if the operating room nurses know the social history of the patients, their illness history, and the plan of care designed by the preoperative nurses. A visit to the patients before surgery can be very helpful in beginning a trusting nurse-client relationship.

The preoperative "prep" assists the patients in avoiding infection. "Preps" are often done by paraprofessionals rather than the nurse, but they are under the supervision of the nurse. These "preps" can be done in a manner that dehumanizes patients and may leave small cuts and scrapes that are no threat to the surgery but are an unnecessary source of postoperative discomfort. "Preps" can also be done in a skilled and careful manner. The procedure communicates to patients how they will be treated by operating room personnel during surgery.

Communication occurs on many levels between nurse and patient. It may be biologic in nature, and relayed to the nurse through blood pressure, pulse, or skin color. It may be through touch or eye contact. It may be through voice or body language. Many of these forms of communication continue, even though patients are anesthetized. It is possible that communications to patients and discussions about them or their illness are remembered in the unconscious, even though there is later no conscious recall. These stored memories could have an impact on postoperative recovery and later mental health.

The nurse in the operating room, more intensively than in any other setting, serves as the patients' self-care agent. Patients are totally dependent at this point and must trust those in the operating room to look after their interests and needs. "Minor" details that will not affect recovery from surgery can affect postoperative patient comfort. Poor positioning on the operating room table can cause muscle or joint discomfort after surgery. Some studies indicate that blood stasis in the legs during surgery is related to the development of thrombophlebitis. Cancer patients, even in early stages of the disease, have an increased risk of thrombophlebitis. Utiliza-

tion of elastic stockings, proper positioning of the legs, and careful placement of safety straps over the legs can reduce this risk. The nurse also functions as the patients' advocate in carefully counting sponges and accounting for instruments before closure of the wound. Careful cleansing of the skin and application of the dressing facilitate comfort as well as serving as a deterrent to infection. Careful movement of patients from table to gurney to bed can prevent unnecessary bumps and bruises.

Although many of these activities are performed by other nursing personnel, professional nurses are accountable for supervision of the quality of care. Their regard for the patient as a person and their values related to patient care will be reflected in the care given by others as well as by themselves.

Direct communication between the operating room nurse and the recovery room nurse can facilitate optimum care by relaying the present state of patients, their social and illness history, and the plan of care. This information will promote greater continuity of care.

Postoperative Care

In the recovery room, the patients are still in a state of almost total dependence on the nurse. Nurse-patient communication is similar to that occurring in the operating room. The nurse monitors biologic communication signals and adjusts nursing care and medical treatment to facilitate the patients' optimum response to the trauma. The patients' first responses will be attempts to reorient themselves by touch to their surroundings. They will feel the bed rails, the sheets, and various parts of their body. They will open their eyes and survey the surroundings. Even in this situation, the needs for territoriality are great. The lack of acceptable space and territory is the most troublesome worry of patients in the recovery room period. They will often cover their head or turn away from other patients.

As patients begin to return to consciousness, their first questions will likely be "Was it cancer?" "Did they get it all?" "Did they remove my breast?" "Do I have a colostomy?" Evasive answers are not particularly helpful. Brief, truthful responses are more desirable. However, some answers are not known, and telling the patients that they have cancer is usually considered the physician's responsibility.

Patients recovering from anesthesia fade in and out of consciousness. They do not usually remember what they are told. They will repeat the same question, even after they are told the answer. If they are not told, they may plead, asking the question louder and louder. Nurses who are uncomfortable with relaying the diagnosis of cancer often have difficulty dealing with this situation. Avoidance strategies may begin: the patient will be discouraged from talking; the nurse will monitor physical signs and quickly leave the bedside; and narcotics may be used more liberally to keep the patient asleep. Because of the close working area provided for recovery room nurses, this situation can precipitate outbursts of anger between nurses and a temporary breakdown of nursing teamwork, and can decrease quality of care throughout the unit.

The surgeon may take advantage of the patients' lack of recall as they recover from anesthesia by informing them of the diagnosis at this point and not repeating the information after consciousness has completely returned. This is a strategy used to avoid dealing with the emotional response to the diagnosis. If the recovery room nurse does not tell the surgical unit nurses that the surgeon has told the patient of the diagnosis, they may never know that the patient has been informed and a conspiracy of silence may begin.

Physical care in the recovery room will include the usual coughing, turning, and deep breathing. This will be facilitated by effective preoperative teaching. These lessons seem to remain on the surface of the patients' thinking, even though the patients have not completely returned to consciousness. Those patients who have learned the importance of these procedures and have chosen to participate in this por-

tion of their care will usually be very cooperative, in spite of their semiconscious state.

Because of the increased risk of thrombophlebitis for the cancer patient, leg exercises in the recovery room are very important. Since cancer surgery is often radical, increased bleeding is likely to occur. Dressing checks are important, as are pulse and blood pressure monitoring. Some surgeons now leave orders for the patient to stand by the bedside periodically while in the recovery room. This can promote favorable physiologic responses to the trauma and a more rapid postoperative recovery. Extremely radical surgical procedures on a patient whose preoperative physical condition was poor may require that the patient receive treatment in an intensive surgical care unit for several days after surgery.

Nursing care of the family during and immediately after the operation has usually been inadequate. Often, the only contact that the family members have is with the surgeon. They may be told of the diagnosis of cancer and then left to deal with their feelings alone. They are usually in a strange area of the hospital with little privacy and may be afraid to leave the area to seek privacy or familiar surroundings. Their only support may come from volunteers and other family members. Operating room and recovery room nurses have little time to spend interacting with families. Their focus is on the patient. Recovery room nurses often perceive the family as a necessary nuisance. When visiting time arrives, the nurses withdraw from the patients and interact very little with family members.

Within the current hospital structure, it is difficult to imagine an alternative that would allow provision of adequate nursing care to families during this time. Social workers can assist to some extent, but they do not provide nursing care. Nurses need to work in coordination with social workers without abdicating their responsibilities as nurses. Nurses must never provide physical care only, leaving the psychosocial care to others; it is not possible to provide holistic care in such a manner.

The return of the patient to the hospital

room is a relief to both patient and family. They are in more familiar surroundings again, and the return is interpreted to mean that all is currently going well. Postoperative care of the cancer patient is little different from the care of any surgical patient. As it does with surgical patients, the quality of nursing care makes considerable difference in the speed and completeness of recovery.

Nurses often feel sorry for the patient who has just been diagnosed as having cancer. Because of the emotional trauma that the patient is experiencing, nurses may not be as aggressive as they should be in insisting on coughing, turning, deep breathing, exercising, ambulation, baths, bed-making, and taking fluids. This is not physiologically or psychologically healthy for the patient. The patient and family can interpret this type of care to be a result of a hopeless situation. The nurses may be neglecting the patient as part of an avoidance strategy. To some extent patients may be grateful to be left alone, but they will not recover as rapidly from surgery, and the risk of complications increases.

The complications most likely to occur in cancer patients are infection and thrombophlebitis. Good handwashing techniques are important in avoiding transmission of nosocomial infections. Postoperative cancer patients should *not* be placed in Fowler's position. This position is the most comfortable, but it limits patient movement in the bed and allows pooling of blood in the pelvis and lower legs. (See Fig. 7–3.) This venous stasis increases the risk of thrombophlebitis and pulmonary embolus.

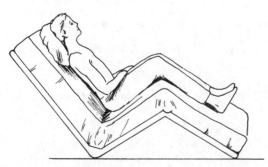

Figure 7–3. Pooling of blood with patient in Fowler's position.

After bowel motility has returned, adequate nutrition should be encouraged. The relationship between good nutrition and recovering from surgery should be explained to the patients in terms meaningful to them.

The diagnosis of cancer or the extent of disease may not be known for several days after surgery when the pathology tissue study is completed. At this point, sometimes the surgeon will stop by the patient's room, announce that the pathology report is back and that the patient does have cancer or that it has spread to the lymph nodes, and then hurry away. Often, the nurses do not even know the patient has been told. They simply walk in the room and discover a patient in an emotional crisis. If the nurses do not know how to handle this, they may also leave hurriedly, leaving the patient and sometimes the family to cope with the diagnosis with little outside support.

The desirable scenario in this situation is that the surgeon and the nurse collaborate. The surgeon tells the nurse that he or she is going to inform the patient and asks the nurse to come along. The surgeon sits down with both the patient and family, explains the results of the pathology study, and discusses future treatment. The patient and family feel free to ask questions and express their feelings. When the surgeon leaves, the nurse remains for a while longer, allowing further expression of feelings. Touching and eye contact are used therapeutically. Thereafter, the nurse will come to the room frequently to provide support and express caring.

Because of the shock of a diagnosis of cancer, patients and families often do not hear all that the surgeon says. If nurses are present, they can repeat the information as needed. This must be done patiently and kindly. The patient cannot honestly remember. Only gradually will the reality of the situation break through the shock and denial and become a part of the patient's world.

A diagnosis of cancer has a marked impact on self-image. If additionally the surgery has been mutilating in some way, self-image problems can be serious. The patient will carefully watch the nurse's face for signs of revulsion, disgust, or rejection. The patient will have difficulty looking at the surgical site, but needs to be encouraged to gradually do so. These patients may feel relatively secure in the hospital environment, but may be afraid to leave the hospital and be exposed to the sometimes harsh reaction of society in general. Family members often have strong reactions to mutilating surgery. They may refuse to look at the site and sometimes may avoid touching the patient. They may cope fairly well when the patient is hospitalized, but may experience increased difficulty when the patient returns home.

Discharge planning is very important for the cancer patient and family. Many of the problems they face will occur after discharge, when there is little opportunity for nursing care. Many nurses have little understanding of the magnitude of problems that cancer patients face. Discharge from the hospital is equated with success by the nurse. Although intellectually nurses may know otherwise, they sometimes believe that the patients "all lived happily ever after" because they seldom see the patient again.

Upon discharge, cancer patients often need referral to a home health care agency. The American Cancer Society can provide volunteer visitors from their programs — Reach to Recovery, the Ostomy Association, or Can Surmount. Supplies for mastectomies, colostomies, and tracheostomies are often available free of charge, as are dressings. Hospital beds, wheel chairs, and other equipment may often be obtained free from the local American Cancer Society chapter.

It would be helpful if hospital nurses would encourage patients and families to call if problems occur after discharge. Patients often have minor problems after they leave the hospital, which can be easily answered over the phone. If the hospital is a comprehensive community cancer center, a clinical nurse specialist in oncology may be available for contact after discharge. If the patient is to receive chemotherapy or radiotherapy in an outpatient clinic associated with the hospital, it is helpful for nurses to assist the patient and family in making contact with the nurses on these units before discharge. Nurse-to-nurse communication and sharing of the nursing history and physical examination and the nursing care plan facilitate continuity of care.

BIBLIOGRAPHY

1. Abeloff, M.: Psychologic aspects of the management of primary and metastatic breast cancer. In *Breast Cancer*, ed. by A. Montague, C. W. Stonesifer, L. Geary, and E. Lewison. Alan R. Liss, Inc., New York, 1977.
2. Allison, S., et al.: The importance of energy source and the significance of insulin in counteracting the catabolic response to injury. In *Metabolism and the Response to Injury*, ed. by A. W. Wilkinson and D. Cuthbertson. Year Book Medical Publishers, Inc., Chicago, 1976.
3. Bahnson, C.: Psychologic and emotional issues in cancer: the psychotherapeutic care of the cancer patient. *Seminars in Oncology*. 2:293–309, 1975.
4. Blues, K.: A framework for nurses providing care to laryngectomy patients. *Cancer Nursing*. 1:441–445, 1978.
5. Buls, J. G., et al.: Women's attitudes to mastectomy for breast cancer. *Medical Journal of Australia*. 2:336–338, 1976.
6. Byrne, N.: Critical care of the thoracic surgical patient. *Cancer Nursing*. 1:135–142, 1978.
7. Carlson, L.: Surgical approaches to cancer management. In *Dynamics of Oncology Nursing*, ed. by P. K. Burkhalter and D. L. Donley. McGraw-Hill Book Co., New York, 1978.
8. Cimprich, B., et al.: A preoperative teaching program for the thoracotomy patient. *Cancer Nursing*. 1:35–40, 1978.
9. Cuthbertson, D. D.: Surgical metabolism: historical and evolutionary aspects. In *Metabolism and the Response to Injury*, ed. by A. W. Wilkinson and D. Cuthbertson. Year Book Medical Publishers, Inc., Chicago, 1976.
10. Davies, J.: Aetiology and treatment of disorders of fat metabolism. In *Metabolism and the Response to Injury*, ed. by A. W. Wilkinson and D. Cuthbertson. Year Book Medical Publishers, Inc., Chicago, 1976.
11. DeVita, V., et al.: Combination versus single agent chemotherapy: a review of the basis for selection of drug treatment of cancer. *Cancer*. 35:98–110, 1975.
12. Fell, G., et al.: The importance of zinc and other essential elements after injury. In *Metabolism and the Response to Injury*, ed. by A. W. Wilkinson and D. Cuthbertson. Year Book Medical Publishers, Inc., Chicago, 1976.
13. Fisher, B.: The changing role of surgery in the

treatment of cancer. In *Cancer: A Comprehensive Treatise*, ed. by F. F. Becker. Plenum Press, New York, 1977.

14. Fleck, A.: The influence of the nature, severity and environmental temperature on the response to injury. In *Metabolism and the Response to Injury*, ed. by A. W. Wilkinson and D. Cuthbertson. Year Book Medical Publishers, Inc., Chicago, 1976.

15. Genzdilov, A., et al.: The role of stress factors in the postoperative course of patients with rectal cancer. *Journal of Surgical Oncology.* 9:517–523, 1977.

16. Gritsman, J.: About oncological operations. In *Cancer: Pathophysiology, Etiology, and Management,* ed. by L. C. Kruse, J. L. Reese, and L. K. Hart. C. V. Mosby Co., St. Louis, 1979.

17. Guthrie, T., et al.: Surgical nursing intervention in patients with hematologic malignancies: an overview. *Cancer Nursing.* 2:353–358, 1979.

18. Hofland, S.: Post mastectomy lymphedema: a study of incidence and etiological factors. *Proceedings – Fifth Annual Congress of the Oncology Nursing Society.* A 68, p. 50, 1980.

19. Johnson, J., et al.: Sensory information, instruction in a coping strategy and recovery from surgery. *Research in Nursing and Health.* 1:4–17, 1978.

20. Kinney, J.: Surgical hypermetabolism and nitrogen metabolism. In *Metabolism and the Response to Injury,* ed. by A. W. Wilkinson and D. Cuthbertson. Year Book Medical Publishers, Inc., Chicago, 1976.

21. Kinney, J.: Surgical diagnosis, patterns of energy, weight and tissue change. In *Metabolism and the Response to Injury,* ed. by A. W. Wilkinson and D. Cuthbertson. Year Book Medical Publishers, Inc., Chicago, 1976.

22. Kuhn, T.: *The Structure of Scientific Revolutions.* University of Chicago Press, Chicago, 1970.

23. Lazare, E.: Changing attitudes in the management of cancer of the breast. *Surgery.* 84:441–447, 1978.

24. Levenson, S.: Influence of injury on vitamin metabolism. In *Metabolism and the Response to Injury,* ed. by A. W. Wilkinson and D. Cuthbertson. Year Book Medical Publishers, Inc., Chicago, 1976.

25. Levenson, S.: Nutrition. In *Fundamentals of Wound Management,* ed. by T. K. Hunt and J. E. Dunphy. Appleton-Century-Crofts, New York, 1979.

26. Luckmann, J. and K. C. Sorensen: *Medical-Surgical Nursing: A Psychophysiologic Approach.* W. B. Saunders Co., Philadelphia, 1980.

27. Marcinek, M.: Stress in the surgical patient. *American Journal of Nursing.* 77:1809–1811, 1977.

28. Meakins, J.: Sepsis in surgical patients. *Hospital Topics.* 56:36–37, 1978.

29. Morris, T., et al.: Psychological and social adjustment to mastectomy. *Cancer.* 40:2381–2387, 1977.

30. Nealon, T., et al.: Surgical principles. In *Clinical Oncology,* ed. by J. Horton and G. Hill. W. B. Saunders Co., Philadelphia, 1977.

31. Patterson, W., et al.: Surgical oncology at the crossroads. In *Cancer: Pathophysiology, Etiology and Management,* ed. by L. C. Kruse, J. L. Reese, and L. K. Hart. C. V. Mosby Co., St. Louis, 1979.

32. Peacock, E. E. and W. Van Winkle: *Wound Repair.* W. B. Saunders Co., Philadelphia, 1976.

33. Rudolph, B.: Lymphedema following a radical mastectomy. *Oncology Nursing Forum.* 6:13–16, 1979.

34. Schain, W.: Prophylaxis, therapy and rehabilitation for the psychosocial concerns of breast cancer patients: a stage related approach. *Breast.* 4:23–27, 1978.

35. Schneider, W.: Nutrition in head and neck cancer: nursing implications. *Oncology Nursing Forum.* 6:5–11, 1979.

36. Sission, G.: The philosophy underlying the treatment of recurrent cancer of the head and neck. In *Cancer: Pathophysiology, Etiology and Management,* ed. by L. C. Kruse, J. H. Reese, and L. K. Hart. C. V. Mosby Co., St. Louis, 1979.

37. Stoner, H.: Changes in the central nervous system and their role in the metabolic response to injury. In *Metabolism and the Response to Injury,* ed. by A. W. Wilkinson and D. Cuthbertson. Year Book Medical Publishers, Inc., Chicago, 1976.

38. Thomas, S.: Breast cancer: the psychosocial issues. *Cancer Nursing.* 1:53–60, 1978.

39. Todd, A., et al.: Ego defenses and affects in women with breast symptoms: a preliminary measurement paradigm. *Journal of Medical Psychology.* 51:177–189, 1978.

40. Turns, D.: Psychological problems of patients with head and neck cancer. *Journal of Prosthetic Dentistry.* 39:68–73, 1978.

41. Wilkins, S., Jr.: Current concepts in cancer surgery. In *Cancer: Pathophysiology, Etiology and Management,* ed. by L. C. Kruse, J. L. Reese, and L. K. Hart. C. V. Mosby Co., St. Louis, 1979.

42. Wirsching, M.: Results of psychosocial adjustment to longterm colostomy. *Psychotherapeutic Psychosomatics.* 26:245–256, 1975.

8

Radiotherapy

INTRODUCTION

Radiation is viewed by health professionals and lay people alike as mysterious, magical, and frightening. Radiation is associated with burning, mutilation, sterility, pain, loss of social acceptance, and death.[1, 37] Individuals may consider the treatment itself to be like a pagan ritual of sacrifice.[25] Many people think that the person receiving external radiation is radioactive and can cause harm to others if close contact is made. Radiation is so generally thought of as being given only to those who are going to die of cancer that it may be perceived as the signal of a death sentence. These factors make some patients more afraid of x-ray therapy than they are of the disease itself.[3]

Radiation therapy for cancer began shortly after the discovery of x-rays at the turn of the century. The first type of cancer treated with radiation was skin cancer. Since that time, research has greatly expanded the knowledge and development of radiation as an effective treatment modality for cancer. The field of radiotherapy is now so complex that it requires a thorough understanding of physics, radiobiology, and medicine. Physicians qualified in this field are called radiation oncologists or radiotherapists. These physicians have had education and training beyond the M.D. in radiotherapy, have passed an extensive examination, and are certified in therapeutic radiology by the American Board of Radiology.

Many people confuse these specialists with radiologists, physicians whose field of knowledge and practice is in the area of diagnostic radiology. Radiologists specialize in the use of radiant energy such as x-rays and scans in the diagnosis of abnormalities. Earlier in the century when the field of radiotherapy was less developed, radiologists administered radiation therapy. Sometimes the radiologists left the actual treatment to inadequately trained technicians.[1] As treatment became more complex and precise, requiring much greater knowledge, fewer radiologists continued to give radiation therapy.[21]

Nurses often have a minimal background in physics and mathematics and find radiotherapy concepts difficult to understand. Basic nursing education programs explain safety precautions and nursing care, but offer little about the physics of radiation therapy or its biologic consequences. This is generally viewed as "nice to know, but not necessary" information. With this knowledge, however, nursing interventions can be more intelligently planned. The nurse who plans to specialize in the field of oncology needs to make the extra effort required to become more thoroughly acquainted with radiotherapy.

HOW RADIATION THERAPY WORKS

Physics

The field of radiation physics has a number of commonly used terms that make up its technical vocabulary. An understanding of these terms is essential in order to communicate with those practicing in the field of radiation oncology or to understand the literature. (See Table 8–1.)

Types of Ionizing Rays

Ionizing rays are a type of electromagnetic or particulate energy. The rays differ

Table 8-1. Terms Used in Radiotherapy

Curie (Ci) – a unit of measure that indicates a specific number of radioactive disintegrations occurring in a specific unit of time.

Decay – the destruction of a radioactive substance as a result of the constant loss of matter and energy through emissions it gives out.

Electromagnetic radiation – x-rays and gamma rays.

Electron – a particle with negative charge that revolves around the nucleus of an atom.

eV (electron volt) – a measure of radiation energy.

Half-life – the length of time that it takes for radioactivity to decay to one-half of its original activity.

Ion – an atom that has an electrical charge. Ions can be created when electrons are released from their orbit in the atom.

Ionization – the process of supplying energy to release the electron from its orbit.

Ionizing radiation – all electromagnetic and particulate radiation that can produce ions, either indirectly or directly, as it passes through matter.

Isotopes – atoms of an element that differ in the number of neutrons in the nucleus and therefore differ in atomic weight. Most of these elements are stable.

Microcurie (μCi) – 1/1,000,000 of a curie.

Millicurie (mCi) – 1/1000 of a curie.

mRe (milligrams of radium equivalent) – the therapeutic strength of a source compared with an equivalent amount of radium.

Neutron – an electrically neutral or uncharged particle that makes up part of the nucleus of the atom.

Particulate radiation – alpha particles, beta particles, neutrons, or protons.

Proton – a positively charged particle that makes up part of the nucleus of the atom.

rad (radiation absorbed dose) – a measure of the absorbed dose of ionizing energy; the amount of radiation absorbed by the tissue.

Radioactivity – the emission of radiation that accompanies nuclear disintegration.

Radioisotope – an unstable isotope that emits radiation.

Relative biological effectiveness (RBE) – the ratio of the number of cells killed by a dose of cobalt measured against an unknown radiation.

rem (roentgen equivalent man) – the amount of radiation that has the same RBE as 1 rad of x-rays.

Roentgen (R) – the amount of radiation in a beam of rays measured in the air.

Specific activity – the number of curies in each gram of radioactive material.

---

in the size and shape of the particle or in their wave lengths, frequencies, and velocities.[33] This is really not as mysterious as it seems. These waves or rays are similar to radio waves or light rays; however, ionizing waves have much shorter wave lengths. The particles in the waves are elements of atoms such as electrons, protons, or neutrons. Atoms are essentially electric in nature and electricity is essentially atomic in structure.[43] Electrons are the basic units of electricity. In fact, an electric current is basically a stream of electrons.

There are several kinds of ionizing rays.

Alpha (α) Particles. Alpha particles are large particles made of two protons and two neutrons with positive charges. These particles can be easily blocked with a piece of paper and can travel only a short distance in the air. They cannot penetrate the skin, but they are intensely ionizing for the short distance they travel. Alpha particles can be damaging to tissues if a substance containing them is absorbed. Because of this, alpha particles are not used in radiotherapy.

Beta (β) Particles. Beta particles are fast-moving electrons. They are more penetrating than alpha particles, but can be blocked by aluminum. They can travel only

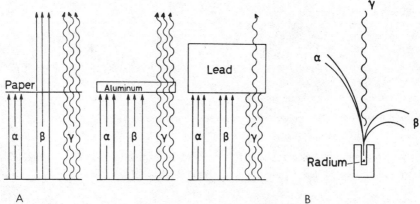

Figure 8–1. *A*, Schematic representation of the penetrating power of alpha, beta, and gamma radiations. *B*, Deflection in a magnetic field. (From Young, M. E. J.: *Radiological Physics*, 2nd ed. London: H. K. Lewis and Co., Ltd., 1967. Used by permission.)

a short distance in the soft tissues of the body. Iodine-131, gold-198, and phosphorus-32 are beta emitters.

Gamma (γ) Rays. Gamma rays are a form of electromagnetic energy and have the same diffusion characteristics as light. Gamma rays can penetrate more deeply into body tissues and thus are of greater value in treating many cancers. Gamma rays are the same as x-rays. When emitted from radioactive substances such as radium, they are called gamma rays; when generated by electrical machines, they are called x-rays. (See Fig. 8–1.)

Neutrons. Neutrons are particles that have no electric charge. Neutrons can be emitted as by-products of atomic reactors. Californium-252 is a neutron source that is being used in interstitial or intracavitary therapy.

Negative Pi-mesons (π⁻). Negative pi-mesons are negatively charged particles. They are 273 times larger than electrons.[33]

Radiation Equipment

The equipment used to administer external radiation therapy has become more complex as engineering and physics, working together, have improved the capacity of radiation therapy. Some of the more common types of equipment are described below.

Orthovoltage X-ray Machine. This machine consists of a glass vacuum tube with a filament that, when heated, releases accelerated electrons. These electrons hit a tungsten target, and x-rays are produced. (See Fig. 8–2.) X-rays are usually in the 200 to 400 kvp range. This is fairly low-voltage radiation. Because of the low-voltage doses, these x-rays do not penetrate deeply into the body. Maximum ionization occurs at the skin level, causing rapidly developing skin damage even with moderate doses of radiation.[33] For many years, this was the machine commonly used to give radiation treatments.

Cesium-137 and Cobalt-60 Teletherapy Units. These machines have a shielded head that houses a radioactive source, a collimating device, an electric circuit, and an off-on system. The radiation is stored in these machines all of the time. The off-on system simply provides an opening that allows the rays to escape from the housing. The rays are aimed in a specific direction by the collimating device. The radiation from these machines is more penetrating than that from the orthovoltage machines, causes less skin damage, and can reach deeper tissues.[33] The half-life of cobalt-60 is 5 years; thus the radiation source for the machine has to be replaced every few years. As the cobalt-60 decays, the treatment time must be lengthened to administer the same amount of radiation.

Linear Accelerators. These machines produce radiation from electricity. They do not have a radiation source inside of them. Linear accelerators can produce either high energy electrons or x-rays. The beam penetrates fairly deeply within the body, and the maximum dose is below the skin

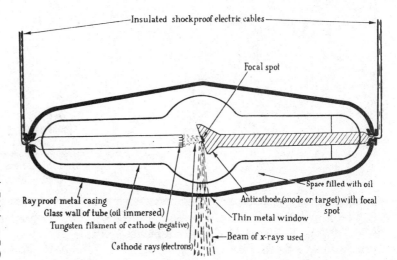

Insulated shockproof electric cables

Focal spot

Space filled with oil

Anticathode,(anode or target)with focal spot

Ray proof metal casing

Glass wall of tube (oil immersed)

Thin metal window

Tungsten filament of cathode (negative)

Cathode rays (electrons)

Beam of x-rays used

Figure 8-2. Schematic diagram of an x-ray tube. (From Walter, J.: *Cancer and Radiotherapy: A Short Guide for Nurses and Medical Students.* New York: Churchill Livingston Inc., 1977. Used by permission.)

surface, thereby decreasing skin damage. The dose is more homogeneous than that from the cobalt-60 unit, since there is no radioactive source to decay.[33]

Betatron. The betatron accelerates electrons, which can hit a target, producing x-rays. It is different from conventional machines because activity takes place in a circular tube. This machine generates high energy x-ray beams with the point of maximum ionization 4 cm below the skin. The betatron is excellent for radiating deep tumors. Its disadvantages are that it does not produce a lot of radiation and can radiate only a small space through a small portal.

Skin-Sparing Effect

Radiation rapidly loses energy when it enters body tissues, so that the tumor within the body does not receive the strongest dose of radiation. With the orthovoltage machine, the strongest dose was received by the skin. Thus the skin was the tissue most severely damaged from radiation. When skin damage became severe, radiation had to be discontinued.

In newer machines, the maximum amount of radiation occurs below the skin. This allows the patient to receive higher doses of radiation with less skin damage. Unless the tumor is shallow, however, the maximum dose of radiation still does not reach the tumor.

Effect of Radiation on Body Tissue Atoms

We often visualize radiation as a beam that travels directly from the machine through the body to the tumor. Actually, the beam is not a single source of energy, but a series of chain reactions. When the radiation beam strikes an atom, it frees electrons from that atom. This is ionization. The process of releasing those electrons requires energy; thus the radiation beam loses energy. The energy has been transferred to the newly released electrons. These freed electrons strike other nearby body atoms and cause further ionizations until their energy has been depleted. In this way, one single ionization disrupts many neighboring atoms. This process continues as the transfer of energy penetrates deeper into the body, eventually involving the atoms of the tumor. The disruption of atoms interferes with cellular function. It is believed that the greater the number of disrupted atoms in a cell, the greater the cell damage; although to some extent this will depend on what structures in the cell have been affected.

Dosimetry

Dosimetry is the measurement and calculation of radiation dosage. This calculation is an exact science, much more so than calculation of drug dosages. These calcula-

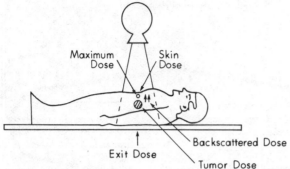

Figure 8–3. Examples of various types of doses commonly used in radiation therapy. See text for detailed information. (From Horton, J., and Hill, G. J. II: *Clinical Oncology.* Philadelphia: W. B. Saunders Co., 1977. Used by permission.)

tions have, in the past, been handwritten by a radiologic physicist. Calculation of the dose for one patient's therapy might require almost a day's work. Now, computers are being utilized for these calculations, allowing for much more complex treatment patterns and providing dosage patterns 2 to 3 minutes after entry of the data into the computer.

The radiation dosage to various parts of the irradiated site will vary considerably. Radiation to each part must be carefully calculated to ensure adequate tumor dose and to avoid overexposure of normal tissues. In order to do this, the dose is examined in several ways. (See Fig. 8–3.)

Air dose is used for radiation below 400 kvp. It indicates the number of roentgens delivered at a given distance measured in the air.[33]

Backscatter dose is the amount of radiation caused by electrons released by irradiated body tissue atoms, which move backward to the skin surface.[33]

Surface dose is the amount of radiation absorbed by the superficial layers of the skin. This dose is calculated only if orthovoltage equipment is used.[33]

Maximum dose usually occurs several millimeters below the skin surface. This is the point at which the maximum number of ionizations occurs. This dose is expressed in rads.[33]

Central axis per cent depth dose expresses the distribution of radiation in body tissues as a percentage of the surface or maximum dose.[33]

Tumor air ratio is the ratio of the absorbed dose to the dose that would have been measured at that same point in free air.[33]

Tumor dose is the minimal amount of radiation absorbed in or around the tumor.[33]

Integral dose is the total absorbed radiation delivered to all body tissues during radiation exposure.[33]

Radiation Biology

The primary purpose of radiation therapy is to kill the cancer cells and avoid damage to normal tissues. However, this is only an ideal. The mechanism by which radiation kills cells and damages tissues is not completely known, although theories explaining it abound. Studies are being conducted to increase knowledge of this process.

Cell Damage

Radiation kills cells by causing damage to them. Many people think that cell death happens at the time of radiation. Actually, very few cells are directly killed by the radiation.[43] The damage may be severe enough, though, that cell death will occur hours or days later. Several different kinds of damage may take place.

Lethal damage occurs when the cell loses its ability to divide. This may not be immediately evident since cells may continue to divide as many as five or six cell divisions after radiation. Eventually, however, all of the cell progeny will die.[33] Although the cell death may occur within hours of radiation, it may not happen for days, weeks, or even years — particularly if the cell is a slowly dividing normal tissue cell. Some cells are "sterilized" so that, although they continue to live, they never again attempt to enter mitosis. This is called premature aging. Cancer cells that are "sterilized" are harmless, since they cannot reproduce.[43]

Potentially lethal damage is less severe, and the cell may be able to recover from the damage. However, altering the environment (by drugs, for example) will interfere with repair and the cell will die.[33]

Sublethal damage can be repaired by the cell, but the cell displays a slowed growth rate.[33]

Indirect effects of the radiation can also cause cell death. The local blood supply may be damaged, cutting off nutrients and causing cells to die. Damaged cells may be weakened to such an extent that the body's immune responses can destroy them.[43]

Sites of Damage in the Cell

For a number of years, it has been thought that deoxyribonucleic acid (DNA) damage caused cell death after radiation. Now the cell membrane, in addition to DNA, is thought to be a fatal target site. It is not known whether a single hit will cause cell death or whether it requires multiple hits of target sites.

In addition to direct hits on the cells, radiation causes ionization in the water surrounding the cells. The ionization of the water may result in the production of H^+, OH^-, $H_2O_2^-$, and HO_2^-. Some of these substances will enter the cell and cause further metabolic interactions. These metabolic alterations have not been clearly identified and cannot be predicted; however, they may contribute to the cell damage.[25, 33]

Hypoxic Cells

Within a solid tumor, some of the malignant cells are hypoxic. This does not occur in normal cell populations. It is believed that the hypoxic cells are a result of rapid cell division that outpaces the development of new blood vessels.

Hypoxic cells are much more resistant to radiation than well-oxygenated cells, for reasons not yet understood. Because normal cells are well oxygenated, they are more easily damaged by radiation than tumor cells. As long as there are hypoxic cells in the tumor, some malignant cells will escape destruction by radiation and allow tumor regrowth.

Many strategies have been designed to oxygenate the malignant cells so that a larger proportion could be destroyed by each radiation treatment. Attempts to provide adequate oxygenation to all tumor cells just prior to radiation have been relatively unsuccessful, although both hyperbaric oxygen and oxygen by inhalation have been attempted. Research suggests that vascular constriction secondary to the administration of oxygen may be preventing a more beneficial effect. Researchers continue to explore effective ways to accomplish adequate oxygenation of malignant cells.

Alteration of Tumor Kinetics

Impact on the Cell Cycle. Cells within the cell cycle that are exposed to radiation are delayed in their progress through the cycle (see Chapter 2). The greater the amount of radiation, the greater the delay. Cells accumulate in the G_2 phase and are blocked from entering mitosis. Cells that are in mitosis and the early S phase are more sensitive to radiation and are more likely to be destroyed. Therefore, the tumor population after radiation will have a greater number of cells in G_1 and G_2 phases.

The Repair Process. *Repair of sublethal injury* is believed to involve enzyme repair of damaged structures inside the cell. But cell contact with other cells and extracellular activities may also affect this process. If this is true, cancer cells would be at a disadvantage since they have little contact with the cells around them. Rapid repair within a few hours of radiation can occur, although repair of malignant cells seems to be slower than that of normal cells. Normal cells seem to have a greater capacity to repair sublethal damage than

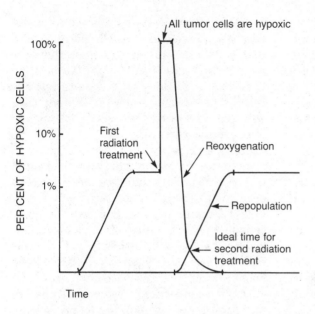

Time

Figure 8–4. The pattern of oxygenated and hypoxic cells during radiotherapy.

tumor cells.[12] Hypoxic cells and cells not in the cell cycle seem to have more difficulty repairing sublethal damage.

Repair of potentially lethal damage (PLD) seems to occur best in starved cells that are not in the cell cycle. Starved cells may be those most distant from tumor capillaries. It is possible that an adequate nutritional status promotes movement of the cell into the cell cycle before repair is complete. The cell would then be destroyed because repair was not complete at the time of mitosis.[12]

Slow repair requires at least 1 week and seems to be dependent on a delay in entry into the cell cycle. Slow repair may be a major factor in normal tissue survival from radiation.

Redistribution. As the damaged cells die and are carried away by body fluids, the remaining cells are redistributed within the tumor. Hypoxic and malnourished cells that have been distant from capillaries move to more favorable positions.

Reoxygenation. As cells are redistributed, they achieve a greater level of oxygenation and nutrition. These cells then enter the cell cycle at a more rapid rate. (See Fig. 8–4.)

Repopulation. Recruitment of cells into the cell cycle becomes greater in the tumor. The rate of movement through the cell cycle increases; thus tumor growth at this point is more rapid than before radia-

tion.[20] But tumor cells are also more susceptible to further radiation. As the tumor regrows, hypoxic cells reappear and sensitivity to radiation again diminishes.[12]

Response to a Single Dose of Radiation

Radiation is administered to patients in fractionated doses. However, in order to study the responses of various types of cells to radiation, animals have been exposed to one measured dose of radiation. Studies reveal that most cells die at the time of mitosis after radiation. One exception to this is lymphocytes, which can die rapidly after radiation without attempting mitosis. The death of other cells, particularly those in normal tissues, is more dependent on the rate of mitosis. After the administration of 1000 rads, radiation damage is expressed within 12 hours in the intestine, within 4 to 5 days in the skin, and many weeks later in tissues such as liver, lung, and kidney.[12] Cells that do not die as a consequence of the radiation are slower in moving through the cell cycle or suffer a loss of proliferative capacity.

Effects of Radiation on the Immune Response

The behavior of a tumor is very greatly influenced by host-tumor interactions. Any treatment that alters the tumor may alter the host responses. Any treatment that affects the normal tissues of the body in a way that alters their interaction with the malignant cells may cause changes in the tumor. However, studying these changes is difficult because of their complexities. Specific and nonspecific immunity and cellular and humoral immunity must all be considered; each one may have very different radiation responses. The type of radiation, the dose, and the previous immune response of the patient will affect the immune changes. Studies in this area are limited and results are often contradictory.[20]

THE EFFECTIVENESS OF RADIOTHERAPY

Radiosensitivity

According to Abramson, "An organ or type of cell or a tumor is deemed radiosensitive if it is quickly destroyed by moderate doses of radiation that are well tolerated by surrounding tissues."[1] The sensitivity of a tumor is usually similar to the sensitivity of the tissue of origin. Lymphoid tissue is the most radiosensitive in the body, followed by epithelial, gastrointestinal, and skin tissues. Vascular, connective, and nervous tissues are relatively radioresistant. The more anaplastic or undifferentiated a tumor is, the more sensitive it is to radiation.

Radiosensitivity is not the same as radiocurability. Radiosensitivity is certainly an important factor in radiocurability, but other variables (including cell type, size of the tumor, extent of its spread, and its vascular supply) also have an impact on the ability of radiation to destroy the tumor. All cancers can be destroyed by radiation if a large enough dose is given to a large enough area of the body. However, radiation doses are limited by the possibility of normal tissue destruction and the risk of death of the host. A delicate balance must be achieved by giving as much radiation as is possible to destroy tumor cells without causing irreparable damage to surrounding normal tissues. Destruction of normal tissue can make the treatment

worse than the disease. Some tissue damage always occurs with radiation, and there are always risks of severe complications that must be taken in the attempt to destroy the tumor. However, these risks must be minimized as much as possible.

Approaches to Radiation Therapy

Cure. The effectiveness of radiation therapy is dependent on a number of factors. In general, if the malignancy is to be cured, the tumor must be localized. Radiation can destroy local spread to the lymph nodes but will have no effect on distant metastases or small nests of malignant cells that may be undetectable at the time of treatment. Radiotherapy alone is not as effective with large tumors as it is with small tumors. With some specific types of very radiosensitive malignancies, radiotherapy is more effective than chemotherapy.

Adjuvant Therapy. Radiotherapy is being used less as a sole therapy than as an adjunct to other treatments. A tumor may be irradiated before surgery in order to shrink the tumor and destroy the rapidly proliferating cells on the surface of the tumor as well as the malignant cells that may have invaded lymph nodes or adjacent normal tissues. Some clinicians believe that this strategy increases the possibility of surgically removing the entire tumor.

Radiotherapy is also utilized after surgery in an attempt to prevent possible local lymphatic invasion by malignant cells. It is thought that this approach can maintain or increase cure rates without requiring extremely radical surgical approaches that may be mutilating and may interfere more with body functions.

Both radiotherapy and chemotherapy may be utilized at various stages in the treatment of a malignancy. This needs to be planned jointly by the radiotherapist and the chemotherapist at the time of institution of treatment. If this approach is planned, radiation is usually limited to small doses and very localized sites. Radiotherapy tends to permanently destroy some of the capacity of the bone marrow to produce blood cells. Limitation of the bone marrow reserve by radiotherapy alone would probably not seriously affect the patient. However, chemotherapy is temporarily very destructive to bone marrow. If the reserve capacity of the bone marrow has been reduced by radiotherapy, effective doses of chemotherapy may be contraindicated. Chemotherapy will also further increase the permanent chronic damage to the bone marrow, thereby diminishing bone marrow capability.[33]

On the other hand, a patient who is receiving chemotherapy and has decreased numbers of blood cells may not be a good candidate for radiotherapy. Some chemotherapy drugs greatly increase the response of both normal and malignant cells to radiotherapy. Although this effect is being studied to determine ways of more effectively destroying tumor cells, the effect on normal tissues can be very harmful.

Tumor Control. Radiotherapy may be utilized to control the growth of a malignancy, thus giving the patient added weeks or months of meaningful life. Radiotherapy can also decrease unpleasant symptoms that interfere with the quality of life or even shorten life. This approach may not necessarily prolong life, but it does provide the patient with a measure of comfort. This approach is used to treat obstructions, bone metastases, and pain from masses causing pressure on strategic sites such as nerves.

Treatment Effects

Tables showing cure rates from radiotherapy must be carefully qualified in terms of stage of disease and radiation dosage. (See Table 8–2.) It may be more meaningful to examine control rather than cure of the disease. Figure 8–5 describes the comparative levels of 80 per cent tumor control from various types of malignancies. The usual fractionated dose of radiation administered in the treatment of cancer ranges from 3500 to 7500 rads.[21]

Table 8–2. Five-Year Survival from Several Types of Cancer Treated with Radiotherapy*

Type or Site of Cancer	Approximate Representative 5-year Survival (%)		
	1950–1955	1970–1975	
Hodgkin's disease, all stages	35	60	
Early			80
Late			50
Cancer of cervix, all stages	50	60	
Stage I			90
Stage II			65
Stage III			40
Stage IV			10
Cancer of nasopharynx, all stages	30	60	
Stage T1			85
Stage T2			70
Stage T3			50
Stage T4			30
Cancer of breast, all stages	50	50	
Early			80
Late			20
Cancer of bladder, all stages	20	30	
Stage T1, T2			40
Stage T3			25
Stage T4			6
Cancer of prostate	10	60	
Brain tumors	20	30	
Testicular tumors			
Seminoma	–	90	
Teratoma	–	25	

*From Fowler, J. F., and Denekamp, J.: Radiation effects on normal tissue. In *Cancer: A Comprehensive Treatise*, edited by Becker, F. F. New York: Plenum Press, 1977. Used by permission.

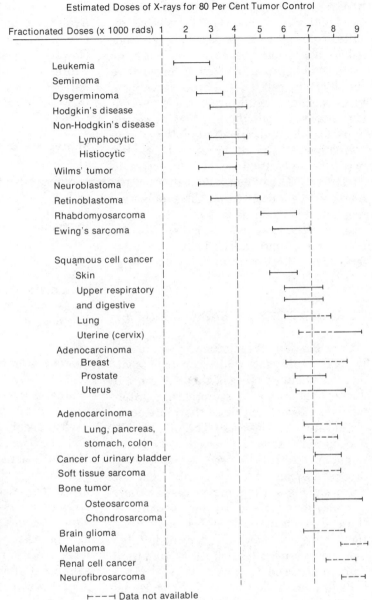

Figure 8–5. Rough estimate of fractionated doses necessary to achieve 80 per cent tumor control in relatively small tumors, in a variety of anatomical locations and histological types. Derived from available data and clinical experience. (From Horton, J., and Hill, G. J.: *Clinical Oncology.* Philadelphia: W. B. Saunders Co., 1977. Used by permission.)

New Approaches to Radiotherapy

Since the greatest problem in radiotherapy is the hypoxic cell, most new approaches are designed to more effectively destroy the hypoxic cell or to provide adequate oxygenation to it. Tailoring the fractionation schedule so that radiation treatments are given when reoxygenation is occurring is being attempted. This procedure is not presently an exact science, since it is not known when reoxygenation occurs in a specific tumor. However, changes are being attempted to improve tumor destruction and include changing the dose per fraction, giving multiple small fractions per day,[42] varying the size of the fraction, or using split course treatment.[20]

Another approach being used is treatment with high linear energy transfer (LET) radiation. High LET radiation produces a dense ionization that is especially effective in destroying hypoxic cells. This approach is still experimental and not available to most patients.[14, 17]

Methods are being attempted to improve

hypoxic cell oxygenation. Although previous studies have not shown effective results, hyperbaric oxygen is still being studied as a possible therapy.[20, 47] Chemicals are now being used to attempt to sensitize the hypoxic cell to radiotherapy. Some types of chemotherapy are being given concurrently with radiotherapy to increase the hypoxic cell's radiosensitivity.[2, 14, 20]

Another treatment being tried is hyperthermia. Heat alone is destructive to tumor cells. Use of heat and x-ray therapy increases cell destruction. The effectiveness of this treatment seems to be increased if the heat is administered about 1 hour after radiation. The heat may interfere with cell repair in tumor cells.[19, 27]

COMPLICATIONS OF RADIOTHERAPY

Complications of radiotherapy are usually divided into those that occur upon treatment (immediate effects), those that occur during or shortly after radiotherapy (intermediate effects), and those that may occur years later (late effects). The effects will depend on the radiation dosage, which fractionation schedule is used, which tissues are radiated, and whether whole organs or only portions of them are radiated. Many complications of radiotherapy, particularly those that only subtly affect body functions, have not been well identified. Table 8–3 shows some of the effects of radiation on normal tissue.

Radiation therapy is actually more destructive to normal cells than to malignant cells because of the high number of hypoxic cells in tumors. Normal cells have a greater capacity for repair, but some damage to normal cells is slow to manifest itself because highly differentiated cells have a very slow rate of mitosis. Therefore, damage to normal tissues can appear years after exposure to radiation.

The dose of radiation required to destroy a major portion of the tumor is dangerously close to the dose that will cause serious side effects. If the dose is increased by 10 per cent, the number of serious complications in patients will rise from 7 to 20 per cent.

This increased dose will also raise the number of cases in which local control of the tumor occurs from 59 to 69 per cent. However, most radiotherapists are not willing to administer doses that will cause patients more than a 5 to 10 per cent increase in serious complications.[15]

Immediate Effects

The most immediate reactions to radiation involve the mucous membranes, the skin, and the blood-forming tissues. The immediate effect resembles an inflammatory response, with increased vascularity, edema, and infiltration of leukocytes occurring.[9] The symptoms will depend on the site of radiation and may include mucositis, epidermitis, nausea, diarrhea, bone marrow depression, and fatigue.

Mucous Membranes

Mucositis will occur in any mucous membrane within the irradiated area: the oral cavity, esophagus, trachea, gastrointestinal tract, cervix, vaginal wall, or bladder. Mucositis usually begins after 2 to 3 weeks of fractionated radiotherapy. The mucous membrane will initially have increased redness, which will progress to yellowish-white patches. These patches will eventually become a pseudomembrane covering large areas of the mucosa. The mucous and salivary glands are inhibited. The patient may experience soreness, pain on swallowing, hoarseness, dryness, or loss of sense of taste if the related membrane is affected.

If the gastrointestinal tract is in the irradiated field, the patient may experience nausea, vomiting, or diarrhea. Because the gastrointestinal tract is very sensitive to radiation, gastrointestinal malignancies are not usually treated by radiation. If even small portions are in the field of radiation, tissue damage and symptoms will occur.

Radiation of the neck or thorax will often affect the esophagus, causing painful swallowing, dryness, and spasms. Abdominal irradiation is frequently associated with

Table 8–3. Radiation Effects on Normal Tissue*

Organ	Transient During Therapy	Early Injury	Late Injury
Small intestine	Diarrhea, colic, malabsorption	6 mo–1 yr, obstruction	1–11 yr, obstruction may require surgery
Colon and rectum	Diarrhea, colic	6–12 mo, diarrhea, necrosis	2–3 yr, slow stenosis, fibrosis, and induration
Stomach	Anorexia plus nausea, reduced acidity	1–2 mo, superficial ulcers	Chronic atrophic gastritis
Esophagus	Pain on swallowing	–	1–5 yr, stenosis
Oral mucosa	Mucositis, moist desquamation	2–3 mo, atrophy	6 mo–1 yr, fibrosis 1–5 yr+, ulcers, deep necrosis, atrophy
Skin	Erythema, desquamation	6–8 wk, desquamation plus healing pigmentation	6 mo–5 yr, atrophy, ulcers, deep fibrosis
Lung	Pneumonitis at end	0–3 mo, pneumonitis	8 mo–2 yr, fibrosis
Kidney	None	6–12 mo, nephrosclerosis	1.5–>3 yr, chronic radiation nephritis with vascular sclerosis
Liver	Changed liver function (rose bengal scan)	–	7 mo–1 yr, changed liver function
Ureters	None	–	1–2 yr, fibrosis and obstruction
Bladder	Cystitis	–	7–8 mo, contraction – 1 yr+, atrophic ulcers
Spinal cord	None unless tumor present	Edema, compression, pain if tumor is present	Transverse myelitis: 6–12 mo, reversible 1–2 yr, paraplegia
Brain	Edema	6 mo–1 yr, reversible effects	1–2 yr, necrosis
Heart	None	–	1–2 yr, pericarditis
Major blood vessels	None	Arterial fibrosis	Seldom seen unless involved with tumor
Eyes	None	–	>2 yr, cataract even at low doses

*From Fowler, J. F., and Denekamp, J.: Radiation effects on normal tissue. In *Cancer: A Comprehensive Treatise,* edited by Becker, F. F. New York: Plenum Press, 1977. Used by permission.

nausea, which is usually low grade. However, greater exposures can cause vomiting, abdominal cramping, and diarrhea. This can lead to electrolyte imbalances, dehydration, and weight loss.

Pelvic irradiation frequently damages both the bladder and the rectum. Dysuria, accompanied by pain and urinary frequency, may occur. Damage to the rectum may cause irritation, tenesmus, and passage of mucus and blood.[43] Mucositis begins to decrease during treatment and is fully healed several weeks after treatment is completed.[21]

Skin

Epidermitis or radiodermatitis usually begins about 2 weeks after the onset of treatment. It reaches its peak of severity near the completion of treatment. The reaction of skin to radiation is often used as a measure of the sensitivity of other normal tissues. Skin reactions were more severe when orthovoltage radiation was being used, and treatments sometimes had to be discontinued because of the severe damage to skin. With the advent of megavoltage, which produces its maximum dosage below the skin, this has not been such a problem.

Skin reaction is an inflammatory response that results from the breakdown of basal cells in the epidermis. The reaction is divided into four stages or degrees of severity.[43]

First Degree.   This is called the epilation dose because of its destructive effect on hair roots. Hairs become loose and fall out spontaneously. The hair regrows in 2 to 3 months.[43]

Second Degree. This is characterized by a bright red erythema limited to the irradiated area. The sweat glands are inhibited and may be permanently destroyed. The hair falls out and may or may not grow back. After the reaction subsides, there is often a permanent residual pigmentation. The patient may experience itching and a temporary dry peeling of the skin may occur; this is called dry desquamation.[43]

Third Degree. The erythema at this stage is purplish and deeper. Blisters will form, coalesce, and burst, forming superficial ulcers that exude serum. This is called moist desquamation. If the skin is left exposed, a scab will form. Healing is rapid and usually complete in 2 to 3 weeks. Hair loss is permanent and sweat glands are destroyed.[43]

Fourth Degree. This is classified as radiation burn or acute necrosis. Technically, it should not occur, because it is the consequence of an overdose. At this stage the erythema is very dark, blisters are deep and involve the whole skin, not just the epidermis. Blisters may be deeper than the skin. The entire surface eventually sloughs and may be very painful. Healing may occur, but it is a long and uncertain process because blood vessels in the area have been destroyed.[43] Areas of the skin folds often have more severe reactions than the rest of the skin. The skin in the groin, under the arm, and in the folds of the obese abdomen may have an erythema with moist desquamation.[9]

Blood-Forming Tissues

Bone marrow and lymphoid tissues are highly radiosensitive. The greatest effect is on the parent cells of lymphocytes, leukocytes, and platelets. Red blood cells are less sensitive. The effect on the blood count varies with the size of the area being irradiated. There is usually a decrease in total white count and in platelets. If the field under radiation is very large, the extent of treatment may be limited by the effect on the blood counts. Treatment may be stopped for a few days or completely discontinued. The lower limits of the cell counts are a matter of medical judgment. As a rough guide, Walter considers 2000 white blood cells or 80,000 platelets to be danger signals.[43] When the count drops below these points, there is a greater risk of infection and hemorrhage. It must be remembered that the blood count will continue to drop for a period of time after radiation is stopped.[1]

General Body Reaction

Generalized symptoms that commonly appear during radiation treatment are fatigue, weakness, headache, nausea, anorexia, and emotional depression. These symptoms are more frequently discussed in nursing literature than in medical literature. The etiology of these symptoms is not well understood. One suggested cause of generalized symptoms is the rapid breakdown of cells destroyed by the radiation. Cell breakdown would release toxic metabolites and end products that accumulate faster than they can be excreted.[18] Walter suggests that these chemicals may act as toxic foreign proteins, causing some degree of shock.[43] Others suggest that it is an attempt by the body to restore homeostasis or that it is a result of impaired aerobic mitochondrial metabolism.[18] Some authors believe the generalized body reaction is primarily an emotional response. However, Haylock and associates have conducted a study of fatigue levels reported by patients receiving localized radiation. Fatigue levels were lowest on Sundays, when radiation was not administered. Fatigue levels tended to rise throughout the treatment period and were highest toward the end of treatment.[18] Welch has found that nausea and vomiting increased among patients being treated for recurrent disease and those receiving treatment of either short or long duration. Nausea and vomiting were not restricted to those patients whose gastrointestinal tract was irradiated.[46]

Intermediate Effects

Damage to many normal tissues may not appear immediately after radiation. This latent period is a result of longer mitotic intervals in many normal tissues. However, every organ in the body that is exposed to radiation is affected to some extent.

Nervous System. Acute changes in the brain and spinal cord are a result of edema and are transient. Lhermitte's sign, a transient effect on the spinal cord, may occur several weeks after radiation. The symptoms are electric-like shock sensations radiating along the spinal cord and into the extremities. Most of the time this reaction is reversible.

Eye. The eye is very sensitive to radiation. The most sensitive area of the eye is the lens. Even small doses of radiation to the lens will cause cataract formation. Doses of 5000 to 6000 rads will cause severe eye inflammation and pain. Necrosis or perforation may occur, requiring enucleation. Lacrimal gland secretion is also suppressed, which may cause secondary problems.[33] The nasolacrimal duct may become obstructed because of desquamation, causing an overflow of tears onto the cheeks. If the radiation dose is high enough, the damage can be permanent.[9, 43]

Ear. Otitis media may occur after radiation to the ear because of hyperemia and swelling of the membranes and the eustachian tubes. Meniere's disease and dizziness may also occur, possibly because of increased lymphatic pressure as a result of edema and vasculitis.[33]

Salivary Glands. Radiation of the salivary glands alters the characteristics of the saliva. Less saliva will be produced; it will be thick and sticky and less effective in preventing dental caries. This ineffective saliva will also cause atrophic changes in the gingivae. Altered taste because of damaged taste buds will be aggravated by the salivary changes.[33]

Liver. The liver is sensitive to radiation and will begin to show damage at 3500 to 4000 rads. Children develop radiation hepatitis from doses as low as 2000 rads. The extent of liver changes is dependent on the dose. The changes manifested are weight gain, liver enlargement, and ascites. Liver function tests will be abnormal.[33]

Lung. Acute radiation pneumonitis may be asymptomatic or cause a hacking cough or mild chest discomfort. If 75 per cent of lung tissue is exposed to 2000 rads or more, severe respiratory distress, elevated temperature, and shortness of breath may result. The patient may die of respiratory insufficiency or cor pulmonale. With moderate levels of radiation, acute changes may subside after 3 or 4 weeks, but large doses will often cause permanent changes.[33]

Heart. Heart injury depends on the dose, fractionation schedule, and portion of the heart exposed. Pericarditis may result from doses of 5000 rads. Patients may also develop endocardial and myocardial damage. Some young people have developed myocardial infarctions as a result of radiation. Adequate shielding of the heart can decrease the incidence of these complications. Irradiation of the heart can increase the cardiac toxicity caused by doxorubicin hydrochloride (Adriamycin).[33]

Kidney. Acute radiation nephritis usually appears 6 months after radiation doses of 2300 to 2500 rads to the kidneys. Symptoms include lassitude, headaches, shortness of breath, nocturia, vomiting, and edema. Blood pressure is elevated, and abnormal changes of the retina occur. Urinalysis will show albuminuria and a low specific gravity. Hematuria is seldom present. This condition usually progresses to chronic nephritis.[33]

Gonads. The germinal cells of the testes are very sensitive to even small doses of radiation. Small doses will cause temporary halting of sperm production. One thousand rads will probably cause permanent sterility. The secretion of testosterone is not affected; thus sexual characteristics are unchanged. Doses of radiation of 200 rads will destroy many ovarian cells. Larger doses may cause menopausal symptoms and sterility. Estrogen production is diminished. Small doses of radiation to either testes or ovaries will cause numerous chromosomal abnormalities in the germ cells.[33]

Breast. The adult breast is resistant to radiation, but the young person's breast is very sensitive. The changes that occur from radiation are irreversible and do not respond to hormones.[33]

Bone and Cartilage. Exposure of the bones of children to radiation will cause bone growth abnormalities. Some recovery will occur after small doses, but damage is permanent if the dose is higher than 2000 rads. Damage to adult bone and cartilage may occur with doses higher than 6500 rads. This damage may cause necrosis or fractures.[33] Cartilage necrosis can occur in the outer ear, the nose, or the larynx.[43]

Thyroid Gland. Radiation of the thyroid gland can result in hypothyroidism.

Late Effects

Late effects of radiotherapy are directly related to the dosage and fractionation schedules. These effects may appear as early as a few months after therapy or may not occur until years after treatment. The effects are usually tissue necrosis, fistulas, and fibroses. The conditions are chronic and bear little relationship to previous immediate or intermediate reactions of the same tissues. Treatment of these conditions is usually conservative.[29] Malignancies may also develop as a result of old radiation injuries.

Brain irradiation may occasionally result in necrosis of the brain. Spinal cord damage may cause myelitis, resulting in motor and sensory changes or sometimes complete paraplegia and anesthesia, because of total transection of the spinal cord. These permanent changes are caused by capillary degeneration, necrosis of the small arterioles, necrosis of neurons, and demyelination of the white matter.

Loss of hearing may occur as a result of sclerosis of the ossicles and degenerative changes in the cochlea. The esophagus may be reduced in caliber and develop severe fibrotic strictures. Large doses of radiation may cause permanent ulceration in the intestines. These lesions may cause stenosis or perforation with the formation of fistulas. Chronic pulmonary fibrosis can occur after lung irradiation. If the radiated area is small, the condition may be asymptomatic. Chronic nephritis usually appears about 18 months after treatment. Patients with this condition may die of chronic uremia, renal failure from malignant hypertension, cerebral vascular accident, or congestive heart failure from elevated blood pressure.[1]

Permanent chronic changes occur in bone marrow when even small segments are irradiated. Repopulation is prevented by vascular degeneration and fibrosis. Late skin changes include fibrosis of the dermis, telangiectasia, pigmentation, and atrophy of the skin. Ulceration, necrosis, and induced carcinoma rarely occur as a result of overdose.[9, 33, 43]

APPROACHES TO TREATMENT

External Radiotherapy

External radiotherapy involves directing a source of x-rays or gamma rays outside of the body at a tumor site within the body. Treatment by ionizing radiation is very precise and must be very accurate. External radiotherapy is generally used for large tumors and those located deep within the body.

Planning for Radiotherapy

Before radiotherapy can begin, a detailed diagnosis of the type of malignancy and extent of its spread must be made. In almost all instances, a biopsy must be performed to provide data about the histology of the tumor. This will give the physician information about the usual behavior and radiosensitivity of that type of tumor.

The exact size and location of the tumor and the extent of local spread must be determined as accurately as possible. Diagnostic studies should be done to determine the existence of detectable metastatic disease. In other words, a very careful clinical staging must be done. In order to determine the exact location, shape, and size of the tumor, several types of diagnostic procedures may be used: x-ray studies, lymphangiograms, computerized axial tomography (CAT) scans, radioisotope scans, and sonograms. These procedures will also provide important information about the exact location of adjacent organs.

Preparing for Treatment

Before treatment begins, the ports (areas of skin through which radiation is aimed at the tumor) must be carefully selected and delineated. A simulator is used for this process. A simulator is a diagnostic x-ray tube housed in a unit that has the capacity for duplicating all of the movements and fields of a treatment unit. Films are taken from two planes to measure the length, breadth, and width of the tumor. Markers that will appear on the film are placed on the skin.

For some patients, devices to immobilize a portion of the body must be designed; these devices may be shells or casts. The purpose of immobilization is to ensure that the body can be placed in exactly the same position for each treatment.

Calculating the Dose

The next step is to decide the number of treatment fields, their sizes and positions. The purpose of this is to give a maximum dose of radiation to the tumor and to minimize the exposure of normal tissues. In order to do this, treatment will often be given through several ports, rather than just one. This will diminish skin damage and destruction of body organs.

The circumference of the body is measured from the point of the center of the tumor. Within this outline, the tumor and vital organs are indicated. This process may be done on paper, or more recently, by computer. The next step is to determine the number of fields, their angulation, and their sizes. This is planned to distribute the radiation dose. Isodose charts are then developed to indicate the total dosage for each portion of the body from all of the radiation fields.

At this point, the final ports are selected and the skin is marked with indelible ink or by tiny tattoos. In some cases, plastic templates may be placed over the patient's skin with the ports marked. It is important that some system be used to clearly delineate the treatment position. Patients are cautioned not to remove the markings since they will be used throughout the treatment program.

The fractionation schedule must then be calculated for the patient. Fractionation is, at this point in time, an inexact science. Before it can be most effective, more must be learned about tumor cell kinetics. Presently, fractionation is based on the clinical judgment of the radiotherapist. Doses are usually administered Monday through Friday for a period of several weeks. Sometimes a split course is used, particularly if the patient is debilitated. In this procedure, treatments are given regularly for a period of time, then the patient does not receive treatments for 2 or 3 weeks, and then treatments resume. Sometimes, two periods of rest are provided. This seems to permit normal tissues to repair and allows debilitated patients a greater chance to complete treatment.

Finally, check films are taken with the patient lying in treatment positions. This can be done with the simulator or the treatment unit. Check films will verify that calculations of tumor location and angulation of treatment doses will provide the tumor with the maximum dose. The patient is then ready for treatment to begin.

Administering the Treatment

For the treatment, the patient is carefully positioned on the table and instructed to lie very still. The x-ray machine is exactly aligned with the port markings on the patient's skin. Sand bags may be used to help immobilize the patient. If an immobilization device has been made for the patient, it is now applied. At this point, all personnel leave the room. This can be a very frightening time for the patient. Although x-rays cause no pain — in fact, the patient feels nothing at all — the machine makes noises, and the feeling of aloneness is usually intense. Both voice and visual contact with the patient are maintained throughout the treatment.

Internal Radiotherapy

Unsealed Sources

Unsealed sources are the least commonly used type of radiotherapy. They are liquids that may be administered orally or injected intravenously or into a body cavity. These sources usually have a very short half-life. They will be administered either by the nuclear medicine department or by the radiation therapy department of the hospital. The liquids usually contain a dye of some type so that if the substance escapes from the body through vomit or leakage from the injection site, contamination can be detected more easily.[25]

The three substances most commonly used in unsealed sources are iodine-131, phosphorus-32, and gold-198. Iodine-131 is used to treat cancer of the thyroid and is sometimes used to treat hyperthyroidism. Phosphorus-32 and colloidal gold-198 are injected into body cavities to decrease the production of pleural effusions or ascites. The use of these two substances has decreased in recent years because chemotherapy drugs are just as effective, without the risk of radioactivity.[25] The half-lives of these substances are: iodine-131 — 8.08 days, phosphorus-32 — 14.3 days, and gold-198 — 2.7 days.[25]

Sealed Sources

Sealed sources are radioactive substances that are encased in metal capsules. These capsules are then mechanically positioned within the patient at the site of the tumor. There are several advantages to this strategy of administering radiotherapy. Using this technique, it is possible to expose the tumor to high doses of radiation with minimal exposure of normal body tissues. Even patients who have received the maximum dose of external beam therapy can receive radiation from mechanically positioned radiation. It is possible to position the sealed sources within the tumor so that all portions of the tumor will receive equal levels of radiation.

One of the disadvantages of this treatment modality is the greatly increased risk of radiation exposure to other people by contact with the patient or by escape of the encapsulated source from the patient's body. There is also an increased risk of necrosis of normal tissues near the site of insertion. The tumor must be located near the surface of the body to allow access.

The capsule containing the radiation source must be designed in such a way that gamma rays can penetrate it, but that beta rays cannot. The capsule must be thin; therefore, a very dense metal must be used. An alloy of platinum and iridium is commonly used for this purpose.

Common Sealed Gamma Ray Sources. *Radium needles* are thin hollow tubes of various lengths with one sharp end designed to penetrate tissues. The other end has an eyelet through which silk is threaded. A thin-walled cell filled with a powdered form of radium occupies the center of the needle. Special forceps are needed for insertion of radium needles.

Radon seeds contain radon, a daughter product of radium. It is a gas that has the same radiation emission as radium. However, its half-life is 3.8 days rather than the 1600 years of radium. In past years, radon encased in short, thin tubing was widely used. Because of the possibility of gas escaping from the capsule and the high risk of necrosis of normal tissues, radon seeds are considered an outmoded therapy and have been replaced by other techniques.

Gold grains are frequently used as a replacement for radon seeds. These grains contain gold-198, which has a half-life of 2.7 days.

Cobalt-60 needles, tubes, spheres, rings, and beads are now being produced, allowing more versatility in the placement of cobalt-60 within or near a tumor. The half-life of cobalt-60 is 5.3 years.

Cesium-137 needles and tubes are also

available. Cesium has a half-life of 30 years. The gamma rays from cesium are less penetrating than those of radium. This means that the protection of others is increased.

Iridium-192 is also being used as a replacement for radium because of its less penetrating gamma rays. Iridium has a half-life of 74 days. It is used in vaginal applicators and is available in wires that are flexible and can be easily shaped or cut into desirable lengths. This allows its use in awkward sites such as the eye, the bladder, the back of the tongue, and the anal canal.[43]

Afterloading. One of the serious problems with the use of sealed sources of radiation is the exposure of health care personnel at the time of insertion. Because this procedure must often be implemented in the operating room, it has the potential of exposing large numbers of people. In afterloading, the container that will hold the radiation source is put into place during surgery, but the actual radiation source is inserted later, in a setting designed to diminish radiation exposure. This procedure is most commonly used in the treatment of cervical or uterine cancer.

Radiation Safety

Radiation safety is not a concern in caring for patients who are receiving external beam therapy; radiation is not being released by their body after treatment. However, patients who have sources of radiation within their body, in either sealed or unsealed forms, are a radiation hazard. Precautions must be taken to protect health care givers, family, and other patients. Hospitals that have an extensive program of radiation therapy may have specially designed facilities for patients who are sources of radiation. These facilities may have strategically placed lead shields. Patient beds will be placed in a way that diminishes exposure of others to radiation. Health care givers will wear radiation badges to measure their exposure level.

Some people unconsciously believe that these badges are a form of protection against radiation, and they may be less cautious when wearing one. The badge provides no protection at all; it simply measures exposure. The badge usually contains film that becomes increasingly cloudy as it is exposed to greater amounts of radiation. The employee who has received the maximum exposure allowed for a given period of time must be transferred to another unit.

Time, Distance, and Shielding. Three factors are important in taking adequate radiation precautions: time, distance, and shielding. The longer one stays near a radioactive patient, the greater the exposure. Therefore, time must be carefully utilized. Doubling the distance between the patient and the nurse will reduce the radiation exposure to one-fourth of the original exposure. (See Fig. 8–6.)

It is helpful to remember that gamma rays travel in straight lines. Walls, doors, and furniture, may provide some, but not complete, protection against gamma rays.

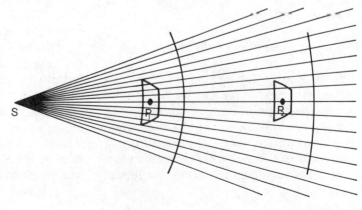

Figure 8–6. The inverse square law. Points P_1 and P_2 are at different distances from the source. The number of particles or photons crossing a small area will be the same, but for P_2 they are spread over a larger area and so the intensity at P_2 is less than at P_1. If P_2 is twice as far away from S as P_1, the intensity at $P_2 = \frac{1}{4} \times$ the intensity at P_1. (Reprinted by permission of Faber and Faber Ltd. from *A Concise Book of Radiotherapy*, by P. A. Barnes and D. J. Rees. 1972.)

Thus patients in adjoining rooms are at risk of some exposure. Lead aprons are generally not considered good protection against gamma rays. The lead is not thick enough to prevent penetration of the rays. The weight of the apron causes the person wearing it to take longer to accomplish the task and also gives the wearer the illusion of safety, thus encouraging carelessness.

On rare occasions implants become dislodged and radioactive liquids occasionally leak from the patient's body. The nurse must frequently check the patient for this possibility. Lost sources should never be touched. Forceps must be used to place the sources in a container, and the radiation safety officer and the physician must be notified.

It must be remembered that radiation precautions are not the same as nursing care. They simply constitute a parameter around which nursing care must be planned and implemented. Nursing care must be organized in such a way that care can be given quickly. Only essential care can be provided. Patients must be encouraged to do as much as possible for themselves. The room should be arranged so that most items are within the patient's reach. If the radiation source is in the patient's pelvis, as many nursing activities as possible should be done from the foot or head of the bed rather than from the side of the bed. Conversations should be held with the nurse standing in the doorway, not at the bedside.[25]

NURSING CARE OF THE PATIENT RECEIVING RADIOTHERAPY

External Radiotherapy

Preparing the Patient for Therapy

Traditionally, the setting in which the nurse prepared the patient for radiotherapy was the hospital. Increasingly, however, nursing care is occurring in outpatient radiation clinics, home care settings, or doctors' offices. The role of the nurse in this capacity is taking on an increasing importance.

As previously mentioned, patients and family members often have primitive or illogical fears and notions about radiotherapy, which need to be identified in order to be dealt with. Patients may believe they will become radioactive. They may expect to experience pain when the radiation enters their body. Radiation is mysterious and frightening. Explanations that describe what the patient will experience during radiation will be helpful.

Since the patients' physical condition at the time of radiotherapy affects their response to treatment, patients should be encouraged to maintain an adequate nutritional level and take care of themselves. They need to be given the information necessary to take care of themselves responsibly during the period when they are receiving radiotherapy. Although this information will usually have to be repeated throughout the treatment period, it is important that teaching begin prior to therapy.

Patients need to be assured that they will have access to a nurse consistently during the therapy period. Studies indicate that patients do not perceive radiotherapists or radiation technologists as persons with whom they can discuss problems. The patient traditionally turns to the nurse for support, guidance, and care.

Physiologic Support

Nutrition. Maintaining a good nutritional state during radiotherapy is important. Well-nourished tumor cells are more easily destroyed by radiation. It can be difficult for patients to sustain good nutrition. Patients often experience low-grade nausea, anorexia, and fatigue during radiotherapy. They may also be emotionally depressed. Achieving adequate nutrition within this framework requires some ingenuity. Most patients can usually tolerate six small feedings better than three large meals a day. With close questioning, it is sometimes possible to detect a pattern of nausea throughout the day, with the nausea decreasing at certain periods, particularly if the radiotherapy is given at a consistent time each day. Feedings should be scheduled during these periods.

Foods should be selected from those that particularly appeal to the patient. Family members often think that since nutrition is important, patients should be made to eat the "right" foods. If they don't eat their meat and vegetables, they should not be allowed to eat dessert. If patients want dessert six times a day, feed it to them. Just make it nourishing. There are many strategies for doing this; they will be discussed in more detail in Chapter 11.

Rest. As mentioned before, patients receiving radiotherapy experience fatigue. The cause for this is not well understood. Some authors believe it to be the result of an accumulation of uric acid and other waste materials from destroyed cells. Others believe fatigue to be psychologic in origin. Haylock and associates, using a self-report scale, found that radiation patients experienced more fatigue during the week, when they were receiving therapy, than they did on weekends. The fatigue progressed as the therapy progressed.[18] In the author's experience, this fatigue is often accompanied by depression.

Patients and family members often interpret fatigue to mean that the patient is getting worse — that the cancer is growing. They are usually very relieved to learn that fatigue is an expected side effect of radiotherapy. With some suggestions for minimizing the fatigue, patients can usually handle it well.

The patients' activities should be planned around frequent rest periods during the day. If patients are already debilitated, this may mean bathing them and then allowing them to rest before changing their beds. Patients need to be taught to recognize signs of fatigue and to rest when they occur. They need to avoid physical activities just before mealtimes.

Patients sometimes feel that the fatigue and depression mean that they are not fighting the disease — that they are not trying to get well. They will fight the fatigue and make themselves do things they do not feel like doing. They may feel that they need "permission" from the nurse to let themselves rest. Conversely, they need to feel free to do whatever they have the energy to do, without being constrained by others. Patients are the only ones who know how they feel and should be the ones who decide what activities are appropriate.

Fluids. If the patients' fatigue is due to an accumulation of waste products from cell breakdown, extra fluids may speed up the excretion process. If extra fluids are not contraindicated, they should be encouraged. If nourishment is a problem, the fluids should contribute to that nourishment.

Skin Care. Skin injury from radiotherapy will not usually begin until the second or third week of therapy. However, skin care is begun at the initiation of treatment in order to minimize the degree of damage. Very little research has been done on the effect of various approaches to skin care on the extent of skin symptoms. Physicians usually establish a regimen based on their own clinical experience. Some physicians insist that the skin within the port area remain dry; water is not even allowed. Other physicians allow the use of soap and water.

It must be remembered that the surface of the skin is not being replaced as rapidly as usual. If the skin surface is rubbed enough to release surface skin cells, these will not be replaced immediately. Therefore, brisk scrubbing with a washcloth or towel is contraindicated. Patients should not wear clothing that rubs or fits tightly against the port area. They should be cautioned against exposing the port to sun, strong winds, or excessively hot or cold water.[25]

Ointments, creams, powders, or other substances should not be put on the skin without specific approval by the physician. Many substances designed for the skin contain heavy metals. When radiation strikes them, these heavy metals function like little mirrors in the skin. The radiation scatters through the surface of the skin, causing much more severe skin damage. Other substances can also cause skin irritation; for example, substances containing alcohol.

When patients are cautioned not to put

anything on the skin within the port area, they may interpret "anything" in a different way than the nurse. The patient may not consider soap, water, deodorant, or perfume to be "anything." Therefore, instructions must be specific. Explanations can help patients to understand the consequences of their actions and give themselves proper care. Because the patient is usually being bombarded with information and instructions at this point, it is wise to give written instructions for skin care. The skin should be checked daily for problems. Continuous assessment should be made of how well the patient is following instructions. These instructions may have to be repeated several times, especially since the patient may see no immediate consequences of not following them.

Some patients have serious body image problems about not bathing or not using soap or deodorant. They feel dirty or think that they have an offensive odor, even if they do not. At this point, they may be more concerned about cleanliness, odor, body image, and the change in daily rituals than they are about the tumor or the radiation. Women unable to wear a bra may be similarly affected. These patients may begin to withdraw from others as a reaction to these feelings.

Psychologic Support

Any division of nursing care into its physiologic and psychologic components is necessarily artificial. The problems of depression and altered self-image have already been mentioned. Some of the effective interventions for these problems may involve alterations in physical care. Another important factor in psychologic care is accessibility. Patients need to know how to contact the nurse if they need help. The opportunity for patients to express feelings and describe experiences is important. Patients may need to consider alternative coping strategies, since they are faced with a situation that they have never before experienced. Opportunities to talk with other patients undergoing radiotherapy are often beneficial. These patients and their families can often provide very helpful mutual support.

Supporting Significant Others

Family members, neighbors, and friends also need support during the therapy period. Often, someone from this group must be responsible for transporting the patient daily to and from treatments. This requires time and may disrupt job responsibilities. (See Chapter 1 for a discussion of the primary caretaker role.) Although actions must not be taken to rescind control from the patient and give it to others, it is important for these significant others to be included, to be informed, and to be provided with emotional support.

Internal Radiotherapy

Preparing the Patient for Therapy

Patients who are to receive internal radiotherapy need careful, detailed explanations of the treatment and care afterward in order to responsibly participate in that care. They need to know what they will experience when the radiation source is applied or administered. The reasons nursing care is planned for minimal exposure time need to be explained. At this point, patients can plan how they will participate in their own care. Any restrictions on physical activities need to be explained and planned around.

The skin should be examined carefully for pressure areas that may break down under low mobility conditions. Aged patients or those with a history of respiratory difficulties may develop pneumonia.[25] The patient may need to be taught deep breathing exercises or plans may need to be made for intermittent positive pressure treatments. Some patients with head and neck tumors will have tracheostomies performed when the implant is made. Care for these patients must be carefully planned at this time.[25]

Physiologic Support

Patients receiving iodine-131 or phosphorus-32 require few physiologic nursing care measures. The primary concern is the risk of vomiting within 4 hours after administration of the radioisotope. If this occurs, decontamination procedures must be implemented to include everything contaminated by the vomitus — patient, nurses, equipment, floor, walls, and furniture. Iodine-131 is excreted in urine, sweat, and saliva. Patients receiving this radioisotope should wear hospital gowns. These gowns, bed linens, and towels should be saved and checked by the radiation officer. The patient should be fed on paper plates and plastic utensils that should also be checked by the radiation officer for radioactivity. Because of the short half-life of these substances, precautions are necessary only for the first 4 days.[25]

After the implantation, patients with vaginal implants may be placed on a low residue diet and given medication to decrease the possibility of a bowel movement while the implant is in place. The patient will be on complete bed rest, and movement is very restricted. The patient can usually be logrolled. The head of the bed cannot be elevated.[25] The patient will often have a urinary catheter inserted. Head and neck cancer patients may be receiving tube feedings. Mouth care will be a primary concern, and tracheostomy care will need to be provided. These patients are usually allowed to ambulate in the room.[25]

The same complications that are common to postoperative cancer patients occur with patients with implants: thrombophlebitis; infection; pulmonary embolus; pneumonia; and hemorrhage.[25] The patients will usually have a local inflammatory reaction from the radiation 8 to 10 days after the implant. This reaction will reach its peak 10 to 15 days after the implant is removed. Patients with vaginal implants may experience urgency, frequency, and burning on urination.[25] This is part of the inflammatory reaction and will not usually be a permanent problem.

After the implant is removed, patients with vaginal implants will need to be treated to restore normal bowel evacuation. Soothing vaginal douches are sometimes given to decrease the symptoms of vaginal inflammation. Head and neck cancer patients will usually have their tracheostomy removed, tube feedings will be discontinued, and normal eating may resume. Patients will usually be discharged at this point and followed on an outpatient basis.[25]

Patients should be cautioned to avoid exposure of the skin to sun and extreme water temperature changes.[25] Although this caution is commonly given to patients receiving external radiation, it is often overlooked in instructions given to the patient receiving internal radiation. Patients with vaginal radiation should be informed that they may experience some staining of vaginal discharge from the endometrium for 3 or 4 days after removal of implants. After consultation with treating physicians, patients may usually resume sexual intercourse when their physical condition allows this activity. In fact, resumption of sexual activity may prevent vaginal wall stenosis.[25]

In the past, nurses have had little opportunity for contact with patients during the period in which late effects develop, unless the patients were hospitalized. Now, however, many more nurses are maintaining patient contact in radiation outpatient clinics, home health care agencies, occupational health settings, rural health clinics, and offices of medical oncologists.

The most commonly observed late effects of internal radiotherapy are infection, necrosis, fistulas, stenosis, and fibrosis.[25] Medical intervention for these conditions is usually conservative: necrotic tissue is debrided; stenotic areas are dilated; fistulas are packed; and surgery is seldom used.[25]

Nursing care is symptomatic and designed to provide physiologic support and allow the patient to continue functioning with the least possible interference with life activities. One of the most difficult problems for patients who have had internal radiotherapy is a foul odor that frequently accompanies late effects. If dressings are being used, they must be changed frequently. Zinc peroxide packs may be used in the oral cavity to eliminate odors and stimulate healing. Water soluble chlorphyll derivatives can be used as a deodorizer. Secondary infections in necrotic areas or fistulas cause many problems and are often difficult to treat. Many of the problems can be avoided by detecting the infection early and beginning treatment at once. Therefore, patients should be assessed by the nurse and taught to observe themselves for any changes in odor or any unusual drainage.[25]

Psychologic Support

In addition to experiencing fears related to the radiation treatment itself, the patient receiving internal radiotherapy will have to cope with a brief period of social isolation. Although measures must be taken to minimize exposure of all hospital personnel to radiation, nursing care should be planned in such a way that communication is maintained and the patient feels supported. The nurse can accomplish this by frequent, brief stops at the doorway of the patient's room or by providing care at intervals throughout the day, rather than giving it all at one time and then staying away for the rest of the shift. Although touching must be diminished, eye contact can be increased, thus providing a type of psychologic touching.

Patients who have internal sources of radiation are usually very sensitive to the fact that they can cause harm to others. This causes an increase in anxiety, especially since they have no way of detecting that this harm is occurring. They are also anxious about the harm the radiation is doing to their own normal tissues. This anxiety can be decreased by explaining controls designed to protect others. It is also important for patients to know that they are no longer radioactive when the source has been removed.

Supporting Significant Others

Family members often have a difficult time during internal radiotherapy because of the enforced separation. They frequently need increased information, support, and sometimes touching by nurses. The radiation may be so fearful that some family members will avoid the patient completely. Explanations of safeguards and limiting time of contact can be helpful to these family members. If they are still reluctant to go near the patient, telephone communication can be encouraged.

BIBLIOGRAPHY

1. Abramson, N.: Radiation therapy — what is it? In *Cancer: Pathophysiology, Etiology and Management*, ed. by L. C. Kruse, J. L. Reese, and L. K. Hart. C. V. Mosby Co., St. Louis, 1979.
2. Adams, G. E.: Hypoxic cell sensitizers for radiotherapy. In *Cancer: A Comprehensive Treatise*, ed. by F. F. Becker. Plenum Press, New York, 1977.
3. Bahnson, C. B.: Psychologic and emotional issues in cancer: The psychotherapeutic care of the cancer patient. *Seminars in Oncology*. 2:293–309, 1975.
4. Barkes, P.: Nursing care of patients undergoing treatment from unsealed radio-active sources. In *Cancer Nursing: Radiotherapy*, ed. by R. Tiffany. Farber and Farber, Boston, 1979.
5. Blake, D.: Ultrasonography in the practice of radiotherapy. *Applied Radiology*. 8:112–114, 1979.
6. Bloomer, W. D. and S. Hellman: Normal tissue responses to radiation therapy. In *Cancer: Pathophysiology, Etiology and Management*, ed. by L. C. Kruse, J. L. Reese and L. K. Hart. C. V. Mosby Co., St. Louis, 1979.
7. Champagne, E.: Teaching program for patients receiving interstitial radioactive iodine[125] for cancer of the prostate. *Oncology Nursing Forum*. 7:12–15, 1980.
8. Cox, S.: Nursing care of patients undergoing treatment from sealed radio-active sources. In *Cancer Nursing: Radiotherapy*, ed. by R. Tiffany. Farber and Farber, Boston, 1979.
9. Crown, V.: Biological effects of radiotherapy. In *Cancer Nursing: Radiotherapy*, ed. by R. Tiffany. Farber and Farber, Boston, 1979.
10. Crown, V.: Planning for treatment. In *Cancer Nursing: Radiotherapy*, ed. by R. Tiffany. Farber and Farber, Boston, 1979.
11. Crown, V.: Principles of radiotherapy. In *Cancer Nursing: Radiotherapy*, ed. by R. Tiffany. Farber and Farber, Boston, 1979.
12. Denekamp, J. and J. F. Fowler: Cell proliferation kinetics and radiation therapy. In *Cancer: A Comprehensive Treatise*, ed. by F. F. Becker. Plenum Press, New York, 1977.
13. Elkind, M. M. and J. L. Redpath: Molecular and cellular biology of radiation lethality. In *Cancer: A Comprehensive Treatise*, ed. by F. F. Becker. Plenum Press, New York, 1977.
14. Fowler, J. F.: New horizons in radiation oncology.

British Journal of Radiology. 52:523–535, 1979.

15. Fowler, J. F. and J. Denekamp: Radiation effects on normal tissues. In *Cancer: A Comprehensive Treatise*, ed. by F. F. Becker. Plenum Press, New York, 1977.

16. Greenfield, L., et al.: Radiation safety precautions with ^{131}iodine therapy. *Cancer Nursing.* 1:379–384, 1978.

17. Hall, Eric J.: High-LET radiations. In *Cancer: A Comprehensive Treatise*, ed. by F. F. Becker. Plenum Press, New York, 1977.

18. Haylock, P., et al.: Fatigue in patients receiving localized radiation. *Cancer Nursing.* 2:461–467, 1979.

19. Hill, S., et al.: The response of six mouse tumours to combined heat and x-rays: Implications for therapy. *British Journal of Radiology.* 52:209–218, 1979.

20. Kallman, R. F. and S. Rockwell: Effects of radiation on animal tumor models. In *Cancer: A Comprehensive Treatise*, ed. by F. F. Becker. Plenum Press, New York, 1977.

21. Kaplan, H. S.: Present status of radiation therapy of cancer: An overview. In *Cancer: A Comprehensive Treatise*, ed. by F. F. Becker. Plenum Press, New York, 1979.

22. Kaplan, H. S.: Basic principles in radiation oncology. In *Cancer: Pathophysiology, Etiology and Management*, ed. by L. C. Kruse, J. L. Reese, and L. K. Hart. C. V. Mosby Co., St. Louis, 1979.

23. Kramer, S.: The study of the patterns of cancer care in radiation therapy. *Cancer.* 39:780–787, 1977.

24. Kramer, S.: Definitive radiation therapy. In *Cancer: Pathophysiology, Etiology and Management*, ed. by L. C. Kruse, J. L. Reese, and L. K. Hart. C. V. Mosby Co., St. Louis, 1979.

25. Leahy, I. M., J. M. St. German, and C. G. Varricchio: *The Nurse and Radiotherapy: A Manual for Daily Care.* C. V. Mosby Co., St. Louis, 1979.

26. Luckmann, J. and K. C. Sorensen: *Medical-Surgical Nursing: A Psychophysiologic Approach.* W. B. Saunders Co., Philadelphia, 1980.

27. Manning, M. R.: Hyperthermia: renewed interest in an old treatment for cancer. In *Cancer: Pathophysiology, Etiology and Management*, ed. by L. C. Kruse, J. L. Reese, and L. K. Hart. C. V. Mosby Co., St. Louis, 1979.

28. Mitchell, G.: Cancer patients: Knowledge and attitudes. *Cancer.* 40:61–66, 1977.

29. Ogi, S. S.: Radiotherapy, cancer and the nurse. In *Dynamics of Oncology Nursing*, ed. by P. K. Burkhalter and D. L. Denley. McGraw-Hill Book Co., New York, 1978.

30. Onuska, R.: The interaction of the occupational health nurse and the employee receiving chemotherapy and/or radiation therapy. *Occupational Health Nursing.* 26:34–37, 1978.

31. Parker, R.: Cancer management: A changing scene. *Radiologia Clinica et Biologica.* 44:214–226, 1975.

32. Parker, R.: Basic radiation physics and protection. In *Cancer Nursing: Radiotherapy*, ed. by R. Tiffany. Farber and Farber, Boston, 1979.

33. Perez, C. A.: Principles of radiation therapy. In *Clinical Oncology*, ed. by J. Horton and G. J. Hill. W. B. Saunders Co., Philadelphia, 1977.

34. Potter, J. F.: Preoperative irradiation and surgery for certain cancers. In *Cancer: Pathophysiology, Etiology and Management*, ed. by L. C. Kruse, J. L. Reese, and L. K. Hart. C. V. Mosby Co., St. Louis, 1979.

35. Powers, W.: They're measuring the quality of patient care. *Impact.* 22:4–5, 1979.

36. Rotman, M.: Supportive and palliative radiation therapy. In *Cancer: Pathophysiology, Etiology and Management*, ed. by L. C. Kruse, J. L. Reese, and L. K. Hart. C. V. Mosby Co., St. Louis, 1979.

37. Rotman, M., et al.: Supportive therapy in radiation oncology. *Cancer.* 39:744–750, 1977.

38. Shalek, R. J.: Physics of radiation therapy. In *Cancer: A Comprehensive Treatise*, ed. by F. F. Becker, Plenum Press, New York, 1979.

39. Smith, D., et al.: Nursing care of patients undergoing combination chemotherapy and radiotherapy. *Cancer Nursing.* 1:129–134, 1978.

40. Smith, L. L., et al.: Social work services for radiation therapy patients and their families. *Hospital and Community Psychiatry.* 28:752–754, 1977.

41. Starling, G.: Radiopharmaceuticals in clinical oncology — an overview. *Canadian Journal of Radiography, Radiotherapy and Nuclear Medicine.* 10:7–17, 1979.

42. Svoboda, V. H. J.: Further experience with radiotherapy by multiple daily sessions. *British Journal of Radiology.* 51:363–369, 1978.

43. Walter, J.: *Cancer and Radiotherapy: A Short Guide for Nurses and Medical Students.* Churchill Livingstone Inc., New York, 1977.

44. Webb, P.: Nursing care of patients undergoing treatment by teletherapy. In *Cancer Nursing: Radiotherapy*, ed. by R. Tiffany. Farber and Farber, Boston, 1979.

45. Webster, J. H., A. M. Danahon, and B. A. Coles: The doctor, nurse and technician work together in radiotherapy. *Proceedings of the National Conference on Cancer Nursing.* American Cancer Society, 1973.

46. Welch, D.: Assessment of nausea and vomiting in cancer patients undergoing external beam radiotherapy. *Cancer Nursing.* 3:365–371, 1980.

47. Windeyer, B.: Hyperbaric oxygen and radiotherapy. *British Journal of Radiology.* 51:875–894, 1978.

9

Chemotherapy

INTRODUCTION

The use of drugs to cure or control the growth of cancer is relatively new in comparison with the utilization of surgery or radiotherapy. Although potassium arsenite and Coley's toxin were used in the late 1800s to treat cancer, the use of drugs has generally been considered ineffective. Modern drug therapy for cancer began in 1942 as a result of an accident with nitrogen mustard gas, which was being studied for possible military use. Individuals exposed to this gas were found to have a decreased white blood cell count. The incident generated an idea: if this substance destroyed white blood cells, what would happen if it were administered to a patient who had an abnormally high white blood count resulting from cancer?

The first patient to receive nitrogen mustard as a medical treatment had advanced lymphosarcoma.[26] He had a dramatic though very brief response to the drug, but his response gave impetus to a field of exploration that has spanned over a quarter of a century. This field of study, beginning in such a serendipitous way, is now an intense, organized, scientific endeavor.

About the same time that drugs began to evolve as a means of treating cancer, many scientists were recognizing that surgery and radiotherapy had probably reached their limits in ability to cure cancer. More time, money, and energy began to be spent on chemotherapy research. Scientists and the public both had high hopes of a "magic bullet," which when discovered would dramatically destroy all cancer. This hope stemmed from the very recent discovery of antibiotics to treat infections. Large amounts of money were generated from both public and private sources to fund research in this area.

The "magic bullet" has not been found. Because cancer includes such a diverse and complex group of diseases, it is unlikely that a single treatment will be found to cure all of its types. In spite of this disappointment, systematic research has made great inroads into the treatment of previously untreatable types of cancer. Some can now be cured and others can now be controlled, slowing the tumor's growth and allowing the patient a longer, more meaningful, and productive life.

HOW CHEMOTHERAPY WORKS

When cancer chemotherapy began, there was scant understanding of how it worked because there was only a minimal knowledge of cellular physiology and cell kinetics. Chemotherapy was considered a potion: mysterious, magical, and frightening. Although much still remains to be understood about cell functioning, some of the processes can now be explained. Because cancer chemotherapy is so dependent on new knowledge in this field, further major developments in chemotherapy may have to await more extensive discoveries in this important area of science.[3]

Mechanisms of Action

Most chemotherapy drugs act by affecting cellular enzymes or the substrates upon which enzyme systems act. These enzymes and substrates are usually involved in deoxyribonucleic acid (DNA) synthesis or function. DNA synthesis occurs only when cells are progressing through the cell cycle. Therefore, most chemotherapy drugs can destroy only actively dividing cells.[11]

Chemotherapy and the Cell Cycle. Many chemotherapy drugs will affect only cells that are in a specific phase of the cell cycle. (See Chapter 2.) These drugs are called cell cycle–specific or phase-specific. Drugs that will affect any actively dividing cell are called cell cycle–nonspecific or phase-nonspecific. Chemotherapy drugs are generally ineffective against resting cells or differentiated cells. This means that chemotherapy is more likely to be effective on tumors that have a large portion of their cells undergoing active division.[6]

Chemotherapy and the Growth Fraction. The number of cells in the cell cycle is called the growth fraction. Because many of its cells are in the cell cycle, the growth fraction in a small, young tumor is usually very high. Because relatively few of its cells are dividing, a larger, older tumor usually has a lower growth fraction. Thus, chemotherapy is generally more effective on smaller, younger tumors.

Malignancies that are characterized by undifferentiated rapidly dividing cells, such as oat cell carcinoma of the lung and some leukemias and lymphomas, initially respond very well to chemotherapy. Many of the cells are rapidly destroyed. However, on many occasions the remaining malignant cells are able to develop resistance to the chemotherapy and again grow rapidly, eventually killing the patient.

Doubling Time. Doubling time is the length of time required for the tumor to double in size. A tumor's doubling time is determined by the size of its growth fraction and the percentage of cell loss (the loss of dividing cells). Cells may be "lost" by differentiation, cell death, exfoliation, or spread to metastatic sites. The cell loss in the average human tumor is over 50 per cent and may be as great as 90 per cent. Chemotherapy increases cell loss, thus lengthening the doubling time. Mathematically, this can be very significant in terms of survival time.

The Gompertzian Growth Curve. In the eighteenth century, a mathematician named Benjamin Gompertz developed an equation that has been applied to the rela-

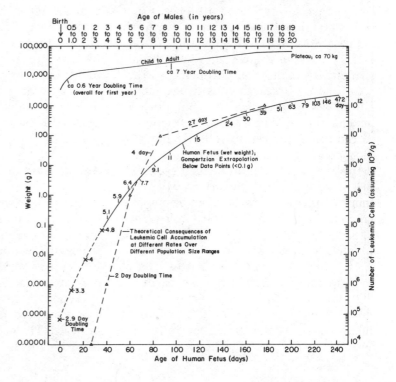

Figure 9-1. Human fetal and childhood growth as a gompertzian process, and the theoretical consequences of accumulation of leukemic cells at different rates over varying population ranges. (From Skipper, H. E., and Perry, S.: Kinetics of normal and leukemic leukocyte populations and relevance to chemotherapy. *Cancer Research.* 30: 1883, 1970. Copyright 1970, The Williams & Wilkins Company, Baltimore. Used by permission.)

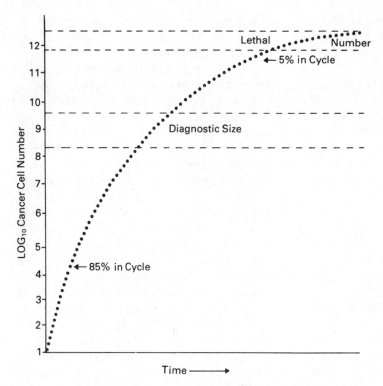

Figure 9–2. Cancer growth in vivo. (From Apple, M. A.: New anticancer drug design: past and future strategies. In *Cancer: A Comprehensive Treatise, Vol. 5, Chemotherapy,* edited by F. F. Becker. New York: Plenum Press, 1977. Used by permission.)

tionship between doubling time and growth fraction. Biologic growth that conforms to his formula is called gompertzian growth. As knowledge of cell kinetics has increased, it has been possible to compare observed growth patterns of cells with the gompertzian growth curve. It appears that both normal and malignant cell growth follows the gompertzian pattern.[11] (See Fig. 9–1 for the gompertzian growth pattern and its application to tumor growth.)

Cell Kill. Chemotherapy drugs cannot kill all of the cancer cells in a single dose. Instead, they will kill a certain fraction or percentage of the cancer cells. This occurs because only a given fraction or percentage of the cancer cells are in the cell cycle and at a phase that leaves them sensitive to the drugs. This cell kill pattern can be put on a graph and is usually expressed in logarithmic terms. (See Fig. 9–2.) A person with an advanced cancer may have a tumor burden of 10^{12} cells. This is equivalent to 1 kg of body weight. The most effective exposure of the tumor to chemotherapy drugs will result in 2 to 5 logs of cell kill. Therefore, to achieve even partial tumor control, many doses of the drug must be given.

THE DEVELOPMENT OF NEW DRUGS

Selecting chemicals that may be successful in treating cancer has formerly been done by trial and error. Now, there is more knowledge of both the classes of chemicals that are effective and the specific cellular actions needed for the chemical to be of use. Although some drugs that are discovered to have properties useful in cancer treatment were first tested for treatment of other disorders, most chemotherapy drugs are now developed through detailed, planned laboratory research.

Animal Studies

After a potential drug has been identified, it is administered in doses of varying amounts to healthy animals. Pharmacologic effects (such as side effects and changes in metabolic pathways, excretion patterns, and absorption rates) are studied. The drug is then given to animals with cancer. Various doses and patterns of administration are used. The animal is then sacrificed and the drug effects on tumor growth are determined. If the drug shows some success and its side effects are acceptable, specific animal tumor models are studied to determine the types of malignancy against which the drug may be effective. Because metabolic pathways are not always identical in animals and humans, these tests can be conducted only to indicate potential usage. The drugs must eventually be tested on humans.

Clinical Trials

The use of experimental drugs on human beings is very carefully controlled. Even if the drug holds considerable promise, it cannot be given to a patient for whom other treatments are available. Therefore, the selection of patients for clinical trials involves both ethical and legal questions and requires careful medical judgment. The patient must always give free and informed consent for the use of an experimental drug. The consent forms for these drugs are lengthy and describe known side effects and other risks in detail. In spite of this, it is difficult to know whether or not patients actually feel free to refuse to participate. Do they feel that they will not be cared for if they refuse? There are also differences of opinion about the extent of informed consent. Should patients be kept informed throughout treatment or is it sufficient to inform them only at the beginning of treatment? Are patients aware of the alternative treatments available to them?

Nurses are becoming increasingly involved in these clinical trials. This is not nursing research; these nurses are assisting in medical research. However, the nurse has an important nursing role in these studies. The nurse may be the person most involved in communicating with the patient. In addition to functioning as a data collector and ensuring that treatment procedures remain consistent from patient to patient, the nurse must often function in the role of patient advocate. Sometimes the patient as a person can get lost in the focus on the patient as an experimental subject. The nurse is often in an ideal position to see that the personhood of the patient is kept foremost in the minds of all members of the research team.

Phase I Trials. Phase I trials are designed to determine the toxicity and optimum dosage of a drug in humans with cancer. The pharmacologic effects of the drug are also studied at this point. Only cancer patients with advanced disease for whom there is no other treatment available can be used for these studies. Patients need to understand that there is little chance that the drug will be helpful to them by either prolonging their life or providing a possibility of cure. Most patients who agree to these studies do so out of a desire to help others. They often feel that this adds meaning to their dying. It may be seen as a contribution lasting beyond their own lifetime. However, they must not be made to feel guilty or selfish if they choose not to participate.

Treating the advanced cancer patient is not the ideal way to determine the effectiveness of a new drug. Many very useful chemotherapy drugs have little or no effect on tumor growth during the late stages of the disease. It is therefore possible to dismiss as ineffective a drug that might have a more pronounced effect on earlier disease states. This risk, however, is more tenable than the risk of causing harm or loss of life to patients who might have a longer period of life before them.

Phase II Trials. Phase II trials are only conducted if the Phase I studies have indicated that the drug shows some effect. The patient is given a dose of drug that is known to be effective in human cancers and whose pharmacologic action and toxic effects have been established. In these studies, attempts are made to determine drug effects on specific types of cancer. This is divided into two effects: partial remission and complete remission. Partial remission is defined as a greater than 50 per cent reduction of measurable tumor masses lasting longer than 1 month. A complete remission means complete disappearance of all evidence of the tumor and a return by the patient to a normal performance status.

Phase III Trials. Phase III trials are conducted to compare the effects of the experimental drug with those of existing drugs currently used to treat a specific type of cancer. There are two particularly important questions to be answered. Is tumor response more effective with the new drug? Will tumors that have developed resistance to established drug therapies respond to the new drug?

When the drug has been found to be effective with a specific type of cancer, treatment with the drug is begun early in the course of the disease and coordinated with other therapies such as surgery or radiotherapy. The drug may retain its experimental status for some period of time. This places some restrictions on its use but allows continued accumulation of data on drug effectiveness and toxicity. Only oncologists who belong to a cancer research group will be allowed to prescribe the drug. They have a responsibility of reporting patient response to the drug to the research group.

Studies of Drug Combinations. When several drugs have been identified as active against a particular type of cancer, their use in combinations is considered. Combinations of drugs can often have unexpected and harmful effects. The drugs may be synergistic or they may counteract each other. Sometimes combining drugs does not produce a better result than giving one drug alone, but may increase the risk and severity of side effects.

The combination of drugs used to treat a specific type of malignancy must be carefully selected. Ideally, each drug should destroy cells in different phases of the cell cycle. Because of the serious side effects of cancer chemotherapy, only drugs that have differing side effects or those whose side effects are likely to occur at varying times must be combined. Absorption, metabolic activation, cell binding, and excretion patterns of each drug must be considered in order to avoid conflicts with another drug in the same category.

Because of these potential problems, a combination of chemotherapy drugs must be tested in Phase I, II, and III trials just as

a single new drug is. In order for its use to be justified, the combination must have a greater effect than established methods of treatment, or it must be used to treat patients who are not responding to demonstrated therapies.[11, 25]

THE THERAPEUTIC RESPONSE TO CANCER CHEMOTHERAPY

The response of malignancies to cancer chemotherapy is not predictable. Some types of malignancies have a dramatic response and a high cure rate. In other cancers, there is little benefit. Even patients who have histologically similar tumors may respond in very different ways to chemotherapy. The response to chemotherapy is dependent on many factors relating to both the tumor and the host or patient.[26]

Tumor Variables

Size. As with surgery and radiotherapy, chemotherapy is most effective in the early stages of a malignancy, when the tumor cell burden is small and there is a larger growth fraction. Therefore, if chemotherapy is given early in the course of the disease, before metastases become evident, there is a decrease in the incidence of recurrence.

Type of Cancer. The response of various types of cancer to chemotherapy is changing rapidly, owing to the discovery of new drugs and new treatment regimens. Types of tumors that formerly had no response to chemotherapy may respond to new drugs. As Kennealey and Mitchell point out, "there are probably no tumors with intrinsic resistance to all therapeutic agents, but simply tumors for which the effective agent has not yet been found."[26] Unfortunately, the most common cancers (such as lung and colon cancers) are the ones that have failed to respond well to present chemotherapy drugs. Current research is focused on finding chemicals to which these target tumors will respond more effectively.

Statistics showing the responses of various types of tumors to chemotherapy are helpful in identifying the usual response, but they are often based on research that is several years old. The drugs and treatment strategies for chemotherapy have often changed in ways that have improved cancer response rates. It is important, therefore, to take into account the year that the table was first published when considering the data presented. Table 9–1, which was published in 1981, presents current statistics on the responses to drug therapy.

Tumor Location. The location of the tumor is significant both in terms of immunologic response and accessibility to chemotherapy. The least accessible sites are those that are relatively avascular. Both chemotherapy drugs and immune substances usually require blood transport. Sites that are relatively avascular are the necrotic centers of tumors and portions of the body such as bone or fat. The blood-brain barrier also presents a problem in chemotherapy treatment. A drug must be lipid soluble to cross this barrier, otherwise it must be administered intrathecally. These sites are often labeled "privileged sites" or "sanctuary sites." Tumor cells may be destroyed in the rest of the body, but metastatic lesions in "sanctuary sites" may survive and continue to grow and spread.

Host Variables

There are many factors affecting the patient's chances of receiving chemotherapy and his or her response to the treatment. These variables include prior therapies, physical health, and psychosocial factors.

Prior Surgery. Many surgeons have been very reluctant to seek chemotherapy for their patients immediately after surgery because of concerns about the effect of chemotherapy on surgical convalescence. One immediate consideration is its effect on wound healing. However, research seems to indicate that chemotherapy does not adversely affect wound healing. Medical oncologists are more concerned about the physical and emotional consequences of aggressive cancer surgery. Patients are often physically debilitated. Those who have had head and neck surgery or gastrointestinal surgery may have serious nutritional problems. These consequences interfere with the patient's ability to tolerate effective levels of chemotherapy. Additionally, many patients who have undergone extensive ablative surgery have such severe emotional problems that further treatment with chemotherapy is impossible.[26]

Radiotherapy. The damage to normal tissue that results from radiotherapy can seriously alter the patient's ability to tolerate chemotherapy. The most serious effect is the permanent destruction of normal bone marrow tissue. Radiotherapy patients must be given smaller doses of chemotherapy over a longer period of time. These smaller doses may be less effective in preventing disease recurrence. Recent studies have indicated that radiotherapy can cause a serious and long-lasting lymphopenia involving primarily the T lymphocytes. These are the thymus-derived white blood cells thought to be responsible for cell-mediated immunity. Their decrease could heighten the risk of disease recurrence. Also, since most chemotherapy causes a temporary leukopenia, it may not be possible to give adequate doses of chemotherapy to these patients.[26]

Prior Chemotherapy. Patients who have received chemotherapy and have failed to respond to it or have relapsed present a serious problem. These patients have usually received the most effective drugs known for their particular type of cancer. They have probably had both surgery and radiotherapy, and their normal tissues may be seriously compromised. They are often in a debilitated state.

The medical oncologist must give these patients "second-line" chemotherapies. These drugs are usually less effective and more toxic. If experimental drugs are used, little may be known about their toxicity. Therefore, the probability of effective treatment decreases and the risks increase.[26]

Table 9–1. Advanced Neoplastic Diseases That Respond to Chemotherapy*

Type of Cancer	Useful Drugs	Response Rate (Per cent)	Survival of Responders (Per cent)
Prolonged Survival or Cure			
Gestational trophoblastic tumors	MTX, Dact, VLB	70 CR†	Cured
Burkitt's tumor	CTX	50 CR	Cured
Testicular tumors: Seminoma Other	CTX, RT PDD, Bleo, Dact, VLB	45 CR, 45 PR 90 CR	30 cured 40 cured
Wilms' tumor	Dact with Surg & RT, VCR (C)‡	30–40 CR	Cured
Acute lymphoblastic leukemia	6MP, MTX, Daun, PDN, L-Asp, BCNU, VCR (C)	90 CR	50 cured
Histiocytic lymphoma	CTX, Adria, VCR, PDN	30 CR	30 cured
Non-Hodgkin's lymphoma (children)	Same as acute lympho-blastic leukemia (C)	90 CR	50–80 cured (depending on stage)
Hodgkin's disease Stages IIB, IIIB, & IV	HN₂, VCR, Procarb, PDN or Adria, Bleo, VLB, DTIC	65–85 CR	50–70 cured
Rhabdomyosarcoma (children)	VCR, Adria, CTX	50–90 CR	20–90 cured (depending on stage)
Palliation and Prolongation of Life			
Prostate carcinoma	Estrogens	70	Questionable increase
Breast carcinoma	Alk. agents, 5FU, MTX, Adria, Androgens, Estro-gens, PDN, NFX, TMX, VCR (C)	60–80	Moderate increase
Acute myeloblastic leukemia	Ara-C & 6TG, Daun, PDN (C)	65	Increase 12 months
Chronic lymphocytic leukemia	Alk. agents, PDN	50	Probable increase
Lymphosarcoma (adults)	Alk. agents, Nitro-soureas, PDN (C)	50	Probable increase
Osteogenic sarcoma	MTX-CF, Adria (C)	20	Increase
Lung, small cell	CTX, Adria, VCR, PDN	70–80	Increase 12–14 months

*From Krakoff, I. H.: Cancer chemotherapeutic agents. *CA—A Journal for Clinicians.* 31:132–133, 1981. Used by permission.
†CR = Complete response; others partial response.
‡(C) = Combination chemotherapy shown to be effective.

General Physical Health. The patients' responses to chemotherapy are directly related to their general health. Patients who are debilitated as a consequence of their disease, its treatment, or other unrelated physical conditions will usually not respond well to chemotherapy. Patients in good physical condition may respond well to chemotherapy, even though their disease is advanced. The aged patient will often have a decreased bone marrow reserve that will require lower doses of drugs. The medical oncologists sometimes elect not to give chemotherapy to aged or debilitated patients.[26]

Nutrition. The cachexia that often occurs as a result of the malignant processes may prevent or limit the administration

Table 9–1. Advanced Neoplastic Diseases That Respond to Chemotherapy *(Continued)*

Type of Cancer	Useful Drugs	Response Rate (Per cent)	Survival of Responders (Per cent)
Palliation with Uncertain Prolongation of Life			
Chronic granulocytic leukemia	Alk. agents, 6MP, HU	90	3 years
Multiple myeloma	Alk. agents, PDN, BCNU, VCR (C)	60	
Ovary	Alk. agents, CPDD, Hex, Adria (C)	30–40	
Endometrium	Progestins	25	
Neuroblastoma	CTX, Adria, Procarb, VCR (C)	30	10–80 surg cures, depending on age and stage
Uncertain Palliation — No Demonstrable Prolongation of Life			
Lung	Alk. agents	30–40 brief responses	
Head and neck	Alk. agents, MTX-CF, Bleo, CPDD	20–30 brief responses	
Large bowel	Ara-C, 5FU, Mito, MeCCNU	15–20	
Stomach	Ara-C, 5FU, Mito (C)	30	
Pancreas	5FU, Adria, Mito (C) (Islet cell: STZ)	<10 (80 in treatment of hypoglycemia)	
Liver	5FU	<10	
Cervix	Alk. agents, Bleo	20	
Melanoma	Alk. agents, DTIC, VLB	20	
Adrenal cortex	o, p'-DDD	Relief of cushingoid syndrome	
Soft tissue sarcoma	MTX-CF, Adria	20	
Local Chemotherapy			
Intracavitary injection for recurrent effusion	Alk. agents, 5FU, Quinacrine, Tetracycline	50 effusions controlled	
Intrathecal injection for meningeal leukemia	Ara-C, MTX	80 brief improvement (also part of combination therapy for acute leukemia)	
Extracorporeal perfusion for cancer of extremities	Alk. agents	Irregular and uncertain	
Continuous infusion for cancer of head and neck, liver and pelvis	5FU, MTX-CF	Irregular and uncertain	

of chemotherapy. If chemotherapy is administered, nutritional deficiencies may actually interfere with the ability of the drugs to destroy the malignancy. If nutritional problems become severe during the course of chemotherapy, treatment may have to be discontinued. Therefore, nutritional maintenance prior to and during chemotherapy is essential to the continuity and maintenance of treatment. Intravenous hyperalimentation is being used more frequently both prior to and during cancer chemotherapy to ensure an adequate nutritional base.[18]

Immunologic Factors. In addition to being important in the prevention of cancer, the immune system seems to be important in the response to treatment. Patients who have a strong immune response are much more likely to respond well to chemotherapy. Patients who have an impaired immune response often do not respond as well to chemotherapy. In fact, in these patients the disease tends to take a rapid, downhill course and they die more quickly, regardless of what treatment is used. Studies are now being conducted using combinations of chemotherapy and immunotherapy to attempt to alter this response.

An effective immune response is very important to tumor control and cure. Thus, the impact of chemotherapy on the immune system has been a serious concern. Because of the damage that most chemotherapy drugs do to the bone marrow, it is often believed that general immunity is severely hampered; however, this is not actually the case. Although immunity is temporarily suppressed at the time of the administration of drugs, there is often a reaction shortly afterwards that stimulates the immune system to rebound at a higher than normal level. Figure 9–3 illustrates the effect of chemotherapy on the immune system.

Psychosocial Factors. Cancer patients have usually known or heard of other persons who have had chemotherapy. Sometimes these people have had very neg-

ative experiences, or they may have died of their disease. As a result, patients may have very negative reactions to the suggestion that chemotherapy be used to treat them. Sometimes they will refuse treatment. If they agree to treatment, they anticipate many problems that may never occur.

The side effects of chemotherapy are often devastating. Some patients will elect to discontinue treatment because to them the side effects are more frightening than the disease itself. Providing information and support may be decisive in determining whether or not the patient elects to continue therapy. Adequate support systems for the patient, whether family or community based, can also facilitate continuity of therapy.[46]

Cancer patients who consider themselves passive recipients of therapy do not respond as well to treatment. Therefore, it is important to include patients in planning and carrying out their care, by encouraging them to participate in related decisions, by keeping them informed about their response to treatment, and by encouraging them to take responsibility for as much of their care as possible.

Financial Factors. The cost of chemotherapy is high. Physicians are sometimes reluctant to inform the patient about chemotherapy as an option because of costs. Even if the care is being paid for by a third party, the patient and family must still pay for many costs (often including medication) not covered by insurance. A single dose of some chemotherapy drugs can cost from $200 to $500. Frequent doctor visits, blood tests, and x-ray studies on an outpatient basis can add up quickly. The cost of aggressive inpatient treatment can be overwhelming.

The patients' concern about costs can lead to their refusal to accept treatment. If they agree to costly treatment, the emotional distress about finances can impair the treatment response.[26] The long-term consequences for the family can be devastating. Some families have sold their house, their car, and other financial assets to provide chemotherapy for a family

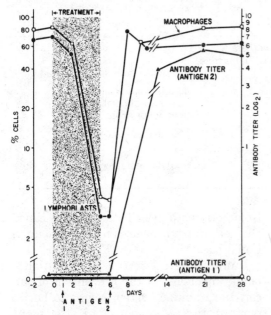

Figure 9–3. Effects of intensive intermittent chemotherapy on host defense mechanisms. (From Hersh, E.: In *Cancer Therapy,* edited by Holland, J. F., and Frei, E., III. Philadelphia: Lea and Febiger, 1973, p. 681. Used by permission.)

member. Although the treatment may prolong the patient's life, the family may be in financial straits for years afterwards.

Treatment Support Facilities. Aggressive treatment with chemotherapy causes serious side effects. Adequate facilities must be available to treat side effects, or doses must be reduced to diminish them. The side effects of greatest concern are the consequences of bone marrow depression. Platelet transfusions and granulocyte transfusions must be available, if needed. A competent laboratory must be available to diagnose severe infections that may occur, and a source of radiation therapy must be nearby to treat brain, spinal cord, or bone metastases.[26]

Some people believe that cancer treatment should take place only in a cancer research center. The treatment there is usually free, and many believe that the care is better. But there are transportation and hotel and meal costs involved in traveling to a research center that can be as great as medical costs. The patient will be away from family and friends — perhaps for long periods of time. Kennealey and Mitchell take the following position:

Because cancer chemotherapy at times requires intensive supportive care, it has recently been suggested that cancer can be treated competently only at a medical center. Robinson (1976), in a widely read popular magazine, has stated that "the average cancer patient is likely to be misdiagnosed by his local doctor and maltreated at his local hospital." While treatment at a medical center may be appropriate, or even necessary in some cases, we believe that in a majority of cases, the difficulty and expense of travel do not justify a transfer of care to a cancer center. The number of well-trained oncologists in private practice has increased considerably in recent years, and will continue to increase in the near future.[26]

The Development of Drug Resistance

One of the most frustrating problems in cancer chemotherapy and a major cause of treatment failures is the development of drug resistance. This occurs after the patient has been receiving a drug that is very effective in reducing the tumor size. Somehow, the tumor becomes resistant to the drug and begins growing in spite of the drug therapy. How drug resistance occurs is not well understood. Much of what is suggested is hypothetical, not based on research. It has been difficult to find ways to conduct research on the causes of drug resistance.

It is possible that the drug destroys all of the cells that were originally sensitive to that particular agent. Other groups of cells within the tumor continue to grow when the drug is given. In this situation, it would appear clinically that the tumor had been responding to the drug and then suddenly stopped responding.

Some researchers believe that the malignant cell develops "repair" enzymes that can mend the DNA damaged by the drug. Other proposed reasons involve changes in the metabolic pathways or in the cell structure itself, perhaps due to the derepression that may occur as the malignant cell progresses to an increasingly abnormal state.

Resistance seems to occur more rapidly when a single chemotherapy drug is given. Combinations of drugs remain effective for longer periods of time. But sooner or later, unless all the cells are destroyed, resistance will develop. If other drugs that are effective against that specific type of malignancy are available, the oncologist will switch to them. But eventually resistance will develop to those drugs, and if no other therapies are effective, the patient will die.[54]

PHARMACOLOGY OF ANTINEOPLASTIC DRUGS USED IN CHEMOTHERAPY

Until very recently, little was known about the pharmacology of the antineoplastic drugs. Studies are now being conducted to further our understanding of the activity of these drugs after administration. This knowledge is needed in order to predict the patient's physiologic responses to the drug. It will also be helpful in the development of new drugs.

Absorption. If the drug is administered orally, it is important to know how much of the drug is absorbed and how fast.

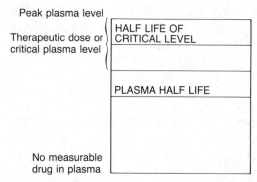

Figure 9–4. Significant points of drug plasma levels.

In other words, how much time is required for the drug to reach its peak blood level? As with many other drugs, the therapeutic response to some antineoplastic drugs is dependent on the drugs' reaching a critical blood plasma level. The length of time this critical level is maintained may also be important. Thus, studies are now being conducted to determine the plasma half-life of a drug. The plasma half-life is the time required for the plasma level of the drug to drop to 50 per cent of the peak drug level. If a critical plasma level of a drug is required, the half-life of the critical level will also be identified. At this point, drug levels have dropped to 50 per cent of the therapeutic dose. See Figure 9–4 for an illustration of plasma levels.

Protein Binding. Several types of proteins normally float in the blood plasma. These proteins have sites on their surface to which drug molecules can attach. Once attached, the drug molecule is very gradually released again into the plasma.

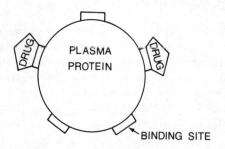

While the drug molecule is protein bound, it is not active. A specific portion of the calculated drug dosage is expected to be protein bound. If this does not occur, the drug plasma level will be higher than expected, possibly increasing the risk of toxic reaction. Sometimes other drugs that have been administered prior to the cytotoxic drug will take up the available binding sites. If the patient's total serum protein level or serum albumin level is below normal, sufficient protein may not be available for binding.

Biotransformation. Many antineoplastic drugs are not in an active form when they are administered. These drugs must be changed into active metabolites by the liver before they can destroy cancer cells. In this situation, the drug disappears from the plasma because it is being converted into metabolites by the liver. Some drugs are converted by the liver into inactive forms, which may then be excreted through the bile. If the liver is not functioning properly, these processes may not occur or may occur more slowly. This may seriously alter drug action and increase toxicity. If other drugs that must undergo biotransformation in the liver are also being given, the possibility of drug interactions increases greatly.

Excretion Patterns. The most common route of drug excretion is through the kidneys. Some drugs are excreted in the form in which they were administered. Others must be transformed by the liver before excretion can take place. If renal function is impaired, drug excretion may occur more slowly, or the drug may cause further kidney damage. Slower excretion may mean higher toxicities. Excretion may also occur in bile, feces, sweat, saliva, respiration, and breast milk.

COMMONLY USED DRUGS

The chemotherapy drugs are generally classified according to their chemical characteristics. The primary classifications are alkylating agents, antibiotics, vinca alkaloids, antimetabolites, and hormones. As with most drug groupings, there is a miscellaneous classification of drugs that do not easily fit into any other category.

Table 9–2. Specific Agents Used in Cancer Chemotherapy: Polyfunctional Alkylating Agents*

Agents	Principal Route of Administration	Usual Dose	Acute Toxic Signs	Major Toxic Manifestations
Methylbis β-Chloroethyl Amine HCl (HN₂, Mustargen)	IV	16 mg/m² single or divided doses	N & V†	Therapeutic doses moderately depress peripheral blood cell count; excessive doses cause severe bone marrow depres-
Chlorambucil (Leukeran)	Oral	6–12 mg/day	None	sion with leukopenia, thrombo- cytopenia and bleeding. Maxi- mum toxicity may occur 2
Melphalan (Alkeran)	Oral	6–10 mg/day 2–4 mg/day maintenance	None	or 3 weeks after last dose. Dosage, therefore, must be carefully controlled. Alopecia
Cyclophosphamide (Endoxan, Cytoxan)	IV	600–1000 mg/m²	N & V	and hemorrhagic cystitis occur occasionally with cyclophos- phamide.
	Oral	single dose 50–200 mg/day		
Triethylenethiophosphoramide (TSPA, Thio-TEPA)	IV	0.8–1.0 mg/kg or 0.2 mg/kg/day × 4–5 days	None	
Busulfan (Myleran)	Oral	2–6 mg/day	None	

*From Krakoff, I. H.: Cancer chemotherapeutic agents. *CA – A Journal for Clinicians*. 31:134, 1981. Used by permission.
†Nausea and vomiting.

Alkylating Agents

Alkylating agents have the ability to substitute alkyl groups for hydrogen atoms in certain organic compounds. Although many substances within the cell can be alkylated in this way, the most important target of cancer alkylating agents is DNA. Alkylation of DNA causes breaks in the DNA molecule and cross-linking, thus interfering with replication and transcription processes. When the cell attempts to divide, it dies. This is similar to the process that occurs as a result of radiation. Therefore, alkylating agents are said to be radiomimetic.[11] The alkylating agents as a group are cell cycle–nonspecific. However, there are distinct differences between the drugs in terms of pharmacologic action and clinical use.[11, 34] (See Table 9–2.)

Mechlorethamine Hydrochloride (Nitrogen Mustard, HN₂, Mustargen). Nitrogen mustard is very damaging to skin and mucous membranes; therefore, gloves must be worn during its preparation. It comes in powder form and must be mixed with water just prior to administration. Care must be taken to avoid inhaling the powder. Nitrogen mustard rapidly becomes inactive after mixing and must be administered immediately after preparation. During its administration, caution must be taken to avoid contact with the skin or eyes of either the patient or the health care providers. If exposure occurs, the area should be immediately washed with water.

Nitrogen mustard may be given intravenously or injected directly into a body cavity. If it is administered intravenously, it is usually injected into the tubing of an established free flowing intravenous infusion of normal saline solution. The primary effects of nitrogen mustard occur within seconds or minutes after administration. The drug is rapidly converted to an inactive form within the body. Severe nausea and vomiting may occur at the time of its injection. To diminish this very unpleasant reaction, an antiemetic is often given prior to the nitrogen mustard. If vomiting is still severe, a sedative may be effective in reducing symptoms.[11]

Cyclophosphamide (Cytoxan). Cytoxan is usually administered orally, but is also available in an intravenous form. It must undergo biotransformation in the liver before becoming active. Approximately 50 per cent of its active metabolites become protein bound. The metabolites of Cytoxan have a plasma half-life of 4 to 6½ hours after an intravenous dose, but some can still be detected in the plasma several days later. The drug is primarily excreted through the kidneys, although small amounts may be found in the cerebrospinal fluid, breast milk, sweat, and saliva. In addition to the common side effects of alkylating agents, Cytoxan can cause a severe hemorrhagic cystitis because of accumulation of the metabolites in the bladder. This can usually be avoided by maintaining a high fluid output. Another side effect usually occurring with high doses of Cytoxan is impairment of water excretion. This is called the syndrome of inappropriate antidiuretic hormone (ADH) secretion. These patients will experience hyponatremia, weight gain, and concentrated urine during and after drug administration. Cardiac decompensation can occur with a fluid overload in susceptible patients.[11, 59]

Chlorambucil (Leukeran). Chlorambucil is given orally and is relatively slow acting. It requires 3 to 4 weeks to achieve the desired effect, after which a lower maintenance dose is given. Toxic effects occur only after prolonged therapy. Its primary use is in the treatment of chronic lymphocytic leukemia.[11]

Melphalan (Alkeran, Phenylalanine Mustard, L-PAM, L-Sarcolysin). Melphalan is administered orally. Frequency of treatment is usually dependent on the patient's white blood count, since the drug can cause severe unpredictable myelosuppression. Its most common use is in the treatment of multiple myeloma.[11]

Busulfan. Busulfan is given orally. Its main effect is on the granulocytes of the white blood cells. The toxicities of the drug are almost completely hematopoietic. It is used chiefly to treat chronic myelocytic leukemia.[11]

Triethylenethiophosphoramide (Thio-TEPA). Thio-TEPA has toxicity patterns and clinical uses almost identical with those of nitrogen mustard. The doses are generally double those of nitrogen mustard. Thio-TEPA is more stable than nitrogen mustard and does not have to be prepared immediately before administration. It is not destructive to skin and seldom causes nausea. However, for the most part, Cytoxan is preferred to thio-TEPA for most clinical uses.[11]

Dacarbazine (DTIC). DTIC is administered intravenously. It is inactive and must undergo biotransformation. Exposure of this drug to light may alter its effectiveness. It causes only minimal immunosuppression. The nausea and vomiting it promotes often cease after 2 or 3 doses. DTIC is used to treat malignant melanoma, sarcomas, and lymphomas.[11]

Nitrosoureas (Carmustine [BCNU], Lomustine [CCNU], Semustine [Methyl-CCNU]). Nitrosoureas must undergo biotransformation to become active. This biotransformation leads to a variety of biologic effects, some of which are unusual for carcinogenic drugs. One of these effects is that nitrosoureas may cause greater damage to resting cells than to those in the cell cycle. The nitrosoureas are lipid soluble and cross the blood-brain barrier. Peak blood levels of the metabolites occur 1 to 6 hours after oral administration. They are excreted primarily through the kidneys, although the liver is also involved. On injection, BCNU causes local pain that is difficult to control. Methyl-CCNU is very unstable at room temperatures, and bottles of the drug kept at room temperature may explode.

Antibiotics

The antibiotics used to treat cancer are natural products of the soil fungus *Streptomyces*. They have both antibiotic and tumoricidal effects. They act by directly binding to DNA and as a result inhibit DNA and ribonucleic acid (RNA) synthesis. They are cell cycle–nonspecific in their action.[11, 21] (See Table 9–3.)

Doxorubicin (Adriamycin) and Daunomycin. Adriamycin and daunomycin are very closely related. Both are administered intravenously and must undergo biotransformation in the liver. A large por-

Table 9–3. Specific Agents Used in Cancer Chemotherapy: Antibiotics*

Agents	Principal Route of Adminis- tration	Usual Dose	Acute Toxic Signs	Major Toxic Manifestations
Adriamycin	IV	50–75 mg/m² in single or divided doses every 3 weeks	N & V†	Stomatitis, GI disturbances, alopecia, bone marrow depres- sion. Cardiac toxicity at cumulative doses over 500 mg/m².
Bleomycin (Blenoxane)	IV SC	10 mg/m²/day × 5–7 days Maintenance: 1.0–2.0 mg/day	N & V, chills, fever	Mucocutaneous ulcerations, alopecia, pulmonary fibrosis in approximately 5% patients.
Dactinomycin (Cosmegen)	IV	0.04 mg/kg weekly	N & V	Stomatitis, GI disturbances, alopecia, bone marrow de- pression.
Daunorubicin‡	IV	Total doses never to exceed 25 mg/kg	N & V, fever	Bone marrow depression with leukopenia and thrombocyto- penia, alopecia, stomatitis, cardiac toxicity at cumulative doses over 25 mg/kg.
Mithramycin	IV	25 micrograms/kg every other day × 3–4 days	N & V	Bone marrow depression particularly thrombocytopenic bleeding, hypocalcemia, hepatic toxicity at large doses.
Mitomycin C (Mutamycin)	IV	0.06 mg/kg 2 × weekly	N & V	Bone marrow depression.

*From Krakoff, I. H.: Cancer chemotherapeutic agents. *CA—A Journal for Clinicians.* 31:135, 1981. Used by permission.
†Nausea and vomiting.
‡Available for experimental use only.

tion of the metabolites become protein bound, are excreted in the bile, and remain in the plasma for long periods. Drug inter- actions are very likely to occur with these drugs because of the extensive biotrans- formations occurring in the liver.

Both Adriamycin and daunomycin are highly toxic. They cause severe bone mar- row suppression and severe nausea and vomiting. Cardiac toxicity, which is dose related, can occur and result in arrhythmi- as or delayed congestive heart failure. Therefore, the recommended lifetime total dosage is 550 mg/m².

Adriamycin has a red color and patients should be told that their urine may turn pink or red shortly after administration. It is sometimes referred to as the "Red Devil" because of the severe vomiting it causes. Adriamycin will also sensitize tissues to radiation if radiation is administered con- currently. Tissues that have previously been irradiated may react by a "recall phenomenon," in which previous reactions to the radiation may recur. Adriamycin is used with a wide variety of malignancies.

Daunomycin is still considered an experi- mental drug and is essentially restricted to the treatment of leukemia. Both Adri- amycin and daunomycin cause severe tis- sue damage if extravasation occurs at the site of injection.[11, 21, 50]

Actinomycin D (Dactinomycin, Cos- megen). Actinomycin D is given intrave- nously, usually through a free flowing infu- sion. It has a plasma half-life of 36 hours and much of the drug becomes protein bound. After 9 days, only about 30 per cent of this drug will have been excreted through urine and feces. Actinomycin D is a radiosensitizing drug and can cause "re- call phenomenon." Severe tissue damage and necrosis may result from extravasa- tion.[11, 21]

Bleomycin (Blenoxane). Bleomycin may be administered intravenously or in- tramuscularly. It has a plasma half-life of 2 hours and becomes highly concentrated in skin, lung, kidney, peritoneum, and lym- phatics. Bleomycin is degraded by an en- zyme found primarily in tumor cells, kid- ney, and liver. The enzyme is not present in skin and lung, the two organs most vulnerable to the drug. The development of tumor resistance seems to be related to the enzyme's increased ability to degrade the drug.

Bleomycin is excreted primarily through the kidneys and doses must be greatly reduced in patients with renal failure. The drug seldom causes bone marrow depression. Its primary toxic effect is a pulmonary dysfunction that occurs in 10 per cent of the patients who receive it. The first reaction is dyspnea with fine rales. In 1 per cent of treated patients, this progresses to a fatal pulmonary fibrosis. This is more common in patients receiving a total dose of more than 400 units, in patients receiving single doses greater than 26 units/m^2, in patients with a previous history of pulmonary disease, and in patients above 70 years of age.[11, 21]

Mithramycin (Mithracin). Mithramycin is administered intravenously. Little is known about its pharmacology, other than that the drug has severe toxicities that make many clinicians reluctant to use it. These toxicities include severe hemorrhagic diathesis, arterial occlusions, central nervous system reactions, hepatorenal dysfunctions, hypocalcemia, and stomatitis.[11, 21] Because these toxicities can be unpredictable and life threatening, it is recommended that mithramycin be administered only to hospitalized patients.

Mitomycin-C (Mutamycin). Mitomycin-C is usually administered intravenously and has a plasma half-life of 10 to 15 minutes. It is metabolized and inactivated by the liver and to some extent by renal clearance. Mitomycin-C is extremely toxic and causes a delayed myelosuppression that is cumulative and sometimes fatal. Patients who have had previous radiotherapy or chemotherapy are particularly susceptible. Mitomycin-C is used with a number of adenocarcinomas, head and neck cancer, and chronic myelogenous leukemia. Unfortunately, it has a short duration of response, usually from 1 to 3 months. Therefore, it is not generally used as a first-line treatment for any tumors.[11, 21]

Vinca Alkaloids

The periwinkle plant is the source of two very useful antineoplastic drugs, vincristine and vinblastine. (See Table 9–6.) These drugs bind to cellular microtubular proteins, preventing proper development of the mitotic spindle in dividing cells and thus leading to mitotic arrest. They are cell cycle–specific.

There are several other plant products currently under active investigation. Some of these are the May apple derivatives called epipodophyllotoxins (labeled VM-26 and VO-16-213). Another is maytansine.[11, 13]

Vinblastine (Velban). Vinblastine is given intravenously and local extravasation will cause tissue damage. It has a half-life of about 20 hours. Vinblastine is extensively protein bound. It is in active form when injected, but is partly metabolized by the liver to another active form. About 80 per cent is excreted in the bile and 20 per cent is excreted in the urine as unchanged drug. Toxicity increases when the drug is given to patients with liver damage. Bone marrow suppression is vinblastine's most dangerous toxic effect.[11]

Vincristine (Oncovin). Vincristine is given intravenously and will cause local tissue destruction from extravasation. The pharmacology of vincristine is identical to that of vinblastine. It becomes extensively protein bound and is slowly excreted through the liver and kidneys. Vincristine will slowly cross the blood-brain barrier and will bind with the microtubules of the nervous system.

The most important toxic effect of vincristine is a mixed autonomic and motor-sensory neuropathy. The earliest indication of neurotoxicity is depression of the Achilles tendon reflex. This is followed by paresthesias of the fingers and toes. Patients begin having difficulty in dressing themselves and particularly with tasks such as buttoning, zipping, and snapping. Muscle pain, weakness, and progressive sensory impairment will occur if drug use is continued. Eventually the patient will develop severe, generalized motor weakness. Autonomic nervous system damage is reflected by severe constipation and, rarely, ileus. Most of these neurologic changes can be reversed by withdrawing the drug, but some symptoms may continue for 6 months after the drug is discontinued. The motor weakness that has developed may be irreversible.[11]

Many oncologists discontinue drug therapy if any motor weakness occurs at all. The easiest test of motor weakness is to ask patients to attempt to walk on their heels. The patients' inability to do this is considered a sign of dangerous neurotoxicity.

The constipation resulting from vincristine can be severe and requires constant nursing attention. Patients can develop fecal impactions in spite of stool softeners, cathartics, and daily enemas. These patients should be checked regularly for impactions if they are bedfast, even if they are having regular bowel movements.

Antimetabolites

Antimetabolites are structurally very similar to some of the normal metabolites that are required for cell functioning and replication. Because they appear to be essential metabolites, antimetabolites are able to enter the cell. They then interact with cellular enzymes and damage the cell. The cell's normal metabolic pathways are disrupted, and the cell cannot function or replicate properly. Many antimetabolites have been developed and tested in the past 30 years, but only five are commercially available and widely used. (See Table 9–4.) With the exception of 5-fluorouracil, the antimetabolites are cell cycle–specific.

Methotrexate (MTX, Amethopterin). Methotrexate can be given either orally or intravenously. It works by strongly competing for the folate binding site of an enzyme called dihydrofolate reductase (DHFR). This binding blocks the metabolic pathway that leads to the synthesis of thymidine and purine nucleotides, thus completely suppressing DNA synthesis. The development of resistance to methotrexate may be related to increased production of DHFR or to cell membrane changes that block the entrance of methotrexate into the cell.

The cytotoxicity of methotrexate can be reversed by leucovorin (citrovorum factor;

Table 9–4. Specific Agents Used in Cancer Chemotherapy: Antimetabolites*

Agents	Principal Route of Administration	Usual Dose	Acute Toxic Signs	Major Toxic Manifestations
Methotrexate (Methotrexate)	Oral IV IV	2.5–5.0 mg/day 25–50 mg 1–2 × weekly 200 mg–10 gm with CF rescue	None	Oral and digestive tract ulcerations; bone marrow depression with leukopenia, thrombocytopenia and bleeding. Toxicity enhanced by impaired kidney function.
6-Mercaptopurine (6-MP, Purinethol)	Oral	100 mg/m²/day	None	Therapeutic doses usually well tolerated; excessive doses cause bone marrow depression.
6-Thioguanine (6-TG, Thioguan)	Oral	80 mg/kg/day	None	
5-Fluorouracil (5-FU, Fluorouracil)	IV	12 mg/kg/day × 3 days; smaller dose, 1–2 × weekly for maintenance	None	Stomatitis, nausea, GI injury, bone marrow depression.
Arabinosylcytosine (Ara-C, Cytosar)	IV	1.0–3.0 mg/kg/day × 10–20 days	N & V†	Bone marrow depression, megaloblastosis, leukopenia, thrombocytopenia.

*From Krakoff, I. H.: Cancer chemotherapeutic agents. *CA—A Journal for Clinicians.* 31:134, 1981. Used by permission.
†Nausea and vomiting.

5-formyl tetrahydrofolate). How leucovorin works is not completely understood. Theoretically, it should bypass the blockage of DHFR. However, it is possible that methotrexate and leucovorin may share the same cell membrane active transport system. The leucovorin would then prevent the entrance of methotrexate into the cell. It is sometimes necessary to administer methotrexate in lethal doses in order to achieve effective tumor response. Leucovorin is then given to block the effect of methotrexate on normal cells. This is called high dose methotrexate with leucovorin rescue.[1]

The effectiveness and toxicity of methotrexate are dependent on the length of time that the cells are exposed to critical concentrations of the drug. After intravenous infusion, there is a rapid initial plasma clearance, but the critical therapeutic concentration remains. The critical plasma level begins to diminish 12 to 36 hours after administration. The half-life of this critical phase is 8 to 12 hours.

Fifty to 70 per cent of methotrexate becomes bound to serum albumin. If the serum albumin level is low or if other drugs that have been given have bound to the albumin's protein binding sites, there is an increased uptake of free methotrexate into the cells. This will cause a concurrent increase in toxicity. Aspirin and sulfonamides are particularly apt to interfere with the protein binding sites required by methotrexate.

Normal intestinal flora partially degrade methotrexate if it is given orally. If methotrexate is administered intravenously, portions of it are exposed to intestinal flora when it enters the enterohepatic circulation. If antibiotics that destroy the normal intestinal flora are given, methotrexate toxicity will increase.

Many drugs alter the ability of methotrexate to enter or leave the cell; for example, cephalothin and hydrocortisone interfere with the entrance of methotrexate into the cell. A high blood level of vincristine enhances the transport of methotrexate into the cell.

The speed of renal clearance also affects the serum level of methotrexate. Methotrexate is insoluble in acidic liquids. If the urine is alkaline, renal clearance is much more rapid. Any decrease in renal function will also increase toxicity. Some drugs, such as probenecid, inhibit the secretion of methotrexate and thus increase its toxicity.[9, 11]

5-Fluorouracil (5-FU). 5-FU is administered intravenously. It diffuses rapidly into all tissues of the body, including the nervous system. Within 10 to 20 minutes, 50 per cent of the drug is cleared from the plasma, and within 3 hours the drug is not measurable in the plasma. However, both 5-FU and its metabolites may be present for long periods of time in some tissues.

5-FU must be converted to an active metabolite in order to be effective. This conversion occurs within the cell, where two active metabolites are formed by the action of several enzymes. The most effective metabolite, 5-fluorodeoxyuridylate, functions as an irreversible inhibitor of the enzyme thymidylate synthetase. The formation of 5-fluorouridylate, which inhibits RNA synthesis, is probably a less desirable consequence.

5-FU is degraded in the liver and in some other tissues. These degrading enzymes are present in high concentrations in carcinomas of the gut, but not in carcinomas of the colon. This may explain the sensitivity of colon cancer to 5-FU. Eighty per cent of 5-FU is degraded by the liver; the rest is excreted by the kidneys. The chief toxicities of 5-FU are to the bone marrow and gastrointestinal tract.[11, 37, 57]

Nucleoside Analogues. Nucleoside analogues are both antineoplastic and antiviral. They are transported very readily into rapidly dividing cells and are easily activated by a single metabolic step. These drugs are cell cycle–specific. The two drugs in this category are immunosuppressive and are primarily used to treat acute myeloid leukemia.

Cytarabine (ara-C, Cytosine Arabinoside, 1-β-D-Arabinofuranosylcytosine, Cytosar). Cytarabine is administered intravenously and functions by inhibiting DNA polymerase. The plasma half-life of the drug is 2 to 2½ hours. The drug is inactivated by enzymes present in plasma and in some cells. The inactive metabolite of the drug is excreted in the urine. The toxicity of cytarabine involves primarily the bone marrow and gastrointestinal tract.[11, 37]

5-Azacytidine (NSC-102816). 5-Azacytidine may be given intravenously or subcutaneously. It undergoes biotransformations similar to those of cytarabine. Its plasma half-life is 3½ hours, and within 24 hours of administration 90 per cent of the drug is excreted in the urine. 5-Azacytidine is usually given by continuous 24-hour infusion for 5 days. It is reconstituted with sterile water and then mixed with Ringer's solution. This drug decomposes in solution and must be freshly prepared every 3 or 4 hours.[11, 37]

Purine Analogues. Preformed purines or those made within the cell are essential components of RNA, DNA, and coenzymes. The two purine antagonists that are antineoplastic were developed in 1952 and are still considered useful today. Although it is not antineoplastic, allopurinol (another purine analogue) is a useful drug in oncology.[11, 31]

6-Thioguanine (6-TG, Thioguanine). 6-TG is given orally and requires metabolic activation for cytotoxicity. What appears to be its chief mechanism of action is its ability to ultimately incorporate into DNA as a false purine base. 6-TG is used primarily in the treatment of acute leukemia and is considered cell cycle–specific. It is usually given in combination with other drugs. The major toxic effect is myelosuppression, which may be delayed and severe.[11, 31]

6-Mercaptopurine (6-MP, Purinethol). 6-MP is very similar to 6-TG in pharmacology, toxic effects, and clinical uses. However, the enzyme xanthine oxidase is essential to degrade 6-MP. If the patient is receiving allopurinol, which inhibits xanthine oxidase, the dose of 6-MP must be decreased by 60 to 70 per cent. 6-MP is usually used to treat acute lymphocytic leukemia.[11, 31]

Allopurinol (Zyloprim). Allopurinol is not an antineoplastic drug. It is used to treat gout and is also effective in lowering the elevated serum uric acid levels that may develop in the aggressive treatment of leukemias, lymphomas, and some other types of cancer. It is administered orally and reaches its peak plasma level 2 to 6 hours after administration.[11, 31]

Hormones

The effectiveness of hormone therapy for cancer is dependent on the fact that some cancer cells retain their responsiveness to normal regulating mechanisms. However, as malignant cells become more undifferentiated and anaplastic, they may be less responsive to such controls. The endocrine regulatory system is very complex and can be manipulated at many levels, from the target receptor sites on a diseased cell membrane to the release of hormone secretion at sites distant from a malignancy.[10]

Since tumors vary in their responsiveness to hormone therapy, research is being conducted to carefully determine the patients for whom hormone therapy will be appropriate. For example, it is now possible to identify the breast cancer patients who will be most likely to respond to hormone therapy.[10]

There are several strategies employed to alter the hormonal environment of the cancer cell and thus interfere with cell functioning. One approach is to surgically remove or destroy the gland that secretes the hormone or the gland controlling the production and secretion of that hormone. Hormone secretion can be suppressed by the administration of a drug that interferes with hormone synthesis or secretion. It is sometimes possible to reduce the effectiveness of a hormone that stimulates cancer cell growth by administering a drug that competes with the hormone for receptor sites on the cancer cell membrane or a drug that alters the cancer cells' response to the hormone. An example of this approach is current use of antiestrogens. Research is now being conducted to find ways to utilize hormones to sensitize the cancer cells to

Table 9–5.   Specific Agents Used in Cancer Chemotherapy: Steroid Compounds*

Agents	Principal Route of Adminis- tration	Usual Dose	Acute Toxic Signs	Major Toxic Manifestations
Androgen				
Testosterone propionate	IM	50–100 mg 3 × weekly	None	Fluid retention, masculiniza-
Fluoxymesterone (Halotestin)	Oral	10–20 mg/day		tion.
Estrogen				
Diethylstilbestrol	Oral	Breast: 1.5 mg 3/day	Occas.	Fluid retention, feminization.
		Prostate: 1 mg/day	N & V†	Uterine bleeding.
Ethinyl estradiol (Estinyl)	Oral	Breast: 0.1–1.0 mg 3/day Prostate: 0.1 mg/day		
Progestin				
Hydroxyprogesterone caproate (Delalutin)	IM	1 gm 2 × weekly		
6-Methylhydroxyprogesterone (Provera)	Oral IM	100–200 mg/day 200–600 mg 2 × weekly	None	
Adrenal Cortical Compounds				
Cortisone acetate	Oral	20–100 mg/day	None	Fluid retention, hypertension,
Prednisone (Meticorten)	Oral	15–100 mg/day		diabetes, increased suscepti-
Dexamethasone (Decadron)	Oral	0.5–4.0 mg/day		bility to infection.
Methylprednisolone sodium succinate (Solu-Medrol)	IM IV	10–125 mg/day		
Hydrocortisone sodium succinate (Solu-Cortef)	IV	100–500 mg/day		

*From Krakoff, I. H.: Cancer chemotherapeutic agents. *CA—A Journal for Clinicians.* 31:135, 1981. Used by permission.
†Nausea and vomiting.

chemotherapy drugs or to actually transport chemotherapy drugs into the cancer cells.[10]

The adrenocorticosteroids are the most widely used hormones in cancer treatment, although there is controversy among researchers about their appropriate use. (See Table 9–5.) The way in which they function in cancer therapy is not well understood. Steroids have multiple side effects that can be serious; for example, the hypothalamic-pituitary-adrenal axis of the endocrine system may be suppressed long after the therapy has been discontinued.[11]

Estrogens.   Two neoplastic diseases are known to respond to estrogen treatment: carcinoma of the breast in postmenopausal women and carcinoma of the prostate. Its mechanism of action is not well understood, but probably involves abrogating androgen in cancer of the prostate and estrogen receptor sites in breast cancer.[11]

The most commonly used estrogen in chemotherapy is diethylstilbestrol (DES). It is potent, relatively long-lasting, can be administered orally, and is inexpensive. For prostate cancer, the usual dose is 1 mg

daily. Higher doses have been associated with an increased risk of death from cardiovascular disease. For postmenopausal breast cancer, the usual dose is 5 mg three times a day. The response is dose dependent, with higher doses more effective than lower doses. However, higher doses cause an increase in toxic effects.[11]

Side effects of estrogen therapy are dose related and include nausea and vomiting; salt and water retention; libido changes in women and impotence in men; aggravation of uterine fibroids, endometriosis, chronic cystic mastitis, and migraine; a low risk of hypertension, thrombophlebitis, and embolism; liver dysfunction at high doses; urinary stress incontinence in women; and hypercalcemia in patients with breast cancer. Other than hypercalcemia, the side effects do not usually require that treatment be stopped. Gynecomastia may develop in men, but may be prevented by a single 900 rad dose of radiation therapy to the breasts before treatment is initiated. Gynecomastia is difficult to treat after it occurs.[11]

Antiestrogens.   Three drugs are included in this classification: clomiphene (Clomid), nafoxidine, and tamoxifen (Nolvadex). Clomiphene is available to treat anovulatory sterility; however, only tamoxifen is available in the United States for the treatment of cancer.[11] All three of these drugs bind to estrogen receptors on the cell membrane, thus depleting the available estrogen receptor sites. In postmenopausal women, mild estrogenic effects such as uterine bleeding may occur.[11]

The antiestrogens are given orally. Widely varying doses have been found to be effective. A dose-response relationship is not evident. Optimal doses and treatment schedules have not been defined. However, the recommended dose of tamoxifen is 10 mg twice a day. The antiestrogens are cleared very slowly from the body. The estrogen antagonism from a single dose may last for many weeks.[11]

The side effects of the drugs are not always the same. All may cause nausea and possible vomiting. Hot flushing occurs with clomiphene and tamoxifen, skin reactions with nafoxidine, visual blurring with tamoxifen and clomiphene, and mild thrombocytopenia with tamoxifen. A severe diffuse, reversible cerebral dysfunction with memory loss and intellectual deterioration can occur with clomiphene.[11]

Progestins. Naturally occurring progestins are not used in chemotherapy. However, synthetic derivatives are commonly used as antagonists of estrogens, androgens, and gonadotropins. The two most commonly used progestins are hydroxyprogesterone caproate (Delalutin) and megestrol acetate (Megace). Delalutin is given intramuscularly, its dosage ranging from 1 gm twice a week to 5 gm weekly. Megace is given orally in doses ranging from 40 to 320 mg per day for endometrial cancer and 160 mg per day for breast cancer.[11]

Progestins have no toxic side effects, but will produce changes in the acinar cells of the breast and in the epithelium of the female genital tract. Their metabolic patterns are not known.

Androgens. The most common use of androgens in chemotherapy is for meta-

static breast cancer in postmenopausal women. How androgens exert their effect on the malignancy is not well understood. If the breast cancer cells have estrogen receptor sites, there will be a greater response rate to androgen therapy.[11]

The parenteral androgen commonly used is testosterone propionate given intramuscularly in a dose of 100 mg three times a week. The oral forms are fluoxymesterone (Halotestin) and testolactone (Teslac). Halotestin is given in divided doses of 10 to 40 mg per day. Teslac may be given intramuscularly at a dose of 100 mg three times a week, or orally at a dose of 250 mg four times a day. The effects of this therapy may not appear for 6 to 12 weeks.[11]

Female patients receiving androgens will experience deepening of the voice, hirsutism, amenorrhea, and clitoral enlargement. The extent of these effects is dependent on the drug used, the dose, and the length of treatment. Changes in libido and personality may also occur. Fluid retention may be a problem. Severe hypercalcemia occurs with this drug in 10 per cent of women with metastases to the bone.[11]

Adrenocorticosteroids. Cortisone and its synthetic derivatives are very commonly used as a component of combination chemotherapy. According to Cline and Haskell, their use is controversial and their mechanism of action in malignancy is not well understood.[11]

There is a wide variation in the potency of the many available corticosteroids. They can be divided into two groups: those with a short duration of action and those with prolonged action and greater potency. Cortisol and prednisone are weak and have a short duration of action. Dexamethasone has a long duration of action and is more potent.[11]

The side effects of short-term therapy include potassium loss, sodium and water retention, psychosis, and exacerbation of diabetes mellitus. The side effects of long-term therapy are extensive and involve most body systems. They include myopathy, osteoporosis, aseptic necrosis of bone, pancreatitis, peptic ulcers, pseudotumor cerebri, glaucoma, cataracts, hypertension, obesity, hyperlipidemia, immunosuppression, impaired wound healing, growth failure, amenorrhea, and suppression of the hypothalamic-pituitary-adrenal axis.[11]

Because of the risk of these serious side effects, cancer patients are treated with large doses for as brief a time as possible to obtain a clinical response. If the treatment period is longer than 7 days, withdrawal of the drug must be gradual.[11]

Miscellaneous Drugs

Almost any grouping of drugs includes some that do not neatly fit into any category; cancer drugs are no exception. Some of the following drugs are still considered experimental and their pharmacology and mechanisms of action have not been as thoroughly studied as drugs that have been utilized over a longer period of time. (See Table 9–6.)

Procarbazine. Procarbazine is administered orally and must undergo biotransformation before becoming active in cancer cell destruction. This transformation occurs rapidly after administration. Procarbazine is cell cycle–nonspecific, although its mechanism of action is not understood. It easily crosses the blood-brain barrier. The major portion of its metabolites have been excreted (primarily through the kidneys) within 24 hours.

Procarbazine causes nausea and vomiting, bone marrow toxicity, and neurotoxicity. One third of the patients treated experience disorders of consciousness such as somnolence, depression, agitation, or psychosis. Peripheral neuropathies may also occur. The fact that procarbazine is a weak monoamine oxidase inhibitor may be the source of its neurotoxic effects. Administration of other drugs (including other monoamine oxidase inhibitors, antihypertensive drugs, phenothiazines, barbiturates, narcotics, sympathomimetic agents, and alcohol) may potentiate the neurotoxicities. Alcohol will cause a flushing syndrome similar to that seen with Antabuse. Foods high in tyramine, such as ripe cheeses, will also potentiate neurotoxicities.[11, 29, 40]

Hydroxyurea (Hydrea). Hydrea is administered orally. Its peak plasma level occurs 2 hours after administration. The half-time of plasma clearance is about 1½ hours. Hydrea is converted to urea by the liver and should be used cautiously in patients with kidney or liver dysfunctions.

Hydrea acts by inhibiting an enzyme essential to DNA synthesis. It is cell cycle–specific, destroying cells in the S phase of the cycle. Its most serious side effect is bone marrow depression.[11]

Mitotane (o,p′DDD, Lysodren). Mitotane was developed from the insecticide DDT. It is given orally. Only about 40 per cent of the dose is absorbed, but that amount is heavily deposited in fat tissues and can be measured in the blood months after the drug is discontinued. Some of the drug is converted to a water-soluble metabolite and is excreted in the urine.

Mitotane is used primarily to treat inoperable adrenal cortical carcinoma. It causes necrosis and atrophy of the adrenal cortex and also inhibits the conversion of cholesterol to steroids. Thus it acts to suppress adrenal function and reduce blood levels of cortisone.

Responses to this drug may not occur until as long as 3 months after treatment is started. Side effects include gastrointestinal problems, central nervous system changes, and skin reactions. The patient must be closely observed for signs of adrenal insufficiency. If the patient experiences severe trauma or shock, steroids must be administered and treatment discontinued. Central nervous system problems may include depression, drowsiness, lethargy, and vertigo. Therefore, the patient must be cautioned to avoid activities requiring mental alertness.[11]

Streptozotocin (NSC-85998). Streptozotocin is an experimental antibiotic with a half-life of 40 minutes. It is administered by injection and is excreted by the kidneys. It chiefly inhibits DNA synthesis, but also inhibits some of the major enzymes involved in gluconeogenesis, which can result in damage to pancreatic islet cells. Approximately two thirds of treated patients develop hepatic or renal dysfunction. The hepatic damage is rarely serious, but

Table 9–6. Specific Agents Used in Cancer Chemotherapy: Miscellaneous Drugs*

Agents	Principal Route of Adminis-tration	Usual Dose	Acute Toxic Signs	Major Toxic Manifestations
L-Asparaginase	IV	200–1000 IU/kg 3–7 × weekly for 28 days	N & V†, fever hyper-sensitivity reactions	Anorexia, weight loss. Somnolence, lethargy, confusion. Hypoproteinemia (including albumin and fibrinogen). Hypolipidemia, abnormal liver function tests, fatty metamorphosis of the liver. Pancreatitis (rare). Azotemia. Granulocytopenia, lymphopenia, and thrombocytopenia (usually mild and transient).
1,3-bis (β-Chloroethyl)-1-nitrosourea (BCNU)‡	IV	100 mg/m² every 6 weeks		
1-(β-Chloroethyl)-3-(4-methylcyclohexyl)-1-nitrosourea (MeCCNU)‡	Oral	120–150 mg/m² every 6 weeks	N & V	Bone marrow depression with leukopenia and thrombocytopenia.
Streptozotocin‡	IV	1 gm/day	N & V	
o,p'-DDD (Mitotane)	Oral	2–10 gm/day	N & V	Skin eruptions, diarrhea, mental depression, muscle tremors.
Dimethyl imidazole triazeno carboxamide (DTIC)	IV	2–4 mg/kg/day × 10 days	N & V	Bone marrow depression.
Hydroxyurea (Hydrea)	Oral	20–40 mg/kg/day	None	Bone marrow depression.
Tamoxifen‡	Oral	10 mg bid	None	Mild bone marrow depression.
Cis-Platinum®(II) diamine dichloride‡	IV	1 mg/kg every 3 weeks 3 mg/kg every 3 weeks with mannitol diuresis	N & V	Bone marrow depression, renal tubular damage, deafness.
Procarbazine (Matulane)	Oral	50–300 mg/day	N & V	Bone marrow depression with leukopenia and thrombocytopenia, mental depression.
Quinacrine (Atabrine)	Intra-pleural	100–200 mg/day × 5 days	Local pain, fever	
Vinblastine (Velban)	IV	0.1–0.2 mg/kg weekly	N & V	Alopecia, areflexia, bone marrow depression.
Vincristine (Oncovin)	IV	0.015–0.05 mg/kg weekly	None	Areflexia, muscular weakness, peripheral neuritis, paralytic ileus, mild bone marrow depression.

*From Krakoff, I. H.: Cancer chemotherapeutic agents. *CA — A Journal for Clinicians.* 31:136, 1981. Used by permission.
†Nausea and vomiting.
‡Available for experimental use only.

may cause problems if streptozotocin is combined with drugs that are metabolized by the liver. Proteinuria is usually the first sign of renal toxicity, which may progress to renal failure and death. Streptozotocin is used to treat pancreatic islet cell carcinoma and has a 60 per cent response rate. It is also being studied for the treatment of other tumors.[11]

Hexamethylmelamine (HMM, NSC-13875). Hexamethylmelamine is an experimental drug that is structurally related to the alkylating agents. However, its primary mode of action does not appear to be alkylation. The mechanism of its cytotoxic effect is unclear. It is administered orally, achieving peak blood levels in 1 hour and plasma clearance half-time in 13 hours. It is demethylated in the liver: the melamines are excreted by the kidneys and the methyl groups are oxidized to carbon dioxide. Its toxicities are not severe, but include nausea and myelosuppression. The drug has antitumor activity in a wide variety of human tumors and holds promise for future therapies.[11]

Platinum Complexes (DDP, Cisplatin, Platinol). DDP is given intravenously. Ninety per cent of the drug becomes protein bound. The drug may persist in body tissues for as long as 4 months. It is excreted by the kidneys. DDP has many toxic reactions, resulting from even a single dose. Nausea and vomiting almost always occur. Twenty-five per cent of patients develop renal dysfunction; 30 per cent develop tinnitus or high-frequency hearing loss. Mild bone marrow suppression sometimes occurs. Toxicities that rarely occur include anaphylactic reactions, peripheral neuropathy, taste loss, and seizures.

Nephrotoxicity is the most serious side effect and limits use of the drug. It has recently been found that mannitol diuresis at the time of drug administration may protect the kidneys. DDP is used primarily in the treatment of nonseminomatous testicular tumors. Other tumors also respond to DDP, but its optimal use is still under study.[11, 19]

L-Asparaginase (Elspar). L-Asparaginase can be administered intravenously or intramuscularly. The drug is very slowly cleared from the plasma and is removed from the body by the reticuloendothelial system. L-Asparaginase is an enzyme that is thought to work by destroying extracellular L-asparagine. Cancer cells, which lack the ability to make this amino acid, in turn die. Normal cells, which can manufacture the amino acid, are spared.

L-Asparaginase causes many toxic reactions, including allergic reactions, depression of clotting factors, central nervous system dysfunction, liver dysfunction, nausea and vomiting, pancreatitis, disordered glucose metabolism, and immunosuppression. Anaphylaxis is the greatest risk to the patient. Presently, this drug is only used to treat acute lymphoblastic leukemia.[11, 56]

CALCULATING DRUG DOSES

Calculating the dose of an antineoplastic drug is a complex process, because the dose must be specifically designed for a particular individual. Therefore, it is not possible to have a table listing the usual doses of each drug. This makes it very difficult for the nurse to know that the ordered dose is the appropriate one. However, it is possible to make better judgments in this area if the nurse has some understanding of the method used to calculate the dose and the rationale behind the calculations.

Many factors must be considered in determining drug dose, including: type of malignancy; body weight; body proportions of bone, muscle, fat, and body fluid; age of patient; liver and kidney function; and method of administration. Drug protocols for treatment of a particular type of cancer will usually recommend a specific drug dosage based on kilograms of body weight or body surface area per meter squared (m^2). Meter squared is believed to be the most accurate calculation, because this method takes into consideration the proportion of bone, muscle, fat, and fluid. The meter squared method of calculating drug doses is probably the least understood by nurses, since it is relatively uncommon. It requires the use of a nomogram table. (See Figs. 9–5 and 9–6.)

The following examples may be helpful in calculating drug dose:

The usual dose of Adriamycin is 50 mg/m^2. The patient weighs 150 pounds and is 60 inches tall. Using the nomogram table, it is possible to determine that the body surface area of the patient is 1.65 m^2. (See Fig. 9–7.)

$$1.65 \times 50 = 82.5$$

The patient would receive 82.5 mg of Adriamycin.

The usual dose of bleomycin is 0.25 mg/kg/day. The patient weighs 150 pounds. To determine the weight in kilograms, divide the weight by 2.2; thus, the patient weighs 68.18 kg.

$$0.25 \times 68.18 = 17.045$$

The patient would receive 17 mg of bleomycin.

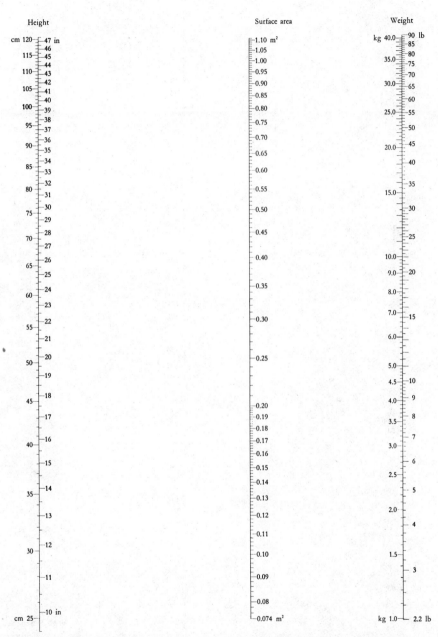

Figure 9–5.   Nomogram for the assessment of body surface area of children. From the formula of Du Bois and Du Bois, *Archives of Internal Medicine.* 17:863, 1916. S = W$^{0.425}$ × H$^{0.725}$ × 71.84, or log S = log W × 0.425 + log H × 0.725 + 1.8564 (S = body surface in cm^2, W = weight in kg, H = height in cm). (From *Documenta Geigy, Scientific Tables,* 7th edition, with supplement. CIBA–GEIGY Ltd., Basle, Switzerland. Used by permission.)

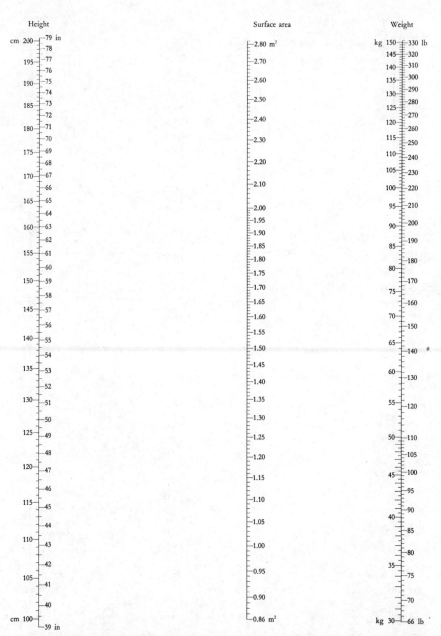

Figure 9–6. Nomogram for the assessment of body surface area of adults. From the formula of Du Bois and Du Bois, *Archives of Internal Medicine.* 17:863, 1916. $S = W^{0.425} \times H^{0.725} \times 71.84$, or $\log S = \log W \times 0.425 + \log H \times 0.725 + 1.8564$ (S = body surface in cm^2, W = weight in kg, H = height in cm). (From *Documenta Geigy, Scientific Tables,* 7th edition, with supplement. CIBA–GEIGY Ltd., Basle, Switzerland. Used by permission.)

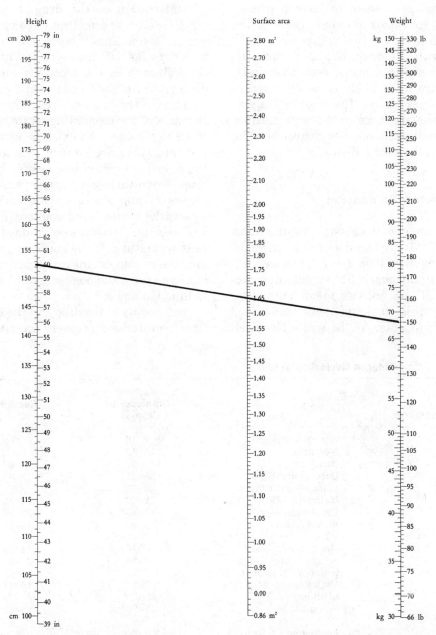

Figure 9–7. Nomogram for the assessment of body surface area of adults. The body surface area is given by the point of intersection with the middle scale of a straight line joining height and weight. From the formula of Du Bois and Du Bois, *Archives of Internal Medicine.* 17:863, 1916. S = W$^{0.425}$ × H$^{0.725}$ × 71.84, or log S = log W × 0.425 + log H × 0.725 + 1.8564 (S = body surface in cm^2, W = weight in kg, H = height in cm). (From *Documenta Geigy, Scientific Tables,* 7th edition, with supplement. CIBA–GEIGY Ltd., Basle, Switzerland. Used by permission.)

DRUG TOXICITIES

Drugs used to destroy malignant cells also cause damage to normal cells. However, normal cells seem to have a greater capacity to repair damage than cancer cells. The toxicities that occur vary considerably with the drug, but some toxicities occur commonly. Normal cells that divide rapidly are more likely to be damaged by antineoplastic drugs. The most actively dividing cells are those in the bone marrow, the inner lumen of the gastrointestinal tract, and the hair follicles.

Bone Marrow Depression

Bone marrow depression is the most common toxicity produced by an antineoplastic drug. It is a very serious effect because it can reach life threatening proportions. There are two major manifestations of this toxicity: leukopenia and thrombocytopenia. As the white blood cell level decreases, the risk of infection increases. Of particular concern is the level of granulocytes. The white blood count usually does not drop immediately after administration of the drug; it may not occur for days or sometimes weeks after the drug is given. This is because antineoplastic drugs do not destroy the white blood cells already in the blood stream — they destroy white blood cells in the process of forming in the bone marrow. The average life span of the circulating white blood cell is 12 to 24 days. As existing white blood cells die, there are no new cells to replace them, and the white blood count begins to drop. When the bone marrow recovers and begins to manufacture white blood cells again, the white blood count will still be low, because it takes several days for new cells to mature. If the count is extremely low, the oncologist may do a bone marrow biopsy to see if the bone marrow has begun to function again.

The severity of the drop and the length of time required for recovery vary with the

Table 9–7. Drug-Induced Myelosuppression*

Category†	Drug	Nadir of Granulocytes (Days)	Recovery (Days)
I	Nitrogen mustard	7–15	28
	Melphalan	10–12	–
	Busulfan	11–30	24–54
	Carmustine (BCNU)	26–30	35–49
	Lomustine (CCNU)	40–50	60
	Methyl-CCNU	28–63	82–89
	Cytarabine	12–14	22–24
	Vinblastine	5–9	14–21
II	Cyclophosphamide	8–14	18–25
	5-Fluorouracil (5-FU)	7–14	20–30
	6-Mercaptopurine (6-MP)	7	14–21
	Methotrexate (MTX)	7–14	14–21
	Actinomycin D	15	22–25
	Procarbazine	25–36+	35–50+
III	Vincristine	4–5	7
	Bleomycin	–	–
	L-Asparaginase	–	–
	Cis-platinum	–	–
	Hormones	–	–

*From Cline, M. J., and Haskell, C. M.: *Cancer Chemotherapy.* Philadelphia: W. B. Saunders Co., 1980. Modified from Henderson, E. S.: In *Drugs and Hematologic Reactions,* ed. by N. V. Dimitrov and J. H. Nodine. New York: Grune & Stratton, 1974; and from Creaven, P. J., and Mihich, E.: *Seminars in Oncology, 4,* 147, 1977. Used by permission.

†Categories: I, primarily myelosuppressive toxicity; II, myelosuppressive but other toxicities equally important; III, rarely cause granulocytopenia.

Table 9–8. Grades of Myelosuppression*

Toxicity Grade	White Blood Cell Count per μL	· Granulocyte† Count per μL	Platelet Count per μL
Normal Values	4500–10,000	2000–7000	150,000–350,000
0	≥4000	≥1500	≥100,000
1	3000–3999	1000–1499	75,000–99,000
2	2000–2999	500–999	50,000–74,999
3	1000–1999	250–499	25,000–49,999
4	<1000	<250	<25,000

*From Cline, M. J., and Haskell, C. M.: *Cancer Chemotherapy*. Philadelphia: W. B. Saunders Co., 1980. As used in the Division of Hematology-Oncology, Department of Medicine, UCLA School of Medicine. Used by permission.

†Granulocytes include both segmented and juvenile neutrophils.

drug and the dosage. The lowest point the blood count reaches before recovery begins is called the nadir. The nadir may differ somewhat from patient to patient, but is predictable to some degree. Table 9–7 gives the granulocyte nadir and recovery time of some of the more common antineoplastic drugs. Patients receiving combinations of drugs may experience multiple nadirs as the various drugs have their impact on the bone marrow. Physicians usually use some form of classification to determine the severity of myelosuppression caused by a drug. Table 9–8 shows one schema that is used. Patients experiencing severe myelosuppression may have to be hospitalized for observation and may require treatment for infection or bleeding. Further chemotherapy is usually postponed until recovery from the toxicity is complete. The dose and timing of chemotherapy are usually more dependent on the severity of normal cell response than on the optimal timing to destroy the malignancy.

In order to carefully monitor blood counts and other laboratory studies that may indicate liver and renal response to the chemotherapy, these values are often recorded on a flow sheet. (See Fig. 9–8.) Treatment protocols using multiple drugs are usually planned according to a schedule. The day the schedule begins is called "day one." Events such as the administration of doses of various drugs or changes in blood counts are referred to in relation to "day one" of the protocol. For example, a second dose of the drug may be given on

"day eight." The nadir of the granulocyte count may occur on "day fourteen." These references have no relation to the calendar date. "Day one" will be marked on the flow sheet as well as the calendar date. When the drug protocol schedule is initiated again (for example, a month or 6 weeks later), it will again be referred to as "day one." Comparisons can then be made between responses that occur between one month and the next, or four months later. Some drugs — particularly some of the alkylating agents — cause a cumulative myelosuppression, so that the nadir may be lower each time the treatment is implemented.

Gastrointestinal Toxicity

The most unpleasant reactions experienced by patients receiving chemotherapy are those that affect the gastrointestinal tract. These include anorexia, nausea, vomiting, stomatitis, and diarrhea. Anorexia, nausea, and vomiting usually occur at the time of drug administration and for a few hours or days afterwards. However, they may be severe enough to cause malnutrition, dehydration, and electrolyte imbalance. Antiemetics are not always effective in controlling these symptoms. Marijuana derivatives seem to be more effective, but cause side effects that may be equally unpleasant. Further research will be necessary before this drug or its derivatives are widely utilized in clinical practice.

Date no./Day									Year: 19 Page:
Day on study									
Course no.									Name:
Drugs									Diagnosis:
									Ht:
									Wt:
									BSA:
XRT									Remarks:

Hgb Gm %							
Hct Vol %							
Plate × 10³							
WBC × 10³							
Bands %							
Polys %							
Monos %							
Lymphs %							
Eos %							
Basos %							
Blasts %							
Pro-M %							
Myelo %							
Meta-M %							

Chemistry							

Parameters							
Weight							

Toxicity							

Figure 9–8. Flow sheet for recording information.

The gastrointestinal symptoms can be severe enough to compromise the patient's nutritional status and may alter the tumor's response to the chemotherapy. In a nutritionally impaired person fewer cells are progressing through the cell cycle. Malnutrition may also slow the rate of repair of normal tissues, thus delaying the administration of the next scheduled treatment.

Stomatitis usually develops about the same time as the white blood count begins to drop. It can range from one or two ulcers in the mouth to severe, extremely painful ulcers that interfere with eating. Proper mouth care can decrease the severity of this problem. The patient with stomatitis is also very susceptible to oral infections.

The ulcers that are seen in the mouth can extend throughout the gastrointestinal tract. The esophagus, stomach, and bowel may be involved. Swallowing may be difficult and painful. Diarrhea may result, causing further nutritional problems and, if severe, causing electrolyte imbalance and dehydration.

Alopecia

Alopecia (hair loss) often does not begin until the fourth or fifth month of drug therapy. The drugs most likely to cause hair loss are Cytoxan and Adriamycin. The loss may vary from thinning or patchy loss to loss of all hair. Hair may begin to regrow after 2 or 3 months even though chemotherapy is continued. Hair loss is very seldom permanent. The hair will regrow after drug therapy is discontinued, although the hair may be somewhat different in texture or color.

There are two main causes of hair loss. First the drug may cause enough damage to the hair follicle that the hair falls out. Second, the cell turnover rate of the hair bulb is normally 24 hours. The administration of an antineoplastic drug can temporarily inhibit cellular activity. This will cause a constriction in the hair shaft, making the shaft weak at the point of constriction. As the hair again begins to grow, it may break, causing a patchy hair loss.[8]

Mutagenicity

Many of the antineoplastic drugs are mutagenic, teratogenic, and carcinogenic. Some of the drugs, principally the alkylating agents, can cause sterility. Women treated with methotrexate or an alkylating agent during the first trimester of pregnancy may give birth to an infant with congenital malformations. There is an increased frequency of second malignancies in patients successfully treated with antineoplastic drugs. This has been most apparent in patients treated for Hodgkin's disease and multiple myeloma. The second malignancy usually occurs many years after chemotherapy. In the future, drugs must be selected more carefully for those patients with a good chance for cure.

NURSING CARE OF THE PATIENT RECEIVING CHEMOTHERAPY

In 1980, Wandelt differentiated between the job of nursing and the practice of nursing.[59] The job of nursing involves activities by the nurse that are done to meet institutional demands or to implement medical care. These may be viewed as the demands of the health care system within which nursing occurs. These activities may or may not be to the patient's advantage. Many of these activities could and sometimes are done by personnel other than the nurse. The job of nursing may interfere with or limit the practice of nursing either by demanding so much of the nurse's time that no time is left to practice nursing or by actually conflicting with a philosophy of nursing practice. However, the activities may also provide a supportive framework within which quality nursing practice can occur. They provide the nurse with access to the patient and can facilitate the interdependence of nursing practice and medical practice. The job of nursing gives the nurse an opportunity to manipulate the environment of the patient in a health promoting way, which is also a part of nursing practice. Manipulation of the environment may involve skills in politics, public relations, management and supervision, assertiveness, teaching, and counseling. Therefore, these skills must be considered a part of both the job of nursing and the practice of nursing.

The practice of nursing has as its goal maximizing the health potential of the patient. In order to accomplish this, the nurse must have a thorough knowledge of disease processes in cancer and of medical treatment practices. However, the nurse's concern is not with the cancer in and of itself or its treatment, but with facilitating the patients' coping with their illness in such a way that movement toward greater health is facilitated. Movement toward greater health involves an interaction of biologic, psychologic, sociologic, and spiritual processes. Treating or curing the disease alone will not accomplish this.

The nurse is concerned with the totality of patients, their quality of life, and the effectiveness of their coping strategies. Coping involves biologic, psychologic, social, and spiritual responses interacting to influence each other. Coping is not the same as adaptation. The goal of adaptation is to maintain the status quo (homeostasis) or to accept and to adjust to a situation. The goal of coping is to use problem-solving strategies to achieve a higher level of health. (See Chapter 12.)

Health exists apart from the presence or absence of disease states. Therefore, it is possible for patients to have cancer or to be dying and to achieve a high level of health for that time in their life. It is also possible for patients to have no evidence of disease but to have a low level of health.

Nurses working in cancer chemotherapy are often so engulfed in the job of nursing that the practice of nursing may be extremely limited. It is possible for nurses to become so involved in implementing medical practice procedures that in the process they adopt the beliefs, values, and perceptions of the patient that are common to medical practice and lose sight of the practice and goal of nursing.

This section of the chapter will discuss both the job and the practice of nursing. The job of nursing will tend to be task oriented and institutionally centered. The practice of nursing will be goal oriented and patient centered. However, a task may be a vehicle for the practice of nursing. The task (for example, administration of chemotherapy) may be perceived as a way of facilitating biologic coping. Administration of chemotherapy alone is not nursing. But while the medication is being administered, the nurse may use the time to interact with the patient in the hope of facilitating psychologic, sociologic, and spiritual coping.

Baseline Nursing Assessment

The practice of nursing always begins with assessment. The nursing assessment may take place quickly and only within the mind of the nurse or it may be a more thorough, planned process that is written down to share with other nurses. When the nurse first encounters a patient who is to receive chemotherapy, a complete nursing assessment should be done. This will establish a baseline against which to measure the patient's functioning during drug therapy. Areas that should be particularly noted are the patient's nutritional status, skin condition, mouth condition, degree of mobility, general physical condition, functional status, psychosocial status, and knowledge of the treatment plan.

Nutritional Status. Nutritional status is a key factor in determining whether or not the patient will be able to tolerate chemotherapy and the effectiveness of the chemotherapy in destroying cancer cells. Physical examination should include an accurate measurement of body weight and an assessment of muscle tone, skin turgor, and skin color. During the physical assessment, patients are often asked to tell their weight. However, nurses themselves should take the patients' weight at the time of assessment. An accurate weight is an extremely important determinant in calculating drug dose. Cancer patients can and often do lose weight without realizing it. Therefore a weight, even from last week, may not be accurate.

An assessment of eating patterns is important and should include the times of day the patient eats, the foods usually eaten, and amount of food eaten. Food likes and dislikes should be noted. The patient should be questioned about changes in sense of taste.

Skin Condition. A thorough head to toe examination of the skin should be performed, looking for skin lesions, infections, unhealed incisions, or wounds. There may be some disruption of the healing process for a few days after administration of chemotherapy. Because of temporary disruption in immune response and the subsequent drop in white blood count, skin infections can become more severe if not treated before therapy begins.

Mouth Condition. A careful examination of the mouth is essential in order to determine the presence of oral irritation, bleeding gums, poorly fitting dentures, or poor oral hygiene. Patients should be asked about their oral hygiene practices. Cancer frequently results in anorexia and rapid weight loss, which cause the oral mucosa to function poorly or to decrease production of saliva. These conditions may increase the oral toxicity induced by the chemotherapy drugs.

Degree of Mobility. Mobility in cancer patients may be impaired for many reasons: fatigue, muscle weakness, the presence of a bulky tumor, bony metastasis, or other unrelated conditions such as arthritis. Sometimes, the patient's response to drug therapy can be evaluated in terms of improvements in mobility. In other cases, drugs such as vincristine may impair mobility. If mobility has not been well assessed before drug therapy, it will not be possible to determine how much of this impairment is a consequence of the therapy itself.

General Physical Condition. General body functioning needs to be assessed, including liver and renal functioning. The skin should be examined for jaundice. Solid tumors should be measured and recorded. The rim of the liver should be palpated. If it is palpable, the size should be measured at two points: number of fingerbreadths below the ribs at the substernal notch and number of fingerbreadths below the ribs at the midclavicular line. The patient should be examined for enlarged nodes. Extremities should be inspected for lymphedema. It is important to detect the presence of fever. If the patient has received previous chemotherapy, toxicities from that treatment must be searched for. Laboratory tests and x-ray studies are vital indicators of the patient's current physical status. It is the nurse's responsibility to know the results of these tests and what the results mean in relation to the patients and the treatment they are to receive.

Functional Status. There is a strong correlation between functional status and response to chemotherapy. Patients who have a low functional status usually tolerate chemotherapy poorly. Patients who have a high functional status usually respond well to treatment. Several scales have been developed to evaluate a patient's functional status, the most well known being the Karnofsky Scale. (See Table 9–9.) This scale has been modified in the Eastern Cooperative Oncology Group Performance Status. (See Table 9–10.) The functional status grade will probably be a factor in determining whether or not patients will receive chemotherapy and can also be used to evaluate response to treatment.

Psychosocial Status. It is important to assess the patients' attitude toward receiving chemotherapy and their level of anxiety. Careful questioning can elicit their usual coping strategies. The nurse should attempt also to ascertain the patients' social support groups and significant others. It is also useful to determine the roles, relationships, and dynamics within the patient's family. If family members are present, this is an effective time to assess each member's attitudes and concerns related to chemotherapy and the patient's illness. The coping strategies of the family should also be assessed.

Notations should be made of the patients' personality characteristics and emotional state. Various emotional reactions can occur as a result of the patients' attempt to cope with their disease. These

Table 9–9. Karnofsky Scale*

Grade	Scale	Status
1	100%	Normal; no complaints, no evidence of disease.
2	90%	Able to carry on normal activity; minor signs or symptoms of disease.
3	80%	Normal activity with effort; some signs or symptoms of disease.
4	70%	Cares for self. Unable to carry on normal activity or to do active work.
5	60%	Requires occasional assistance, but is able to care for most of his needs.
6	50%	Requires considerable assistance and frequent medical care.
7	40%	Disabled; requires special care and assistance.
8	30%	Severely disabled; hospitalization is indicated, although death is not imminent.
9	20%	Hospitalization necessary; very sick, active supportive treatment necessary.
10	10%	Moribund: fatal processes progressing rapidly.

*From Kennealey, G. T., and Mitchell, M. S.: Factors that influence the therapeutic response. In *Cancer: A Comprehensive Treatise, Vol. 5, Chemotherapy,* ed. by F. F. Becker. New York: Plenum Press, 1977. Used by permission.

need to be recognized and dealt with. However, the nurse must distinguish between changes that may result from the drug therapy and those that are emotional responses to a stressful situation.

Knowledge of the Treatment Plan. The patients' understanding of the diagnosis, the treatment to be used, and expectations of treatment results should be determined. The patients' perception of their role as patient must also be assessed.

Planning Care

After sufficient data are collected from the nursing assessment, nursing diagnoses and a plan for care should be made in collaboration with the patients and their family. The plan should include interventions with the family. Chemotherapy is often administered in an outpatient clinic or doctor's office. Planning nursing care in these settings is often not as formalized as in hospitals, but it is still as important. Some record of the nursing plan should be developed, even if it must be jotted on a plain sheet of paper and kept in a separate file.

Nursing Interventions Prior to Chemotherapy

Before chemotherapy is administered, patient teaching must be given. The pa-

Table 9–10. Eastern Cooperative Oncology Group Performance Status

Grade	Status
0	Fully active, able to carry on all predisease performance without restriction. (Karnofsky 90–100)
1	Restricted in physically strenuous activity, but ambulatory and able to carry out work of a light or sedentary nature, e.g., light housework, office work. (Karnofsky 70–80)
2	Ambulatory and capable of all self-care, but unable to carry out any work activities. Up and about more than 50% of waking hours. (Karnofsky 50–60)
3	Capable of only limited self-care, confined to bed or chair more than 50% of waking hours. (Karnofsky 30–40)
4	Completely disabled. Cannot carry on any self-care. Totally confined to bed or chair. (Karnofsky 10–20)

*From Kennealey, G. T., and Mitchell, M. S.: Factors that influence the therapeutic response. In *Cancer: A Comprehensive Treatise, Vol. 5, Chemotherapy,* ed. by F. F. Becker. New York: Plenum Press, 1977. Used by permission.

tients should know what drugs they are receiving and the usual side effects.[58] The role of patients as active participants in their care should be discussed with patients and their family. Patients need to decide whether or not they are willing to be active participants. The implications of this role need to be considered, including an increased responsibility for learning about the disease and its treatment and an avoidance of the passive, dependent patient role. The consequences of taking on the passive, dependent patient role may need to be explored, including poorer response to therapy, loss of control, and avoidance of responsibility. This role may also provide a greater feeling of security for some patients. Patients who have used ineffective coping strategies in the past and patients with poor mental health may be unwilling or unable to function completely in the active participant patient role.

If the patients elect to function within the active participant role, family members must be prepared to accept that role. Often family members attempt to keep patients in the passive, dependent role; they feel that this is what they should do. Altering the patient role may change all of the family roles in an illness situation. The family must receive support from the nurse to function in a new capacity.

Patients will need to accept the responsibility of observing side effects of the drug therapy and reporting them to the health care team. This may include taking their own temperature on a schedule. The importance of taking oral medications on schedule must be discussed. Many patients have a pattern of low compliance with drug prescription directions. The serious results of not following directions for antineoplastic drugs need to be explained. Mechanisms for ensuring treatment compliance must be discussed with the patient.

The nurse and patient need to consider ways the patient can take an active role during the months of drug therapy. Since nutrition is of paramount importance, the patient needs to experiment with ways to diminish nausea and vomiting and must take responsibility for adequate mouth care. The patient must be assertive in avoiding people with infections and must be willing to contact the health care team when problems occur.

In general, nurses are not accustomed to taking care of patients functioning in the active, participant role. When patients exercising this role are admitted to the hospital, the nurses and other hospital personnel may feel a loss of power and control, become defensive or perhaps angry, and attempt to direct the patient into the passive, dependent patient role. The patient may refuse to function in that role, but he or she must have support in order to do this.

Administration of Antineoplastic Drugs

The administration of cancer chemotherapy agents carries with it greater risks and responsibilities than occur with most other drugs that the nurse administers. Some hospitals require that physicians give the more dangerous drugs. However, nurses are being given greater responsibilities for administering these drugs. Although the technique remains the same, the nurse will encounter different problems when administering drugs in a hospital unit, an outpatient clinic, or a physician's office.

Drug Preparation

As with all drugs, preparation time is crucial to proper administration of the chemotherapy drug. Since an incorrect dose can cause the death of a patient, the careful preparation of antineoplastic drugs is vital. Drug preparation should occur in a quiet place. Interruptions should not be allowed.[4] Although this may seem impossible in some settings, it is essential to devise some means to accomplish it. Some chemotherapy drugs have very similar names. Their usual doses are not as easily recognized as in other drugs. Because of these factors, it is prudent to check the original order written by the physician. The name of the patient, the name of the drug, the dose, the route of administration, and the time of administration should be checked. The dose of the drug can easily be misread because of poor handwriting or it may actually be incorrectly written.

Nurses are legally responsible for knowing the usual doses of drugs that they administer. To ensure that the dose is within a reasonable range, they can refer to the pharmaceutical package insert. If the dose to be administered is not the same as the dose specified by the pharmaceutical company, dosage should be carefully calculated and checked with another nurse.

The drugs should always be mixed with the diluent recommended in the package insert. If mixed with another diluent, precipitation may occur. The amount of diluent used is very important. If the drug is too concentrated, it may be more likely to cause adverse reactions. Miller recommends diluting Cytoxan, Adriamycin, and nitrogen mustard beyond the manufacturer's recommendations.[41]

If the patient is receiving more than one drug, each syringe should be labeled as soon as it is prepared. This will prevent confusion in three possible situations if two or more colorless drugs in unlabeled syringes are administered: (1) if one of the drugs extravasates, it is not possible to know if the drug is one that is destructive to local tissues; (2) if the patient has an immediate reaction to a drug, it is not possible to determine which drug caused the reaction; (3) if one drug is to be administered intravenously and another intramuscularly, it is possible to accidentally switch the two drugs.[41]

Preparation of drugs for administration should also include having drugs available for emergencies such as anaphylactic reactions or extravasation. Miller recommends a portable basket or tray containing Benadryl, Adrenalin, Solu-Cortef, sodium thiosulfate, and hyaluronidase.[41] Patients receiving chemotherapy drugs should have written standing orders on their charts that allow the nurse to initiate the appropriate treatment immediately. This can save a life in patients with anaphylaxis or minimize tissue damage if extravasation occurs.

Patient Identification

Correct patient identification is essential in the administration of all drugs; however, errors in giving antineoplastic drugs have the potential of creating more serious consequences than most other drugs. It is essential that some means be developed to ensure correct patient identification. With hospitalized patients, this can be accomplished by checking the wrist identification band. Patients in the outpatient clinic or doctor's office cannot be as easily identified.

One possible approach is to ask patients to repeat their name and check this against the chart or medication order. Addressing patients by name is a very poor method of patient identification. Patients will often respond positively to any name because they are in a stressful situation. Some outpatient clinics use wrist identification bands that are applied each time the patient arrives. Miller suggests the use of the driver's license.[41]

Selection of Equipment

Decisions about needles and types of equipment to be used to administer antineoplastic drugs should be based on considerations of minimizing damage to veins, diminishing the risk of extravasation, and decreasing the probability of phlebitis. The most ideal needle for this purpose is the butterfly needle. The gauge of the needle is small but the bore is relatively large. The butterfly tabs allow the needle to be secured in such a way that stability is increased. These needles are also small enough to discourage too rapid an injection of the drug.

Larger needles commonly used to give intravenous infusions cause greater damage to the blood vessel wall, thus increasing the risk of extravasation. Some physicians, however, believe that giving sclerosing drugs into a larger vein in the antecubital space with a large needle decreases damage to the inner wall of the vein. They believe that the more rapid blood flow carries the drug away more quickly, thus decreasing contact of the drug with the vein wall.[41] However, if greater dilution were needed, this seemingly could be accomplished by further diluting the drug before administration.

The use of plastic cannulas for the administration of antineoplastic drugs is generally ill-advised. They are associated with a high incidence of phlebitis. They do decrease the number of vein sticks that have to be done, but the tradeoff does not seem to be favorable.

Heparin locks, on the other hand, seem to be an effective way of decreasing the number of vein sticks with little increase in phlebitis. However, caution must be used in ensuring continued patency of the vein before drugs are administered. Extravasation is still a risk.

Gever cautions against using equipment containing aluminum when administering cisplatin, since cisplatin reacts with the aluminum. The result is usually a black precipitate. The reaction also causes the drug to lose potency.[20]

To a great extent, techniques of intravenous injection are part of the art, rather than the science, of medical and nursing practice. Very little clinical research has been conducted in this area. Judgments about the best way to perform a specific technique are based primarily on clinical experience and observation.

Vein Selection

Patients who are receiving chemotherapy will usually be getting intravenous drugs over a long period of time. Thus, it is essential to maintain the patency of their veins by careful selection and skilled techniques of needle insertion.

As a rule, intravenous administration should be initiated in the veins on the back of the hand or low on the forearm. However, some prefer not to use the back of the hand because damage from extravasation can be severe. During the weeks or months of chemotherapy, veins higher on the forearm can be used.

The antecubital space should *not* be used. Extravasation in this site can be extensive before it is detectable and can cause severe, irreparable damage to ligaments, tendons, and the elbow joint. Utilization of an already existing intravenous site is not wise because of the greatly increased risk of extravasation. Patients who have had a mastectomy should not have injections in the arm on which side the surgery was done. Leg veins should never be used because of the high incidence of phlebitis occurring after utilization of these sites for antineoplastic drugs.

Patients generally know which veins are sclerosed and which are difficult to enter. This information should be carefully considered in selecting a site. In selecting the injection site, both arms should be carefully examined. This is easily done with hospitalized patients; however, outpatients are usually fully dressed. Shirt or dress sleeves may cover a large portion of the arm. Watches or bracelets block the view and constrict the veins.

Sleeves should be rolled above the elbow or clothing should be removed for drug administration. This will prevent selection of a vein that has been damaged by previous injections higher on the arm. It will also allow the nurse to more carefully observe for hives or erythema that may occur along the venous pathway during injection.[41] Miller reports evidence of erythematous skin reactions under watchbands. Patients experienced itching and a sensation of heat in the skin under the watchband during injection of drugs. She advises removal of jewelry for the injection period.[41]

Skin preparation before injection should be thorough. Various agencies have established specific protocols for skin preparation. Whatever the protocol, careful attention should be given to maintaining sterile technique. The immune response of many of these patients will be compromised by the drugs to be administered. The disease may also have altered the immune capacities. Therefore, these patients are at higher risk of infections from poor technique.

Needle insertion should be careful and skilled. This procedure is best done by nurses who regularly perform venipuncture. It is a skill that must be performed frequently to maintain competence. Certainly nurses not experienced in this capacity must perform this procedure in order to gain the skill. However, the practice of using large numbers of nurses who are assigned temporarily to this activity may meet the needs of the institution, but certainly not of the patient. Some type of evaluation of the nurses' skill in venipuncture should be made before assigning them to this responsibility. Training programs should be conducted for those not yet skilled.

After a successful venipuncture has been performed, the needle should be carefully secured with tape to avoid being dislodged. Forceful infusion of drugs can displace the needle. The patient should be informed of the risk of extravasation and the consequences. Symptoms of extravasation will often be evident to the patient before they are to the nurse.

Many institutions now have established protocols for the type of dressing to be applied to a venipuncture site. These may include the application of an ointment and a protective dressing. This dressing should not be applied while sclerosing antineoplastic drugs are being administered. Extravasation usually occurs at or immediately above the needle insertion site,[4] and must be detected quickly.

Drug Injection

Drugs may be injected in one of several ways. They may be given undiluted with a syringe and injected directly into the venous blood. This is often referred to as "IV push." They may be injected into the tubing of a free flowing intravenous infusion. This may be referred to as "piggyback." Special equipment is used for this purpose. This approach decreases the risk of extravasation. The drug may also be added to intravenous infusion solution and given over a period of hours.

Drugs administered by IV push should not be injected rapidly. Slow, even pressure should be used to inject the drug. The usual rate is 1 ml per minute. The patency of the vein should be checked with 5 to 10 ml of normal saline before drug injection is begun. If resistance is felt after drug injection is begun, injection should be stopped and the cause investigated. Needle repositioning may be the solution. Increasing the force of injection may cause a small, weak vein to burst. It can also cause venous spasm and pain. Patients may also experience unnecessary, immediate nausea if the injection is too rapid. Vein patency should be verified by checking for blood return every 3 to 4 ml. Absence of blood return does not mean the needle is outside the vein. The needle bevel may be against the vein wall. But infusing should be continued cautiously.[41] If more than one drug is to be given, 3 to 5 ml of normal saline should be injected between drugs. The drugs should never be mixed together in one syringe. The risk of drug incompatibilities is too great. After drug injection is complete, 20 ml or more of flushing solution should be injected to ensure that the drugs have been moved out of the peripheral circulation into the systemic blood flow.[41]

Tissue-toxic drugs being given piggyback or by IV push should be checked every 2 to 3 minutes. Some institutions require the constant attendance of a nurse in these situations. If a second nurse must replace the first nurse, a detailed report and examination of the injection site and the general condition of the patient should be given before the first nurse leaves. The patient should not be allowed to leave the area for any reason while the drug is infusing. This may conflict with needs of other departments (such as laboratory, x-ray, or physical therapy), but must be insisted upon.[41]

The patient should be closely observed during and immediately after drug injection for signs of anaphylactic reactions. These may include lightheadedness, pain, generalized pruritus, tingling, or shortness of breath. If any of these symptoms occur, drug injection should be stopped immediately. The intravenous site should be kept open with normal saline as a potential route for the administration of emergency drugs, which should be in the room whenever antineoplastic drugs are being administered.[41]

The existence of extravasation is not always easy to determine. Slow leaks can allow penetration of the drug into deeper subcutaneous tissues without surface evidence of infiltration. In other situations, typical signs of infiltration are present. If extravasation is suspected, injection should be immediately discontinued. Various approaches are being used to decrease tissue damage from extravasation of tissue-toxic drugs. Some professionals immediately remove the needle. Others infiltrate the area with large amounts of normal saline. Others aspirate any possible remaining antineoplastic drug in the needle and tubing before giving possible antidotes.[41]

Antidotes differ for each drug. It is the responsibility of nurses to be familiar with the antidote for the drug they are administering. Hyaluronidase (Wydase) 150 U is used for the vinca alkaloids. Sodium thiosulfate is used for nitrogen mustard. Hydrocortisone sodium succinate (Solu-Cortef) and sodium bicarbonate are also recommended antidotes for some drugs.[41]

The chemotherapy research nurses of the Medical Branch, National Cancer Institute (NCI) have studied the use of local corticosteroids after extravasation of Adriamycin. They found that injection of Solu-Cortef 100 mg through the IV tubing before removing the needle and an ice pack for 24 hours decrease damage. However, they were able to achieve a greater reduction of complications by intradermal and subcutaneous injection of Solu-Cortef and the application of the ice pack immediately after needle removal. Solu-Cortef 100 mg/vial was then injected both intradermally and subcutaneously with 25-gauge needles. Multiple injections were given to include the entire affected area. A 1 per cent hydrocortisone cream was applied to the skin and a sterile dressing secured with paper tape. An ice pack was kept in place continuously for 24 hours. The steroid cream was applied twice a day until the erythema had disappeared. Patients were encouraged to exercise the arm or hand. The patients treated in this manner retained venous patency and complete function of the extremity.[5] Although the sample used in this study was very small, the results are nonetheless important to nursing care.

There is some controversy about whether heat or ice should be applied after extravasation. There is physiologic rationale for the use of either, but research has not been conducted to clinically determine differences in effectiveness. Heat is expected to increase the blood supply, improve dispersion of Wydase into subcutaneous tissues, promote healing by increasing blood supply, and improve absorption of the tissue-toxic drug by vasodilation. Those opposed to the use of heat believe that the tissue-toxic drugs damage the metabolic mechanisms of the cells. Heat increases the metabolism in the area and thus may increase the cellular destruction. The expected effect of ice is to decrease the blood supply and decrease absorption of the drug into the subcutaneous tissues. Pain is minimized. The drug pools in local tissues because absorption and diffusion are decreased, thus minimizing the number of cells exposed to the drug. The ice is believed to decrease enzymatic actions, slow metabolic rates, and improve the survival of marginally injured cells.[41]

After drug injection is successfully completed, the needle should be removed, an adhesive bandage applied, and pressure applied to the site for 3 to 4 minutes. Because these sites may be crucial for future drug injections, the risk of hematomas must be minimized. Many chemotherapy patients have an increased clotting time as a consequence of thrombocytopenia. Patients are often anxious to leave and may attempt to persuade the nurse to omit this step. Patients should also be assessed for general physical condition before leaving. Antiemetics or antihistamines given with the antineoplastic drugs may cause drowsiness, making driving unsafe.[41]

Detailed records should be kept of drug

administration. These should include data about the IV site, needle size, flushing solutions, and side effects as well as name of drug and amount of dose. Extravasation and treatment of it should also be noted.

Miller recommends calling the patient the day following the first drug treatment. This provides an opportunity for the patient to ask questions and allows the nurse to determine the patient's response to the drug therapy. This time can also be used to remind the patient of indications of adverse effects and timing of oral medications.[41]

Assessment of Drug Effect

Tumor Growth. In order to provide effective nursing interventions, it is important for the nurse to continually assess the effect of the drugs on tumor growth. There are several means for the nurse to determine this. X-ray reports will often indicate changes in tumor size. If the tumor is palpable, a tape measure can be used to measure size. A decrease in the size of the liver may be an indication of improvement. Therefore, palpation of the rim of the liver becomes important. An increased mobility and a decrease in pain are both signs of progress. If signs of a decrease in tumor growth are found, the nurse can begin to encourage more independence in activities, while continuing to evaluate the patient's tolerance for increased physical exertion.

Many patients are now receiving chemotherapy as adjuvant therapy. They have no sign of recurrent disease, but are at high risk for recurrence. These patients should be observed for signs of recurrence as well as drug side effects. The nurse should be familiar with recurrence patterns of the patient's type of tumor.

Side Effects. The nurse should check hospitalized patients daily for side effects of chemotherapy. Outpatients should be assessed on each visit. The nurse should be familiar with the results of laboratory studies and with the implications of those results. Such results affect not only medical care, but also nursing care.

The patient's skin should be examined for signs of infection. The most common sites are warm, dark, moist areas of the body. Sites that should be closely checked include the outer aspect of the nares, the corners of the mouth, the underside of pendulous breasts or a pendulous abdomen, the pubic area, and the anus. *Pseudomonas* infection of the skin begins very innocuously as a small, black, circular area on the skin. This lesion can become a systemic infection in a very short period of time. Other infections may appear as small pustular areas, cracks, or breaks in the skin. If the patient is immunologically compromised, these infections can become life threatening if not treated quickly. The skin should be palpated for enlarged lymph nodes, particularly in the areas of the neck, underarm, and groin.

Examination of the mouth is important. This should include notation of amount and consistency of saliva, color of oral mucosa, presence and extent of oral lesions, and signs of infection.

Auscultation of the chest should be performed. Fine rales may indicate bleomycin toxicity or respiratory infection. Alterations in heart sounds may be an indication of cardiac toxicity if Adriamycin is being given.

If the patient is receiving vinca alkaloids, neurologic status should be determined. If the patient is ambulatory, the patient's ability to heel walk should be assessed.

The patient should be questioned concerning eating patterns, bowel elimination, urinary excretion, occurrence of nausea or vomiting, and neurologic functioning. The Karnofsky Scale can again be used to determine the patient's functional state.

Nursing Interventions After Chemotherapy

Nausea and Vomiting

The nausea and vomiting that occur after chemotherapy are not easily controlled by the common antiemetics.[48] If vomiting is severe immediately after chemotherapy, a combination of antiemetics and sedatives may be used. In this case, the patient may sleep most of the first day after chemotherapy. Most patients prefer this to severe vomiting. Derivatives of marijuana have shown some promise in relieving the nausea of chemotherapy, but at this time are still experimental.[2] Severe vomiting for several days can cause fluid and electrolyte imbalances. Loss of hydrogen and chloride may result in hypochloremic alkalosis.

The nausea that occurs after chemotherapy is usually not consistently severe throughout the day. With careful questioning, it is often possible to identify periods of time when nausea is at a minimum. This is the time to provide food. These times often are not consistent with the usual serving times of the dietary department. An understanding dietitian is a valuable resource. Unfortunately, many dietary departments are very inflexible in their ability to provide food at unusual hours. Attempts should then be made for other sources, such as family members, to provide food.

John was a 17-year-old being treated for Hodgkin's disease. He had severe nausea and vomiting throughout the day for several days after his chemotherapy. However, he could eat at night. The dietary department at the hospital closed at 7 PM and was only able to provide food for night use that did not appeal to John. The nurse and John's parents decided to bring in food. Each night John happily ate pizza, hamburgers, French fries, and milk shakes. He sat up all night eating, watching TV, and reading. During most of the daytime hours, he slept. This required some adjustment of the nursing routine, which was carefully planned not to disrupt John's pattern.

Stomatitis

Stomatitis usually develops at the same time that bone marrow suppression occurs, that is, about 2 weeks after chemotherapy. However, it may occur earlier with aggressive chemotherapy. Mouth care for stomatitis should be instituted the day after chemotherapy is given. The nurse should not wait until oral lesions appear. An oral mucosa that is in a healthy state will have less damage from the drug therapy than an oral mucosa that is dry, pale, and bleeds easily.

The major principle of effective mouth care is to give it every 4 hours, around the clock. After 6 hours without mouth care, the oral mucosa begins to deteriorate.[47] Hospitalized patients on chemotherapy usually have their vital signs checked every 4 hours, even at night. It takes very little extra time to give mouth care at this time.

Nursing research has failed to clearly indicate the most effective chemicals to use for mouth care. Currently, normal saline or hydrogen perioxide seems to be the most effective. Lemon juice and glycerin should *never* be used. Glycerin is drying to the oral mucosa and lemon juice changes the pH of the saliva and can be damaging to the teeth. (For a thorough review of oral care and substances currently in use see Daeffler, references 14 to 16.)

If severe discomfort is experienced during eating, Xylocaine Viscous may be used as a mouthwash before meals to provide local anesthesia to the oral mucosa. A bland diet may also be helpful. Patients should be asked to report bleeding gums and discomfort or a burning sensation when they drink acidic liquids.

Both outpatients and hospitalized patients should be taught the reasons for conscientious mouth care and be given as much responsibility as possible for their own care. Most patients will be living at home and caring for themselves during most of their treatment time, even if they are hospitalized for acute periods.

Diarrhea

Diarrhea or abdominal cramps may be indicators of hypermotility of the intestinal tract due to cellular damage. Damage similar to the stomatitis may exist throughout the gastrointestinal tract. The frequency of episodes indicates the extent of tissue destruction. If the diarrhea is severe, it can lead to electrolyte imbalance and dehydration, with the loss of sodium, potassium, chloride, and bicarbonate resulting in acidosis. A bland or low residue diet may be helpful. Drugs acting to decrease motility may also be used. It is important to record the frequency, amount, and consistency of stools.

Increased Risk of Infection

Suppression of white blood cell production by the bone marrow results in a decrease in the body's defense against infection. This is usually the most life threatening consequence of chemotherapy. If the suppression is severe, patients are usually hospitalized for observation. Careful nursing planning is required to decrease the risk of infection and detect infections in their early stages when they are most treatable.

Careful handwashing technique is a must with the leukopenic patient. Handwashing is such a simple, basic part of early nursing education that its importance is often discounted. However, when the patient's natural defenses are compromised, the nurse must become a part of that defense system rather than adding to the environmental assault upon the patient's weakened resistance. The nurse's hands are the major transporter of infection and should be washed before each contact with the patient. This means washing them before preparing the patients' medication, before bringing them food, and before touching patients or their bed. If two patients are in the same room, the nurse's hands should be washed after contacting the other patient. After a dirty procedure hands should be washed before performing a clean procedure on the same patient. Cancer patients can get an infection from bacteria being transferred from one part of their body to another.

Patients should be taught careful handwashing technique and be encouraged to wash their own hands before eating and after urination or defecation. Family members should also be taught good measures of cleanliness, but family members do not usually pose the same threat to the patient as the nurse does.

The nurse's uniform, lab coat, or sweater carries large numbers of bacteria. We are not as careful as we used to be about having clean apparel each day. The same lab coat or sweater may be worn for many days. Because we come in contact with so many patients who have disease-causing pathogens, these garments can be the transporters of serious illness or death to a cancer patient. The sleeves of lab coats in particular seem to be easily contaminated. If lab coats or sweaters are worn, they should be washed daily, as should the uniform.

Patients with low white blood counts are usually having their temperature taken every 4 hours. An infection can occur in these patients without an elevation of temperature, so that patients must be closely observed for other symptoms of infection. If the patient's temperature reaches 101° F, it is a sign of a dangerous infection. White blood cells are required to cause the usual temperature elevation with infection. Since these cells are decreased, the infection will be in more advanced stages before the temperature is able to reach 101° F.

When the temperature reaches this point, the physician must be notified immediately, no matter what time it happens. Night nurses in a hospital are understandably reluctant to call physicians unnecessarily in the night. However, this situation is serious. Severely leukopenic patients can die of infection within 6 hours after their temperature reaches 101° F, if treatment is not begun. Treatment usually consists of broad-spectrum intravenous antibiotics.

These patients can also develop systemic fungus infections. *Candida albicans,* which normally occupies the gastrointestinal tract, is a common cause of these infections. Blood and urine cultures may both contain *Candida.* Amphotericin B is usually used to treat this infection. Patients sometimes refer to this as the "silver bullet" because the drug is light sensitive and the intravenous solution and tubing must be wrapped with aluminum foil. The solution is usually administered over a 6 hour period and causes many unpleasant and frightening symptoms. Patients may be given Benadryl, steroids, and sometimes a sedative to decrease the symptoms. They may experience severe chills and fever, severe chest pain, headache, gastrointestinal cramping, and muscle pain. Patients need to be warned of these side effects. The symptoms should subside within 2 to 4 hours after the infusion is complete. If the drug is administered too rapidly, cardiovascular collapse can occur. The drug can cause severe renal damage.

Severely compromised patients are susceptible to *Pseudomonas* infections. The microorganisms can be transmitted by respiratory therapy equipment or air conditioning ducts, or they may already be harbored in the patient's body. Treatment of these infections is difficult, requires very toxic intravenous antibiotics, and is not always successful.

Patients who have severe granulocytopenia may be placed in reverse isolation. To some degree, this will protect the patients from the hospital environment, but it cannot protect them from bacteria harbored within their body. Reverse isolation will increase the social isolation that the patients experience and may cause emotional responses that could increase their susceptibility to infection.

Increased Risk of Bleeding

Thrombocytopenia is the second greatest life threatening consequence of chemotherapy. The nursing goals for this condition are to decrease the risk of bleeding and to promptly detect any bleeding that does occur in order to diminish blood loss. Patients are usually hospitalized for observation. Platelet transfusions may be given. These are more successful for some patients than for others. The platelets must be very compatible or the patient's body will destroy them shortly after infusion.

These patients bruise very easily. Bed rails should be padded with blankets. Care must be taken in lifting, turning, or assisting the patient to ambulate. Minor falls or bumping into doorways can cause painful bruises.

Patients may have to stop using a toothbrush; some patients can use a toothette, others must use oral care solutions only. Roughage may be eliminated from the diet. Protective padding may be needed for bony prominences.

Intramuscular injections should be discontinued. If an injection must be given, hemophelic precautions should be used. The injection should be given with as small a needle as possible. The medication should be injected slowly. When the needle is withdrawn, pressure should be applied for 10 minutes. Ice should then be applied for 30 minutes. The patient should be checked every 10 to 15 minutes for bleeding.

Patients should be observed frequently and closely for bleeding. They can bleed from any body orifice: eyes, ears, nose, mouth, urethra, vagina, or anus. Internal bleeding can also occur: abdominal bleeding can be detected by checking abdominal girth; thoracic bleeding will usually result in respiratory difficulty; and severe internal bleeding will usually result in a drop in blood pressure and an increased pulse rate. Transfusions can sometimes be life saving. Patients will sometimes die of intracranial bleeding.

Fatigue

Chemotherapy may cause a rapid breakdown of cancer cells. These destroyed cells are released into the circulatory system and must be excreted by the kidneys. The result may be an elevated blood urea nitrogen (BUN) level and an elevated uric acid level. The low energy level of the patient may be a consequence of hyperuricemia and decreased food intake. Increasing the patient's fluid intake speeds the excretion of uric acid crystals and decreases the hazard of urate stone formation in the kidneys. Accurate intake and output records are essential to monitor kidney function during this period. Occasionally, Zyloprim is given to lower the uric acid levels.

Outpatients will experience their greatest fatigue level about 2 weeks after drug administration or when the blood count drops. They should be encouraged to rest more during this time and pace their activities to avoid undue stress. They need to be assured that the fatigue is physiologic in origin and will disappear as their body recovers from the drug therapy.

Alopecia

Alopecia is certainly not a life threatening consequence of chemotherapy, but can have a serious emotional effect. Patients need to be reassured that their hair will regrow. Patients should be encouraged to purchase a wig before their hair falls out, so that a wig can be selected to match their own hair color and style. Some patients dislike the discomfort of a wig and prefer a cloth head covering, except when going out.

Because the hair shaft is weak, vigorous brushing or teasing of the hair and the use of brush rollers will increase hair loss. Hair that has been lost on the bed or floor should be removed to avoid increasing the distress of the patient.

Scalp tourniquets and ice packs are being used in some clinics to decrease the hair loss. Research studies on these approaches have failed to consistently demonstrate their effectiveness.[47] These strategies will be effective only when used with drugs that are rapidly cleared from the blood plasma. With blood-borne malignancies such as leukemia, there is a risk of trapping a malignant cell in the scalp veins that otherwise would have been destroyed by the chemotherapy.[39]

Evaluating Nursing Care

Tools need to be developed to evaluate the effectiveness of nursing care of the chemotherapy patient. Research in this area is beginning to be conducted. Lum and colleagues have studied the relationships between nursing activities and the subsequent health status of the cancer patient.[35] The study identified a number of variables involved in patient outcomes and generated hypotheses for continued research in this area. Lewis and colleagues have developed an instrument designed to measure patient health outcomes during extended courses of chemotherapy.[32] Their study indicated that the instrument holds promise, but needs further development.

BIBLIOGRAPHY

1. Akahoshi, M.: High-dose methotrexate with leucovorin rescue. *Cancer Nursing.* 1:319–325, 1978.
2. Andrysiak, T., R. Caroll, and J. T. Ungerleider: Marijuana for the oncology patient. *American Journal of Nursing.* 79:1396–1398, 1979.
3. Apple, M. A.: New anticancer drug design: past and future strategies. In *Cancer: A Comprehensive Treatise, Vol. 5, Chemotherapy,* ed. by F. F. Becker. Plenum Press, New York, 1977.
4. Bahnson, C. B.: Psychologic and emotional issues in cancer: the psychotherapeutic care of the cancer patient. *Seminars in Oncology.* 2:293–309, 1975.
5. Barlock, A. L., D. M. Howser, and S. M. Hubbard: Nursing management of Adriamycin extravasation. *American Journal of Nursing.* 79:94–97, 1979.
6. Bingham, C. A.: The cell cycle and cancer chemotherapy. *American Journal of Nursing.* 78:1201–1205, 1978.
7. Burns, N.: Cancer chemotherapy: a systemic approach. *Nursing 78.* 8:56–63, 1978.
8. Cadman, E.: Toxicity of chemotherapy agents. In *Cancer: A Comprehensive Treatise, Vol. 5, Chemotherapy,* ed. by F. F. Becker. Plenum Press, New York, 1977.
9. Chabner, B. A. and D. G. Johns: Folate antagonists. In *Cancer: A Comprehensive Treatise, Vol. 5, Chemotherapy,* ed. by F. F. Becker. Plenum Press, New York, 1977.
10. Clifton, K. H.: The physiology of endocrine therapy. In *Cancer: A Comprehensive Treatise, Vol. 5, Chemotherapy,* ed. by F. F. Becker. Plenum Press, New York, 1977.
11. Cline, M. J. and C. M. Haskell: *Cancer Chemotherapy.* W. B. Saunders Co., Philadelphia, 1980.
12. Cool-headed cancer patients keep hair. *Medical World News.* 20:19, 1979.
13. Creasey, W. A.: Plant alkaloids. In *Cancer: A Comprehensive Treatise, Vol. 5, Chemothera-*

py, ed. by F. F. Becker. Plenum Press, New York, 1977.

14. Daeffler, R.: Oral hygiene measures for patients with cancer, I. *Cancer Nursing.* 3:347–356, 1980.

15. Daeffler, R.: Oral hygiene measures for patients with cancer, II. *Cancer Nursing.* 3:427–432, 1980.

16. Daeffler, R.: Oral hygiene measures for patients with cancer, III. *Cancer Nursing.* 4:29–36, 1981.

17. Donley, D. L.: Chemotherapy and the nurse's role. In *Dynamics of Oncology Nursing,* ed. by P. K. Burkhalter and D. L. Donley, McGraw-Hill Book Co., New York, 1978.

18. Englert, D. M. and S. J. Dudrick: Principles of ambulatory home hyperalimentation. *American Journal of Intravenous Therapy.* 5:11–28, 1978.

19. Eustace, P.: History and development of cisplatin in the management of malignant disease. *Cancer Nursing.* 3:373–378, 1980.

20. Gever, L. N.: Crisplatin: a breakthrough for the cancer patient, a nursing challenge for you. *Nursing 80.* 10:53, 1980.

21. Goldberg, I. H., T. A. Beerman, and R. Poon: Antibiotics: nucleic acids as targets in chemotherapy. In *Cancer: A Comprehensive Treatise, Vol. 5, Chemotherapy,* ed. by F. F. Becker. Plenum Press, New York, 1977.

22. Golden, S.: Cancer chemotherapy and management of patient problems. *Nursing Forum.* 14:278–303, 1975.

23. Higgins, N. M.: Nursing implications of *cis*-platinum therapy. *Oncology Nursing Forum.* 5:3–4, 1978.

24. Hildebrand, B. F.: The nursing management of the cancer patient receiving chemotherapy. *The Nursing Clinics of North America.* 13:267–380, 1978.

25. Keiser, L. W. and R. L. Capizzi: Principles of combination chemotherapy. In *Cancer: A Comprehensive Treatise, Vol. 5, Chemotherapy,* ed. by F. F. Becker. Plenum Press, New York, 1977.

26. Kennealey, G. T. and M. S. Mitchell: Factors that influence the therapeutic response. In *Cancer: A Comprehensive Treatise, Vol. 5, Chemotherapy,* ed. by F. F. Becker. Plenum Press, New York, 1977.

27. Krakoff, I. H.: *Cancer Chemotherapeutic Agents.* American Cancer Society, Professional Education Publication.

28. Krakoff, I. H.: *Cancer chemotherapy.* In *Clinical Oncology,* ed. by J. Horton and G. J. Hill, II. W. B. Saunders Co., Philadelphia, 1977.

29. Kreis, W.: Hydrazines and triazenes. In *Cancer: A Comprehensive Treatise, Vol. 5, Chemotherapy,* ed. by F. F. Becker. Plenum Press, New York, 1977.

30. Law, D.: Successful chemotherapy: quality care for the cancer patient. *The Canadian Nurse.* 76:19–22, 1980.

31. LePage, G. A.: Purine antagonists. In *Cancer: A Comprehensive Treatise, Vol. 5, Chemotherapy,* ed. by F. F. Becker. Plenum Press, New York, 1977.

32. Lewis, F. M., S. C. Firsich, and S. Parsell: Clinical tool development for adult chemotherapy patients: process and content. *Cancer Nursing.* 2:99–108, 1979.

33. Luckmann, J. and K. C. Sorensen: *Medical Surgical Nursing: A Psychophysiologic Approach.* W. B. Saunders Co., Philadelphia, 1980.

34. Ludlum, D. B.: Alkylating agents and the nitrosoureas. In *Cancer: A Comprehensive Treatise, Vol. 5, Chemotherapy,* ed. by F. F. Becker. Plenum Press, New York, 1977.

35. Lum, J. L. J., M. Chase, S. M. Cole, A. Johnson, J. A. Johnson, and M. R. Link: Nursing care of oncology patients receiving chemotherapy. *Nursing Research.* 27:340–346, 1978.

36. Machey, C. L. and A. W. Hotetl: Keeping infections down when the risks go up. *Nursing 80.* 10:69–73, 1980.

37. Maley, F.: Pyrimidine antagonists. In *Cancer: A Comprehensive Treatise, Vol. 5, Chemotherapy,* ed. by F. F. Becker. Plenum Press, New York, 1977.

38. Marino, E. B. and D. H. LeBlanc: Cancer chemotherapy. *Nursing 75.* 5:22–33, 1975.

39. Maxwell, M. B.: Scalp tourniquets for chemotherapy-induced alopecia. *American Journal of Nursing.* 80:900–905, 1980.

40. Maxwell, M.: Reexamining the dietary restrictions with procarbazine (an MAOI). *Cancer Nursing.* 3:451–458, 1980.

41. Miller, S. A.: Nursing actions in cancer chemotherapy administration. *Oncology Nursing Forum.* 7:8–16, 1980.

42. Moore, P.: Beyond the protocol. *Oncology Nursing Forum.* 5:12–14, 1978.

43. Nirenberg, A.: High-dose methotrexate for the patient with osteogenic sarcoma. *American Journal of Nursing.* 76:1776–1780, 1976.

44. *Nurse's Guide to Drugs.* Nursing 80 Books, Intermed Communications, Inc., Horsham, Pa., 1980.

45. Ostchega, C. Y.: Preventing — and treating — cancer chemotherapy's oral complications. *Nursing 80.* 10:47–53, 1980.

46. Parker, D. E.: The employee and cancer chemotherapy. *Occupational Health Nursing.* 25:22–24, 1977.

47. Passos, J. Y. and L. M. Brand: Effects of agents used for oral hygiene. *Nursing Research.* 15:196–202, 1966.

48. Pesce, A., et al.: Scalp tourniquet in the prevention of chemotherapy-induced alopecia. *New England Journal of Medicine.* 298:1204–1205, 1978.

49. Rose, K.: The stress of chemotherapy. *The Canadian Nurse.* 74:18–21, May 1978.

50. Saito, T. E.: Adriamycin: a review of its use, and guidelines for administration. *Cancer Nursing.* 1:169–173, 1978.

51. Schertz, G. L. and J. C. Marsh: Applications of cell kinetic techniques to human malignancies. In *Cancer: A Comprehensive Treatise, Vol. 5, Chemotherapy,* ed. by F. F. Becker. Plenum Press, New York, 1977.

52. Scogna, D. M. and R. V. Smalley: Chemotherapy-induced nausea and vomiting. *American Journal of Nursing.* 79:1562–1564, 1979.

53. Shaw, M. T. and R. D. Stebbins: Adjunctive chemotherapy. In *Cancer: A Comprehensive*

Treatise, Vol. 5, Chemotherapy, ed. by F. F. Becker. Plenum Press, New York, 1977.

54. Skeel, R. T. and C. A. Lindquist: Clinical aspects of resistance to antineoplastic agents. In *Cancer: A Comprehensive Treatise, Vol. 5, Chemotherapy,* ed. by F. F. Becker. Plenum Press, New York, 1977.

55. Todres, R. and R. Wojtiuk: The cancer patient's view of chemotherapy. *Cancer Nursing.* 2:283–286, 1979.

56. Uren, J. R. and R. E. Handschumacher: Enzyme therapy. In *Cancer: A Comprehensive Treatise, Vol. 5, Chemotherapy,* ed. by F. F. Becker. Plenum Press, New York, 1977.

57. Valentine, J. and I. H. Krakoff: The antimetabolites — 5-fluorouracil, 6-mercaptopurine, and 6-thioguanine. *Hospital Formulary,* 15:547–551, 1980.

58. Van Scoy-Mosher, M. B.: Chemotherapy: a manual for patients and their families. *Cancer Nursing.* 1:234–240, 1978.

59. Wandelt, M.: "Nurse work: the ideal is possible." Paper presented at the conference of the Texas League for Nursing, San Antonio, Texas, 1980.

60. Zia, P.: Cyclophosphamide: a review of its use, and guidelines for administration. *Cancer Nursing.* 1:83–85, 1978.

10

Immunotherapy

INTRODUCTION

Immunotherapy is the newest approach to the treatment of cancer. It is so new that none of the therapies are yet considered conventional; they are still in the experimental stage.

Current conventional therapies have only a limited ability to cure cancer. One reason for this is their inability to distinguish normal from malignant cells. Destruction or damage to normal tissue limits the intensity of treatment to such an extent that successful elimination of the malignant tissues is often not possible.

There are many immunologic deficiencies in the cancer patient, the number and extent of which progress as the disease progresses. This host defense failure is not addressed by the current conventional therapies. All three of the conventional therapies (surgery, chemotherapy, and radiotherapy) are immunosuppressive to some extent. Radiotherapy seems to cause the most long-lasting damage to immune responses. In chemotherapy, the immune response is at first suppressed, then rebounds at a higher than normal level. It is not known at this time what impact, if any, the immunosuppressive nature of the treatments has on the course of the disease.[2]

The field of immunotherapy is still in its infancy. Theories of immune response in man, such as immune surveillance, have proved to be inaccurate, inadequate, or simplistic as new information has been discovered. The immune functioning of the human body is very complex. Only segments of it have presently been identified. How these segments interact with each other or with the rest of the body is only beginning to be understood. Figures 10–1 and 10–2 present models of the possible interactions operating in tumor immunity within the immune system.[4, 13]

One of the serious limitations to the progress of immunotherapy is the lack of fundamental knowledge of the field of immunology. Immunotherapy must be based on a sound foundation of basic research. To leap from theory to clinical practice without first testing the theory by research is very unwise and may actually delay the search for effective interventions. Currie describes the necessity of further research in immunology.

The immunological aspects of cancer are many and varied and are the subject of intense investigation at present. There is almost universal optimism about the potential value of these studies in detecting, curing and even preventing cancer. It is imperative that such optimism be tempered with a careful appraisal of what we really know and how that knowledge can be applied. We must not discard the usual care and scrupulous investigation which normally precede the introduction of any new clinical approach to a disease in favor of a 'nothing to lose' attitude which has frequently and regrettably been the main characteristic of many previous attempts to employ immunological phenomena for the treatment of cancer patients. . . . Tumor immunology, especially when applied to therapy, is an intellectual minefield; it is so easy to put a foot in the wrong place. It may of course be possible to obtain results in a blind rush, but the odds are against it. Only by cautious progress, by close examination of the ground before each step is taken can reasonable forward progress be achieved.

Cancer research frequently involves a series of intuitive leaps from the crumbling debris of one hypothesis to the scaffolding of the next. This is clearly illustrated by recent progress in the immunology of tumors. With the extensive research into this topic undertaken in recent years, hypotheses have become as numerous and as ephemeral as the mayfly. Any discussion of the current status of such immunological research in the cancer field must, of necessity,

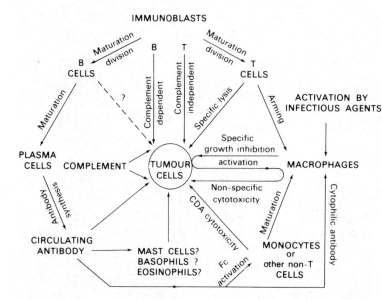

Figure 10–1. Diagrammatic representation of the possible types of specific effector mechanisms operating in tumor immunity, illustrating the apparent complexity of this topic at present. (From Currie, G.: *Cancer and the Immune Response.* 2nd edition, in series "Current Topics in Immunology." London: Edward Arnold [Publishers] Ltd., 1980. Used by permission.)

entail a description of many complex postulates, most of which may eventually be shown to be false.[4]

Cochran also expresses his concern about the intense pressure to apply current levels of knowledge about immunology immediately to clinical practice.

It is easy to be disappointed by the lack of progress in tumor immunology and the lack of major technological advances applicable in the clinic. This reaction, however, is in large measure a result of the quite unreasonable levels of expectation engendered by the intense pressures developed by the anxiety of clinicians, laymen, research administrators, and politicians to apply laboratory results to patient management with minimal delay. These pressures, in addition to overheating our levels of expectation, are counter-productive by endangering the traditional and well-founded "gradualism" by which the advance of scientific knowledge occurs. Specifically accelerated speculation leads to erroneous concepts and the uncritical and unnecessarily prolonged investigation of such concepts, which, in turn, perpetuate central fallacies and myths.

Tumor immunology certainly has its share of middle-aged and elderly myths, but there are some indications that these are now being recognized for what they are and that the subject is presently proceeding on a more strengthened scientific basis. The main priority remains the generation in a variety of laboratories of that scientific atmosphere without which progress is impossible and which permits the generation and *recognition* of the significant unexpected spin-off result. Obviously, we are at the *very beginning* of this whole game and have *barely scratched its surface.* . . . Manipulating the immune response in favor of the cancer patient may or may not be feasible, but we are unlikely to know this answer in the short term.[2]

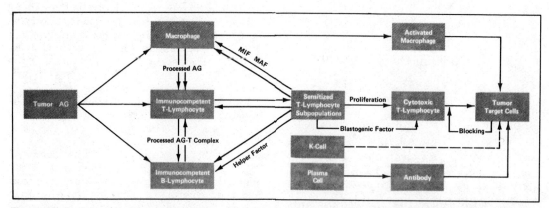

Figure 10–2. Interaction between components of the lymphoid system in tumor immunity. (From McKhann, C.: Cancer immunotherapy: a realistic approach. *CA — A Cancer Journal for Clinicians.* 30:286–293, 1980. Used by permission.)

Much of the current clinical research that has been conducted, particularly with bacillus Calmette-Guérin (BCG), has been poorly designed, using very small samples and often no control groups. There is a tendency to apply the results of these studies to clinical practice. In reacting to this situation, Currie voices concern.

It is a little difficult to see why many of the recent descriptions of these various manipulations are referred to as 'immunotherapy.' Evidence for immunological effects is often absent, and for therapeutic effects even less convincing. A treatment which does not work can hardly be called therapy.[4]

Researchers in the area of immunology have arrived at some empirical findings on which the expectations of the possibility of successful immunotherapy are based. These include:

1. Antigens that are not present on normal cells are commonly found on malignant cells.
2. The host is frequently capable of responding immunologically against a malignancy.
3. In cancer, there is a correlation between immunocompetence and prognosis.
4. Immunologic resistance to the growth of a malignancy can be effected.[4]

It seems reasonable to assume that if the immune system abnormalities were corrected, prognosis would improve. It might also seem logical to propose that if some of the host defenses were elevated above normal, prognosis would improve. These are current hypotheses of immunotherapy. It is possible, however, that the immune abnormalities that occur as cancer progresses are independent factors or may be only indirectly related to the progress of the disease. No cause and effect relationship has yet been identified. Or it is possible that the abnormalities may be the result, rather than the cause, of tumor progression.[10] If so, correcting the immune abnormalities might have no effect on tumor growth or on prognosis.

If immunotherapy is to be effective, its goal must be to control or destroy the malignancy by restoring or amplifying the body's normal mechanisms of defense against disease.[10] This may be accomplished by these objectives:

A. Restoring the immunocompetence of immunodeficient patients
B. Preventing or reversing immunosuppression induced by surgery, radiotherapy, or chemotherapy
C. Inducing or potentiating specific tumor immunity
D. Modulating immune response for selected objectives
   1. Augmenting cell-mediated immunity[7]
   2. Augmenting cytotoxic antibody[7]
   3. Activating macrophages[7]
   4. Increasing reticuloendothelial system (RES) clearance[7]
      a. Reducing blocking or inhibitory factors[7]
      b. Reducing circulating antigen or antigen-antibody complexes[7]

There are seven strategies currently under study that are designed to accomplish these objectives: active nonspecific immunotherapy, active specific immunotherapy, passive immunotherapy, adoptive immunotherapy, immunorestoration, local immunotherapy, and combination immunotherapy.

MAJOR APPROACHES TO IMMUNOTHERAPY

Active Nonspecific Immunotherapy

Active nonspecific immunotherapy functions by increasing general immunocompetence, augmenting cell-mediated or humoral immune responses, expanding the T-lymphocyte population, activating macrophages, and increasing reticuloendothelial system (RES) function. This is the oldest, most researched approach to immunotherapy and is considered at this time to be the most effective.[10]

Coley's Toxin. This treatment began in the 1890s, when Dr. W. B. Coley observed a spontaneous regression of a sarcoma of the tonsil after a streptococcal infection. He then developed a bacterial vaccine made of heat-killed bacteria. Unfortunately, he had inconsistent results and did not set up a research design that could be replicated. Although his vaccine, referred to as Coley's toxin, Coley's mixed bacterial toxin, or mixed bacterial vaccine (MBV), was produced for a while by a pharmaceutical company, the approach soon fell into disrepute. However, more recent studies tend to verify that Coley's observations were valid.[7, 10]

Bacillus Calmette-Guérin (BCG). In 1924, studies indicated that a virulent infection of tuberculosis increased humoral immunity. In 1936, Dienes found that it also strengthened cell-mediated immunity. There has been continued interest and research on the effects of mycobacteria on immune response. In 1956, Freund developed a very successful mixture of killed mycobacteria emulsified in mineral oil. It was used to immunize against tuberculosis. However, the mineral oil caused severe necrosis at the injection site. In an attempt to find a less tissue-toxic substance, BCG was developed in 1959.[2] BCG is a live, nonpathogenic TB bacillus (attenuated). The live TB organisms were considered safe and probably more effective than the killed bacteria.

The first use of BCG was as an immunization against tuberculosis. Then it was reported that children immunized in infancy with BCG to protect against tuberculosis had a decreased incidence of childhood leukemia.[8] Animal research and clinical trials were conducted on the effectiveness of BCG on tumor growth.[2] In 1969, Mathé, in a frequently referenced study, reported that BCG was effective in prolonging the remission of acute lymphoblastic leukemia. This stimulated a flurry of clinical studies on the effectiveness of BCG. However, Mathé's report has been challenged by studies later conducted on childhood leukemia.

BCG has been studied extensively in the treatment of malignant melanoma. In most cases, nodules injected with BCG will completely regress, as will many uninjected nodules. However, there is little or no ef-

fect on visceral spread of the malignancy, no prolongation of life, and no prevention of new skin lesions.[8]

Studies of other malignancies treated with BCG have used very small samples, and in many cases the research design has been questionable.[4, 8] BCG is a controversial therapy. Various scientists have said of BCG that it is "the most important clinical approach to immunotherapy"[10]; that it shows little evidence that it has "any therapeutic effect in man or in animals"[4]; and that "BCG has seen its day."[13]

The use of BCG is not without risk. It can actually enhance tumor growth. With usage, there is an increased incidence of tuberculosis. It may cause ulcers at the injection site, systemic BCG infections, hepatitis, and anaphylactoid reactions.[8]

Corynebacterium Parvum (C. Parvum). *C. parvum* has been shown to be a strong stimulant of the reticuloendothelial system. Its action is similar to that of BCG. *C. parvum* is a killed vaccine and does not have the infective risk of BCG. It is a member of the group of anaerobic corynebacteria, all of which stimulate the reticuloendothelial system.

Studies of *C. parvum* given concurrently with chemotherapy show an extension of the length of clinical response. Patients had fewer viral and bacterial infections. *C. parvum* also decreases the myelosuppression that occurs with chemotherapy. However, these are the results of preliminary studies and must await confirmation from further research.

In early studies, *C. parvum* was administered subcutaneously, causing local pain and swelling and transient systemic symptoms of fever, chills, and malaise. Later, it was administered intravenously. This increased its systemic toxicity; however, preliminary studies show tumor regression with this approach.[8]

Other Bacterial Adjuvants. Many types of bacteria and bacterial products are currently under study for use in immunotherapy. One of the most interesting groups is the bacterial endotoxins or lipopolysaccharides. These substances can either augment the antibody response or become immunosuppressive, depending on the timing of administration. The endotoxins also stimulate the production of tumor necrosis factor.[10]

Viruses, which can directly or indirectly inhibit tumor growth, are also being studied in immunotherapy research. Their mechanism of action is unknown. Fungi and fungal extracts are also under study and have shown antitumor activity.[10]

Synthetic chemicals, which function as interferon inducers, are also generating research interest. These substances augment antibody production and activate macrophages. However, they have an immunosuppressive effect on the T cells and can accelerate rather than retard tumor growth.[10]

Active Specific Immunotherapy

Active specific immunotherapy involves the injection of tumor cells, modified tumor cells, or tumor-cell surface antigens into the cancer patient, usually under the skin.[10] These cells may be autologous (prepared from the tumor cells of the recipient).[11] These cells may be extracts of the cell membranes of the tumor itself. Since the tumor cell membrane contains the antigenic sites, this will be the important factor whether the cells are live or attenuated or whether the cell membrane is extracted. One of the important goals of any of the strategies used to prepare the cells is the exposure of cell antigens, which are believed to be covered in tumor cells within the body.[10]

It may seem strange to take tumor cells from a patient, manipulate these cells in some arbitrary fashion, and then return them to the patient and expect a favorable response. However, this procedure does have clinical effects.[2]

The first studies of active specific immunotherapy were conducted in 1902. Since then further studies have been conducted, many of them using small samples and poor research designs. None of the studies has shown a clear-cut, positive clinical response.[2, 4, 10]

Currie, in addition to studying clinical responses, examined the patient's immunologic response. He found that the procedure he used improved the patient's immunologic response without producing any major improvement in the clinical condition of the malignancy.[4]

Patients with malignant melanoma who are treated in this manner sometimes have a decrease in the size of the tumor; however, the therapy has no effect on distant metastases or overall length of survival. Additionally, there is an increased incidence of local recurrence.[4]

Theoretically, this approach to immunotherapy should be effective, but clinical studies have not demonstrated this. Most of the studies have been done using patients with advanced disease after the failure of other forms of treatment. Active specific immunotherapy has been used as a sole therapy. It is possible that this form of immunotherapy might be of value to patients with minimal residual disease when combined with other treatment modalities.[4]

Passive Immunotherapy

Passive immunotherapy is the transfer of serologic components that have direct or indirect antitumor activity from a donor to a patient with active cancer.[10] Passive immunity confers immunity on the patient for only a short period of time.[11] From a theoretical point of view, this is a very logical approach to treatment. However, research in this area, which has been minimal and poorly designed, has not shown a favorable tumor response. In fact, some of the studies have resulted in tumor enhancement — the tumor grew more rapidly, rather than diminishing in size. What causes this enhancement is not understood.[2, 4, 7, 10]

Passive immunotherapy primarily involves the administration of antibodies obtained from specifically immunized animals or from other animals with the same type of tumor that is in remission or cured. The antibody given in this way can kill tumor cells in the presence of complement.

It can also arm leukocytes and macrophages, which can then kill or inhibit the growth of tumor cells. Antibody can also coat tumor cells and make them susceptible to the activity of lymphocytes or macrophages by increasing their ability to recognize the tumor cells and kill them. Serum from immunized animals or animals with regressing tumors can also have a deblocking effect on animals with growing tumors.[10] Researchers are now attempting to isolate tumor-associated antibodies for administration to humans.[11]

A newer approach to passive immunotherapy is the coupling of radioactive isotopes, toxins, or drugs to antitumor antibody. In some experiments, the drug or the antibody alone has little effect, whereas the combination produced dramatic effects. In other cases, administering the drug and antibody separately but concurrently was also effective.[10]

All of the above findings have been from animal research studies. Only a very limited number of studies in this area have been conducted on humans. Those that have been were so poorly controlled that they are not useful. Advances in this area will require increased understanding of the immune system and extensive, well-designed animal research before clinical studies can be performed.[2, 4, 7, 10]

Adoptive Immunity

Adoptive immunity involves the administration of blood components that provide passive immunity to the patient. These components are then utilized by the patient for the development and maintenance of active immunity.[11] In cancer, the components of importance are those that prevent the growth or cause regression of the malignancy. Theoretically and empirically, it should be possible to transfer specific immunity — either humoral, cell-mediated, or both — from one individual to another.

Adoptive immunity in cancer has been extensively studied in animal models. The studies have explored transfer of immunity using lymphoid cells and other host defense cells and their products such as immune RNA and transfer factor.[10]

Cells. Animal research on the transfer of immune lymphocytes has shown the treatment to be very effective. In some studies, the animal is immunized with tumor cells, then the lymphocytes are given to an animal with a growing tumor. This type of immunity is more effective than active immunization.

Although some studies have been conducted on patients with cancer, it is not possible to conduct extensive human research in this area. Donors would need to be other cancer patients, and they would be unsuitable because of the immunoincompetence caused by their disease. Even if they were immunocompetent, it would not be safe for the donors to lose some of their lymphocytes.

In addition, these transplanted cells would sensitize the human leukocyte antigen (HLA) antigens and rapidly be destroyed. Also, cell collection techniques are difficult, time-consuming, and expensive, thus making the procedure technologically impractical. Future studies will likely focus on subcomponents of these immune cells.[10]

Immune RNA. Studies of immune ribonucleic acid (RNA) began in 1967. The intent was to discover the portion of the cell involved in adoptive immunity. Animal experiments were conducted with RNA extracted from lymphocytes. Significant tumor regressions and one permanent cure resulted. Prolonged survival rates have also been demonstrated with immune RNA. Nonspecific immune RNA and RNA from nonimmune cells are ineffective. Effectiveness requires immune RNA from lymphocytes that have been exposed to a specific type of malignancy.

Clinical studies are beginning to use immune RNA in the treatment of patients with advanced disseminated malignant diseases. There is considerable skepticism about the use of immune RNA in cancer treatment. The area is promising, but one that needs more study.[10]

Transfer Factor. The original studies on the use of transfer factor in cancer began in 1976. The factor has been identified and carefully evaluated. It is a very stable substance that is antigen specific and transfers cell-mediated immunity. If the donor does not have delayed hypersensitivity or cell-mediated immunity to a specific antigen, the recipient will not develop it from the donor's transfer factor. There also seems to be some degree of general immunocompetence-boosting ability in transfer factor. In some cases, treatment with transfer factor has also resulted in a decline in cell-mediated immunity. It has been discovered that transfer factor is complex and actually contains multiple factors. Some of them transfer specific cell-mediated immunity, some transfer nonspecific immunity, and some may even be immunosuppressive. Attempts are now being made to purify transfer factor.

There seems to be a relationship between immune RNA and transfer factor. Immune RNA appears to be a larger, more complete molecule, with transfer factor as a subcomponent containing the specific immunologic information.

Studies have been conducted on humans in the area of transferring immunity to both infectious and malignant diseases. These studies have demonstrated that transfer factor can confer donor immunity on anergic cancer patients. Transfer factor can induce tumor regression in a fraction of patients. Studies continue to further identify transfer factor. Its proper role in immunology for cancer awaits further trials.[10]

Immunorestorative Immunotherapy

Immunorestorative immunotherapy refers to the use of agents that increase the immune response of the individual and particularly the number of mature functional T-lymphocytes. This group of substances might be classed as immunologic stimulants.

Interferon. Interferon is a family of proteins, produced in several body tissues, including lymphoid cells, macrophages, spleen, liver, lung, and thymus.[10] It was first described in 1957 by Isaacs and Lindenmann. Research on interferon has been limited by the substance's inaccessibility. Since it is species specific, it must be extracted from the white blood cells of the same species animal being tested. The method of extraction is complex, and obtaining a minuscule portion of interferon requires large numbers of white cells. In spite of these obstacles, studies have been conducted and many data have been collected about the actions of interferon.

There are at least three varieties of interferon: one produced by leukocytes, another generated by fibroblasts, and a third (called immune interferon) produced by T-lymphocytes. The interferon now being studied is in crude form. Only 1 part to 999 parts is pure interferon. Thus, studies cannot state with certainty that the resulting changes occur as a consequence of interferon.

Experimental data indicate that interferon does exert antitumor effects. It can delay the onset of a neoplastic disease, slow tumor growth, inhibit viral and cellular proliferation, and modulate the immune response. Interferon is also able to control or prevent the viral infections that can be so destructive to cancer patients.

In 1980, the American Cancer Society provided 2 million dollars for clinical research studies using interferon. Research laboratories and pharmaceutical companies are searching for methods to provide a more pure form of interferon for study. Although interferon is not expected to be the "magic bullet" in the cure of cancer, it may be a very effective addition to the existing armamentarium of the oncologist.[6, 10, 17]

Lymphokines. Lymphokines are a group of substances that mediate delayed type hypersensitivity reaction (cell-mediated immunity). These substances include macrophage and leukocyte migration inhibitory factors, lymphotoxins, macrophage-activating factors, chemotactic factors, and lymphocyte blastogenic factors. They are all products of stimulated lymphocytes.[10]

Cancer patients have a defect in lymphocyte-mediated immunity. It is thought that this defect results in the body's failure to release lymphokines. It is also possible that lymphokine inhibitory substances are present in tumors. If this is so, a major immunotherapeutic effect could theoretically be achieved by the administration of lymphokines.[10]

Several research studies have supported this idea. Lymphokines were injected directly into tumor nodules. Tumor regression occurred. In the future, the macrophage-activating factor must be purified and appropriate animal model studies conducted.[10]

Thymic Hormones. The role of the thymus in cell-mediated and humoral immunity was demonstrated in 1967. Since that time, much work has gone into identifying the thymic hormones. Laboratories have identified factors extracted from the thymus or present in the serum that have activities associated with normal thymus functioning.

It has been found that the level of thymic hormone activity declines in the blood with increasing age and that the level is very low in patients with some malignancies. From this discovery developed the hypothesis that decreased thymic hormone and related deficiencies in cell-mediated immunity could be associated with the development or progression of malignancies. If this is true, administration of thymic hormone should correct the deficiencies in cell-mediated immunity and improve the body's resistance to the tumor.

The purified form of thymic hormone is called thymosin. Administration of thymosin does improve the immunologic function of cancer patients. However, giving thymosin to immunocompetent patients may be dangerous. Phase I and II trials (see Chapter 9) are now being conducted.[10]

Levamisole. Levamisole is a unique immunologic reagent. It has shown some activity in the immunotherapy of cancer in both animals and humans. Levamisole was used for years as an anthelmintic agent. It has been found to increase the antibody response to a number of antigens. Levamisole has a variety of immunologic effects. It can restore immunity in immunologically

depressed patients. However, there is some concern that high doses may be immunosuppressive. Tumor enhancement has occurred in animal studies.[10]

Local Immunotherapy

Local immunotherapy involves applying an immunotherapeutic agent directly onto the region of a tumor or injecting it into the tumor. Theoretically, local or regional administration of an immunotherapeutic agent has a systemic effect and, for a local effect, is dependent on systemic immunocompetence. There are three types of local immunotherapy. Topical treatment entails placing the agent directly over an intradermal tumor (by applying it to the surface of the skin) or using scarification or intradermal injection. In intratumoral inoculation, the agent is injected directly into the tumor. This treatment is used for intradermal or subcutaneous tumors. Regional immunotherapy involves placing the immunotherapeutic agent in the region of a tumor by either scarification or intradermal injection. This may be done before or after the tumor is surgically removed or irradiated. Theoretically, an interaction between the agent and the tumor cells occurs within the lymphatic drainage or in regional lymph nodes.

The important consequence of local immunotherapy is a delayed hypersensitivity reaction: tumor cells are killed by a bystander effect of delayed hypersensitivity. Studies indicate that the major cell involved in this activity is the activated macrophage. Another less understood interaction occurs between the immunotherapeutic agent and the cancer cells or tumor antigens. This theoretically results in the appearance of tumor antigen in the lymph nodes, vigorous sensitization of the host; and the development of systemic tumor immunity. Distant metastases will be challenged or may regress.[10] Not all researchers agree that a systemic reaction occurs. Often visceral metastases will continue to grow, even when local control is effective.[2, 4]

In order for this treatment to work, the

tumor must be small and the host must be immunocompetent. Agents that have been used in local immunotherapy include BCG, *C. parvum,* vaccinia virus, BCG cell-wall skeleton, methanol extracted residue (MER), dinitrochlorobenzene (DNCB), triethyleneaminobenzoquinone (TEIB), purified protein derivative (P.P.D.), streptokinase-streptodornase, nitrogen mustard, 5-fluorouracil (5-FU), Adriamycin, the nitrosoureas, and the lymphokines.

Combination Immunotherapy

Combinations of the approaches just described may be used in treatment. Theoretically, this should result in greater effectiveness than the use of a single modality. For example, using active specific and active nonspecific immunotherapy together should be more effective than using either alone. This speculation has yet to be proved. The immunologic defects that occur in cancer have not been well identified. Until they are, selection of approaches to therapy will to some extent remain arbitrary.

COMPLICATIONS OF IMMUNOTHERAPY

Immunotherapy with BCG. The most frequent problems encountered in immunotherapy are a consequence of the use of BCG.[4] Most patients experience influenza-like symptoms that begin 12 to 24 hours after receiving the BCG and usually subside within 48 hours. The usual symptoms are malaise, shivering, low-grade fever, nausea, and anorexia. Local problems with intradermal BCG are rare, although scabbing, scarring, and depigmentation can cause body image problems. The mixture of BCG and tumor cells or intralesional BCG can cause abscess formation and large amounts of pus over a period of weeks or months. These abscesses contain live BCG organisms and drainage must be handled with caution. Exposure of immunodepressed individuals to these organisms could be disastrous.[2]

Many patients receiving BCG develop some degree of liver dysfunction that may alter liver function tests. Some patients develop tuberculoid granulomas in the liver and granulomatous hepatitis.

A mycobacterial bacteremia follows the administration of BCG and is viewed by some as a necessary and desirable event. The mycobacteria spread from the injection site into the draining lymph nodes and may cause lymph node enlargement. Some researchers have reported persistent lymphadenopathy and mycobacterial abscesses of the lymph nodes.

A generalized progressive infection with BCG is rare, but does occur and can cause death. Early detection is essential. Early use of antituberculosis therapy will resolve the condition. Anaphylactic reactions and death may occur after BCG administration. Resuscitation equipment should be available when BCG is to be given.[2]

Immunotherapy with C. Parvum. *C. parvum* almost always produces a febrile reaction. Subcutaneous and intralesional injections cause pain. Intralesional injection causes severe local inflammation and sometimes abscess formation. Systemic reactions are more common if *C. parvum* is administered intravenously and may include hepatotoxicity, mild cardiovascular changes, and transient hypotension or hypertension. There is concern that intravascular coagulation, thrombocytopenia, and nephrotic syndrome may develop in a small number of patients.[2]

Immunotherapy with Levamisole. The side effects of levamisole are most common in patients with rheumatoid arthritis, perhaps because some components of the immune system are operative in this disorder. Some patients have developed skin rashes. High doses of levamisole may cause gastrointestinal symptoms. Granulocytopenia may occur and there have been several reports of agranulocytosis.[2]

Active Specific Immunotherapy. No major problems have been observed to be associated with the injection of tumor cells. These cells are rendered incapable of replication before injection. There is a theoretical risk of introducing oncogenes, or oncogenic viruses. Most patients who are treated in this manner have advanced malignancies and do not live long enough for these problems to arise.[2]

Passive Immunotherapy. The major problems that occur with passive immunotherapy are anaphylaxis, serum sickness, and glomerulonephritis. Graft-versus-host disease may occur if foreign immunocompetent cells are given. Passive immunotherapy has been used so infrequently that there has not been sufficient opportunity to identify many complications.[2]

Potential Dangers of Immunotherapy. The greatest hazard of immunotherapy is tumor enhancement. This is a risk that may occur in all forms of immunotherapy. The mechanism by which this occurs is not understood.

Another problem that may occur if active immunotherapy is given over a long period of time could be the effects of overstimulation of the reticuloendothelial system. This could lead to amyloidosis, autoimmune disease, or the development of malignant reticuloses.[4]

THE EFFECTIVENESS OF IMMUNOTHERAPY

Measurement of the effectiveness of immunotherapy is difficult and has not been well done, according to the reports of many research studies.[2, 4] Some researchers have conducted studies on the level of immunocompetence of the patient and consider an increase in immunocompetence a success. Others have judged regression of the tumor at a local site as successful, even though distant malignancies continue to grow.

If, as some propose, immune deficiency in cancer is an effect, not a cause, of tumor progression, immunocompetence could be completely restored and yet have no effect on the disease process. This would be like the intern who insisted that all of his patients die in electrolyte balance.

It would seem necessary to use the same measures of effectiveness that are used in evaluating other therapies for cancer: number of cures, increased length of life, increased disease-free intervals, and de-

gree of regression of tumor masses. These must be demonstrated in quantifiable terms so that comparisons can be made with other studies and therapies.

Table 10–1 shows the types of cancer that have shown responses to various types of immunotherapy.

THE PROCESS OF IMMUNOTHERAPY

Assessment of Immunologic Status

To determine the level of immunocompetence of the patient, most therapists conduct skin tests before administering immunotherapy. The anergic patient will not respond to some types of immunotherapy. It is a risk to administer some types of immunotherapy to the patient who is already immunocompetent.[12]

In order to evaluate the patient's immune response, the following tests are often performed. A total and differential white blood count is obtained and the percentage of T and B cells is measured. The white blood cells are examined for proliferative capacity. This test is usually performed using phytohemagglutinin (PHA) and mixed leukocyte culture (MLC) test. Delayed hypersensitivity response is measured by a battery of cancer skin test antigens. Commonly used preparations include intermediate strength P.P.D., *Candida albicans* extract, mumps antigen, and streptokinase-streptodornase.[8] If all of these are nonreactive, the patient is anergic. DNCB is also used to determine the patient's ability to react to a new antigen.[3]

The patient's humoral immunity may be assessed with serum samples. Tests that will assist in this analysis are total protein determination, quantitative immunoglobulin assays, protein electrophoresis, immunoelectrophoresis, and baseline antibody titers.[12]

The nurse may be responsible for performing the skin tests and reading the skin test responses. Since the testing will require multiple injections, some measure may be used to anesthetize the skin.[12] The

Table 10–1. Immunotherapy of Human Solid Tumors*

Approach	Agent	Mechanisms	Disease in Which Activity Demonstrated
Systemic active nonspecific	Immunoadjuvants or immunopotentiators BCG C. parvum Mycobacteria extracts (MER, CWS)† Pseudomonas vaccine Mixed bacterial vaccines	Increased general competence, increased reticuloendothelial activity	Malignant melanoma Lung cancer Malignant melanoma Breast cancer Colon cancer
	Immunorestorative Levamisole	Restores immuno-competence	Head and neck cancer
Systemic active specific	Unmodified tumor cells Modified tumor cells Tumor antigens	Increase tumor specific cellular and/or humoral immune response	Malignant melanoma Lung cancer
Local	Haptenes (DNCB) Virus BCG Bacterial antigens	Active macrophages destroy tumor by bystander effect, induce tumor immunity	Skin cancer Malignant melanoma Breast cancer
Adoptive	Lymphocytes Immune RNA Transfer factor	Transfer specific immunity	Malignant melanoma
Mediators and hormonal	Lymphokines Interferon Thymosin Tumor necrosis factor	Not well under-stood; under study	Osteogenic sarcoma‡
Passive	Allogeneic or xenogeneic antibody	Transfer cytotoxic or opsonizing antibody couples with chemotherapy	?Melanoma
	Plasmapheresis	Removal of tumor antigen and antigen-antibody complexes	None for certain

*From Guttermann, J. U., Mavligit, G. M., Schwartz, M. A., and Hersh, E. M.: Immunotherapy of human solid tumors: principles of development. In *Immunological Aspects of Cancer,* ed. by Castro, J. E. Baltimore: University Park Press, 1978. Used by permission.

†Methanol extracted residue, cell wall skeleton.

‡For interferon.

skin should be cleansed with alcohol and allowed to dry. Skin tests are given by intradermal injection in a predetermined order. It is important to space the injections 3 to 4 cm apart to avoid overlap of responses. The site of each injection should be marked with indelible ink.[12]

The skin tests are read at 24 and 48 hours. It is wise to double-check reactions by having two nurses check the site. The lesions should be evaluated for erythema and induration. Measurements of both the horizontal and vertical dimensions of the site should be recorded in millimeters.[12]

DNCB skin testing is performed somewhat differently. A high dose of 2000 mcg and a low dose of 50 mcg of DNCB are given. Most commonly, the volar surface of the forearms is the site of injection. Croft recommends routinely giving the high dose on the left arm and the low dose on the right arm. This standardization will ensure correct reading of skin responses.[3]

The skin is prepared with acetone to remove oil. A plastic ring is placed on the skin. Croft recommends using color-coded rings so that the same ring is always used for the high-dose side. DNCB can adhere to the ring and, if the ring is later used for a low dose, may distort the results.

The arm is placed in a level position. The DNCB is dropped on the skin within the ring and the ring rocked gently to evenly distribute the DNCB. None of the drug should be allowed to leak outside the ring, since any skin exposed to the chemical will react.[3]

As soon as the DNCB is dry, the ring is removed and the site is covered with a Telfa patch and a wide strip of occlusive tape. The dressing must be kept dry for 24 hours, after which the dressing is removed and the patient can begin bathing. The skin reaction is read and recorded daily by the patient or a family member.[3]

A red, itching, blistered site indicates an initial positive reaction. A secondary flare will occur in the immunocompetent patient 7 to 14 days later. A flare on the low-dose arm is a 4+ reaction and a flare on the high-dose arm is a 3+ reaction. If the patient does not have a secondary flare, this is considered a 2+ reaction, or a negative response.

The patient can apply an ice pack to the area to reduce itching and should be cautioned not to scratch the area. DNCB under the fingernails can sensitize any other part of the body with which it comes in contact. Healing will take place over the course of a month. The skin will peel and the new epidermis will often be more deeply pigmented than the normal skin.[3]

Timing of Immunotherapy

There is a specific time during which immunotherapy will be maximally effective. This is when the tumor level is small. Ideally this would be immediately after primary therapy or after treatment of the first recurrence. Patients with advanced disease are unlikely to respond effectively. There is a period of immunosuppression that occurs following surgery, radiotherapy, and chemotherapy. This is not an appropriate time to administer immunotherapy. However, administration of immunotherapy just before or during these treatments may reduce the amount of immunosuppression that occurs. It may also decrease bone marrow suppression and thus diminish the risk of infection and bleeding. This may allow for more successful doses of radiation or chemotherapy. During chemotherapy, the period of the postimmunodepression "overshoot" may be the ideal time to administer immunotherapy. Studies of the timing of therapy have not been conducted because of differences in animal model and human response patterns. See Figure 10–3 for suggested timing of immunotherapy.[2]

Factors That Influence the Effectiveness of Immunotherapy

There are a number of factors that can influence the effectiveness of immunotherapy. The performance of any adjuvant will vary greatly with the route of administration. The most effective route will vary with the type of tumor, its site, and the adjuvant used. The dose is also an important factor. Too high a dose may be toxic or may cause a different effect. Too low a dose may be ineffective. Doses of immunotherapy agents are not as easy to determine as doses of drugs. A high dose may cause no toxic reaction, but may not be as effective in producing the desired immune reaction as a low dose.[16]

Because this type of treatment is only effective against small numbers of cells, tumor volume will influence the outcome of immunotherapy. Combining immunotherapy with conventional therapy may be effective against larger tumors.[16] The location of the tumor is also an important factor. Some body sites, such as the nervous system, are not easily accessible to immunologic reactions.

If the patient is severely immunosuppressed or anergic, immunotherapy may not be as effective and may be more likely to cause tumor enhancement.

Administering Immunotherapy

Since the entire field of immunotherapy is still considered experimental, most immunotherapy is currently being conducted at medical research centers. Some of the treatments are administered by physicians. Others are administered by nurses who are participating in medical research and have special preparation in immunotherapy. Very few nurses working in general hospitals would be asked to take on these responsibilities.

The primary area of nursing responsibil-

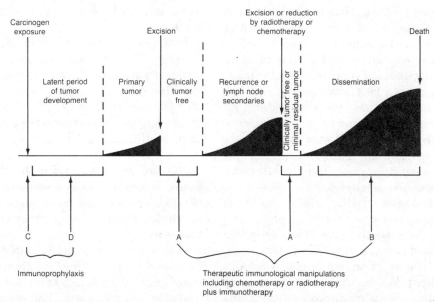

Figure 10–3. The timing of immunotherapy. *A,* Therapeutic immunological manipulation when a clinically detectable tumor is absent or minimal. *B,* Therapeutic immunological manipulation when tumor burden is considerable. *A* and *B* may be combined with radiation therapy or chemotherapy. *C,* Immunoprophylaxis. Immune manipulation at the time of carcinogen exposure or (in animals) at time of tumor transplantation. *D,* Immunoprophylaxis. Immune manipulation during latent period between carcinogen exposure (or tumor transplantation) and emergence of a clinically detectable tumor. (With permission from Cochran, A. J.: *Man, Cancer, and Immunity.* Copyright: Academic Press Inc. [London] Ltd., 1978.)

ity that requires different skills is the administration of active nonspecific immunotherapy agents, particularly BCG. BCG is administered in many ways, including scarification and intralesional, intracavitary, intravesical, intrapulmonary, intradermal, and oral administration.[3]

Scarification. Scarification can be done by scratching the skin or by using the tine technique. It may be necessary to teach the patients and their family to perform this procedure at home.

Scarification by Scratching. An area of skin 5 cm by 5 cm is selected. The area should be cleansed with acetone. The skin is drawn taut and the skin is scratched just deeply enough to break it, using a 21-gauge needle. Each scratch should be 5 cm long. The result will be a cross-hatched grid. A carefully measured amount of BCG is dropped on the broken skin and spread over the entire 5 cm by 5 cm area with the side of the needle. The area is then dried with a hairdryer on the lowest setting (heat will destroy the BCG). The hairdryer should be held 6 inches from the skin.

When the area is dry, the skin will look glazed and feel tacky. The grid may then be covered with a plastic wrap, such as Saran wrap, cut to the size of the grid. The plastic film is then taped with occlusive tape. A folded gauze pad may be placed at the lower edge of the plastic to absorb any seepage.[3] Some physicians prefer that the site remain open to the air and instruct the patient to keep it dry for 24 hours.[3]

The Tine Technique. The area is cleansed with acetone. A measured amount of BCG is placed on the skin and spread over a 2 inch by 1 inch area with a sterile gloved finger. The tine, a grid square with 36 prongs attached to a magnet holder, is pressed into the skin through the liquid with a firm, downward pressure. The pressure should be maintained for a moment to allow the skin to rebound against the tine. The tine should not be rocked or twisted. Two side-by-side punctures are made. The BCG is then reapplied. The site will be cared for in the same manner as in the scratch method.

The patient should be informed about

common side effects that may occur, such as malaise, bone and joint aches, fever and chills, and enlargement of lymph nodes. Symptoms may be treated with aspirin or acetaminophen and increased fluid intake. Patients should be encouraged to call the physician if unusual symptoms occur. As additional scarification is done, patients should be aware that old sites may flare up, causing redness and itching.[3] Scarring and hyperpigmentation may remain after the treatments are concluded.

Intralesional BCG. BCG injection into a tumor is usually done by a physician. Because the potential side effects are more serious and can result in death within 24 hours of the injection, patients are usually hospitalized. During this time the patient should be closely monitored. Vital signs and state of consciousness should be checked frequently. The body temperature may rise to 105° F. The pulse and respiration rates may increase. The blood pressure may decrease. Cyanosis may become evident. The patient may become lethargic. Patients who have brain metastases may have seizures. Nursing interventions should include maintaining hydration and decreasing the temperature elevation.[3]

Intracavitary Instillation. BCG may be injected into the abdominal or pleural cavity after paracentesis or thoracentesis. Injection into the pleural space is a greater risk and causes complications similar to those of intralesional BCG. After instillation, the patient should be asked to turn from side to side and back to front every 5 minutes to distribute the BCG.[3]

Patients who receive this type of treatment usually have multiple nursing problems. They are usually cachectic patients with advanced cancer. They are in negative nitrogen balance, have just had more protein withdrawn in the removal of body fluids, and have received BCG. Nursing measures should be similar to those given to the patient with intralesional BCG.

Intravesical Instillation. Patients who have cancer of the bladder may have BCG instillations in the bladder. Urine cytologies are usually done before and after completion of the treatments. Instillations are usually done on a weekly or bi-weekly basis.

Patients are first asked to empty their bladder. The urethral meatus is prepared with an antiseptic. Xylocaine jelly may be instilled several minutes before the catheter is inserted. The BCG is dissolved in 5 to 10 ml of sterile water just before instillation. Instillation is followed with 30 to 50 ml of sterile water or normal saline. Patients are asked to retain the fluid for 3 hours before voiding.[3] Excessive drinking of fluids during this period should be discouraged. Patients may experience chills and fever.

Intrapulmonary BCG. BCG can be delivered into the lungs by aerosol. Treatments are given once a week for 12 weeks and then once a month. The initial dose is very small, and the dose is increased if the patient has no adverse reaction. Visitors should be asked to leave the room during the treatment.

Both patient and nurse should wear a mask during the treatment. After treatment is begun, the nurse should leave the room. Some patients will require assistance in order to coordinate the mechanics of the equipment or to maintain a sitting position. Some patients may need to be reminded to inhale and exhale properly.

Croft suggests checking the P.P.D. reaction of health care personnel administering aerosol BCG every 1 to 3 months. She also proposes monitoring a record of the nurse's exposure time with each treatment. There is a risk to the nurse of chest x-ray abnormalities or hypersensitivity reactions.[3]

After the treatment, the equipment should be rinsed with tap water, placed in a plastic bag, and labeled "Isolation" before being sent to central services. Patients have very few side effects from this treatment.

Intradermal BCG. BCG is given intradermally, primarily to convert a negative P.P.D. to a positive P.P.D. A patient with a positive P.P.D. is more sensitive to immunologic stimulation with BCG. The injection will cause the development of a raised, pustular lesion that will heal, leaving a small scar.[3] The drainage will contain live BCG from which other patients and small children should be protected. A clean dressing should be worn by the patient until the wound heals.

Oral Administration. BCG is given orally to patients with gastric, hepatic, or pancreatic tumors. Croft suggests mixing the BCG with cranberry juice. The only side effect that may be experienced is nausea during the first 24 hours.[3]

Monitoring and Evaluating Immunotherapy

Patients receiving immunotherapy should be monitored for side effects and the effect of the treatment on immune functioning and tumor growth. The nurse should keep careful records of the symptoms that the patients experience. Patients should be regularly assessed for signs of changes in their functional state or the state of their tumor. Palpable tumors should be measured and recorded. Changes in size of lymph nodes should be noted. Location of the rim of the liver should be measured. The Karnofsky Scale would be a useful tool for assessing the patients' functional state.

The physician may do serial studies of the immunologic status of the patient in order to determine changes. However, improvement in immunologic functioning cannot be the final rule for judging the success of the treatment. Success must be based on the patients' increased length of life or increased length of remission.

NURSING IMPLICATIONS

Much of the nursing literature seems to view the role of the nurse in immunotherapy as one of performing technical duties and counseling patients in such a way that they accept and comply with the medical treatment plan. Some references are made to the need to assist patients in their attempt to cope with the impact of the medical treatment on their lifestyle.

Although all of these roles are commendable and important, they seem to narrow the focus and diminish the impact that nursing practice could have on the level of the patient's health. We must learn to look at why we do things and the impact of our actions on the patient's health. Health must be viewed in a broader sense than changes in physiologic status alone.

The practice of nursing must develop a more scientific basis. We are very inclined to jump on someone's bandwagon (or theory) with little empirical data to justify our actions. We then decide that everyone who is a "good nurse" functions according to that theory.

The hypotheses on which immunotherapy is based have not yet been adequately tested. They include the belief that immunologic functioning in an individual changes with states of health and perhaps with life events, that deficient immunologic functioning may have a role in the etiology of cancer, and that diminished immunologic functioning causes the cancer to grow faster and thus contributes to or hastens the patient's death. It is believed that the functioning of the immune system is possibly increased through therapeutic interventions. This improvement is expected to alter the course of the disease by curing it or by slowing down tumor growth. The patient who has dormant nests of malignant cells is thought to have controlled the tumor growth by an effective immune response that may, when it fails at some later date, allow regrowth of the malignancy.

If these beliefs are true, there are many significant implications for nursing practice. We do not yet know the effect of specific nursing actions on the patient's immune response. Could it be possible that forcing the patient into a passive, compliant role decreases effective immune functioning? There are many factors very much within the realm of nursing that could alter the immune response. These include nutrition, vitamin intake, stress, relaxation, emotional state, self-esteem, interpersonal relationships, support systems, beliefs, and physical activity.

Nursing research needs to be conducted to determine the relationships between these variables and immune functioning. If there are relationships and if immune functioning does make a difference in the course of cancer, nursing interventions could be planned with a predicted patient response. Nursing actions could play a significant role in controlling the patients' response to their disease and helping them move toward a higher level of health.

Nursing interventions could have an impact on many aspects of the cancer situation: the at-risk patient, the patient receiving medical treatment for cancer, the patient in remission, the patient just completing medical therapy such as chemotherapy, or the education of groups and communities. But at this point, this is only an ideal. Let's not jump on the bandwagon until we have sufficient data.

BIBLIOGRAPHY

1. Carroll, R. M.: BCG immunotherapy by the tine technique: the nurse's role. *Cancer Nursing.* 1:241–246, 1978.
2. Cochran, A. J.: *Man, Cancer and Immunity.* Academic Press Inc. Ltd., London, 1978.
3. Croft, C. L.: BCG administration and nursing implications. *American Journal of Nursing.* 79:315–319, 1979.
4. Currie, G.: *Cancer and the Immune Response.* Year Book Medical Publishers, Inc., Chicago, 1980.
5. Donley, D. L.: Immunology and immunotherapy: new frontiers in nursing. In *Dynamics of Oncology Nursing,* ed. by P. K. Burkhalter and D. L. Donley. McGraw-Hill Book Co., New York, 1978.
6. Grasser I.: Antitumor effects of interferon. In *Cancer: A Comprehensive Treatise, Vol. 5, Chemotherapy,* ed. by F. F. Becker. Plenum Press, New York, 1977.
7. Guttermann, J. U., G. M. Mavligit, M. A. Schwartz, and E. M. Hersh: Immunotherapy of human solid tumors: principles of development. In *Immunological Aspects of Cancer,* ed. by J. E. Castro. University Park Press, Baltimore, 1978.
8. Harris J.: Tumor immunology. In *Clinical Oncology,* ed. by J. Horton and G. J. Hill, II. W. B. Saunders Co., Philadelphia, 1977.
9. Herrmann, C.: Immunology: the method to our madness. *Cancer Nursing.* 2:359–363, 1979.
10. Hersh, Evan M., G. M. Mavligit, J. U. Gutterman, and S. P. Raichman.: Immunotherapy of human cancer. In *Cancer: A Comprehensive Treatise, Vol. 6, Radiotherapy, Surgery and Immunotherapy,* ed. by F. F. Becker. Plenum Press, New York, 1977.
11. Luckmann, J. and K. C. Sorensen: *Medical-Surgical Nursing: A Psychophysiological Approach.* W. B. Saunders Co., Philadelphia, 1980.
12. McCalla, J. L.: Immunotherapy: concepts and nursing implications. *Nursing Clinics of North America.* 11:59–71, 1976.
13. McKhann, C.: Cancer immunotherapy: a realistic appraisal. *CA — A Cancer Journal for Clinicians.* 30:286–293, 1980.
14. Morton, D. L.: Cancer immunotherapy: an overview. *Seminars in Oncology.* 1:297–310, 1974.
15. Prager, M. D.: Experimental specific immunotherapy. In *Immunological Aspects of Cancer,* ed. by J. E. Castro. University Park Press, Baltimore, 1978.
16. Sadler, T. E. and J. E. Castro: Experimental non-specific immunotherapy. In *Immunological Aspects of Cancer,* ed. by J. E. Castro. University Park Press, Baltimore, 1978.
17. The big IF in cancer. *Time,* March 31, 1980, pp. 60–66.

The Nursing Management of Cancer

11

Nursing Care Related to Physiologic Conditions

INTRODUCTION

The process of nursing is not simple. It involves more than just identifying a problem, applying a nursing intervention, and thus eliminating the problem. This is a very simplistic view of the patient and of nursing. In this view, the problem is somehow extracted from the patient, is examined scientifically and objectively, a nursing intervention is applied, and (if you are a good nurse) the problem should be solved (see Fig. 11–1).

A problem cannot be isolated and treated as if it has no relationship to the patient. Patients cannot be isolated and treated as if they have no relationship to their world. Patients, their health situation, and their world form a totality that cannot truly be disconnected into parts.

And yet, in nursing it is necessary to temporarily place labels on portions of this totality in order to facilitate its movement in the direction of health. This process must involve identification of as much of the totality as it is possible for the nurse to determine, including problems, strengths, realities, ways of being, perceptions, values and beliefs, physiologic functioning, and the relationships among all of these parts. This is the nursing assessment. Although it is impossible to ever know the patient's entire situation, the more that the nurse does know, the more likely that interventions will be effective.

Effective nursing care requires the utilization of multiple interventions to various aspects within the patient's totality, sometimes simultaneously, sometimes in a carefully planned sequence, and sometimes in response to dynamic changes within the totality. (See Fig. 11–2.)

This and the following chapter will discuss specific aspects of the cancer patient's totality that may have a negative effect on the patient's health. Specific interventions are suggested for each aspect. However, these interventions must be utilized in coordination with others that focus on different aspects of the totality in order to maximize the patient's movement toward health.

CACHEXIA

Pathophysiology

Cachexia is a complex pathophysiologic process characterized by anorexia, significant weight loss, weakness, anemia, fluid and electrolyte abnormalities, increased basal metabolic rate, abnormalities in the senses of taste and smell, and a reduced dietary intake.[81] In one study, 25 of 35 cancer patients experienced a decrease in taste perception (hypogeusesthesia). Sixty-four per cent had an aversion to meat. Changes in the sense of taste caused patients to refuse to eat meat, fish, poultry, eggs, fried foods, tomatoes, and tomato products. Foods rejected were described as tasting rancid or spoiled. A persistent salty, sour, bitter, or metallic taste was also noted. This is referred to as dysgeusia (a perversion of the sense of taste). Some cancer patients are unable to tolerate sweet tastes. To some, sweet foods no longer taste sweet, and they will seek foods that are extremely sweet. The response to sweet foods may vacillate during the course of the illness.

The patients with hypogeusesthesia complained that their food was tasteless.

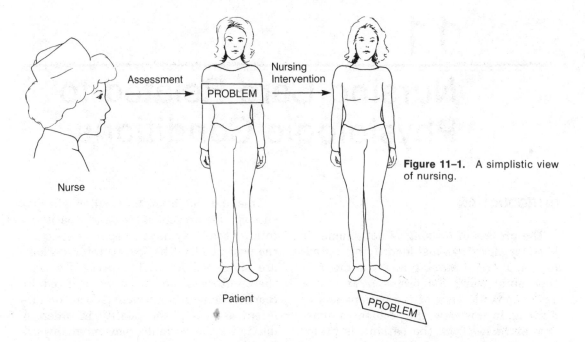

Figure 11–1. A simplistic view of nursing.

They often compared eating to chewing and swallowing sawdust or flour paste. Aversion to protein was selective and progressive. Beef and pork were disliked most, followed by fish and poultry, and then eggs and cheese.[22, 65] Disorders of the body's central hunger-satisfying mechanisms caused patients to become satisfied after eating a small amount of food and to stop eating.[33] Psychosocial factors that are common in cancer also interfere with the maintenance of adequate nutrition.[57] Patients are often depressed, anxious, fearful, and in pain.[81] As the malignancy progresses, the cachexia becomes more severe. In fact, cachexia is one of the major causes of death in many cancer patients.[81]

The effects of cancer on body metabolism were discussed in Chapter 2. The major

points will be reviewed because they are so necessary to effective nursing.

In cachexia, there are changes in the metabolism of all of the major nutrients. All but 10 per cent of the body's stored fat may be lost. Body tissues and organs lose nitrogen, which is transferred from body tissues to the tumor. The patient is often in negative nitrogen balance. Glucose is converted to lactate before being metabolized. The tumor uses anaerobic rather than aerobic processes of metabolism. The serum insulin level is low. The patient has hypoalbuminemia and elevated uric acid and blood lactate levels.[8, 57]

There is an increase in the water content of body tissues and retention of both water and sodium, but since the tumor takes up the sodium, the patient may actually be sodium poor. This, in addition to the tumor's growth, often causes an increase in body weight. Unlike conditions in starvation, hypertrophy of the liver occurs.[57, 81] The core temperature of the body rises; the basal metabolic rate increases, and there is an increased energy expenditure in spite of a caloric deficit. There are changes in the lumen of the gastrointestinal tract, accompanied by atrophy, decreased patency, and decreased gastrointestinal secretions.[57]

Scientists differ in opinion about the

Figure 11–2. Holistic nursing care.

cause of these changes. Theologides proposes that cachexia is a result of changes in body enzymes, with some being deactivated, some activated, and some altered; these changes throw the body metabolism into chaos.[81] Costa believes that cachexia is caused by anatomic alterations created by the malignancy and by paraneoplastic syndromes.[16]

In addition to the consequences of the malignancy, the treatments for cancer often have a serious effect on the patient's nutritional status. Surgical procedures may alter the structure and function of the gastrointestinal tract, thus causing nutritional depletion. The side effects of chemotherapy and radiotherapy — anorexia, nausea and vomiting, oral pain, diarrhea, and fever — have an impact on nutrition. Dysfunction of body organs caused by chemotherapy may impair the patient's nutritional status. Radiation to the gastrointestinal tract may cause serious long-term nutritional consequences.[52]

Other pathophysiologic processes in cancer also affect the patients' nutritional state. Cancer patients often have a diminished immune response and a high risk of infection. There is a synergistic interaction between infection and malnutrition. Malnutrition diminishes the immune response and thus the body's response to infection. Infection alters the nutritional status by increasing the metabolic rate and decreasing the appetite.[13]

Improving the nutritional status has been shown to improve the patient's response to the malignancy and to treatments. Enhancing the patient's nutritional standing will restore both humoral and cell-mediated immunity.[13] Patients who return to an adequate nutritional level before surgery are able to tolerate more extensive procedures with fewer complications. The cancer cells of patients with good nutrition are more easily destroyed by both radiotherapy and chemotherapy, perhaps because more of the cells are in the cell cycle.

Such patients are better able to tolerate the chemotherapy and have fewer side effects. They have a more effective response to the chemotherapy and are more likely to be able to continue their treatments. Recovery from chemotherapy is usually shorter, allowing for more frequent doses. In one study, patients receiving effective nutritional therapy during chemotherapy had decreased gastrointestinal toxicity, an improved sense of well-being and performance status, and weight gain.[13] Effective nutritional management may allow some cancer patients who otherwise would not tolerate chemotherapy to take the treatments.

Nutrition has historically been primarily within the territory of nursing. Florence Nightingale, for example, placed heavy emphasis on the importance of nutrition in nursing care. In recent years, this area has sometimes been considered an unimportant nursing duty that has been relegated to nurse aides or other hospital personnel. Although some nutritional interventions such as total parenteral nutrition (TPN) are medical therapies, the nursing care given during this and other means of nutritional support may have a major impact on patient response to therapy or on the patient's overall health.

Assessment

History. Careful questioning can elicit much helpful information about the patients' eating patterns: the times of day at which they eat and types and amount of foods eaten. Food likes and dislikes are important, but may change during the treatment period. The patient's present response to sweets and to beef, pork, and other proteins should be determined. Sometimes patients have stopped eating meats, but do not realize that their taste has changed. Values and cultural patterns related to food should be determined. Knowledge of social and family patterns of eating can be helpful in planning effective nursing interventions; for example, does the patient usually have a cocktail before dinner or wine or beer with the meal? Is there any valid reason why this should not be continued?

Physical Examination. Body weight, although only a gross measure of nutritional status, is important and must be accurate. Because of fluid retention, weight may appear to have been maintained when it has not been. The mid-arm muscle circumference and the triceps skin-fold are good indicators of fat and muscle reserve.[57]

To measure the triceps skin-fold thickness (TSF), use Lange or Harpenden calipers. Identify the mid-arm circumference point. Lift the skin-fold at that point and measure the skin-fold about 1 cm below the pinched skin-fold. The TSF measures the body's caloric reserves. It is decreased in malnutrition.[69] (See Table 11-1.)

To measure the mid–upper arm circumference (MUAC), allow the arm to hang freely. At the mid-point of the upper arm, measure the circumference.

The arm muscle circumference (AMC) is a measure of the state of muscle protein. This measure is obtained by a formula that uses the two previous measures: AMC = MUAC − 0.314 × TSF. The resulting score can then be compared with normal values. The AMC will be decreased in patients with protein malnutrition. This indicates that muscle protein is being burned by the body for energy.[69] Skin turgor can indicate the level of hydration. The liver should be palpated to determine alterations from normal. Other less specific clues to nutritional status are skin and mucous membrane condition, vital signs, behavior, speech, the presence of edema, and the ability to chew and swallow.[24]

Laboratory Data. Serum protein levels (particularly of serum albumin and serum transferrin), electrolyte levels, and types of anemia may be helpful in indicating nutritional problems.[24] Total lymphocyte count and skin tests to measure immunoreactivity are also helpful.[57]

Observations. If patients are hospitalized, it is helpful to carefully record types and amounts of foods eaten. If they are at home, patients or family members can be encouraged to keep a diary of eating patterns. Careful nursing observations can give an indication of the level of depression, anxiety, fear, and pain that the patient is experiencing. The nurse should carefully note patient responses to social situations related to eating. Do they eat better when family members are with them? Does the presence of the nurse alter their eating? Do they consider some specific foods to be reward foods or nurturing foods? How do patients respond to food odors? Under what conditions do patients reject food?

Planning

In order to adequately plan alterations in the patient's food intake, it is valuable to know the patient's nutritional needs. As reported by Mullen and Hobbs, Blackburn and colleagues have developed a mechan-

Table 11-1. Normal Values of Muscle Mass and Fat Stores*

Test	Sex	Standard	Percentiles of Population			
			90%	80%	70%	60%
Triceps skin-fold	Male	12.5 mm	11.3	10.0	8.8	7.5
	Female	16.5 mm	11.9	13.2	11.6	9.9
Mid-upper arm circumference	Male	29.3 cm	26.3	23.4	20.5	17.6
	Female	28.5 cm	25.7	22.8	20.0	17.1
Arm muscle circumference	Male	25.3 cm	22.8	20.2	17.7	15.2
	Female	23.2 cm	20.9	18.6	16.2	13.9

*From Blackburn, G. L., et al.: *Manual for Nutritional/Metabolic Assessment of the Hospitalized Patient.* Paper presented at the Sixty-second Annual Clinical Congress of the American College of Surgeons. Chicago, Oct. 11–15, 1976. Used by permission.

ism for calculating the patient's nutritional requirements.[57] The basal energy expenditure is calculated based on weight, height, and age. The patient's intake should be 1.5 times the number of calories required for basal energy expenditure. If parenteral feedings are being used, they should provide 1.7 times the calories needed for basal energy expenditure. The amount of protein in grams must be 1.5 times the patient's weight in kilograms.[57] This should give the nurse some standard against which to evaluate the adequacy of the patient's food intake.

Presently, TPN is the only strategy that has been found to be effective in reversing the cachexia of advanced cancer, and it is effective only when used concurrently with other medical treatments. When used alone, it will reverse the cachexia for only a short period of time.

The nurse needs to be realistic in setting goals and objectives for nutritional interventions. Since cancer is a complex disease with multiple metabolic derangements, force-feeding patients is not going to cure their disease. However, effective nutritional interventions coordinated with other nursing measures can facilitate the best possible response that the patients can make within their health situation. Such interventions may improve their response to treatment, improve their sense of well-being, and improve their functional status.

Interventions

As with most treatments for cancer, the ideal time to begin nutritional intervention is early in the course of the disease. Patients and family members need to have the knowledge necessary to understand and deal with nutritional problems. Many patients and families believe that weight loss and anorexia are inevitable consequences of cancer and make no attempt to correct them. The cancer beliefs of hopelessness, despair, and resignation may be quite evident in their response to this situation.

The same attention that is now given to the nutritional aspects of diabetes needs to be given to the nutritional aspects of cancer. Patient and family teaching programs need to be developed and information needs to be prepared and distributed.[60] Diets need to be carefully planned and dietary records kept. Vitamin and mineral supplements should be considered. (*Note:* patients receiving methotrexate should not take multiple vitamins containing folate.) The diet planned should be high in protein and high in calories (unless the patient is overweight), and should contain adequate amounts of fruits and vegetables.

Patients should be cautioned to be alert to changes in their sense of taste and adjust their protein intake accordingly. Some patients cannot tolerate beef or pork, but can eat fish, poultry, eggs, cheese, and peanut butter. Legumes and beans are good sources of protein if meats are not well tolerated.

Patients and family members should be helped to understand the impact of nutritional status on the effectiveness of and the patient's tolerance to cancer therapy. The therapies further interfere with nutritional maintenance, thus requiring even more careful attention to nutritional strategies. Surgery for cancer may interfere with the actual intake of food or may alter digestive and absorption processes. Chemotherapy and radiotherapy may cause anorexia and nausea. Stomatitis or infection from chemotherapy may further disrupt eating patterns.

Attempts must be made to control nausea so that the patient can eat. There is some evidence that the time of day that chemotherapy or radiotherapy is administered affects the extent of nausea. The severity of the nausea usually fluctuates throughout the day. With careful questioning, periods of diminished nausea can be identified, and meals should be served at those times. Patients should be fed whatever foods they tolerate best.

If the patient is hospitalized, the nurse should attempt to control the physical, psychologic, and social environment in such a way as to support a positive response to eating. The patient's room should be clean and orderly. Dressings that may cause an odor should be changed. Activities that cause fatigue or pain should be completed at least 1 hour before meals or postponed until after eating. If the patient is weak or easily fatigued, energy should be conserved for eating. This may require that the nurse help with some activities that the patient is able to do, such as bathing.[24]

Attempts should be made to ensure that patients are pain free at mealtime, if pain medication does not cause drowsiness. Mouth care should be performed before meals. If severe stomatitis is present, Xylocaine viscous can be swished in the mouth 5 minutes before eating. Comfort is also important. The patients' hands and face should be washed and the bed linens straightened. Placing patients in a sitting position will lessen the energy required for eating. If necessary, pillows can be used for support.[24]

Nurturing and nourishing are activities that, for most people, are very closely related. It is possible that nurturing will enable patients to get the greatest amount of nourishment possible from the food they eat. This requires the gentle caring and provision of time that seem to have been lost in the modern nursing unit.

The reaction of the nurse to patients and to their food has an important impact on the patients' response to the food. The way in which the tray is carried, the way in which it is placed on the table, eye contact with the patient, a smile, and warm, caring words are all actions that can influence the patients' response to food.

The food should be arranged on the tray to allow easy access by the patient. Covers should be removed by the nurse and packages and containers should be opened. Food should be cut into bite-sized portions. If the plate has a cover, removing it before entering the room may avoid overwhelming the patient with food odors. After the patient has eaten, the tray should be removed from the room quickly. There is nothing as offensive to an anorexic patient as cold, leftover food sitting nearby.

Patients who are cachectic should be fed five or six small meals a day. Bringing in large amounts of food will often cause them to completely reject eating. Dietary departments are inclined to serve nutritionally poor foods, such as gelatin and fruit juice, between the regular feeding times. To avoid this, the dietary request should indicate high protein, high caloric meals.[24] It is helpful to be able to work with an understanding dietitian.

Patients will often respond better to food that has been prepared at home. The family can be encouraged to bring favorite dishes from home whenever possible. Teenagers will sometimes prefer hamburgers, pizza, and French fries.

Patients will often eat better if they have someone to eat with. Although group dining areas are rare in hospitals, patients can sometimes be placed in small groups at mealtimes. Family members can be encouraged to stay with patients for meals or eat with them.[24]

Nurses can sometimes offer special treats, such as Popsicles, ice cream, or food supplements, between meals to increase caloric intake. Although many patients find food supplements served straight from the can unacceptable, nurses have developed recipes for making the supplements more palatable. Welch suggests mixing Ensure with ice cream, instant breakfast, milk, ice cubes, and an egg for a tasty drink.[85] This can be prepared in several flavors. Food supplements can be frozen and served with ice cream toppings or heated and served as a hot drink. Liqueurs, hard liquor, or wine can be added to the supplement and may also function as an appetite stimulant. Liqueurs or instant coffee will mask the metallic taste of supplements, about which patients sometimes complain.[85]

Some patients cannot be given alcohol because of the risk of drug interactions. However, beer or wine with meals or before meals can function as an appetite stimulant and will also provide calories. Some hospitals have maintained a very puritanical attitude toward the consumption of alcohol. Such an attitude seems unnecessary and, in some cases, may be detrimental to the best interests of the patient.

Fruit juices or milk can be served in the place of water if the patient is severely anorexic. Instead of water, small cups of some nourishing beverage may be offered with medications.[24]

Patients who are being cared for at home usually have less difficulty with eating than hospitalized patients. However, family members are usually grateful to receive helpful hints from the nurse or recipes that may tempt the reluctant eater. Family members who understand the importance of the high protein, high caloric diet often devise many clever strategies for increasing the nutrition of the patient's diet.

Nursing interventions related to psychologic conditions present with cachexia will be discussed in Chapter 12. Effective interventions in this area are essential to the maintenance of adequate nutrition.

Total parenteral nutrition (TPN) is a relatively new medical treatment that can greatly improve the nutritional status of the patient. It is a method of administering a hypertonic solution of amino acids, fats, glucose, vitamins, and minerals into the subclavian vein. This is the only strategy presently used that can effectively reverse the cachectic process. It is effective only when other treatments for the cancer are being used.[11, 13, 57, 73]

The most serious complication of TPN is sepsis, although thrombosis, hyperglycemia, acidosis, hypophosphatemia, and hypercalcemia can occur. Skilled nursing management is required to administer the hypertonic solution and care for the catheter site. A hyperalimentation team consisting of a physician, a nurse, a pharmacist, and a dietitian should exist to provide the care needed during this procedure.[52] TPN is most safely given in cancer care centers, where nurses have had adequate instruction in administering it. In less adequately prepared hospitals, the incidence of complications is much higher.

Careful sterile technique must be used to prepare the solution, since it is an excellent medium for bacterial growth. Some institutions use laminar air-flow rooms for solution preparation. Because the catheter will remain in place for a long period of time, the catheter insertion site must be carefully managed using skin-defatting agents, antibacterial cleansers, antibiotic ointments, and sterile dressings. The risk of infection increases with the length of time that the catheter is kept in place.[24] Administration of the solution must be carefully monitored. Although the infusion rate is usually controlled by a pump, there is a risk of air embolism if the bottle runs dry.

Patients receiving TPN may have difficulties with the amount of glucose being administered. Insulin may have to be added to the solution. Urine should be tested every 4 to 6 hours for urine sugar. A sudden increase in the infusion rate can cause severe hyperglycemia. Because of the risk of drug incompatibilities, drugs should not be added to the infusion. Solution bottles should be changed every 8 hours.

Techniques and equipment have now been developed that enable TPN to be administered at home. A permanent catheter is used, a vest has been designed to hold the infusion container, and the pump is battery powered. Patients and family are taught the necessary procedures for mixing infusions, changing dressings, and monitoring conditions. This approach increases the patients' quality of life and greatly decreases the cost of treatment.

Evaluation

The most significant measures of success in interventions related to nutrition are weight gain or maintenance of weight and improvement in measures of TSF, MUAC, and AMC. Other measures that may reflect improvements in nutritional status are improved scores on the Karnofsky Scale and an improved sense of well-being. In evaluating care for the patient with advanced cancer, maintenance of current status may be a major success. Even though patients may continue to decline physically, nutritional interventions may slow that decline and provide a greater sense of comfort: these things are difficult to measure.

PAIN

Factors Influencing the Pain Experience

The experience of pain is a very complex process that is not well understood. There are several theories of pain, the most recent and most complex of which is the gate control theory (to be discussed later in chapter).[52] The nerve pathways and physiologic processes involved in the experience of pain, however, cannot be completely explained at present.[37, 45-47] Additionally, pain is a subjective experience that can be verified only by the person experiencing it.[26, 45-47] Pain involves not only physiologic processes, but also has psychologic, intellectual, interactional, and spiritual components.[26, 35, 36, 56] Pain does not arise from only one of them. Interrelationships among the components can be found in the cause of pain, the experience of pain, and the consequences of experiencing pain.

The most quoted definition of pain is that of Richard Sternbach, a psychologist. He defines pain as an "abstract concept which refers to (1) a personal, private sensation of hurt; (2) a harmful stimulus which signals current or impending tissue damage; (3) a pattern of responses which operate to protect the organism from harm."[35]

One factor that often is not considered in definitions of or expected behaviors with pain is whether the pain is chronic or acute. This is an important consideration because both the way in which the pain is experienced and the behavior elicited by the pain differ with acute and with chronic pain.

Acute pain is usually intense, sharp, and localized and may last from 1 second to several months. It is usually caused by injury or illness and subsides as healing progresses. It is a warning signal from the body and usually stimulates actions to eliminate or relieve the causes of the pain.

A person usually reacts to acute pain with sympathetic nervous system responses such as increases in pulse rate, blood pressure, respiration, and muscle tension. The person may moan or groan or in some way openly communicate the experience of pain.[24, 37, 45-47] Acute pain is associated with a high level of anxiety.

Chronic pain may begin with acute pain, or its beginnings may be more insidious. It may recur regularly, or it may be continuous. It may vary in intensity or always remain the same. The cause of the pain may be known, but treatment or healing may not be possible. The pain becomes something that must be lived with. If the person is unable to get pain relief with treatment, the pain is referred to as intractable. Chronic pain is often a duller pain or ache that may be described by the person as a discomfort rather than a pain.[24, 37, 45-47]

Living with chronic pain has been described as a nightmare. Everything about the person's life is shrouded in pain. There is an utter senselessness to the pain. The person experiences anger, but there is no exernal force at which to direct it. People with this type of pain tend to become introverted, withdrawn, and depressed.[24, 35, 37]

For centuries, philosophers and theologians have sought to explain the meaning of chronic pain. It has been viewed as punishment for past sins or a means through which people can strengthen their character or possibly find a way to God. Pain may be seen as an experience that forces people to seek a meaning to existence outside of their own self.[24]

Chronic pain does indeed sometimes have some of the effects just mentioned. Whether chronic pain is the only pathway to these experiences can be debated. Chronic pain is a physical, emotional, and financial strain on the individual. Contrary to common beliefs, the individual does not become accustomed to chronic pain, but suffers more as the pain continues to cause physical and mental depletion.[37]

Cancer patients may experience both acute and chronic pain. In the early stage of cancer, the patient may experience insidious pain that is often treated by the patient with analgesics, antacids, laxatives, or vitamins. These undefinable symptoms may eventually stimulate the patient to seek medical care. Because of their vague character, early symptoms may be treated by the physician with analgesics, antispasmodics, and tranquilizers.[44]

Acute pain is frequently experienced as a result of surgery. Because of the anxiety, uncertainty, and implications of a diagnosis of a malignancy, the cancer patient may experience a greater amount of suffering than the average surgical patient.[44]

In the intermediate stage of cancer, chronic pain may be the result of the disease process, but may also occur because of scarring from surgery or radiation. Late stage cancer pain is often magnified by psychosocial factors that frequently accompany an advanced disease.[44]

Pain is not usually manifested in cancer as a consequence of the disease process until late in the course of the disease. Even then, not all cancer patients experience pain. Bonica states that 60 to 80 per cent of hospitalized cancer patients have severe pain.[10] According to Twycross, about 50 per cent of cancer patients experience no pain, 40 per cent have severe pain, and 10 per cent experience moderate pain.[82] Patients, their family, and some health care providers frequently expect extreme, uncontrollable pain to occur as the disease progresses. This expectation will often influence the patient's responses to early experiences of pain.

The growth of cancer does not, in and of itself, cause pain. Pain occurs when the growth of the malignancy intrudes on normal tissues. Pain may then occur because of pressure on nerves or obstruction of hollow tubes such as the trachea, gastrointestinal tract, or ureters. Occlusion of blood vessels will cause tissue ischemia, necrosis, and sometimes infection, and with these, pain. Obstruction of lymphatic flow can cause tissue edema. If the tumor is encased in a capsular organ, pain will occur when the capsule begins to stretch. If surgery or radiotherapy has caused scarring in the area of the tumor, the pressure of the growing tumor on the nonelastic scar tissue will increase the amount of pain experienced by the patient. Bone tissue is relatively insensitive to pain, but periosteum is extremely sensitive to pain; thus, most bony metastases are very painful.[44, 74]

Emotional factors are involved in all phases of the pain experience — cause, occurrence, and consequence. Pain may hold for the patient deep fantasies from early childhood and produce the unconscious fear of punishment by an angry parent and of consequent abandonment. Pain generates desires to be good, to repent, to call for help. If the pain continues, the patient may feel unloved and abandoned.[1, 24]

A person's past experiences with pain will often influence responses to present pain. A person who has very negative beliefs about cancer may respond to the pain of cancer more intensely. The emotional pain from the social isolation that frequently occurs in cancer can only add to the physical experience of pain. Closely akin to this is the pain of knowing that one has a potentially fatal illness and that remaining life may be short. Added to these emotional reactions may be cachexia, with its accompanying fatigue and depression.

These emotional factors that accompany physiologic changes increase the patient's level of stress and result in tension, anxiety, and anger. These factors may increase the level of pain, which in turn may result in feelings of helplessness, dependency, introversion, depression, and anxiety. These emotions may very well work to increase the rate of the patient's physical deterioration. All of these factors act then to increase the levels of pain and stress and reinforce the negative, destructive aspects of the cancer. This experience takes the form of a vicious circle. (See Fig. 11–3.)

Severe chronic pain may have serious physiologic consequences. Patients who have chronic pain often avoid moving, particularly the portion of the body in which pain is experienced. The resulting immobility can be a factor in causing decubiti,

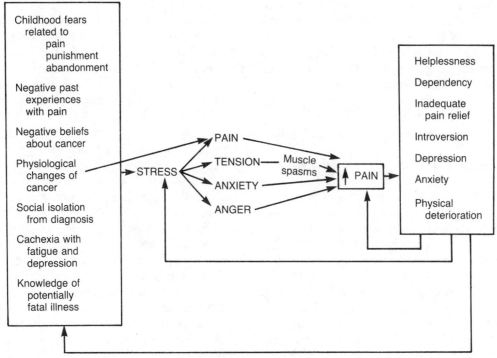

Figure 11–3. The dynamics of the experience of pain in cancer patients.

muscular weakness, diminished circulation, poor ventilation, constipation, and contractures. The immobility may become more severe as the pain causes depression, lassitude, fatigue, loss of sleep, and further muscular weakness. Bone decalcification, osteoporosis, and renal calculi may occur. Anorexia and nausea from the pain may further deplete the patient's nutritional state. The apathy of the patient may result in poor hygienic measures that may cause further deterioration of the oral mucosa, skin, and perineum. The patient's general appearance may be neglected, demonstrating a low morale that may progress to despair.[24]

People who experience chronic pain often change their values. They tend to focus on the things that seem to be central to their existence and may completely ignore what they consider to be trivialities. If the pain can be relieved or diminished, these people may achieve an inner peace and calm.[24] If the pain continues relentlessly, it may destroy the person. Patients with chronic, unrelieved pain are consumed by their pain; it dominates their life. Perception

may be narrowed to an awareness of the pain and nothing else: no feelings, no ideas, no desire to interact with others. This lack of connectedness weakens the ego and encourages regression back to the helplessness and dependency of childhood.[24] Some patients become angry, hostile, and very irritable, exaggerating even minor annoyances. Other patients have suicidal tendencies.

Thus, the effective relief of pain can have far-reaching implications for the cancer patient. It means a higher quality, and perhaps a more prolonged life. More important, it will allow the patient to continue functioning as a responsible, valuable person who can relate meaningfully to family, friends, and health care givers.

Assessment

In the pain situation, the values, beliefs, and attitudes of the nurse will determine to a great extent what data are gathered, what is observed and perceived, and what conclusions are drawn from this information. Nurses have many preconceived ideas about patients and their pain. Many nurses feel so helpless and anxious about patients in pain that they use distancing as a strategy to decrease their own anxiety. They discount the amount of pain that the patient is experiencing.[20] In addition, as Charap has found, physicians and nurses have a poor understanding of the pain process and how to relieve pain effectively.[14]

In order to assess pain effectively, some terms must first be defined. Pain researchers distinguish between the terms sensation and reaction. In very simple terms, a sensation is the electrical impulse that travels up the nerve pathways to the central nervous system and becomes a recognized pain perception. A reaction is a secondary response to the sensation. The pain threshold is the level of stimuli necessary for the individual to experience the sensation of pain. The pain threshold is essentially the same for all people. Pain tolerance is the length of time or intensity of pain that the individual will tolerate before responding with an overt expression of pain. The difference between the pain threshold and pain tolerance is sometimes called the pain sensitivity range. The pain threshold is primarily dependent on physiologic factors; pain tolerance is more dependent on psychologic factors.[36]

Before the pain assessment is discussed, its purpose needs to be clarified. The author concurs with McCaffery that the patient is the only authority on the fact that pain is being experienced.[45-47] This avoids the necessity of the patient's legitimating the pain, as described by Fagerhaugh and Strauss.[26] Legitimating puts the onus on the patient to use strategies, tactics, and measures to prove that pain is actually being experienced. The nurse should begin the assessment with the conviction that the patient is experiencing pain. The purpose of the assessment is to determine the nature of the pain in order to more effectively relieve it. The major portion of the pain assessment involves careful questioning and astute observation.

Pain Characteristics. Johnson identifies four factors that must be assessed in order to measure the sensation of pain experienced by the patient: location, intensity, quality, and chronology of the pain experience.[37] Questions designed to elicit this information should be carefully phrased to avoid influencing the patient's response.[37] The patient, in the desire to be helped, may see the nurse as a powerful person and tend to agree with whatever the nurse says. This type of game playing, which frequently occurs in hospitals, will interfere with the nurse's ability to get the needed information.[26] Until some sense of trust is established between the nurse and the patient, it may be difficult to convince the patient that honest communication can and will result in pain relief.

Patients experiencing chronic pain have more difficulty describing pain characteristics than those with acute pain. The source of the pain will also influence the sensory characteristics. The three most common pain sources are cutaneous, which includes skin and subcutaneous tissues; deep somatic, which includes nerve, bone, muscle, and the tissues that support these structures; and visceral, which includes the body organs.[37]

Location. Pain is experienced in relation to a specific body part or, in the case of a phantom limb, a previous body part. The pain location should be specifically identified and should include the areas of the body where the pain spreads. Identification can usually be accomplished most effectively by asking the patient to point to the areas of the body where pain is felt. There are several terms that may be useful in describing the pain: localized pain is felt only in the site where the pain originated; projected pain travels along the course of nerve pathways; radiated pain extends out in several directions from the original site; and referred pain occurs in some parts of the body not related to the cause of the pain.[37]

Acute pain is more easily defined by the above parameters. Chronic pain tends to be diffuse and, because the pathology of cancer is usually progressive, may vary in terms of extent, making it difficult for the patient to consistently identify painful areas. In addition, intense pain is likely to be very dispersed, sometimes enveloping the entire body.[37]

When the cancer patient experiences pain, it is not wise to assume that the pain is due to the malignancy and will be in the usual place. Cancer patients sometimes have problems not directly related to the malignant growth, such as ulcers, muscle spasms, abscesses, and constipation, which could cause pain. These conditions may require many different interventions to provide effective pain relief. Patients who have experienced pain for a long time will sometimes fail to differentiate one pain from another.

Though not cancer related, one clinical situation in which the author was involved may illustrate this point.

Mrs. M. was a 45-year-old woman who had surgery 3 weeks previously for a hiatus hernia. I was functioning as a clinical instructor with new nursing students who were learning to administer medications. Because of the illness of another instructor, I was supervising students on a nursing unit with which I was unfamiliar. A nursing student and I entered Mrs. M.'s room with oral medications. Mrs. M. asked if we had her pain medication. I said no, I did not know that she had asked for something for pain. Mrs. M. began to cry.

Mrs. M. was sitting on the side of the bed. I sat down on the bed beside her and reached for her hand. I told her she seemed frightened to me and asked if she felt afraid. Words began tumbling out rapidly: she had had surgery 3 weeks ago, she was receiving injectable analgesics every 4 hours, she was still having pain.

She was afraid she had not healed inside. She was afraid the surgery had not solved her problem and she would continue to have pain. I asked her to show me her incision. It was well healed. I assured her that operative sites usually healed from the inside out, so it looked as though she was healing well. I asked her to show me where she felt the pain. She pointed to the thoracic area of the back. When I felt the muscles, they were very tight. I told her that although the pain from a hiatus her-

nia was often felt in that area, it was possible that her current pain was due to muscle pain coming from her body's attempt to splint itself at the incision site and also because of her tension.

I suggested that she lie on her stomach and let me give her a backrub. As I rubbed her back, I pointed out to her how tight her muscles were and asked if the pain she felt came from that area. She affirmed that it did. I also suggested that if her wound was not healed, she would have great difficulty lying on her stomach.

I continued to massage her back muscles and talked soothingly to her. I told her that when I was a staff nurse, I had put most of my patients to sleep with backrubs and that I seldom gave my patients sleeping pills. I talked about relaxing and suggested that she imagine herself as a limp, wet dishrag. When I felt a muscle in her back relax, I expressed my pleasure at the feel of that soft muscle. From continued gentle stroking and the sound of a soothing, relaxing voice, Mrs. M. fell asleep. I left the room and continued my other responsibilities.

This event occurred on Friday. The following Monday, as I entered the hospital, the head nurse from the unit came rushing down the hall toward me. "What did you do to Mrs. M?" she asked. "After you left, she never asked for another pain injection and went home on Sunday." "I gave her a backrub," I replied.

Intensity. Pain intensity is a completely subjective experience and is therefore difficult to assess. It is a combination of the experienced sensation and the distress that occurs with the sensation. Some of the distress is a consequence of the pain sensation and some is a result of other factors in the patient's health situation. Most people are able to tolerate severe pain for short periods of time better than less severe pain for prolonged periods.[37]

When pain becomes chronic, the perception of the sensation changes, thus increasing the difficulty of assessing its intensity. Cancer patients will often describe the sensations that occur with ascites, shortness of breath, abdominal pressure, and lymphedema as uncomfortable, not painful. However, they will often say that the sensation was painful when it was first experienced.[37]

The nurse's information about the intensity of the pain can come only from the person experiencing the pain. Asking patients to compare the present pain with other pain that they have experienced can sometimes be helpful. Johnson has developed two scales that can be used to determine the intensity of the sensation and the distress. (See Fig. 11–4.)

The situation of Mrs. W. (described in Chapter 5) presents a clinical problem related to pain intensity in which the author was involved. In this situation, the nurses' assessment was that Mrs. W. was not experiencing the amount of pain that she claimed to have.

Quality. A great variety of words are used in our culture to describe pain. However, similar sensations are usually described in fairly consistent terms. These descriptions can be very useful in identifying the pain source. Acute pain is usually defined in precise terms; chronic pain is more difficult to define. Patients may use terms such as constant ache, discomfort, or soreness to describe their experience.

Chronology. Identifying the relationship between the pain experience and its chronology is often very important in planning effective nursing interventions. Johnson suggests five factors that should be assessed in this area: "(1) the mode of onset, (2) precipitating factors, (3) variations in time of occurrence, (4) variations in character, and (5) duration of the pain

experience."[37] Pain can sometimes be insidious in its onset. It may also begin as another type of sensation, such as pressure or tingling, that gradually changes to pain.[37]

Identification of precipitating factors may be important in planning interventions to diminish or relieve the pain. Variations in time of occurrence may sometimes be related to distractions (to be discussed later in chapter). Changes in the character of pain may be related to changes in pathology. The pain muy be constant and steady, throbbing, intermittent, increasing and decreasing in a cycle, or progressively more intense. Pain may last a second or a lifetime. If the pain begins to recede, this may mean changes in the pathology, changes in the psychologic factors that make up part of the pain perception, or damage to nerve pathways.[37]

Pain Responses. Responses to the pain stimulus are very much a part of the pain experience. They are very complex and reflect a sequence of events involving physical, behavioral, and emotional components. Responses to acute pain are similar to instinctual fight, flight, or withdrawal patterns designed to protect the individual. Responses to chronic pain may reflect more learned patterns of coping with the pain.[37] Johnson lists six factors that will affect the pain response: (1) integrity of the central nervous system, (2) level of consciousness, (3) training and previous experience in pain control, (4) attention and distractions, (5) fatigue, and (6) anxiety.[37]

Physical Responses. The autonomic nervous system is activated in response to

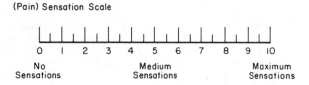

(Pain) Sensation Scale

Figure 11–4. Johnson's sensation and distress scales. (Courtesy of J. Johnson) From Stewart, M. L.: Measurement of clinical pain. In *Pain: A Source Book for Nurses and Other Health Professionals,* edited by Jacox, A. K. Boston: Little, Brown and Company, copyright 1977. Used by permission.)

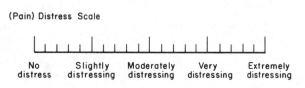

(Pain) Distress Scale

the pain stimulus. Sympathetic stimulation is the most typical, but does not occur consistently and may be mixed with parasympathetic stimuli. Similar responses may be initiated by emotions. Cutaneous pain is more likely to evoke response from the sympathetic system. Deep pain or prolonged severe pain is more likely to stimulate the parasympathetic system.[37] See Table 11-2 for common autonomic responses to pain. As pain becomes chronic, these autonomic responses will change or diminish so that they are less evident. Since these symptoms are often used by the nurse to determine if patients are experiencing pain, patients with chronic pain may be judged not to have pain or to be experiencing less than they express.

Pain Behavior. People commonly respond to pain with gross motor activity, voluntary behavior, and verbal expressions of pain. Flexion and withdrawal are typical motor behaviors. Deep pain may be accompanied by spasm of smooth or skeletal muscle, which occurs as a splinting or protective action. This may actually increase the amount of pain.

Voluntary behaviors are usually attempts to decrease the pain and may involve rubbing or supporting a body area, frequent change of position, pacing or walking, or reduction of activity. The behaviors selected will usually be those that have previously been effective in reducing pain. As pain increases in severity, these activities diminish or cease.[37]

Facial expressions are probably the first thing observed by the nurse when the patient expresses pain. Facial grimaces, dilated pupils, perspiration, a frown, a drawn, pinched look — all present an image of pain. These are often not evident in the patient with chronic pain. Johnson indicates that patients with chronic pain often have a tired, drawn look, or their eyes may be the only indication of the amount of suffering that they are experiencing.[37]

Verbal expressions of pain may include moans, groans, crying, screaming, sighing, word repetition, or statements about the pain. Although the nurse may sense pain from other behaviors and physical responses, the patient's expression of pain is the only available mechanism of verifying pain. Patients may use words other than pain to describe their experience, particularly for chronic pain. Words commonly used include discomfort, soreness, and ache.[37, 45-47]

Emotional Responses. Although almost any emotion can occur with pain, some are more frequent. Depression commonly occurs with chronic pain. Regression may occur, with either aggressive demands for attention or passive responses of crying and dependent behavior. Increased anxiety is frequent and may decrease the patient's pain tolerance, thus intensifying the pain experienced. This situation can develop into a cycle of increasing anxiety and pain that can be altered by decreasing the anxiety level. The patient's normal behaviors may be altered, causing withdrawal or irritability. Ability to learn is decreased, so that patient teaching may be less effective or may require a longer period of time.[37]

Table 11–2. Physiologic Responses That Occur With Stimulation of the Autonomic Nervous System and May Be Useful in Pain Evaluation*

Response	Sympathetic Stimulation	Parasympathetic Stimulation
Pupil size	Dilated	Constricted
Perspiration	Increased	No effect
Rate and force of heartbeat	Increased	Decreased
Blood pressure	Increased	Decreased
Depth and rate of respiration	Increased	No effect
Urinary output	Decreased	No effect
Peristalsis of GI tract	Decreased	Increased
Basal metabolic rate	Increased	No effect

*From Johnson, M.: Assessment of clinical pain. In *Pain: A Source Book for Nurses and Other Health Professionals,* ed. by Jacox, A. Boston: Little, Brown and Company, copyright 1977. Used by permission.

Suffering. The amount of suffering a person experiences with pain is determined by the cultural, psychologic and social history, and environment of the patient. The nurse's assessment of the degree of the patient's suffering may vary with the patient's culture, income, sex, and life situation.[20] It is important for the nurse to be aware of personal biases in order to accurately evaluate the patient's suffering and the meaning the patient places on the pain. This meaning is philosophic and increases in importance as the pain becomes prolonged.[37]

Reactions to the pain may differ depending on whether the patient views the condition as curable, chronic, or progressively destructive. Patients may view pain as useful for personal growth, as punishment, as having religious connotations, or as a challenge. Other patients may see pain as having no meaning. The nurse should not impose personal values on the patient. The patient's ideas should be determined and respected. These perceptions are useful in selecting effective approaches to helping the patient cope with pain.[37]

The questions Johnson presents are valuable in assessing the patient's perception of pain.

The personal meaning that is placed on pain may be influenced by the way in which pain alters the life-style of the individual. These changes can be assessed with pertinent questions. Has the pain hampered physical activities? Does this affect self-care, occupation, leisure activities? How much time is spent up and how much down? Is this change seen as negative or does it have some positive value for the person? Does the pain interfere with personal relationships — in the family, with friends, with co-workers? Does the person associate pain with an uncertain prognosis? Does it mean a disease is becoming progressively more severe, impending death, or eventual loss of function of a body part? Has it changed his self-concept? Does he see himself as less productive, less useful, a drain on others? Or as an individual who can still contribute to life although the method of contribution may be different? Are pain and suffering to be endured — either quietly or not so quietly? Or are they seen as a challenge to be overcome?[37]

Coping Strategies. Assessing the patient's usual methods of coping with pain can be very useful in determining which nursing interventions are most likely to be effective. Observation of patient behavior may give some clues to the coping methods being used by the patient. Denial may be used to minimize or conceal the pain and to maintain a "well" behavior. If the patient verbalizes the use of denial or the nurse verbally describes the behavior to the patient, it may become less effective.[37]

Other strategies that the patient may use include information seeking, focusing, distraction, or careful timing of medication. Diversionary activities involving physical or cognitive activity can be very helpful. The easiest way to determine these strategies is to ask the patient about them.

Some patients use ineffective coping strategies that can actually increase the amount of pain experienced. These may include focusing all attention on the pain, engaging in excessive activity that causes fatigue, and over-preparing for impending pain, which increases anxiety and fear.

The McGill-Melzack Pain Assessment Questionnaire is an effective way for patients to thoroughly assess their pain. (See Fig. 11–5.) The assessment of pain must be an ongoing process because the pathology and the character of the pain can change over time. New causes of pain may develop that can be overlooked. In addition to assessing the pain itself, important information can be gained from determining the number and types of medications required to control pain.

Planning

Planning for pain relief involves more than the selection of an intervention. It requires some consideration of the philosophy of pain relief held by the nurse and by those in the institution within which the patient is being cared for.

In hospitals, pain relief is often a secondary concern. Attention to life and death situations comes first, and pain seldom causes a threat of death. In some situations, the ward routine also comes first.

Patient's name_____ Age_____

Hospital No._____

Clinical category (e.g. Cardiac, Neurological, etc.):_____

Diagnosis:_____

_____

_____

Analgesic (if already administered):

    1. Type_____

    2. Dosage_____

    3. Time given in relation to this test_____

Patient's intelligence: Circle number that represents best estimate.

1 (low)   2   3   4   5 (high)

****

This questionnaire has been designed to tell us more about your pain. Four major questions we ask are:

    1. Where is your pain?

    2. What does it feel like?

    3. How does it change with time?

    4. How strong is it?

    It is important that you tell us how your pain feels now. Please follow the instructions at the beginning of each part.

A

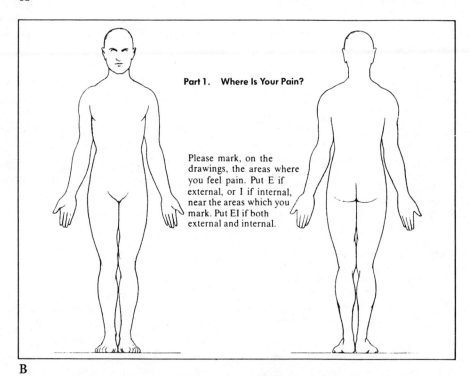

Part 1. Where Is Your Pain?

Please mark, on the drawings, the areas where you feel pain. Put E if external, or I if internal, near the areas which you mark. Put EI if both external and internal.

B

Figure 11–5. McGill-Melzack Pain Assessment Questionnaire. (Courtesy of R. Melzack.) *A,* Cover Sheet. *B,* Part One. *C,* Part Two. *D,* Parts Three and Four. (From Stewart, M. L.: Measurement of clinical pain. In *Pain: A Source Book for Nurses and Other Health Professionals,* edited by Jacox, A. K. Boston: Little, Brown and Company, copyright 1977. Used by permission.)

Illustration continued on opposite page

Part 2. What Does Your Pain Feel Like?

Some of the words below describe your present pain. Circle ONLY those words that best describe it. Leave out any category that is not suitable. Use only a single word in each appropriate category--the one that applies best.

1	2	3	4	5
Flickering	Jumping	Pricking	Sharp	Pinching
Quivering	Flashing	Boring	Cutting	Pressing
Pulsing	Shooting	Drilling	Lacerating	Gnawing
Throbbing		Stabbing		Cramping
Beating		Lancinating		Crushing

6	7	8	9	10
Tugging	Hot	Tingling	Dull	Tender
Pulling	Burning	Itchy	Sore	Taut
Wrenching	Scalding	Smarting	Hurting	Rasping
	Searing	Stinging	Aching	Splitting
			Heavy	

11	12	13	14	15
Tiring	Sickening	Fearful	Punishing	Wretched
Exhausting	Suffocating	Frightful	Gruelling	Blinding
		Terrifying	Cruel	
			Vicious	
			Killing	

16	17	18	19	20
Annoying	Spreading	Tight	Cool	Nagging
Troublesome	Radiating	Numb	Cold	Nauseating
Miserable	Penetrating	Drawing	Freezing	Agonizing
Intense	Piercing	Squeezing		Dreadful
Unbearable		Tearing		Torturing

C

Part 3. How Does Your Pain Change With Time?

1. Which word or words would you use to describe the pattern of your pain?

1	2	3
Continuous	Rhythmic	Brief
Steady	Periodic	Momentary
Constant	Intermittent	Transient

2. What kind of things relieve your pain?

_____
_____
_____
_____

3. What kind of things increase your pain?

_____ _____
_____
_____
_____

Part 4. How Strong Is Your Pain?

People agree that the following 5 words represent pain of increasing intensity. They are:

1	2	3	4	5
Mild	Discomforting	Distressing	Horrible	Excruciating

To answer each question below, write the number of the most appropriate word in the space beside the question.

1. Which word describes your pain right now? _____
2. Which word describes it at its worst? _____
3. Which word describes it when it is the least? _____
4. Which word describes the worst toothache you ever had? _____
5. Which word describes the worst headache you ever had? _____
6. Which word describes the worst stomach-ache you ever had? _____

D

Figure 11-5 Continued

Curing the disease is also considered more important than relieving suffering.

The consequences of the failure to relieve pain are often not evident. However, in acute pain situations, the pain may slow down recovery. In chronic pain situations, the patient's quality of life is drastically reduced. If the pain is effectively relieved, the patient may dramatically improve, physically as well as emotionally.[45-47]

Nurses and physicians often rely almost totally on drugs to relieve pain. If the drugs are not effective, little consideration is given to minimizing the remaining pain with palliative nursing measures.[26]

Because of the complexity of the pain experience, pain relief must be planned to include more than drugs. There are several theories of pain relief. General concepts include altering some of the causes and effects of pain by decreasing anxiety, depression, muscle tension, and fatigue, as well as the pain sensation. Another strategy, based on the gate control theory, uses techniques to prevent pain impulses from being perceived. This may involve cutaneous stimulation, increased sensory input, eliciting behaviors inconsistent with pain responses, or resolving cognitive dissonance (mixed feelings about a situation). Producing physical changes such as relaxation and using physical stimuli such as heat or cold are other effective strategies.[45-47]

In order for the nurse to plan beneficial pain relief, some prerequisites must be considered. In most hospitals, no one on the staff is accountable for pain relief.[26, 45-47] Someone may be responsible for administering drugs for pain, but this person is no way accountable for the effectiveness of the treatment or for taking further measures if the first action does not relieve the pain.

If pain relief is to be maximized, the nurse must be accountable to the patient for pain relief. The patient must also accept some accountability for learning and utilizing the pain relief measures that are offered. The nurse must remain open-minded about measures that may relieve pain. At this point, we understand very little about the process of pain relief. However, we must not limit ourselves to those measures

we can explain. (We cannot actually explain how a narcotic works.) If a strategy works for a patient and causes no harm, the patient should be encouraged to use it.[45-47]

Establishing a nurse-patient relationship is an essential prerequisite to effective pain relief. One very important factor in developing patient trust is for the nurse to believe the patient when pain is expressed. The patient must trust the nurse and feel that the nurse cares about his or her pain. Illness and pain cause the patient to feel very vulnerable. The trust implicit in a nurse-patient relationship can improve confidence in the interventions used by the nurse and thus improve their effectiveness.

Including the patient in the planning process for pain relief will greatly enhance the effectiveness of most strategies. Doing so, however, greatly changes the role of the nurse. Traditionally, nurses have had tremendous power — much more than they generally view themselves as having — in the realm of pain relief. Nurses have been the "keeper of the keys." The patient has been almost totally dependent on the nurse's mercy for pain relief. The nurse could dispense or withhold relief to punish or reward. If the nurse believed that it was good for patients to endure some pain, this theory could be imposed on patients, who were powerless.

Collaborating with the patient for pain relief takes some of the nurse's power away and gives it to the patient. Inherent in this approach is the assumption that the patient knows when pain is being exerienced and which strategies work best to relieve it. This view projects an image of the patient as a responsible, competent adult. It is not presumed that the nurse always knows what is best for the patient. Patients may even be allowed to administer their own drugs.[17] This approach might have prevented many of the serious problems that Mrs. W. had. (See Chapter 5.)

Selecting the pain relief measures to be used is an important planning strategy. A variety of pain relief measures should be included, using at least two at the same time. This provides an additive effect and increases the pain relief. Pain relief measures should be used before the pain becomes severe and, in chronic pain, often before the patient experiences pain. Measures that the patient believes will be effective should be included, if they are not harmful to the patient.[45-47]

In selecting specific methods of pain relief, the nurse must consider the patient's preference to be an active or passive participant in the activity. Some strategies such as guided imagery or relaxation require the patient to play an active role. Cutaneous stimulation, on the other hand, can be used with a patient who prefers to remain passive.[45-47]

There are two basic strategies that can be used in pain relief. One is a method aimed at diminishing or eliminating the sensation of pain. The other is a method aimed at decreasing the suffering that the patient experiences with the pain. Strategies should always include measures to diminish suffering. Even when the pain cannot be relieved, often the suffering can be. General comfort measures can be effective in diminishing suffering. Straightening the bed sheets and pillows, adjusting lights, providing mouth care, brushing the hair, proper positioning, backrubs, and range of motion exercises may not change the intensity of pain, but will decrease the suffering.[45-47]

If the pain is not relieved by selected nursing measures, the nurse should continue attempts to relieve the pain. Even the continued attempt helps to diminish the patient's suffering. Patients in pain feel very alone. They may feel abandoned, rejected, and unacceptable. As Benoliel and Crowley note, staying with the patient can also be very helpful.

"Staying," then, is an additional element in the management of pain: staying in the sense not so much of actual physical presence — though at times this is part of it — but staying in the sense of being open or available to the patient. For the nurse to stay confident that one is helping, that what one does is meaningful to one's self as well as to the patient, that one is genuine, and real, and present when needed is essential.

This is not easy — it will involve a rethinking of many facets of the care and treatment. Not only is pain in another human being anxiety-provoking: it is especially so to stay with a patient as the pain continues. Part of a well established tradition, only recently begun to be questioned, is the idea that somehow, somewhere in the education of the nurse and the physician, something magic happens to free them from personal reaction to pain, mutilation, disfigurement, offensive odors, sights or sounds, while at the same time preserving and, in fact, nurturing an exquisite sense of sensitivity and compassion. In fact, personal reactions to unrelieved pain, disfigurement, and mutilation are a real strain in providing care to such patients. Furthermore the patients whose pains are not completely relieved and the patients whose illnesses cannot be cured are, in some sense, an affront to care and treatment — a reminder of man's finiteness and limited capacity to control his environment.

To stay requires a deep conviction of the worth of what one is doing and an awareness of the help one can bring. The maintenance of such an approach is almost impossible in settings which are organized around cure as the prime goal. Providing person-centered care in such situations involves both recognition of the strains involved and a strong support system for the staff. The capacity for staying means being able to give with no guarantee of return. The patient who is in pain and the patient who is terminally ill are in a limited position to provide feedback that makes one feel good about what one is doing. The strong support system can help to make up for this.[7]*

Interventions

There are many effective medical strategies for the relief of pain in cancer. These include removing the tumor or shrinking its size, surgery to by-pass obstructions, and blocking of nerve pathways. Since the focus of this chapter is nursing interventions, these strategies will not be discussed.

The nurse must believe in the effectiveness of the strategies to be utilized. Patients respond more positively to nurses who have a strong sense of confidence in themselves and in the treatments that they provide. Pain relief will be more effective if it is accompanied by a strong suggestion that the treatment should relieve the patient's pain.[35]

---

*Used by permission of the American Cancer Society, Inc., 1973.

Cognitively based interventions are designed to increase pain tolerance rather than decrease pain sensation. They diminish pain responses. This may seem to be a secondhand approach to pain relief, but these strategies can be extremely effective.

Giving Information

Giving information prior to the pain experience decreases the pain by lessening anxiety and uncertainty. This strategy is more effective when the nurse describes the sensations rather than only explaining the process of a procedure. This approach is the basis for much preoperative teaching and preparation for treatment procedures.[35]

Interpretation of Sensations

If a patient is unsure of the cause of a particular body state, perception of the experience can be manipulated. The patient can be encouraged to interpret the sensation as pleasant rather than unpleasant or to consider it discomfort rather than pain. This strategy has been used primarily in research studies exposing subjects to painful stimuli. Subjects were instructed to deny the pain or to think of it as being pleasurable. These subjects were able to tolerate higher levels of pain.[35] This strategy might be effective with patients experiencing lower levels of short-term pain.

Control Over Events

In experiments, subjects who were allowed some control over the experience of pain were able to tolerate higher levels of pain. They had control over such factors as when the pain began, the intensity of the pain, inflicting the pain themselves rather than having it initiated by the researchers, and participating in activities to distract themselves from the pain. This strategy might be helpful for patients undergoing painful treatment procedures.

Distraction

Distraction functions by focusing the patient's attention on stimuli other than the pain. It increases the clarity of the sensations upon which attention is focused. This process seems to protect the individual from awareness of the pain sensation. Distraction seems to be effective only during the time when it is in use. Total awareness returns as soon as the distraction stops.[45-47]

Some nurses believe that patients who are able to use distraction effectively do not really have very severe pain. This is not true. People apparently may commonly use distraction to relieve pain but are reluctant to tell health professionals about it for fear of disapproval.[45-47]

Distraction works to relieve pain even when the patient is unaware of it. Visitors, an entertaining TV program, or a stimulating conversation with the nurse may temporarily diminish the pain. During this time the nurse may regard the patient as not experiencing pain and may refuse to administer pain medication. This is a serious injustice to the patient and may discourage further use of distraction.[45-47]

Distraction has disadvantages as well as advantages. After the distraction, the patient will experience fatigue, irritability, and an increased awareness of pain. The patient should be given adequate pain relief after a period of distraction. If distraction is planned for a specific period of time, medication for pain can be given 30 to 45 minutes before the distraction is over. Or distraction can be used to help the patient with pain relief after medication has been administered, but before it has taken effect.[45-47]

Distraction can be used with pain that suddenly increases in intensity or with pain from treatment procedures that have an expected time limit. Distraction strategies that are effective for several hours in patients with chronic pain have not yet been developed. However, individual patients do sometimes develop their own individual strategies for relieving chronic pain. It is important for the nurse to recognize that the patient is using distraction and not to underestimate the amount of pain the patient is experiencing. It is helpful to explain this approach to the patient and encourage its use.[45-47]

McCaffery describes a number of distraction techniques and discusses their use in detail.[45-47] These include the use of a visual concentration point, rhythmic massage, slow rhythmic breathing, pant-blow rhythmic breathing, he-who rhythmic breathing, sing and tap rhythm, describing a series of pictures, auditory stimulation via earphones, and humor.

Hypnosis

Hypnosis has not been commonly seen as a nursing intervention, but the technique of hypnosis is not particularly difficult to learn and can be skillfully used by the nurse who has advanced preparation in this area.[5] Contrary to common thought, the patient does not have to be particularly susceptible to hypnosis to achieve a clinically useful hypnotic state. Pain relief can be accomplished by achieving only a "light" state of hypnosis.[5]

Hypnosis can relieve pain without the side effects of other measures. It does not interfere wtih the physical or mental functioning of the patient. In addition to relieving the pain, the hypnosis can be used to promote life-enhancing attitudes and personal growth.[5]

In order to achieve the last goal, the hypnosis needs to be performed by a nurse with additional preparation in the field of psychology. Psychologic counseling or psychotherapy along with hypnosis for pain relief can be very effective in freeing the patient of the anxieties and the sense of helplessness so commonly felt in the cancer situation. The patient's own resources can be supported, resulting in enhanced self-esteem, increased awareness of the inner life, and changes in the patient's experience of self, family, and the disease.[5]

The effective use of hypnosis requires a patient who is willing to be a participant in the activities. Therapy that includes psychologic care always necessitates the active involvement of the patient.[5] Involve-

ment of family members is also important. Patients will usually need to learn self-hypnosis techniques and practice them regularly between hypnosis sessions.

During hypnosis sessions and during self-hypnosis, the hospitalized patient must be provided with privacy. To avoid conflicts, self-hypnosis times can be planned along with medications and treatments. A sign can be posted on the door to prevent interruptions. It is very important that the nurses place value on these sessions.[5]

Hynposis is not magic. It has its limitations and patients need to be informed of them. Hypnosis does not always result in instant improvement. It requires time and practice to be successful.

Scientists still do not understand how hypnosis works. Suggestions that are given during hypnosis not only affect cognition, but also seem to cause physiologic changes. Barber and Gitelson list six strategies that are used in hypnosis to reduce pain:

1. Blocking pain awareness through the suggestion of anesthesia or analgesia.
2. Substituting another feeling for the pain.
3. Moving pain perception to a smaller or less vulnerable area.
4. Altering the meaning of pain to make it less painful and debilitating.
5. Increasing tolerance of pain.
6. Dissociating perception of body from patient's awareness (in extreme cases).[5]

Relaxation

In recent years relaxation has received considerable interest as a strategy for dealing with stress. Relaxation alone will not relieve pain, unless the pain is caused by muscle tension. However, when used concurrently or alternately, relaxation can increase the effectiveness of other strategies. Relaxation decreases muscle tension and lowers the anxiety level. Anxiety and tension often function in a cycle to perpetuate each other. Eliminating one can greatly diminish the other.[45-47]

Multiple techniques are available to induce the relaxation response.[8] Many have been used for thousands of years. Whatever approach is used, teaching relaxation techniques requires time. They should not be introduced at a time when the patient is in severe pain. It is helpful, almost necessary, for the nurse to have experienced the relaxation response before trying to teach the patient. Relaxation as a means of pain relief is different from our usual image of relaxing. It decreases respiration, slows the pulse rate, lowers the blood pressure level if it is high, decreases muscle tension, and increases alpha brain waves.[8, 45-47]

Whether meditation, yoga, Zen, biofeedback, progressive relaxation, autogenic training, or some other relaxation strategy is used, the following common components must be present in order for the strategy to be effective. When learning the technique, the person must be in a comfortable position, either lying down or sitting.[45-47] The hands and feet should not be crossed, and clothing should be loose and comfortable. Some people prefer to remove their shoes. A mental device is used to focus the person's concentration. This may be a mantra (a word or sound repeated silently), concentration on breathing or the heartbeat, staring at an object, or rhythmic rocking or rubbing motions. The mental device tends to block out logical or externally oriented thoughts and can progressively condition the individual so that when the device is used, the relaxation response immediately begins to occur.[45-47]

A passive attitude may be the most important aspect of any relaxation technique. This attitude applies to both what *is* happening and what *will* happen.[45-47] Concentration on happenings is passive. There is no urge or compulsion to will things to happen. The strategy is to let them happen, not make them happen. If distractions occur or thoughts intrude, they are allowed to pass out of awareness. They may be "breathed out" with exhalation or allowed to "flow out" of the body. The patient may experience a feeling of heaviness, warmth, or floating.

Patients usually cannot accomplish the relaxation response on the first attempt. The patient may feel a sense of frustration and may need to be reassured and encouraged to try again at a later time. With each attempt, the patient will be able to relax more deeply.

Patients with chronic pain should establish routine times for practicing relaxation twice a day for 20 minutes. Some patients who practice relaxation experience an increased awareness of pain. In this case, it may help to practice relaxation when little pain is being experienced. Patients may feel a tingling, prickly feeling in their extremities during relaxation. They need to know that this is an expected sensation. Extremely depressed patients probably should not be started on relaxation strategies, which may promote further withdrawal.[45-47]

Patients who have successfully suppressed feelings of sadness and anxiety may begin to experience these feelings when they practice relaxation and may cry or shake with fear. If the patient is willing to discuss the feelings, this should be done before relaxation is continued.

Guided Imagery

Imagery is an ancient healing technique and yet, in modern health care, it is a very new approach. Guided imagery uses a person's imagination to achieve a specific therapeutic goal. This may seem rather illogical and unscientific, but researchers have found that imagining can produce physiologic changes that we are usually unable to control consciously.[45-47]

If the patient and nurse can select an appropriate image, this strategy may result in pain relief. The relief may be a result of physiologic changes that decrease the painful stimuli, as well as a subjective feeling of diminished pain.

The technique of guided imagery is most effective for the patient with chronic pain. The technique is time-consuming and requires the active participation of the patient. Guided imagery is usually preceded by a relaxation technique, since relaxation facilitates concentration upon the image.

McCaffery gives an excellent discussion of the technique of guided imagery. Both McCaffery[45-47] and Donovan and Pierce[24] present scripts that can be used in imagery sessions. The relaxation and imagery script can be tape-recorded for the patient's use on a regular basis, or the patient may wish to learn the procedure and use self-devised images.

Imagery should not be used with a patient who is psychotic or has psychotic tendencies. Also, since some patients experience total pain relief by analgesia or anesthesia in guided imagery, pain may not be present as a warning signal. Patients using this technique should remain under the care of a physician for treatment and regular evaluation of the pain.[45-47]

Cutaneous Stimulation

Cutaneous stimulation involves techniques used to stimulate the patient's skin in order to relieve pain. The effectiveness of cutaneous stimulation varies and is not very predictable. The pain may completely cease, it may be diminished, it may be increased, or it may remain the same. The effectiveness of cutaneous stimulation may last only as long as the stimulation continues or it may last for several hours. The techniques of cutaneous stimulation include the use of heat, cold, pressure massage, vibration, plain and menthol ointments, and transcutaneous electrical nerve stimulation (TENS).[45-47]

How cutaneous stimulation relieves pain is not well understood, although several theories have been proposed. One explanation is suggested by the gate control theory. According to this theory, cutaneous stimulation activates the large-diameter nerve fibers, thus inhibiting pain messages carried by smaller nerve fibers. Other theories posit that the stimulation may balance nerve impulses, cause the release of endorphins, or disrupt the pain-memory process in the central nervous system. Pain relief may also be related to immediate changes in the tissues as a result of the stimulation. These could include muscle relaxation, changes in blood supply, or partial numbness. The touching, nurturing, and interaction that occur with cutaneous stimulation may also have a major role in relieving pain.[45-47]

Cutaneous stimulation techniques are not specific to certain types of pain. The patient should be allowed to select the techniques that feel good to him or her. If the patient has not experienced some of the techniques, they might be offered on a trial basis.[45-47]

Applying pressure is a fairly common, rather automatic response to some types of sudden pain or injury. One type of pressure that has become popular in recent years is acupressure. This is the application of pressure at the traditional acupuncture sites. In some cases it can be very effective.[45-47]

Massage has also been commonly used by those in pain. Hands or fingers may be moved over the area in circles or long strokes, slowly or rapidly. Backrubs can also be very effective in pain relief, combining cutaneous stimulation and relaxation and decreasing the patient's anxiety. Michelsen[54] gives an excellent description of the techniques involved in a backrub.

Vibration can sometimes mask perception of low level pain and in some cases may provide pain relief. It has primarily been used by patients at home. Little research has been conducted on its effectiveness.[45-47]

Heat and cold are both commonly used for pain relief. They both appear to raise the pain threshold. Many sources are available for the application of heat or cold. Their use is so common that their effectiveness is often minimized by health care givers. Some physicians have expressed caution about using heat on the site of a malignancy, fearing that the heat may speed up the growth of the tumor.[45-47]

Over the centuries, ointments, liniments, lotions, and balms have been used for pain relief. Research to validate their effectiveness is contradictory. Some of these contain substances such as menthol that have an odor and also cause various skin sensations. The sensation usually described is one of warmth, although some patients may experience coolness. Some of these substances contain methyl salicylate, which may be absorbed through the skin and result in some systemic analgesia. Some can cause skin irritation and should be tested on a small skin surface before use.[45-47]

Transcutaneous electrical nerve stimulation (TENS) is a fairly new approach to pain relief. Use of this method requires a physician's prescription.[45-47] TENS systems usually consist of a battery that powers a stimulator, lead wires, and multiple electrodes. When attached to the skin, the patient will feel a buzzing, tingling, or vibrating sensation. The intensity of the stimulation can be adjusted. Research has indicated that TENS can provide relief in both acute and chronic pain. However, its mechanism of action is not well understood.

Space does not allow a more extensive discussion of cutaneous stimulation techniques. For a thorough discussion of nursing strategies in this area, see references 45 through 47. These measures may be a very effective supplement when other measures do not completely relieve pain, or, in some cases, in their stead.

Therapeutic Touch

Therapeutic touch is a relatively new nursing care approach developed by Krieger[39] and based on Martha Rogers' theory of nursing.[64] Some of the major concepts of this theory are man as an energy field, man and environment as an open system in constant interaction, and a holistic order to all energy fields. This way of perceiving man and environment seems incompatible with the tenets of Western science and more in keeping with Eastern philosophy.[9]

The effectiveness of therapeutic touch has been difficult to document because it is not easy to scientifically measure energy fields. However, nursing research is currently being conducted in this area. In spite of a lack of scientific explanation for the process, proponents for the theory report its effectiveness in the relief of pain.[9] Heidt also reports that therapeutic touch is effective in relieving anxiety, which could help reduce pain.[34]

The process of therapeutic touch requires some skills that are best learned by working with a practitioner in this field. The first step in the process is centering, which is a meditative state of the nurse. The nurse's energy field is used to alter the energy field of the patient. The nurse's hands are held 2 to 3 inches from the patient's body and movements are made to distribute the energy. The strategy is reported to be effective in relieving both acute and chronic pain. Boguslawski suggests using meditation and guided imagery with therapeutic touch for the most effective results.[9]

Drug Therapy

Drug therapy for chronic cancer pain is often unnecessarily ineffective. There are many reasons for this. Both nurses and physicians have an inadequate knowledge of the pharmacology of analgesics. They may both be misinformed about the risks of addiction and habituation. There are many social interactions involving values, power, and control that may interfere with responsible decisions about the administration of drugs.

Marks and Sachar have demonstrated that hospitalized patients are commonly undertreated for pain.[43] Meperidine, which has an average duration of action of 3 hours, is usually ordered every 4 hours, causing the patient to experience at least 1 to 2 hours of pain before the next dose is given. The dose of drug ordered is usually inadequate to relieve the pain. To make this situation worse, nurses often administer less than the ordered dose. If the drug is switched from injectable to oral administration, the physician often orders the same dose. Since absorption from oral administration is poorer and slower, pain relief will be far less effective.

Physicians and nurses generally have a poor knowledge of the relative effective-

Table 11–3. Narcotic Analgesics: Approximate Equanalgesic Doses of Selected Commercially Available Dosage Forms*

Drug	Route	Dose (mg)	Average Duration of Action (hours)
Hydromorphone	PO	3–4	3–4
(Dilaudid)	PR	3–6	3–4
	IM, SC	2–3	3–4
	IV	2	3–4
Levorphanol	PO	2–3	6–8
(LevoDromoran)	SC	2	6–8
	IV	2	4–6
Meperidine	PO	100–150	3
	IM, SC	75–100	3
Methadone	PO	12.5	6–8
(Dolophine)	IM, SC	10	4–6
Morphine sulfate	PO	15	3–4
	IM, SC	10	4–6
	IV	8	3–4
Oxymorphone	PR	2–5	4
(Numorphan)	IM	1–1.5	4

*From Lipman, A. G.: Drug therapy in cancer pain. *Cancer Nursing.* 3:39–46, 1980. Used by permission of Masson Publishing USA, Inc., New York. Copyright 1980.

ness of various analgesics for the relief of pain. Table 11–3 shows narcotic analgesics and their effective doses compared with 10 mg of morphine. This kind of comparison is called equanalgesic doses and is very useful in planning effective pain relief. Tables 11–4 and 11–5 show the effectiveness of non-narcotic analgesics compared with 650 mg of aspirin.[32]

Aspirin is far more effective as an analgesic than it is usually considered to be. Most of the pain relief of non-narcotic drug combinations is due to the aspirin. As is shown on Table 11–4, 650 mg of aspirin is more effective than 65 mg of codeine.

Two aspirin tablets or two acetaminophen (Tylenol) tablets given at the same time as an injected narcotic will greatly increase pain relief and, because the oral drug reaches peak action more slowly, pain relief may be prolonged.[45-47] This is a very rational approach to pain relief, because narcotic analgesics seem to affect the central nervous system, whereas non-narcotic

Table 11–4. Relative Therapeutic Effect of Oral Analgesics According to Mean Percentage of Relief of Pain Achieved in 57 Patients*

Analgesic Agent	Dose (mg)	Relief of Pain (%)	
Aspirin	650	62	
Pentazocine	50	54	
Acetaminophen	650	50	Significantly superior
Phenacetin	650	48	to placebo (p<0.05)
Mefenamic acid	250	47	
Codeine	65	46	
Propoxyphene	65	43	
Ethoheptazine	75	38	Significantly inferior
Promazine	25	37	to aspirin (p<0.05)
Placebo	–	32	

*Moertel, C. G., et al.: A comparative evaluation of marketed analgesic drugs. Reprinted, by permission of the *New England Journal of Medicine.* 286:814, 1972.

Table 11–5. Comparative Therapeutic Effect of Placebo, Aspirin Alone, and Aspirin Combinations[*]

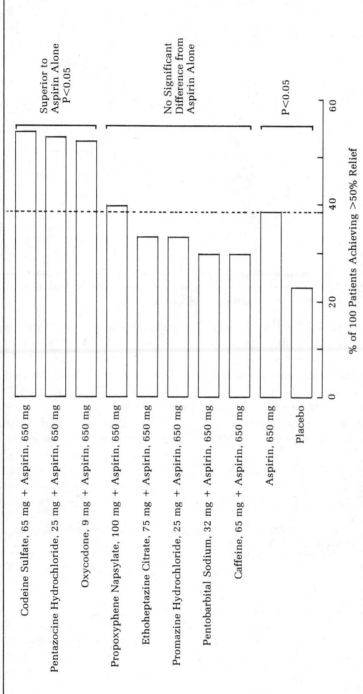

[*]According to the percentage of patients achieving significant (i.e., more than 50 per cent) relief of pain. From Moertel, C. G., et al.: Relief of pain by oral medication. A controlled evaluation of analgesic combinations. *Journal of the American Medical Association*. 229:57, 1974. Used by permission from the Mayo Foundation, who owns the copyright.

analgesics affect the peripheral nervous system — perhaps by inhibiting the synthesis of prostaglandins.[29]

Patients receiving chemotherapy may be unable to take aspirin because one of the side effects of aspirin is a prolongation of the bleeding time. Acetaminophen, however, can be safely used in this situation.

Patients often feel that aspirin is given when the nurse does not believe that they are really experiencing pain. If aspirin is used, either alone or with narcotics, the reason for its use should be explained to the patient. Sometimes, because of the patient's distrust of aspirin's capability, a non-narcotic drug combination may be more effective in pain relief.

Addiction and habituation to drugs for chronic pain are minor, if not negligible, problems. Less than 1 per cent of all hospitalized patients treated for pain ever become addicted. Because pain alters the drug physiology, addiction is highly unlikely. In the dying patient, this is somewhat of a moot issue, anyway.[40, 45-47]

One of the greatest fears of nurses and physicians in caring for cancer patients in pain is that habituation to drugs will make it impossible to relieve increasing pain. Studies by Saunders,[70] Twycross,[82] and Mount[56] indicate that this does not occur. Increased drug demands are usually the consequence of increased pathology. If extremely high doses of narcotics are required for pain relief, they can be safely given without fatal respiratory failure. Respiratory depression does not occur from narcotics given during severe pain.[45-47] If the pain is suddenly relieved, as sometimes occurs with myocardial infarction or renal colic, respiratory depression can occur, but this is not as likely to happen in cancer patients.

Social values, power plays, and the need for control — all of which are a part of the hospital environment in which nursing care occurs — influence decisions about pain control. The p.r.n. order for analgesics can be and is interpreted in many ways. Many dynamics that occur with the administration of pain relief are often mentally unhealthy for the patient, the family, and the health care professionals. Fagerhaugh and Strauss[26] have described this situation in detail.

Because the process of chronic pain is much different from that of acute pain, different strategies need to be used to manage it. The approach to chronic pain should be that of prevention. The patient should not be allowed to experience pain. In order to accomplish this, analgesics are administered on a regularly scheduled basis, rather than p.r.n.

This approach to pain relief began as part of the hospice movement and is now becoming a generally more accepted therapy. If the patient is in severe pain when first seen, large doses of narcotics may be used to relieve the pain. The patient may then sleep for many hours. This is not a sign of drug overdose. Pain is exhausting and patients have often been without sleep for several days. The drug doses are then titrated downward until the patient experiences some pain. The next dose will be slightly increased.[40] (See Fig. 11–6.) This dose will usually continue to control the pain if given regularly until progressive pathology intervenes.

These patients are often given oral liquid narcotics rather than injections. Because of differences in absorption, these doses may seem extremely high. The solutions given to patients may be Brompton's mixture, hospice mix, or liquid morphine. Brompton's mixture contains heroin and cocaine, both of which are illegal in the United States. More recent research has indicated that liquid morphine is just as effective. Patients may also be given liquid phenothiazine to control the nausea caused by morphine and a stool softener such as Peri-Colace to control the constipation.

Family Support During Pain

Family members of a patient with chronic pain also need nursing care. To see a loved one in constant pain is extremely difficult. Family members may feel anxiety, anger, and guilt. Sometimes anger is directed toward the health care profession-

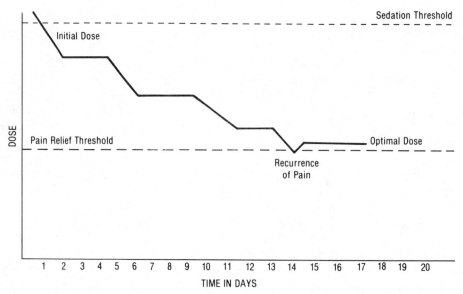

Figure 11–6. Titration of drug dosage for relief of chronic pain. (From Lipman, A. G.: Drug therapy in cancer pain. *Cancer Nursing* 3:39–46, 1980. Used by permission of Masson Publishing USA, Inc., New York. Copyright 1980.)

al and sometimes toward the patient. In addition to these very exhausting feelings, family members often get inadequate rest and do not eat properly. They may have no one to talk to about their feelings.

The nurse can provide opportunities for family members to express feelings. Information about the patient and the planned treatment can sometimes reduce their anxiety. Family members can participate in pain relief measures or in general care. Sometimes family members may develop effective pain relief measures that have not been considered by the nurse. Family members should be encouraged to take care of themselves. In some instances, the family members may not feel that they have a right to take care of themselves because of social expectations. They may need the permission and encouragement of the nurse.

Evaluation of Pain Relief Measures

Evaluation of pain relief measures is often completely neglected. Because nurses are not held accountable for pain relief, this stage of the nursing process is usually not done. Evaluation is likely to consist of the nurse standing in the doorway and asking, "Feeling better?" This type of question is designed to elicit an affirmative response from the patient and is not useful in evaluating pain relief.

Evaluation should examine several parameters. How much time was required for pain relief to occur after administration of the treatment? Was the pain relieved or only diminished? If the pain was diminished, to what extent was it diminished? Did the pain return after a period of time? How long did pain relief last? Was the pain actually relieved or did the patient simply stop expressing pain? Patients can sometimes be so sedated that they are unable to express pain even though it is still being experienced.[45-47]

Answers to these questions should be used to plan further nursing interventions. If pain relief has been incomplete, additional interventions should be used. If an injection for pain lasts for 2 hours and is only ordered every 4 hours, collaboration with the physician is needed. If the physician is unwilling to change the order, other nursing measures should be used.

Since chronic pain control requires that the patient does not experience pain, the patient should be regularly evaluated for the occurrence of pain. This strategy is best implemented by mutual agreement of all health care team members. It certainly requires coordination of pain relief activities by nurses caring for the patient on all three shifts. The p.r.n. orders for pain are often more flexible than nurses consider them to be. This leaves much to the judgment of the nurse. If the nurse's clinical judgment, based on evaluation, is that the patient needs regular administration of drugs for pain, it is within the nurse's prerogative to do this.

INFECTION

The incidence of infection in cancer patients is very high. Infections that could easily be controlled in other individuals may cause death to the cancer patient.[6] (See Table 11–6.) Infections in cancer patients are often caused by organisms that are not normally pathogenic. Most of the treatments for cancer further diminish the patient's resistance to infection. As a result of these treatments, cancer patients are surviving their disease for longer periods of time and, consequently, the incidence of infection has gone up. Because of these factors, nursing measures related to prevention of infection and care of the patient with infection take high precedence. Nursing measures for the patient at high risk of infection because of chemotherapy are discussed in Chapter 9. The discussion will be further expanded here because of its salience for all cancer patients.

Pathophysiology

Cancer patients, in general, have a diminished resistance to infection. The pathophysiologic processes involved in this are not completely understood. Cell-mediated immunity is often decreased in cancer patients. Patients with leukemia, lymphomas, Hodgkin's disease, and multiple myeloma have defects in humoral immunity. As people age, their immune capacity decreases. Since the incidence of cancer increases with age, normal aging processes may be a factor in the incidence of infection. The cancer patient often has nutritional defects and sometimes cachexia, which alter immune responses. Lengthy hospital stays also increase the incidence of infection. Tumor growth may cause tissue damage, which would increase vulnerability to infection.

Patients with cancer are frequently in high stress situations. They may be depressed, hopeless, anxious, or angry. All of these feelings are associated with a decreased immune response. Social isolation, disruption of family and community roles, and dependency may further depress the immune response. Together these factors form the image of a patient at high risk of infection.

The pathophysiology of the infectious process is complex. As with most human conditions, it is multicausal. It is much too simplistic to say that a specific organism "causes" an infection. When infection occurs in the cancer patient, however, physiologic processes normally related to

Table 11–6. Fatal Infections Related to Type of Malignancy*

Malignancy	No. of Clients	Disseminated	% Clients with Pneumonia	Peritonitis	% Dying of Infection
Acute leukemia	366	65	28	0.1	70
Lymphoma	206	53	40	3	51
Genitourinary	208	48	34	10	58
Gastrointestinal	142	45	39	13	49
Lung	104	20	78	2	44
Head and neck	94	19	74	2	46
Melanoma	78	35	59	3	37

*Reprinted with permission from Bodey, G. P., Sr., et al.: Supportive care in the management of the cancer patient. In *Cancer Patient Care at M. D. Anderson Hospital and Tumor Institute,* ed. by Clark, R. L., and Howe, C. D. Copyright 1976, by Year Book Medical Publishers, Inc., Chicago.

infection may be different. Temperature elevation may not occur until late in the infection. The inflammatory process may not occur with local infections. Pus or abscess formation may not occur because of the absence of white blood cells. Open wounds that appear "clean" may be infected. Untreated infections can disseminate rapidly and lead to death.[6]

Most infections are caused by gram negative bacteria. Twenty-five per cent of these are *Pseudomonas*.[55] Infections by opportunistic organisms are common. Fungal infections such as candidiasis are likely to occur. Tuberculosis is not uncommon, particularly in patients with Hodgkin's disease or lung cancer. Viral infections such as cytomegalic inclusion disease, herpes simplex, herpes zoster, and chicken pox occur frequently and are extremely destructive to the cancer patient.[55]

Antibiotics are less effective in patients with low white blood counts. These patients also are inclined to contract repeat infections with the same organism. Many times, multiple organisms may be causing infections in the patient at the same time. Cultures will often show the presence of several infectious organisms in the same site. Superinfection occurs commonly. If the normal intestinal flora are destroyed by antibiotic therapy, overgrowth of other opportunistic organisms — such as *Candida* — may develop and become systemic.[6]

Assessment

Assessment for infection is discussed in Chapter 9. To summarize, a temperature of 101° F or greater is considered an indication of probable infection. If this occurs, routine cultures should be taken from the throat, urine, blood, sputum, stool, or lesions that could be infected. The patient's skin should be thoroughly examined daily for signs of infection, particularly the outside crevices of the nares, the corners of the mouth, under the breasts, the axillae, groin, perineum, and perirectal area, and under folds of fat. The mouth should also be closely examined. *Candida* will appear as white patches in the mouth. The chest should be auscultated for rales. Intravenous sites should be closely checked for signs of inflammation. Infection is very likely to occur in areas with lymphedema or regions where lymph node dissection has been performed.

Planning

Nursing interventions should be planned with two focuses, one aimed at the prevention of infection and one at the optimum supportive care of the patient with an infection. Interventions with these two aims overlap. Since control of the environment is a major factor in the prevention of infection, organizational planning will be as important as the planning of an individual nurse caring for an individual patient. All health care personnel on all shifts must participate in handwashing routines, the wearing of clean uniforms, and other measures designed to protect the patient from nosocomial infections. This may require nursing unit meetings. Equipment and supplies needed for infection control must be available. An attitude that places a high value on infection control measures must pervade the thoughts and behavior of all nursing personnel. This may require some persuasion and positive reinforcement by the nurses in leadership positions.

Interventions

Maintenance of adequate nutrition is very important in the prevention of infection. Factors that seem to be the most important for good body defense are adequate protein and sufficient vitamin intake. Therefore, the nursing measures discussed in the section on cachexia are equally important for prevention or control of infection.

Skin care and protection are important aspects of infection control. The patient's nails should be kept short and well manicured to avoid infections around the nails and from scratching. Toenails should also be well cared for.[24] Patients who are thrombocytopenic are likely to have breaks in the skin and mucosa, allowing entry of microorganisms. Meticulous care should be given to these areas. Patients should be turned frequently to avoid formation of decubiti. Caution should be taken to avoid use of excessive soap during the bath, since this can cause drying and cracking of the skin.

Intravenous needles should be changed regularly.[24] Intravenous catheters should be avoided if possible because of the increased risk of phlebitis. Intravenous sites should be carefully observed. An antiseptic germicidal ointment (for example, povidone-iodine [Betadine]) and a sterile dressing should be used on intravenous sites.[6] Strict aseptic technique should be used in preparing IV solutions, adding piggybacks, and changing IV's. An in-line filter of 0.45 or 0.22 micron pore size should be used if the patient is granulocytopenic. IV tubing should be changed every 24 hours.[42]

Perineal care should be performed regularly. Female patients should be taught how to wipe properly after a bowel movement to diminish the risk of vaginal and bladder infections. If the patient experiences perineal itching or burning on urination, she should be checked for infection. A female patient who is granulocytopenic should have counseling regarding care during sexual activity. Measures should be taken to maintain cleanliness, prevent contamination, avoid excess friction, and utilize sufficient lubrication. Both homosexual and heterosexual anal activity should be avoided since the anus is susceptible to tears or breaks that can easily develop into abscesses. Rectal bacteria can also be transported to other body parts that are susceptible to infection. Enemas, rectal medications, and rectal thermometers should also be avoided in leukopenic patients. If anal cracks or abscesses do occur, they can be treated with sitz baths, antibacterial ointments, and topical anesthetics.

Bladder catheterization adds significantly to the risk of infection. Research indicates that there is a high incidence of bacteriuria after catheterization. If catheterization is necessary, extra care should be used to maintain sterile technique. A small catheter and sufficient lubrication should be used to avoid unnecessary urethral trauma. Indwelling catheters are an even greater risk. After 10 days, 100 per cent of patients have bacteriuria. Sterile drainage systems and a closed system should be meticulously maintained. The system should not be interrupted unless it is absolutely necessary. Catheters should not be irrigated unless occluded. The catheter should be secured to prevent movement in the urethra. Increased fluid intake may decrease the bacteriuria.[24]

Respiratory infections are common in cancer patients and may involve the middle ear, sinuses, throat, upper air passages, or lungs. These infections can be very serious. Measures to prevent pneumonia are important and include mobility, frequent turning, deep breathing, and coughing. Visitors or personnel with respiratory infections should not be allowed near the patient. Respiratory therapy equipment should be carefully cleansed. The mouthpiece and nebulizer should not be used for other patients, even if the equipment is cleaned afterwards. Tracheostomies greatly increase the risk of respiratory infection. Sterile suctioning techniques should be used and the stoma and tracheostomy tube should be kept clean. The patient should be breathing humidified air.[24]

Oral care is an important part of infection control for cancer patients. Mouth care should be given every 4 hours around the clock. Details of mouth care are discussed in Chapter 9.

Many of the infections that cancer patients have are nosocomial. One very effective way to decrease the incidence of infection is to reduce hospital stays as much as possible. Patients and family members can often be taught preventive care, signs of infection, and what actions to take if infection occurs.[24]

Medical treatment of patients who have an infection will usually involve the administration of IV antibiotics. Antibiotics are not as effective for infections in leukopenic patients. Therefore, more potent antibiotics with greater toxicities may be used. The mortality rate for cancer patients with infections is high. Patients receiving antibiotics may develop superinfections of *Pseudomonas* or *Candida* or *Staphylococcus*.[24]

Patients who are severely granulocytopenic may be given granulocyte transfusions. This treatment is used for patients who have received antibiotic treatment that has failed to control the infection. This treatment is given in conjunction with antibiotic therapy. Effects are sometimes dramatic.[30, 62]

Septic shock can occur in cancer patients with systemic infections. Patients with this condition are usually cared for in an intensive care unit. Antibiotics, leukapheresis, and corticosteroids may be used. Vasopressors may be necessary to maintain the systolic blood pressure and adequate renal perfusion. Mechanized ventilating assistance and intubation may be necessary if tissue oxygen perfusion is not adequate. Intensive care measures for cancer patients may seem to be excessive; however, this type of treatment can greatly prolong the patient's life. If the patient has leukemia, it is possible for the patient to recover from the infection and go into remission.[6]

Activities for patients with systemic infections should be minimal, although some activities can be allowed. Patients with local infections may be able to maintain normal activity.

High fever may be a problem for patients with serious infections. If aspirin is contraindicated, acetaminophen can be used. If the fever is dangerously high, alcohol sponge baths or a cooling mattress may be used. When the temperature begins to drop, excessive perspiration may occur. Bed linens and clothing should be changed frequently. The patient should be kept warm and dry. Patients with high fever should wear minimal clothing and be kept in a cool room to promote heat conduction. Fluid intake should be increased as much as possible. Since high fever increases the metabolic rate and causes anorexia, the prolongation of this condition can have serious implications for adequate nutritional maintenance.[24]

Patients who have drainage from infected areas are at risk of cross-contamination. Attempts should be made to confine the drainage to the infected area. Bulky dressings and frequent dressing changes may be required. Proper disposal of dressings is important. It may be necessary for nurses to wear gloves while changing dressings to avoid contaminating their hands.[24]

Odor control may be a problem with some infections. *Pseudomonas,* in particular, has a very offensive odor. Frequent dressing changes and irrigations can help control the odor. Deodorizers can sometimes be helpful. This type of odor is very difficult for the patient to cope with. It may interfere with appetite, self-image, social contacts, and emotional status.

Because infections in cancer patients are so serious, it is sometimes easy to focus on treating the infection but not the person who has it. The patient's emotional state will have an effect on the body's response to the infection. The patient needs to be delegated important responsibilities in fighting the infection. Keeping the patient informed of the situation and treatment plan can be helpful. The nurse should talk and work with the patient in such a way that activities are a cooperative venture.

Evaluation

The most obvious evaluation of nursing measures designed to prevent infection is whether or not infection occurs. However, infection with opportunistic organisms cannot be seen as a failure of nursing activities, but rather as a progression of disease pathology.

Evaluation of the effectiveness of nursing measures designed to prevent infection based on one patient is not very informative. If the nursing unit cares for many cancer patients, it would be more helpful to examine data on groups of patients. For example, what is the incidence of urinary tract infections in patients who have been catheterized? This should be measured 1 or

2 weeks after the procedure for meaningful information. What is the incidence of intravenous site infections, within a given time after insertion? How many patients in the unit develop nosocomial infections? Are there patterns in these patients related to which member of the nursing staff provides the care? If nonthreatening ways could be designed to do this, it would be interesting to take cultures of nurses' hands, lab coat sleeves, or uniforms in spot checks. This type of activity would have to be done in a trusting environment for the purpose of increasing awareness, not for coercive reasons. Otherwise, it could have many negative effects.

INCREASED RISK OF THROMBOPHLEBITIS

Pathophysiology

Cancer patients have an increased risk of developing thrombophlebitis, even in the early stages of the disease. The cause for this is not known, but it may be due to the production of some substance by the tumor, which causes a state of hypercoagulability. Thrombus formation is usually due to venous stasis, hypercoagulability and/or injury to the venous wall. It is believed that at least two of the three must be present for the development of a thrombus.[41, 59] Small thrombi often develop in the pockets of valves in the deep veins. (See Fig. 11-7.) A newly formed thrombus has a "tail" that can become detached and cause pulmonary embolism. About 24 to 48 hours after the thrombus has formed, the "tail" either undergoes lysis or adheres to the vessel walls, thus eliminating the risk of embolism.[41]

Assessment

Patients with a diagnosis of cancer should be examined regularly for thrombophlebitis. The patient should be asked about pain or tenderness in the calves of the legs. Extra warmth may be felt along the pathway of a leg vein; however, in

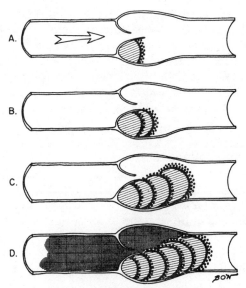

Figure 11-7. Diagrammatic illustration showing propagation of a deep thrombus arising in a valvar pocket with deposition of successive layers (A, B, and C) and retrograde extension of the thrombus after venous blockage by propagation (D). (From Hume, M., Sevitt, S., and Thomas, D. P.: *Venous Thrombosis and Pulmonary Embolism.* Cambridge, Mass.: Harvard University Press, 1970. Used by permission.)

many patients, this sign is not present. The pathway of the deep veins in the calf of the leg and behind the knee should be palpated for tenderness. Homans' sign can be very helpful in detecting thrombophlebitis. To test for Homans' sign, the patient's leg is extended. The nurse's hand is placed on the sole of the foot near the toes. The foot is moved upward, toward the patient's head, in a quick motion. Patients with thrombophlebitis will experience pain with this maneuver.

Cancer patients can also develop thrombophlebitis in the veins in the pelvic area. If this has occurred, deep palpation of the lower abdomen may elicit pain or tenderness.

Planning

Nursing units with large numbers of cancer patients should have established protocols for routinely checking patients for thrombophlebitis. Nursing measures designed to prevent the development of thrombophlebitis should be implemented as a part of the established routine of the unit. Nurses who work in outpatient clinics or physicians' offices should also routinely check patients and teach them and their family preventive measures.

Interventions

Cancer patients should not be placed in Fowler's position. This position allows pooling of blood to occur in both the lower legs and the pelvis and also discourages mobility. (See Fig. 11–8.) The knee gatch should not be raised for patients with cancer.

Patients should be encouraged to move frequently. Ambulation should be encouraged, if permitted by the physician. At home, patients should not sit in one position for long periods of time, particularly not in lounge chairs. Quadriceps exercises should be performed either actively or, if necessary, passively at least 4 times a day.

These measures should be taken on all cancer patients, early postoperative patients as well as patients with metastatic disease. Even if the surgeon thinks "we got it all," the substance produced by the tumor may still be present in the body and able to promote the development of thrombophlebitis.

Care of the cancer patient who develops thrombophlebitis is the same as that for any patient with this disorder. The patient is placed at bedrest with the leg elevated

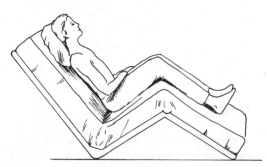

Figure 11–8. Pooling of blood with patient in Fowler's position.

above the level of the heart; the foot should be higher than the knee. After 48 hours, when the risk of embolism is diminished, ambulation may be allowed (provided that the patient wears elastic stockings). Anticoagulant drug therapy may be administered. If pain or swelling is present, heat may be used on the leg.[41]

Evaluation

Evaluation of preventive measures always must consider whether the situation was actually preventable. Sabiston[68] indicates that thrombophlebitis will sometimes occur in spite of a carefully designed regimen. The incidence, however, is decreased with such a regimen. Evaluation should also include determination of the extent to which the preventive actions were done. This can be determined in several ways. Charting of activities should be checked. The patient can be asked if planned activities were performed. The nurse, in self-evaluation, can examine the frequency of activities and the factors that interfered with their implementation. Plans can then be made to deal with those factors.

PULMONARY EMBOLISM

Pathophysiology

Patients with cancer have a high incidence of pulmonary embolism. These emboli usually break loose from the "tail" of thrombi that have formed in the iliac and femoral veins. They travel up the vena cava, through the right side of the heart, and into the pulmonary circulation. The embolus is frequently broken up into multiple small emboli by the churning action of the heart. These emboli then obstruct pulmonary blood flow, increasing venous pressure in the pulmonary artery. A reflex vasoconstriction then occurs, which decreases blood flow to lung tissues surrounding the site of the embolism. It is believed that serotonin is released by platelets in the area, causing the reflex vasoconstriction and pulmonary hypertension.[41, 68]

Pulmonary embolism occurs abruptly. The mortality rate is about 38 per cent. Of the patients who die, one-half die within 30 minutes of the onset, two-thirds within 1 hour, and three-fourths within 2 hours. If the patient survives, spontaneous resolution of the condition occurs over a 2 week period.[41, 68]

Assessment

The symptoms that accompany pulmonary embolism vary. The classic symptoms commonly listed in textbooks are dyspnea, chest pain, hemoptysis, and hypotension. Table 11–7 records the signs and symptoms that Sabiston found in 1000 patients at Duke University Medical Center. Only one-third of the patients had clinically evident thrombophlebitis. This is probably because embolism occurs most frequently soon after thrombus formation.[68]

The physician may order chest x-ray and electrocardiogram studies, blood enzyme level tests, pulmonary angiograms, arteri-

Table 11–7. Clinical Manifestations in 1000 Patients with Pulmonary Embolism at the Duke University Medical Center*

Symptoms	Per Cent
Dyspnea	77
Chest pain	63
Hemoptysis	26
Altered mental status	23
Dyspnea, chest pain, hemoptysis	14

Signs	Per Cent
Tachycardia	59
Recent fever	43
Rales	42
Tachypnea	38
Leg edema and tenderness	23
Elevated venous pressure	18
Shock	11
Accentuated P₂	11
Cyanosis	9
Pleural friction rub	8

*From Sabiston, D. C., Jr.: Pulmonary embolism. In *Davis-Christopher Textbook of Surgery, 12th edition,* ed. by Sabiston, D. C. Jr. Philadelphia: W. B. Saunders Co., 1981. Used by permission.

al blood gas determinations, and a radioisotope lung scan to make the medical diagnosis. The nurse, who is most likely to be present at the onset of symptoms, must make an immediate assessment and take nursing actions based on the best judgment of the situation.

Planning

Because of the rapid onset and extreme urgency of pulmonary embolism, prior organizational planning for such an emergency is essential. Needed equipment and supplies must be readily available. A plan of action will keep confusion and disorder to a minimum and keep the focus on the patient. It will reduce the time needed to provide the patient with immediate care.

Interventions

The nurse is confronted with a patient who has had a sudden onset of severe chest pain, has difficulty breathing, and is coughing up blood. The patient will be anxious, restless, and apprehensive. Multiple actions need to be taken almost simultaneously. The head of the bed should be elevated to 30 degrees to ease breathing. Continuous oxygen should be administered by nasal catheter or oxygen mask. Vital signs should be closely monitored. The physician should then be notified. The patient may require ventilatory assistance with an intermittent positive pressure machine or a respirator. Caution should be taken in using intermittent positive pressure if the patient has a low platelet count from chemotherapy, since the treatment can cause pulmonary hemorrhaging. If shock occurs, treatment with vasoconstrictors such as levarterenol (Levophed) or metaraminol (Aramine) may be necessary.

Some professionals may question using aggressive measures on a patient with cancer when the risk of death from the pulmonary embolism is so high. However, if the patient can be given biologic and emotional support through the crisis period of reflex pulmonary vasoconstriction, recovery from the embolism is much more probable.

The patient should not be left alone because of the high level of patient apprehension and the immediate risk of death. Verbal communications to the patient explaining what has happened and what is being done are important. These communications should be given in a calm, supportive way. Touching the patient in a reassuring manner is important. The patient should be told that the nurse will not leave and that the physician has been contacted.

If family members are present, a nurse should stay with them if possible. In any case, the family should be kept informed of what is being done and that the situation is serious.

The nurse's communications with other health care givers should be designed to provide calmness, support, encouragement, and praise for effective actions. Tension, anxiety, hostility, confusion, and quarreling should be kept at a minimum. In addition to promoting professional development, this behavior will facilitate the best care for the patient.

At this point, the patient may be transferred to an intensive care unit. Anticoagulant and fibrinolytic therapy may be implemented. Physical support activities may be continued for some time. Activities designed to prevent the development of additional thrombi are important. (See section on thrombophlebitis.) Other than these activities, the main focus will be providing excellent supportive care to enhance the environment in which the healing process can be facilitated.

Evaluation

Evaluation of nursing care during the crisis of pulmonary embolism cannot entirely be based on whether the patient lives or dies, since this may be a function of the extent of pathology. Evaluation should consider the nursing actions that were taken. Were all the actions that should have been taken actually done? Were health care givers able to work together effectively? What was the effect of actions that were taken? What factors interfered with effective nursing actions? What can be done to improve future functioning?

Because of the stress of this situation, it is helpful if evaluation can occur in a group discussion. In nursing, judgments of success or failure are often based on patient survival. Group evaluation allows a greater focus to be placed on actual effectiveness of specific nursing actions. It also allows for expression of feelings and mutual support.

HEMORRHAGE OR BLEEDING

Pathophysiology

Bleeding or hemorrhage may occur in cancer patients because of various pathologies. Clotting disorders occur in patients with leukemia. Patients receiving chemotherapy may have decreased numbers of platelets. Patients with altered liver function may not have an intact clotting mechanism. Radiation therapy or surgery may cause the walls of blood vessels to weaken. Tumor growth may invade blood vessel walls and weaken them.

Assessment

Assessment may be a determination of the risk of bleeding or the extent of bleeding that has occurred. Assessment of bleeding in patients receiving chemotherapy is discussed in Chapter 9. The discussion in Chapter 9 is also appropriate to leukemia patients. Knowledge of surgery and radiation treatments will give some indication of the risk of bleeding from weakened vessel walls, as will knowledge of the growth patterns of specific malignancies. Liver function and amount of blood loss can be determined by laboratory tests.

Planning

Planning the care for patients at high risk of bleeding involves nursing interventions that decrease that risk. If bleeding is occurring, the goal is to diminish the blood loss. Another goal is to provide supportive care that increases patient functioning in a state of physiologic stress.

Interventions

Patients who have an increased tendency to bleed must be protected from assaults from the environment that could cause further bleeding. Bed rails should be padded. Intramuscular injections may need to be discontinued. Toothbrushes may have to be avoided. (See Chapter 9 for further nursing measures.)

Emotional stress situations should be avoided when possible. Leukemic patients can have an "intracranial bleed" from a rise in blood pressure. This is a crisis situation that often results in death. However, with excellent supportive care, patients can sometimes recover.

Patients who have lung cancer will sometimes hemorrhage from an eroded pulmonary artery. If the artery is large, death will usually occur within a matter of minutes. This is an extremely frightening experience for both patient and family members. This often occurs when the patient is at home, but will sometimes occur during hospitalization. The patient may cough, sneeze, laugh, or strain at stool, and the hemorrhage begins.

If the hemorrhage is from a smaller vessel, surgery may be able to stop the bleeding. If not, little can be done to save the patient's life. It is important for the nurse to stay with the patient rather than rush out to get help or "do something." The emergency call light can be used to summon other help. The patient should be talked to and touched to avoid feeling alone. Family members will also need support both during and after this traumatic experience. When the situation is over, the nurse will need support from fellow professionals.

One of the most terrifying situations that can occur with cancer patients is a "carotid blowout." This occurs in patients who have had head and neck surgery and possibly radiation therapy for cancer. The wall of the carotid artery may be weakened in the process; sometimes infection has further weakened the wall. A blowout usually takes place with little or no warning. Death occurs rapidly. If by chance the nurse is with the patient when a blowout happens, it is sometimes possible to prevent the massive blood loss and death that are otherwise inevitable. Direct pressure must be applied to the bleeding carotid artery. This requires calmness and quick thinking and is difficult to do. Bleeding obscures the area, making it so slippery that pressure is hard to maintain. Pressure must be continued until surgical intervention can stop the bleeding.

Family members may panic both during and after this experience. A massive loss of blood has a very terrible, primitive meaning to us. Nurses are not immune to this feeling. It may be necessary for another nurse to care for the family while the original nurse takes a moment to get back together emotionally.

Evaluation

Evaluation of nursing actions during bleeding should be based on whether all possible nursing actions were taken. The effectiveness of the action should be evaluated. If the action was not effective, was it because of the pathology or because the nursing action was not well done? What factors interfered with nursing activities? If bleeding precautions were implemented, did bleeding occur because the precautions were not observed?

CONSTIPATION

Constipation can occur in cancer patients as a result of a variety of processes. Vincristine (Oncovin) can cause serious constipation problems (see Chapter 9). Narcotics, particularly opiates, decrease peristalsis and thus cause constipation. Decreased food intake, cachexia, diminished social interaction, decreased mobility, fatigue, depression, pain, and negative beliefs about cancer that result in hopelessness and dependency all interact to reduce normal bowel function and cause constipation. An increasing tumor burden in the abdominal cavity will also interfere with bowel function.

Constipation occurs when the feces is compact, hard, and difficult to evacuate. The longer the feces remains in the lower bowel, the more of the water in the feces is extracted by the bowel wall and the harder the feces will become. If this condition progresses, the patient will develop an impaction. Occasionally, it can progress to an intestinal obstruction.

Assessment

The most obvious symptoms of constipation are a bowel evacuation of hard, compact stool; straining of the patient in the attempt to have a bowel movement; and anal bleeding or pain on evacuation. The patient may express a feeling of fullness or discomfort in the lower colon. Digital rectal examination may show hard, compact stool filling the rectum. The stool may be in a solid, large mass or multiple, small, hard balls. This mass may have reached the point of impaction. Sometimes the impaction is too high to palpate with a digital examination.

Frequency of bowel movement can (with some reservations) be used as a measure of constipation. People have different patterns of bowel evacuation. Some people consider themselves constipated if bowel evacuation does not occur daily. Unless the texture of the feces is altered, this is not constipation. However, if a patient fails to have a bowel movement for several days and this is not the patient's usual pattern, it is reasonable to classify this as constipation and intervene accordingly.

Planning

Hospitalized patients with cancer should be regularly assessed for constipation. Time and character of bowel movements should be recorded on the patient's chart. Since this information is often gathered by nonprofessional nursing personnel, it is essential for the professional nurse to maintain regular surveillance of the activity. Employees who perform this activity well should be rewarded. If the professional nurse places a high value on knowing and intervening in bowel evacuation patterns, other nursing personnel may do the same.

Constipation is a problem that is high on the list of concerns of cancer patients. It may seem minor to health professionals, since it is seldom life threatening, but it seriously affects the patient's quality of life. The patient needs to know that the nurse will give serious attention to this problem until it has been resolved.

Effective strategies used in the past by the patient to relieve constipation should be determined. The nurse and patient together can then plan a program to prevent or treat constipation problems. When the patient has multiple factors that frequently cause constipation, prevention is usually the wisest course of action.

Cancer patients who are being seen on an outpatient basis should also be regularly assessed for constipation problems. The patient may see this as a problem too minor to trouble the health professionals with. Careful planning with the patient and family can prevent much discomfort and concern.

Interventions

Interventions should be designed to alter as many of the variables that interact to cause constipation as possible. We have become so accustomed to rely on medications and treatments that we often forget to use our common sense. The larger goal must be to achieve a greater sense of well being and a higher level of health for the patient. This is not as likely to be accomplished by the achievement of a single bowel evacuation as it is by a program that relieves the existing problem and establishes measures to lessen the probability of further occurrence of the problem. Food intake may need to be increased. (See section on cachexia for strategies to increase food intake.) If possible, additional fiber should also be added to the diet. Increasing the intake of fluids is helpful. Various possibilities should be considered for increasing the patient's mobility and physical activity level. Relieving the patient's pain will increase food intake and mobility as well as improve the emotional outlook. The psychologic and social environments are very important and should be manipulated to be positive and supportive.

Stool softeners or bulk laxatives such as Peri-Colace or Metamucil may be given regularly to help prevent constipation. Retention enemas or suppositories that stimulate peristalsis may be helpful in some cases.

When constipation is already present, laxatives or enemas or both may be required. The nurse should be familiar with the side effects and physiologic effects of the laxative to be administered. The time of day when the laxative is given may alter its effectiveness. Possible sleep disruption should also be considered. Enemas function by increasing the bulk in the bowel, increasing peristalsis, and lubricating the feces, thus allowing easier evacuation. Soapsuds enemas and tap water enemas irritate the bowel wall, therefore further increasing peristalsis. Normal saline will cause less bowel wall irritation.

The art of administering an enema has largely been lost in the excitement of learning challenging new nursing skills. This procedure is now usually delegated to "lesser" hospital personnel. However, the way in which an enema is given greatly influences its effectiveness.

The patient should be encouraged to participate in the procedure by concentrating on relaxing and by informing the nurse of cramping. The nurse should reassure the patient that the fluid will be stopped if cramping occurs or if the patient feels that no more fluid can be retained. Sensations that the patient may experience should be described beforehand and the cause for them explained. This allows the patient some control when in a very awkward, helpless position.

The patient should be lying on the left side with the right leg flexed. The bed should be flat. The patient should be appropriately covered to maintain dignity. During the procedure, the nurse should talk to the patient in a soft, reassuring, and calm voice. The patient should be encouraged to relax. An enema will be more effective if it is administered slowly. The enema container should be held no more than 18 inches above the patient.

One of the main reasons for cramping during an enema is the presence of gas in the bowel. This problem can prevent administration of the amount of water needed to effectively cleanse the bowel. Lowering the enema container below the bed during cramping will allow this gas to escape, stop the cramping, and permit the introduction of more fluids.

After the desired amount of fluid has been administered, the patient should be encouraged to retain the fluid for at least 10 minutes. The patient should turn from lying on the left side to lying on the back for 5 minutes and then turn to the right side for 5 minutes. The bed should be kept flat. This maneuver will cause evacuation from a greater portion of the large bowel.

Evacuation of the enema solution may be delayed by this maneuver and may occur in two stages, with one evacuation occurring shortly after the enema and another 30 minutes to an hour later. Some of the fluid may be absorbed by the patient; therefore, an enema should not be used for patients on limited fluid intake. Patients should be told not to expect a normal bowel evacuation the following day.

Manual removal of an impaction is sometimes necessary and must be done very carefully to avoid injury. This procedure may need to be followed by an enema and measures designed to prevent recurrence of the impaction.

Evaluation

Evaluation of nursing measures for constipation must consider whether the measures were accomplished and whether they actually did result in normal bowel evacuations or a decrease in constipation. Because of progressive pathology and the debility of the patient, constipation is likely to be a continuing problem and should be reevaluated regularly.

DIARRHEA

Pathophysiology

Diarrhea in cancer patients may be a consequence of the disease process, but it is more likely to occur as a result of treatments. Radiation therapy to the abdomen may expose some portion of the large bowel. Pelvic radiation is even more likely to cause diarrhea. Although the diarrhea usually occurs for only a few weeks, the damage can be permanent and cause long-term diarrhea.

Chemotherapy can damage the inner lumen of the intestinal tract, causing diarrhea. The severity of the diarrhea is an indication of the seriousness of damage. The diarrhea ceases when the tissue begins to repair itself, but can be severe enough to cause electrolyte imbalances and malnutrition.

Antibiotics very commonly destroy the normal intestinal flora and cause abdominal cramping and diarrhea. In addition to the discomfort, there is a risk of an overgrowth of *Candida* and an intestinal superinfection causing more prolonged diarrhea.

Patients with an impaction may have diarrhea around the impaction. This often causes the impaction to be overlooked and inappropriate treatment to be used to treat the diarrhea. Patients who have a partial obstruction due to growth of the malignancy may also develop diarrhea.

Assessment

Assessment of diarrhea involves more than observing the instance of a liquid stool. It is important to know how frequent the stools are and the approximate amounts of each stool. This information should be carefully recorded on the patient's chart. Changes in the odor of the stool should also be noted.

Planning

The greatest problem with diarrhea is developing strategies that will ensure consistent observing and recording of stools. This sometimes involves convincing the patient of its importance. Patients are frequently embarrassed by the diarrhea and reluctant to summon the nurse to the room to examine a stool. Since diarrhea is considered even more unclean than a normal stool, the urge is to flush it quickly. Also, nursing personnel do not get their greatest joy from looking at diarrhea and may nonverbally communicate this to the patient. In the hierarchy of nursing responsibilities, this may take a low priority. Nursing personnel should be rewarded for consistent observations and recording of diarrhea.

Interventions

Diarrhea will be treated according to its cause. Alterations in the diet may be necessary, including a decrease in roughage. Raw fruits and vegetables, spices, nuts, and coconut may be eliminated. Patients with radiation diarrhea sometimes benefit from the administration of Metamucil. Patients receiving antibiotics may benefit from adding buttermilk and yogurt to their diet, since these substances will tend to restore the normal intestinal flora. Lactinex tablets are also effective for this purpose. Patients with disseminated cancer should be checked for impaction.

The physician may order medication to slow the peristalsis. If the diarrhea is caused by chemotherapy and is severe, oral intake may be discontinued and total parenteral nutrition (TPN) administered until the bowel has healed.

Patients who have diarrhea usually have excoriation in the anal area. This can be very uncomfortable and can increase the risk of infection in the area. A variety of effective ointments are available and should be used regularly to keep the patient comfortable.

In addition to the discomfort, fatigue, and dietary limitations that usually accompany diarrhea, the patient may feel shame and increased social isolation. Eye contact, touching, and frequent visits by the nurse may be helpful. Special diet surprises may help make the restrictions easier to tolerate.

Evaluation

If the diarrhea is self-limiting, it may be difficult to attribute its cessation to effective nursing measures. However, this must be included in any evaluation. Medical treatment may also be more of a factor in diarrhea control than nursing measures. Patient comfort is an important consideration in evaluating nursing measures. Prevention of additional complications from the diarrhea must also be recognized.

FISTULAS, DRAINING WOUNDS, AND ULCERATING METASTATIC LESIONS

Pathophysiology

Fistulas and draining wounds in cancer patients are usually a consequence of four factors: extensive surgery, radiation damage, infection, and recurrent malignancy. Ulcerating metastatic lesions are a direct manifestation of the disease process. These lesions cause multiple problems: odor, drainage (which is often copious and difficult to contain), excoriated skin from exposure to drainage, infection, severe damage to the patient's self-image, social isolation, depression, and shame.

Assessment

The condition of the lesion should be closely assessed. The skin surrounding the lesion should also be examined for inflammation or excoriation. The drainage should be checked to determine if it is blood, feces, pus, digestive enzymes, urine, serum, or saliva. The color, amount, and odor of the drainage should be noted. If a culture of the lesion has not been done recently, one should be obtained. Factors that could impair wound healing — including nutritional status, circulation, fluid and electrolyte balance, blood urea nitrogen (BUN) and serum protein levels, and hydration — should be assessed.[79]

Planning

Nurses often approach fistulas and open lesions with feelings of helplessness, frustration, and avoidance. Measures commonly used to control drainage and odor are often ineffective. In recent years, enterostomal therapists have developed much more effective means to manage these problems. If such an expert is available, it is wise to consult one. Goals for care should include infection and odor control, improvement of wound and skin conditions, improvement in patient comfort, and maintenance of an environment conducive to good mental health.

Interventions

The first step in managing a lesion that has been improperly cared for is to clean it adequately. Proper cleaning will frequently eliminate the odor problem. One useful strategy is to give extensive irrigations every 4 hours with 1000 ml of a solution made of 1 part ½ normal saline and 1 part hydrogen peroxide, followed by packing the lesion with iodoform gauze. Cautions should be taken to prevent flow of the irrigation fluid into other wounds or drains. Ulcerating lesions can be cleaned by scrubbing with soap or detergent. Soap breaks up surface fat and detergent contains hexachlorophene, which is bacteriostatic. Soap or detergent must be thoroughly rinsed off. A washcloth or gauze sponge may be used for this procedure.[28]

Surface lesions may require debridement, as in decubitus care. Enzymatic agents may be used. Oxidizing agents are also useful. These include Dakin's solution (1 part bleach to 9 parts water), hydrogen peroxide, and potassium permanganate.[28] Bacterial reduction is also important. Oxidizing agents are helpful in reducing bacteria, as are povidone-iodine, Silvadene, and acetic acid. Yogurt, which contains live *Lactobacillus,* is an acid medium that will inhibit the growth of some wound bacteria that cause offensive odors.[28, 87]

Odors are primarily a product of infection. Cleansing and debriding will greatly diminish this problem. If odor is still a problem, other measures that can be taken are baking soda sprinkled between bandage layers; liquid products such as Nilodor, Hexol, or Banish applied sparingly to dressings; and clothing or room deodorants.[79]

The patient with a fistula or draining wound will probably require some method of drainage collection. Collector bags commonly used for ostomy patients can sometimes be used. The skin around the wound may be excoriated and may require treatment before application of a bag. After cleansing the area, skin protectors can be applied to the excoriated area. Maalox liquid is very useful; it is soothing and will prevent an allergic reaction to the collector bag adhesive. The Maalox liquid should be thoroughly dried with a small head fan or an electric hair dryer on a cool setting. Karaya paste is then applied over the dried Maalox next to the wound edges and should be allowed to dry.[79] Karaya paste is available commercially, or it can be mixed by using 2 parts karaya powder and 3 parts glycerin.

Skin-bond cement can then be applied on top of the dried karaya paste. This cement should never be placed directly on excoriated skin. The cement should also be applied around the collector opening. The collector bag should not be attached to the wound until the cement is completely dry. If possible, the collector bag should remain in place for several days before being changed. If drainage is greater than 1 liter in 24 hours, tubing should be attached to the drainage bag and connected to continuous suction. Saran wrap can be pressed over any karaya paste not covered by the collector bag to prevent sticking to the bed linens. If the wound is draining urine, karaya paste should not be used, since the urine will disintegrate it. Stomahesive and skin-bond cement will be more effective.[79]

Relieving the odor and drainage problems will greatly alter the patient's attitude. However, the nurse needs to increase touching and eye contact with the patient. Planning frequent visits to the patient can alter patterns of avoidance.

Family members often react very negatively to patients with these offensive types of lesions. They may stop visiting or in other ways reject the patient; for example, they may resist taking the patient home. Eliminating the odor is the first step in dealing with this problem. If the family sees that there are ways to handle the problem, they may be more receptive. Some family members may be willing to learn how to properly care for the lesion. The family may then be more willing to care for the patient at home.

The patient should be allowed to provide self-care as much as possible. Once the procedure has been established, it can become a cooperative venture.[79]

Evaluation

Evaluation of nursing measures for draining or ulcerating lesions must consider improvements in odor, containment of drainage, and skin condition. The morale of the patient is also a good measure of effective interventions. In patients with advanced cancer, these measures are not likely to result in healing of the lesion.

LYMPHEDEMA

Pathophysiology

Lymphedema in cancer patients occurs most frequently in one of two situations: (1) when part of the lymphatic drainage system has been surgically removed, or (2) when a growing tumor has obstructed the lymphatic flow. The process by which lymphedema develops is complex.

Edema is an excess amount of fluid in the interstitial tissues. The fluid dynamics that usually maintain a steady state are disrupted. The amount of fluid entering the interstitial space becomes greater than the fluid leaving. Four main factors influence fluid movement across capillary membranes: capillary permeability, lymphatic drainage, colloid osmotic pressure (controlled by the amount of serum proteins), and hydrostatic pressure in the capillary.

When lymphatic drainage is blocked, protein collects in the tissue spaces. This causes a rise in the colloid osmotic pressure; fluid collects in the tissue spaces; capillary pressure rises; and the edema becomes more severe.[67]

When edema has developed, it tends to perpetuate itself. Collection of fluid causes a rise in capillary pressure, which draws more fluid into the tissue spaces, which in turn continues to increase the pressure.

Lack of muscle activity will cause lymphostasis and predispose the patient to lymphedema; obesity also seems to aggravate lymphedema. Radiation scarring may contribute to edema, and infection, although not the major cause of lymphedema, can increase its severity.[67]

Assessment

Lymphedema usually goes beyond the point of being measured by the degree of pitting from finger pressure. A tape measure can be used to gauge the circumference of an extremity at a carefully selected point. This measure can be used to compare one extremity with the other or note changes in size from one day to the next. Care must be taken to always measure the extremity at the same place and to exert a uniform amount of pressure on the tape.

Planning

Goals related to lymphedema may be to prevent its development, to decrease its severity, or to eliminate it. The most effective strategy, of course, is prevention. Prevention will require all nursing personnel to try to control those factors in the environment that may increase the risk of lymphedema.

Intervention

Two factors involving the patient's physiology are important to the prevention or management of lymphedema: gravity drainage and the lymph-muscle pump. The extremity of concern should be elevated above the level of the heart, with the distal end of the extremity higher than the proximal part. This can be accomplished with pillows, towels, blankets, or if the extremity is a leg, by elevating the foot of the bed. However, the foot cannot be lower than the knee. This position may allow venous pooling in the pelvic area and an increased risk of thrombophlebitis and pulmonary embolism.

Contraction of muscles is an important factor in the movement of lymph through the vessels. Immobile patients are much more likely to develop lymphedema. Active rather than passive exercises are necessary to accomplish the movement of lymph. Any measures that increase the patient's mobility will be helpful. If the patient is bedfast, quadriceps exercises may decrease the risk of lymphedema in the lower extremities.

Women who have had mastectomies can benefit from hand and forearm exercises. Shoulder exercises are sometimes contraindicated until the wound has healed. Rhythmic clenching of the hand into a fist is helpful. The upper arm can be propped up and the patient can brush her hair or teeth or put on make-up with that arm, using elbow and wrist movement.

Mastectomy patients must not have the blood pressure taken on the affected arm, tourniquets should not be used, injections must not be given, and the laboratory personnel must not be allowed to take blood samples from that arm. This is more difficult to accomplish than it would seem. The nurse cannot stand guard in the patient's room for 24 hours a day. Signs can be placed over the patient's bed, but often they are ignored, particularly by laboratory personnel. The most effective strategy is to involve the patient and her family. If the reasons behind the limits are well understood, they can be vigilant 24 hours a day.

After the patient goes home, shoulder exercises should be started. The patient also needs to be taught how to care for the affected arm. For the rest of her life, she must protect that arm similar to the way diabetics must care for their feet. The American Cancer Society recommends that patients:

1. Push cuticles back, no cutting.
2. Use canvas gloves when gardening, rubber gloves when using steel wool.
3. Use padded gloves when reaching into a hot oven.
4. Use a thimble when sewing.
5. Avoid pressure on the arm; wear jewelry, watch, and sleeves loosely.
6. Carry packages and purse on unaffected arm.
7. No B/P, vaccinations, or injections on affected arm.
8. Use an electric razor on affected arm.
9. Avoid sunbaths, hot baths; no heat to affected arm.
10. Smoke with the unaffected arm.
11. Wash any break in skin or cuts with soap and water and cover with a Band-aid.
12. Contact your Doctor immediately if your arm feels hot, is red, or swollen.
13. Keep your arm elevated when sitting.
14. Do not use hormone beauty creams or drugs without consulting your Doctor.[67]

If the patient has lymphedema, the nurse's concern will be with preventing greater edema or decreasing the edema that is present. In some cases, this may be a battle against progressive pathology; however, without adequate nursing care, the problem will be much more severe. An edematous extremity is at greater risk of local infection. The edema also causes a diminished sense of touch, so that injuries or pressure that cuts off local circulation can occur without the patient's knowledge. The nurse must be observant of this patient deficit in order to protect the patient from further damage.

Evaluation

The tape measure is the most effective tool for determining changes in lymphedema or its prevention. If the lymphedema is caused by tumor obstruction, it is difficult to separate the effects of nursing measures from the effects of the growing tumor. Sometimes maintenance of the status quo is in itself an accomplishment.

PATHOLOGIC FRACTURES

Pathophysiology

One of the most common sites for metastatic lesions is bone. This occurs most commonly in patients with cancer of the breast, lung, or prostate. Bone metastases often cause severe pain that is difficult to control. If the bone fractures, healing is usually not possible. However, if the metastasis is identified before fracture occurs, the site can be irradiated. When the malignancy in the bone is destroyed by radiation, fibrous tissue replaces it, thus strengthening the bone and often preventing a fracture. Irradiation will also eliminate the pain in that site. Chemotherapy is usually not very effective in treating bone metastases because of the poor blood supply to bone.

Assessment

Bone metastases or fractures must be identified medically by x-ray studies or bone scans. An x-ray study will not delineate bone metastasis until 60 per cent of the bone is destroyed, whereas a bone scan will identify it much earlier. If the bone fractures, it may be accompanied by pain or a grating feeling over the area. This is usually verified by an x-ray study. It is important for the nurse to know all sites of bone metastases and fractures in order to adequately plan and implement nursing care.

Planning

Nurses are usually very much afraid of caring for patients with pathologic fractures. The patient generally has severe pain, which is intensified by movement. New fractures will sometimes occur when nursing care is being provided. Nurses sometimes feel responsible for the new fractures and thus feel guilty. Nurses may tend to avoid the patient or may take turns caring for the patient. Because moving the patient causes pain and the risk of more fractures, activities requiring movement are greatly decreased. Consequently, the patient is at greater risk of problems on account of severely impaired mobility.

Nurses caring for these patients need a great deal of support. All of the nurses must recognize that the patient must be moved, that fractures may occur during movement, and that the fractures are due to the pathology. However, nursing care can be designed to minimize these risks. Patients can fracture vertebrae or ribs by coughing, sneezing, or laughing.

Interventions

Positioning is extremely important in order to control pain levels in patients with pathologic fractures. Multiple pillows may be needed to accomplish this. Splinting of fractures may also be helpful.

Patients must be turned at least every 2 hours or hypostatic pneumonia can occur, as well as decubiti and other conditions that will severely diminish the patient's quality of life. This is a very difficult procedure, both physically and emotionally. The patient should have adequate pain medication at the time when turning is to be done. Several nursing personnel should assist in turning, which should be accomplished by a procedure similar to the logrolling of patients with back injuries. Patients will often beg not to be turned or will refuse. The pleading will usually cease if the pain can be controlled. A combination of adequate medication and proper handling during movement will greatly decrease the pain.

Families (and even nurses) sometimes do not understand why the turning is necessary. It seems kinder to leave the patient alone. However, these patients are not usually within a few days of death; they can sometimes live for months in this condition. If, in addition to the fractures and pain, they have bedsores, infection, and impairment of eating and elimination, their agony will be heightened.

Emotionally, this situation is difficult for all concerned: anxiety is high, tempers are on edge, nurses feel inadequate. The nurse who remains calm, reassuring, and supportive can defuse this situation. Patient and family should be allowed to participate as much as possible in the care. The possible complications of inadequate movement should be explained. Tactics to diminish pain should be planned with both patient and family.

Patients who have bone metastases are likely to develop hypercalcemia. This condition can be life-threatening and, if detected early, can sometimes be treated. Early signs of hypercalcemia are excessive thirst and urination, since the elevated calcium level promotes diuresis. If hypercalcemia progresses, the patient may become confused or disoriented.

Evaluation

Evaluation of nursing care for patients with pathologic fractures includes diminishment of pain levels and accomplishment of necessary nursing tasks with a minimum of patient discomfort. A positive response by patient and family to nursing care can also be considered, but should not be an absolute standard.

IMPAIRED MOBILITY

Pathophysiology

Mobility is extremely important to health. In recent years, extensive research has been conducted on the effects of immobility. Most body tissues are adversely affected. Muscle tissue is catabolized, bones lose calcium, blood pressure control mechanisms are altered, peristalsis is slowed, blood circulation is diminished, excretion patterns are poor, and the patient is less responsive to sensory stimuli. Time orientation is changed. The patient becomes less interested in interactions with others and tends to become more introverted. The quality of life is severely diminished.

Assessment

Assessing the patient's level of mobility requires careful observation. Although asking questions and reading the patient's chart can give some information, it may not clearly reflect degree of mobility.

Not only the amount of movement, but also the way that the patient moves must be considered. Does the patient lie still in bed or move around? Is turning mostly a passive procedure or does the patient help? If the patient is ambulating, body movements can be observed. Interactions with objects and individuals can also be assessed.

Planning

Mobility is something that must be valued and emphasized by the entire nursing staff. The consequences of immobility must be thoroughly understood. This may require some nursing education and attitude reversal. Mobility should be a high priority activity in caring for cancer patients. However, nurses often tend to be more lenient with cancer patients, perhaps because they feel sorry for them. (This would be an interesting nursing research study.) Patients and families also seem to believe that less mobility should be required. Therefore, plans should be made to include both patient and family in strategies to increase mobility.

Interventions

Patients and family members need to be taught the importance of mobility and specific ways to increase mobility. It may be necessary to encourage movement at each nurse-patient contact.

Quadriceps exercises and simply moving around actively in bed are helpful. Changes in bed position are also effective. A flat bed promotes more body movement.

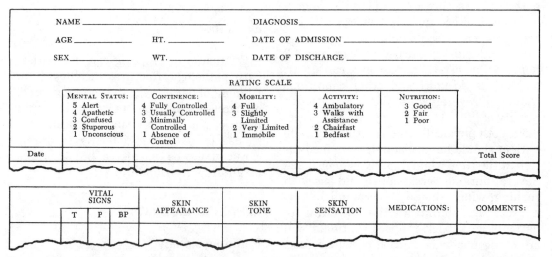

Figure 11–9. Data collection sheets for assessment of patients' potential for pressure sores. (From Gosnell, D. J.: An assessment tool to identify pressure sores. *Nursing Research.* 22:55–59, 1973. Used by permission.)

Bed rails or a trapeze can be very useful in facilitating active changes of position.

Sitting up, standing, or walking can lead to dramatic changes in body functioning and the patient's outlook on life. A little mobility causes changes that will stimulate further movement. These changes also have positive effects on the cancer patient's eating patterns, elimination, circulation, and morale.

Mobility activities should be planned for a specific number of times a day and charted. Since the activities may be performed by nonprofessional nursing personnel, the nurse should check regularly to ensure that they are being carried out. Personnel who value these activities and perform them well should be rewarded.

Evaluation

Evaluation should consider whether the activities were performed as scheduled and whether the patient was able to achieve the desired level of mobility. If it is possible, mobility can then be increased.

Secondary effects of mobility are more difficult to attribute solely to these specific interventions and may be a consequence of other nursing interventions. The absence of complications from immobility can also be used to evaluate the effectiveness of nursing measures.

DECUBITI

Pathophysiology

Decubitus ulcers are caused by pressure on an area, which cuts off the circulation and causes death of the tissues. Decubiti, or pressure sores, are more common in patients in negative nitrogen balance who are underweight, immobile, and incontinent. Once a decubitus has developed, it is difficult to heal. Therefore, prevention is desirable.

Assessment

The patient's skin should be examined regularly for signs of damage from pressure. A reddened area that does not fade quickly should be a source of concern. This is the earliest sign of a pressure sore. A break in the skin will indicate more serious damage. A decubitus is usually rated according to the extensiveness of tissue damage.

It is important also to identify patients who are at high risk of developing a pressure sore. More aggressive nursing measures can then be taken to prevent the development of pressure sores. Gosnell has developed an excellent tool for this assessment. (See Fig. 11–9.) According to Gosnell,[29a] patients at high risk of developing a decubitus ulcer are of either sex, over 65 years of age, and have a circulatory disturbance. Their score on the decubitus assessment scale shows a consistently downward pattern; patients usually have a total score of 11 or less at the time of occurrence of the pressure sore. Mental status is 3 or less and the patient is less than continent, usually with a Foley catheter. Mobility and activity are limited and nutrition is poor. The patient may be on a full liquid diet, has a pulse rate of 80 beats per minute, and has a diastolic blood pressure that is less than 60. The patient usually has had a temperature elevation at some point since admission. Medications being administered include analgesics, cardiotonics, sedatives, and tranquilizers. Touch sensation in the buttocks and the coccyx is decreased.[30]

Planning

Prevention of decubiti requires an all-out effort by all nursing personnel. Patients with advanced cancer are often in a high risk category for decubitus development. Along with aggressive treatment, early detection of pressure signs must be a major goal of nursing.

Interventions

There is an old saying that you can put anything you want on a decubitus to cure it and it will work — as long as you keep the patient off of it. There is some truth to this, but unfortunately the view is a bit simplistic.

The patient should be placed on a circulating mattress or an egg crate mattress. Frequent turning is essential — every 2 hours may not be often enough. Skin care is extremely important. The skin must be kept dry. If the patient is incontinent, linen must be changed frequently. Massage of reddened skin areas may be helpful. Care should be taken to avoid shearing the skin, which occurs when forces pull the skin in two directions at the same time. This can occur in the coccygeal area if the patient is kept in bed with the head of the bed highly elevated. It can also occur during turning.

Treatment of existing decubiti differs in the literature. Debriding agents are often used to get rid of dead tissue. Infection is often present and must be treated locally. The patient must be kept off of the pressure sore to allow healing to occur. Sometimes, if care if not taken, another pressure sore will develop in another site. Healing is slow, very difficult, and expensive. The patient's quality of life is severely affected.

There are many different strategies and many pharmaceutical preparations that may be used to care for decubitus ulcers. The following protocol has been found to be an effective method of treatment.[15, 62a] The protocol changes as the decubitus becomes more severe. Each grade is defined, in order to make assessment and planning of treatment more specific.

Grade I

Involves superficial epidermal and dermal layers. The area is surrounded by a rim of erythematous tissue, heat, and edema, and it usually overlies a body prominence. The skin is not broken.

Treatment:
1. Cleanse skin with soap and water, pat dry.
2. Apply Granulex every 8 hours. Massage gently. Apply heat lamp for 15 minutes twice a day.
3. Turn patient every 2 hours.
4. Pad bony prominences.

Grade II

Involves shallow full thickness skin injury extending into adipose tissue with complete loss of epidermal and dermal layers. The area is surrounded by erythematous tissue, heat, and edema. The skin is broken.

Treatment:
1. Cleanse wound with Betadine. Rinse with normal saline, pat dry.
2. Fill wound ½-inch deep with dry DEBRISAN granules. (May use glycerine to make a paste if the wound is shallow.) Cover with light dressing.
3. Turn patient at least every 2 hours.
4. Check dressing each shift. Repeat treatment when DEBRISAN granules become saturated (normally every 12 hours). Wound *MUST* be irrigated well at each change to remove all old DEBRISAN granules.

   (NOTE: The purpose of DEBRISAN is to absorb the exudate so that the wound can heal. If DEBRISAN is used after the wound is dry, tissue fluid will also be extracted, causing formation of eschar and delaying healing.)
5. After wound is dry, switch to following protocol:
   a. Cleanse wound with Betadine. Rinse with normal saline, pat dry.
   b. Apply Granulex every 8 hours. Massage gently.
   c. Turn patient at least every 2 hours.
   d. Pad bony prominences.

Grade III

Deeper progression into fascial layer with complete loss of epidermal and dermal

DECUBITUS ULCER FLOW SHEET

Name _____ # _____ Age _____ M.D. _____

Date of Onset _____ Before Admission _____ After Admission _____

Location _____ Risk Score _____
                                                                                              (From Form 101)

PARAMETERS	DATES				
Stage					
Reddened only					
Broken skin					
Crater					
Infection					
Description					
Size					
Exudate*					
Odor*					
Inflammation*					
Crater content*					
Treatment					
Turning schedule					
Padding					
Sheep skin					
Air mattress					
Dressings					
Antibiotic-topical					
Antibiotic-systemic					
Debridement-manual					
Debridement-enzyme					
Whirlpool					
Other					
Cultures					
Signatures					

Figure 11–10. Decubitus ulcer flow sheet. (Used by permission of the Knoll Pharmaceutical Company, Whippany, New Jersey. Copyright 1977.)
  *Rate on a scale of 0 to 3; where 0 = none, 1 = slight, 2 = marked, and 3 = severe.

layers. May have serosanguineous drainage. May have large amount of necrotic or eschar tissue. This tissue must be debrided before healing can take place.

Treatment:

1. Debride wound.
   a. Surgical debridement (by physician).
   b. Enzyme debridement: Wound must be free of necrotic tissue for healing to take place. To debride wound using enzymes:
      (1) Obtain debriding ointment (this usually requires a physician's order).
      (2) Cleanse wound using H_2O_2. Rinse with normal saline.
      (NOTE: Use H_2O_2 only when trying to remove necrotic tissue. H_2O_2 is *HARMFUL* to *NEW* granulation tissue. Some debridement ointments are ineffective if Betadine (or iodine solutions) is used. Therefore, Betadine *SHOULD NOT* be used when using Travase, Elase, Santyl, or other such debridement ointments.
      (3) Dry wounds using O_2 for approximately 10 minutes. This helps to destroy anaerobic bacteria. Garamycin ointment can be applied to the rim of the ulcer.
      (4) Apply debridement ointment.
      (5) Spray surrounding healthy tissue with Granulex.
      (6) Apply ABD dressing. Use tape sparingly.
      (7) Repeat treatment three times a day.
   c. Turn patient at least every 2 hours.
   d. Pad bony prominences.
   e. After wound is debrided and dry, switch to the following protocol:
      (1) Cleanse wound with Betadine. Rinse with normal saline, pat dry.
      (2) Apply Granulex every 8 hours. Massage gently.
      (3) Turn patient at least every 2 hours.
      (4) Pad bony prominences.

Grade IV

Most advanced stage. Progression through full thickness of epidermal, dermal, adipose, fascial, and soft tissue layers. Necrosis to point of communication with bones and/or joint. Eschar may be present.

Treatment:

1. Ask physician to trim eschar from edges.
2. Cleanse wound with H_2O_2. Rinse with normal saline.
3. Apply debridement ointment to eschar.
4. Cover with light dressing.
5. Turn at least every 2 hours.
6. Pad bone prominences.
7. When eschar is removed, treat according to Grade II decubitus.

Evaluation

Evaluation of nursing care designed to prevent decubiti is based on whether or not decubiti develop. Evaluation of treatment of existing decubiti must be based on whether or not healing occurs. Severity of the pathology that affects decubitus formation must be considered. A flow sheet may be helpful in evaluating the effectiveness of treatment. (See Fig. 11–10.)

BIBLIOGRAPHY

1. Alexander, L. and J. Barry: Nursing management of the oncology patient in pain. In *Dynamics of Oncology Nursing,* ed. by P. K. Burkhalter and D. L. Donley. McGraw-Hill Book Company, New York, 1978.
2. Armstrong, D.: Life threatening infections in cancer patients. *CA — A Cancer Journal for Clinicians.* 23:138–150, 1973.
3. Armstrong, M. E.: Acupuncture. In *Pain: A Source Book for Nurses and Other Health Professionals,* ed. by A. K. Jacox. Little, Brown and Company, Boston, 1977.
4. Barber, J.: Hypnosis as a psychological technique in the management of cancer pain. *Cancer Nursing.* 1:361–363, 1978.
5. Barber, J. and J. Gitelson: Cancer pain: psychological management using hypnosis. *CA — A Cancer Journal for Clinicians.* 30:130–136, 1980.
6. Bates, M. D., and M. B. Orton: Infection control in clients with acute leukemia. In *Cancer Nursing,* ed. by L. B. Marino. C. V. Mosby Co., St. Louis, 1981.
7. Benoliel, J. Q., and D. M. Crowley: The patient in

pain: new concepts. In *Cancer: Pathophysiology, Etiology, and Management,* ed. by L. C. Kruse, J. Reese and L. K. Hart. C. V. Mosby Co., St. Louis, 1979.

8. Benson, H.: *The Relaxation Response.* Avon Books, New York, 1976.

9. Boguslawski, M.: Therapeutic touch: a facilitator of pain relief. *Topics in Clinical Nursing.* 2:37–38, 1980.

10. Bonica, J. J.: Cancer pain: a major national health problem. *Cancer Nursing.* 1:313–316, 1978.

11. Borgen, L.: Total parenteral nutrition in adults. *American Journal of Nursing.* 78:224, 1978.

12. Budzynski, T.: Biofeedback procedures in the clinic. In *Pain: A Source Book for Nurses and Other Health Professionals,* ed. by A. K. Jacox. Little, Brown and Company, Boston, 1977.

13. Butler, J. H.: Nutrition and cancer: a review of the literature. *Cancer Nursing.* 3:131–136, 1980.

14. Charap, A. D.: The knowledge, attitudes and experience of medical personnel treating pain in the terminally ill. *The Mount Sinai Journal of Medicine.* 45:561–580, 1978.

14a. Cleveland, S. A.: Treating decubitus ulcers: a nursing study comparing a research-based protocol with non-structural protocols. Unpublished master's thesis, University of Texas at Arlington, 1981.

15. Copeland, E. M. III and S. J. Dudrick: Cancer: nutritional concepts. *Seminars in Oncology.* 2:329–335, 1975.

16. Costa, G.: Cachexia and the systemic effects of tumors. In *Cancer Medicine,* ed. by J. I. Holland and E. Frei. Philadelphia, Lee & Febiger, 1973.

17. Coyle, N.: Analgesics at the bedside. *American Journal of Nursing.* 79:1554–1557, 1979.

18. Crasilneck, H. B., and J. A. Hall: Clinical hypnosis in problems of pain. In *Pain: A Source Book for Nurses and Other Health Professionals,* ed. by A. K. Jacox. Little, Brown and Company, Boston, 1977.

19. Davis, A. J.: Brompton's cocktail: making goodbyes possible. *American Journal of Nursing.* 78:610–612, 1978.

20. Davitz, L. L., J. R. Davitz, and C. F. Rubin: *Nurses' Responses to Patients' Suffering.* Springer Publishing Co., New York, 1980.

21. Dewys, W. D.: A spectrum of organ systems that respond to the presence of cancer: abnormalities of taste as a remote effect of a neoplasm. *Annals of the New York Academy of Sciences.* 230:427–434, 1974.

22. Dewys, W. D., and L. Walters: Abnormalities of taste sensation in cancer patients. *Cancer.* 36:1888, 1975.

23. Diggory, G. and R. Tiffany: The use of entonox in the relief of pain. *Cancer Nursing.* 2:279–282, 1979.

24. Donovan, M. I. and S. G. Pierce: *Cancer Care Nursing.* Appleton-Century-Crofts, New York, 1976.

25. Englert, D. M. and S. J. Dudrick: Principles of ambulatory home hyperalimentation. *Ameri-can Journal of Intravenous Therapy.* 5:11–28, 1978.

26. Fagerhaugh, S. Y. and A. Strauss: *Politics of Pain Management: Staff-Patient Interaction.* Addison-Wesley Publishing Co., Menlo Park, Ca., 1977.

27. Fidler, M. R. and A. Whidden: Pathophysiology of pain. In *Pain: A Source Book for Nurses and Other Health Professionals,* ed. by A. K. Jacox. Little, Brown and Company, Boston, 1977.

28. Foltz, A. T.: Nursing care of ulcerating metastatic lesions. *Oncology Nursing Forum.* 7:8–13, 1980.

29. Gebhart, G. F.: Narcotic and non-narcotic analgesics for relief of pain. In *Pain: A Source Book for Nurses and Other Health Professionals,* ed. by A. K. Jacox. Little, Brown and Company, Boston, 1977.

29a. Gosnell, D. J.: An assessment total to identify pressure sores. *Nursing Research.* 22:55–59, 1973.

30. Graham, V. and B. J. Rubal: Recipient and donor response to granulocyte transfusion and leukapheresis. *Cancer Nursing.* 3:97–100, 1980.

31. Greene, R.: Physicians, pain and cancer patients. *Hospital Physician.* 14:36–37, 1978.

32. Guerry, D. IV: Pain management. In *The Cancer Patient: Social and Medical Aspects of Care,* ed. by B. R. Cassileth. Lea & Febiger, Philadelphia, 1979.

33. Harris, J. G.: Nausea, vomiting and cancer. *CA — A Cancer Journal for Clinicians.* 28:194–201, 1978.

34. Heidt, P.: Effect of therapeutic touch on anxiety level of hospitalized patients. *Nursing Research.* 30:32–37, 1981.

35. Jacox, A. K.: Sociocultural and psychological aspects of pain. In *Pain: A Source Book for Nurses and Other Health Professionals,* ed. by A. K. Jacox. Little, Brown and Company, Boston, 1977.

36. Jacox, A. K. and A. G. Robers: The nursing management of pain. In *Cancer Nursing,* ed. by L. B. Marino. C. V. Mosby Co., St. Louis, 1981.

37. Johnson, M.: Assessment of clinical pain. In *Pain: A Source Book for Nurses and Other Health Professionals,* ed. by A. K. Jacox. Little, Brown and Company, Boston, 1977.

38. Krieger, D.: *The Therapeutic Touch: How to Use Your Hands to Help or Heal.* Prentice-Hall, Inc., Englewood Cliffs, N.J., 1979.

39. Krieger, D. and E. Peper, and S. Ancoli: Therapeutic touch: searching for evidence of physiological change. *American Journal of Nursing.* 79:660–662, 1979.

40. Lipman, A. G.: Drug therapy in cancer pain. *Cancer Nursing.* 3:39–46, 1980.

41. Luckmann, J. and K. C. Sorensen: *Medical-Surgical Nursing: A Psychophysiologic Approach.* W. B. Saunders Co., Philadelphia, 1980.

42. Mackey, C. and A. W. Hopefl: Keeping infections down when risks go up. *Nursing 80.* 10:69–73, 1980.

43. Marks, R., and E. Sachar: Undertreatment of medical inpatients with narcotic analgesics. *Annals of Internal Medicine.* 78:173–181, 1973.

44. Mathews, G. J., V. Zarro and J. L. Osterholm: Cancer pain and its treatment. *Seminars in Drug Treatment.* 3:45–53, 1973.

45. McCaffery, M.: Understanding your patient's pain. *Nursing 80.* 10:26–31, 1980.

46. McCaffery, M.: Relieving pain with non-invasive techniques. *Nursing 80.* 10:54–57, 1980.

47. McCaffery, M.: *Nursing Management of the Patient with Pain.* J. B. Lippincott Co., Philadelphia, 1979.

48. McCorkle, R. and K. Young: Development of a symptom distress scale. *Cancer Nursing.* 1:373–378, 1978.

49. McDonnell, D.: Surgical and electrical stimulation methods for relief of pain. In *Pain: A Source Book for Nurses and Other Health Professionals,* ed. by A. K. Jacox. Little, Brown and Company, Boston, 1979.

50. Meissner, J.: Which patient on your unit might get a pressure sore? *Nursing 80.* 10:64–65, 1980.

51. Melzack. R., B. Mount, and J. M. Gordon: The Brompton mixture versus morphine solution given orally: effects on pain. *CMA Journal.* 120:435–438, 1979.

52. Melzack. R. and P. D. Wall: Psychophysiology of pain. In *Pain: A Source Book for Nurses and Other Health Professionals,* ed. by A. K. Jacox. Little, Brown and Company, Boston, 1979.

53. Miaskowski, C.: The Brompton cocktail. *Cancer Nursing.* 1:451–455, 1978.

54. Michelsen, D.: Giving a great back rub. *American Journal of Nursing.* 78:1197–1199, 1978.

55. Minton, J. P.: General factors in cancer management. In *Clinical Oncology,* ed. by J. Horton and G. J. Hill, II. W. B. Saunders Co., Philadelphia, 1977.

56 Mount, B. M., I. Ajemian, and J. F. Scott: Use of the Brompton mixture in treating the chronic pain of malignant disease. *CMA Journal.* 115:122–124, 1976.

57. Mullen, J. L. and C. L. Hobbs: *The Cancer Patient: Social and Medical Aspects of Care,* ed. by B. R. Cassileth. Lea & Febiger, Philadelphia, 1979.

58. Mundinger, M. O.: Nursing diagnoses for cancer patients. *Cancer Nursing.* 1:221–226, 1978.

59. Nathanson, L.: Remote effects of cancer on the host. In *Clinical Oncology,* ed. by J. Horton and G. J. Hill, II. W. B. Saunders Co., Philadelphia, 1977.

60. *Nutrition: Its Special Importance to You.* Adrian Laboratories, Inc., Columbus, Ohio, 1979.

61. Oberst, M. T.: Cancer cachexia. *Cancer Nursing.* 1:402, 1978.

62. Patterson, P.: Granulocyte transfusion: nursing considerations. *Cancer Nursing.* 3:101–104, 1980.

62a. Perkins, S. Personal communication.

63. Rankin, M.: The progressive pain of cancer. *Topics in Clinical Nursing.* 2:57–74, 1980.

64. Rogers, M.: *Introduction to the Theoretical Basis of Nursing.* F. A. Davis Co., Philadelphia, 1970.

65. Rose, J. C.: Nutritional problems in radiotherapy patients. *American Journal of Nursing.* 78:1194–1196, 1978.

66. Rowlingson, J. C.: Management of cancer pain. *Cancer Nursing.* 1:317–318, 1978.

67. Rudolph, B. J.: Lymphedema following a radical mastectomy. *Oncology Nursing Forum.* 6:13–17, 1979.

68. Sabiston, D. C., Jr.: Pulmonary Embolism. In *Davis-Christopher Textbook of Surgery,* 12th edition, ed. by D. C. Sabiston, Jr. W. B. Saunders Co., Philadelphia, 1981.

69. Salmond, S. W.: How to assess the nutritional status of acutely ill patients. *American Journal of Nursing.* 80:922–924, 1980.

70. Saunders, C.: Control of pain in terminal cancer. *Nursing Times.* 72:1133–1135, 1976.

71. Schein, P. S., J. S. Macdonald, C. Waters, and D. Haidak: Nutritional complications of cancer and its treatment. *Seminars in Oncology.* 2:337–347, 1975.

72. Schneider, W. R.: Nutrition in head and neck cancer: nursing implications. *Oncology Nursing Forum.* 6:5–7, 1979.

73. Shabert, J.: Nutrition and cancer. In *Dynamics of Oncology Nursing,* ed. by P. K. Burkhalter and D. L. Donley. McGraw-Hill Book Company, New York, 1978.

74. Shawver, M. M.: Pain associated with cancer. In *Pain: A Source Book for Nurses and Other Health Professionals,* ed. by A. K. Jacox. Little, Brown and Company, Boston, 1977.

75. Shealy, C. N.: Holistic management of chronic pain. *Topics in Clinical Nursing.* 2:1–8, 1980.

76. Silman, J.: The management of pain: reference guide to analgesics. *American Journal of Nursing.* 79:74–78, 1979.

77. Sternbach, R. A.: *Pain: A Psychophysiological Analysis.* Academic Press, Inc., New York, 1968.

78. Stewart M. L.: Measurement of clinical pain. In *Pain: A Source Book for Nurses and Other Professionals,* ed. by A. K. Jacox. Little, Brown and Company, Boston, 1977.

79. Taylor, V.: Meeting the challenge of fistulas and draining wounds. *Nursing 80.* 10:45–51, 1980.

80. Terzian, M. P.: Neurosurgical interventions for the management of chronic intractable pain. *Topics in Clinical Nursing.* 2:75–88, 1980.

81. Theologides, A.: Pathogenesis of cachexia in cancer: a review and a hypothesis. *Cancer.* 29:484–488, 1972.

82. Twycross, R. G.: Disease of the central nervous system: relief of terminal pain. *British Medical Journal.* 4:212–214, 1975.

83. Valentine, A. S., S. Steckel, and M. Weintraub: Pain relief for cancer patients. *American Journal of Nursing.* 78:2054–2056, 1978.

84. Welch, D. A.: Assessment of nausea and vomiting in cancer patients undergoing external brain radiotherapy. *Cancer Nursing.* 3:365–371, 1980.

85. Welch, D. A.: Hi-protein nutritional supplement. *Oncology Nursing Forum.* 7:24, 1980.

86. Wolf, Z. R.: Pain theories: an overview. *Topics in Clinical Nursing.* 2:9–18, 1980.

87. Yates, J. W.: Problems in neoplastic disease: infections. *Seminars in Drug Treatment.* 3:27–35, 1973.

12

Psychosocial Aspects of Nursing Care

INTRODUCTION

Once overlooked, the psychosocial aspects of cancer are being more comprehensively explored in the literature.[12, 15, 22, 28, 34] The problems experienced by cancer patients and the care that they "ought" to be given are usually described in detail; however, the nurse must often make a large cognitive leap to apply that information to clinical practice. This chapter is designed to assist the nurse in that process.

Psychosocial reactions to cancer are usually a consequence of negative beliefs about cancer and physiologic changes that occur during the disease process or as a result of treatment. These reactions are best described as part of a process that begins when cancer is first suspected and continues throughout the course of the disease.[2, 8, 25, 33, 43, 47, 64, 69, 75] The developmental stage of the patient during this process will greatly affect the reactions.[4]

Many of these psychosocial reactions are harmful and can diminish the patient's quality of life. Some health care professionals believe that these reactions can have an effect on whether the patient lives or dies or on the length of survival. Unfortunately, some professionals think that little can be done to alter psychosocial reactions to cancer and, therefore, tend to disregard them. Others believe that only professionals highly skilled in psychosocial interventions (such as psychiatrists or psychologists) can be effective in providing this care.

The last two attitudes could lead health care givers to avoid responsibility and accountability for providing effective psychosocial interventions. Certainly, it is not possible for the nurse to cure the patient's cancer and thus relieve the patient's primary cause for distress. One or 2 years of psychotherapy might promote more positive changes in the patient's mental health than the nurse could ever facilitate. But psychosocial interventions are not an all-or-nothing matter. It is possible to help patients alter their perceptions of the situation, improve their coping strategies, and thus alter their response to the situation. In a way, the patient's condition cannot be changed. But a changed response may mitigate the actual situation.

PSYCHOSOCIAL ASSESSMENT

Before plans can be made for effective interventions, it is necessary to conduct a thorough psychosocial assessment. This assessment requires time and must be preceded by the establishment of a trusting nurse-patient relationship. Patients will usually be more willing to allow a physical examination by a stranger than to reveal their inner self, as is vital to a psychosocial assessment.

This is an area in which institutional forces may interfere with or prevent the provision of adequate nursing care. Since psychosocial assessment and interventions are not usually valued or rewarded by health care institutions, it may be difficult

Table 12–1. List of 122 Psychosocial Problems*

I. *Physical Discomfort*
1. Prehospital physical discomfort
2. Current physical discomfort
3. Side effects—hospitalization
4. Side effects—surgery
5. Side effects—chemotherapy
6. Side effects—radiation
7. Side effects—medication

II. *Upset re: Medical Treatment*
8. Surgery upsetting
9. Chemotherapy upsetting
10. Radiation upsetting
11. Medication upsetting
12. Side effects—hospitalization upsetting
13. Side effects—chemotherapy upsetting
14. Side effects—radiation upsetting
15. Side effects—medication upsetting
16. Future procedures upsetting (surgery)
17. Future procedures upsetting (chemotherapy)
18. Future procedures upsetting (radiation)
19. Future procedures upsetting (medication)

III. *Dissatisfaction with Medical Service*
20. General hospital care
21. House staff
22. Nursing staff
23. Nursing aides
24. Friends/family visiting (due to transportation or finances)
25. Hospital discharge plans
26. Hospital accounting dept.
27. Lack of social service
28. Effectiveness of social service/psychosocial intervention program
29. Lack of physical therapy
30. Effectiveness of physical therapy
31. Lack of counseling
32. Effectiveness of counseling
33. Lack of Reach to Recovery (breast patients)
34. Effectiveness of Reach to Recovery
35. Physician care
36. Getting questions put to M.D. answered
37. Adequate medical advice
38. Ongoing medical care
39. Transportation to medical care
40. Taking time off from home

IV. *Mobility*
41. Personal care of self
42. Physical mobility
43. Limited range of movement (ROM)
44. Carrying, lifting things

V. *Housework*
45. Housework routine
46. Household business (at home)
47. Household business (away)
48. Home maintenance
49. Personal care (helping other adults)
50. Physical changes in home

VI. *Vocational*
51. Taking time off from work/school
52. Responsibilities changing
53. Employer treating patient differently
54. Co-workers treating patient differently
55. Looking for work
56. Employment agencies, employers
57. Acquisition of new skills
58. Not working
59. Loss of time from school
60. School administration treating patient differently
61. Classmates treating patient differently
62. Change in career plans
63. Career planning

VII. *Financial*
64. Finances

VIII. *Family*
65. Change in activities with family
66. Child-related activities (at home)
67. Child-related activities (away)
68. Significant other's (SO's) reaction to illness
69. Change in relationship with SO
70. Family reaction to illness
71. Change in interaction with family (at home)
72. Change in interaction with family (away)
73. Change in interaction with family (phone calls/letters)
74. Change in family role
75. Change in relationship with family members

IX. *Social*
76. Change in activities alone
77. Change in activities with friends
78. Personal solitary activity (at home—active)
79. Personal solitary activity (at home—idle)
80. Personal solitary activity (away)
81. Change in pattern of dating
82. Change in interaction with friends (at home)
83. Change in interaction with friends (away)
84. Change in interaction with friends (phone calls/letters)
85. Friend's reaction to illness

X. *Worry re: Disease*
86. Symptoms affect patient emotionally
87. Past hospital procedures upsetting
88. Routine checkups upsetting
89. Future procedures upsetting (general)
90. Future procedures upsetting (hospitalization)
91. Future procedures upsetting (routine checkups)
92. Worry re: medical condition
93. Watching news media

XI. *Affect*
94. "Hospitalization" upsetting
95. Depression (feeling low, down, or blue)
96. Being irritable, on edge
97. Feelings interfering with daily activities
98. Sleeping
99. Eating
100. Concentrating

XII. *Body Image*
101. Changes in clothing
102. Prosthesis
103. A change in sex life
104. Sex life upsetting
105. Side effects—surgery upsetting

XIII. *Communication*
106. Asking questions of M.D.
107. Employer knowing/not knowing about illness
108. Co-workers knowing/not knowing about illness
109. Telling/not telling prospective employers
110. School administration knowing/not knowing about illness
111. Classmates knowing/not knowing about illness
112. Not talking to SO
113. Talking to SO not being helpful
114. Not talking enough to SO
115. Talking to SO about future
116. Not talking to family
117. Talking to family not being helpful
118. Talking not enough to family
119. Talking to family about future
120. Not talking to friends
121. Talking to friends not being helpful
122. Not talking enough to friends

*From Freidenbergs, I., Gordon, W., Ruckdeschel, M., and Diller, L.: Assessment and treatment of psychosocial problems of the cancer patient: a case study. *Cancer Nursing.* 3:111–119, 1980. Used by permission of Masson Publishing USA, Inc., New York. Copyright 1980.

to find the time to do an adequate assessment, but it is still essential. The assessment need not be completed at one session. Data can be collected over a period of time and recorded in a systematic way.

Several excellent guides have been developed for conducting a psychosocial assessment.[24, 25, 46, 49, 52, 71] Francis and Munjas[24] provide a very thorough assessment that takes 3 hours to complete. Although it is designed for the psychiatric patient, many portions of it can be very useful in assessing the cancer patient and family.

A nursing history and physical examination should proceed or accompany the psychosocial assessment. The assessment should be conducted with the assumption that the patient has an average level of mental health and is presently experiencing a situation that commonly alters affect, social interactions, and behavior. The nurse is therefore not searching for signs of mental illness, but is collecting data to determine the patient's and family's capacity for managing the present situation and to use in nursing interventions that might improve that capacity.

Freidenbergs and colleagues have taken a different approach to the psychosocial assessment.[25] They have attempted to identify the areas that patients perceive as problems. (See Table 12–1.) The severity of each problem is rated by patients on a 10-point scale (1 = mild, 10 = severe). The responses are then used in order to plan nursing interventions. This information can be useful if collected in addition to the previously suggested assessment.

Weisman has developed criteria for assessing the coping strategies commonly used in the cancer situation and determining the person's degree of vulnerability.[69, 71] Through careful research, Weisman has identified coping strategies commonly used by cancer patients. Some of these strategies are much more effective in solving problems than others. (See Table 12–2.) Determining coping strategies is not an easy task and requires some skill in interviewing people and evaluating their re-

Table 12–2. General Coping Strategies*

1. Seek more information (rational inquiry)
2. Share concern and talk with others (mutuality)
3. Laugh it off; make light of situation (affect reversal)
4. Try to forget; put it out of your mind (suppression)
5. Do other things for distraction (displacement/redirection)
6. Take firm action based on present understanding (confront)
7. Accept but find something favorable (redefine/revise)
8. Submit to the inevitable; fatalism (passive acceptance)
9. Do something, anything, however reckless or impractical (impulsive)
10. Consider or negotiate feasible alternatives (if x, then y)
11. Reduce tension with excessive drink, drugs, danger (life threats)
12. Withdraw into isolation; get away (disengagement)
13. Blame someone or something (externalize/project)
14. Seek direction; do what you're told (cooperative compliance)
15. Blame yourself; sacrifice or atone (moral masochism)

*From Weisman, A. D.: *Coping with Cancer.* New York: McGraw-Hill Book Co., 1979. Used by permission.

sponses. Weisman suggests asking the following questions:

1. What problems, if any, do you see this illness creating?

2. How do you plan to deal with them?

3. When faced with a problem you must do something about, what happens? What do you do?

4. How does it usually work out?

5. To whom do you turn when you need help?

6. What has happened in the past when you've asked for help?

7. What kinds of problems usually tend to get you down or upset?[69]

Some people are more vulnerable to distress in the cancer situation; they tend to cope less effectively. If they can be identified, effective interventions can be used to strengthen their coping strategies and lessen their distress. Weisman has developed a tool for determining the patient's degree of vulnerability.[69] (See Fig. 12–1.) Weisman has also identified those factors that correlate with a high level of vulnerability and a low level of vulnerability. He classifies these as higher emotional distress (HED) and lower emotional distress (LED). (See Table 12–3.)

Most of the data needed for this estimation are available from the previously suggested psychosocial assessment.

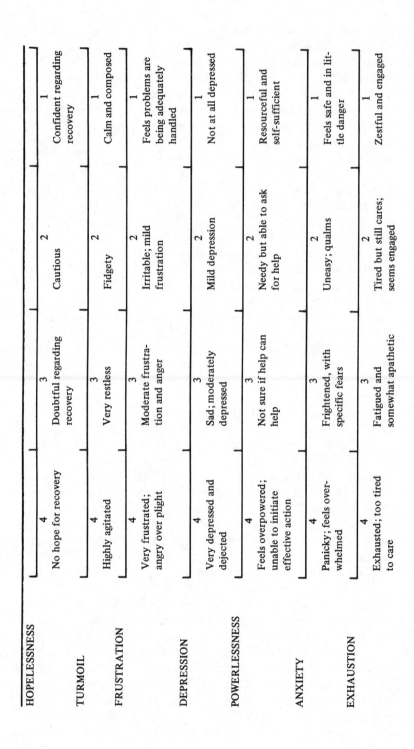

	4	3	2	1
HOPELESSNESS	No hope for recovery	Doubtful regarding recovery	Cautious	Confident regarding recovery
TURMOIL	Highly agitated	Very restless	Fidgety	Calm and composed
FRUSTRATION	Very frustrated; angry over plight	Moderate frustration and anger	Irritable; mild frustration	Feels problems are being adequately handled
DEPRESSION	Very depressed and dejected	Sad; moderately depressed	Mild depression	Not at all depressed
POWERLESSNESS	Feels overpowered; unable to initiate effective action	Not sure if help can help	Needy but able to ask for help	Resourceful and self-sufficient
ANXIETY	Panicky; feels overwhelmed	Frightened, with specific fears	Uneasy; qualms	Feels safe and in little danger
EXHAUSTION	Exhausted; too tired to care	Fatigued and somewhat apathetic	Tired but still cares; seems engaged	Zestful and engaged

	4	3	2	1
WORTHLESSNESS	Worthless; not okay and never will be; undeserving	I'm not okay; feels flawed and inadequate	I'm okay but I goof-up, make mistakes	I'm okay; strong self-regard
ABANDONMENT	Feels abandoned and rejected	Lonely and isolated	Feels somewhat neglected	Feels cared for and well looked after
DENIAL	Avoids speaking word "cancer" or its equivalent	Admits diagnosis and illness, but denies implications	Uncertain or uses euphemism	Correct perception of illness and related problems
TRUCULENCE	Feels victimized, bitter, mistreated by caregivers	Has doubts and serious questions regarding care and treatment	Believes that only "adequate" care is being given	Feels that very good care is received. Very positive attitude to caregivers
REPUDIATION OF SKO	Rejects or antagonizes sources of support	Mild rejection of others; somewhat sullen	Accepts help grudgingly	Gladly accepts sources of help and support
TIME PERSPECTIVE	Closed; no tomorrow	Only a day at a time	Cautious about future; wait and see	Unlimited; foresees future as if no illness

Figure 12–1. Omega vulnerability rating scale. (From Weisman, A. D.: *Coping with Cancer.* New York: McGraw-Hill Book Co., 1979. Used by permission.)

Table 12–3. Correlates of Vulnerability*

Higher Emotional Stress (HED)	Lower Emotional Stress (LED)
1. Pessimistic, including outcome of illness	1. Optimistic attitudes in general
2. Regrets about past	2. Fewer regrets, if any
3. History of psychiatric treatment or suicidal ideation	3. Less entensive psychiatric treatment, if any
4. High anxiety; low ego strength (MMPI)†	4. Low anxiety; high ego strength
5. Marital problems prior to cancer	5. Few marital problems, if any
6. Lower socioeconomic status	6. Higher socioeconomic status
7. More alcohol abuse	7. Abstinence or use, not abuse
8. Multiproblem background	8. Few problems in background
9. Little or no church attendance	9. Church attendance
10. More physical symptoms	10. Fewer physical symptoms
11. Cancer at advanced stage	11. Less advanced cancer stage
12. Expects little support from others	12. Expects adequate support
13. Doctor seen as less helpful	13. Doctor's help is adequate at least
14. More current concerns of all kinds	14. Fewer current concerns
15. Feels more like giving up	15. Fewer giving up feelings
16. Poor problem resolution	16. Better problem resolution
17. More Cope 4, 8, 12, 13, 15‡	17. More Cope 6, 7, 14‡
Not significant: age, marital status, lagtime until diagnosis, life stress events	

*From Weisman, A. D.: *Coping with Cancer.* New York: McGraw-Hill Book Co., 1979. Used by permission.
†Minnesota Multiphasic Personality Inventory.
‡See Table 12–2.

NURSING GOALS

Nurturing the Patient

The patient must feel cared for and cared about before psychosocial nursing interventions can be effectively utilized. The first step in the process is the establishment of trust within a nurse-patient relationship. Such trust, however, does not emerge fully developed; it increases over time as a result of the patient's positive experiences with the nurse.

Nursing behaviors that tend to increase trust are genuineness, openness, expression of a desire to help, a moderate amount of touching and eye contact, expression of acceptance of the patient, nonjudgmental behavior, a moderate amount of self-revelation, communication of competence, and successful nursing interventions. The development of trust is also dependent on the patient's general ability to trust others and any previous experiences with nurses and the health care system. To some extent, trust is a two-way process. The nurse must also be willing to trust the patient. This trust is involved in believing what the patient says and in the mutual planning process.

Nurturing involves a feeling on the part of patients that the nurse is acting in their best interests. It does not necessarily require that patients function in the passive, dependent role. However, it does require feeling cared for and cared about. (Warmth and friendliness are essential characteristics that must accompany competence in effective nursing care.) This type of nursing care is possible in outpatient clinics and home care as well as in hospital settings. In the hospital, control of the environment is an essential part of caring.[30] The nurse's behaviors related to nourishment, pain relief, comfort care, frequency of contact, and attempts to relieve symptoms indicate that the patient is cared for. If the patient interprets the nurse's behavior as rejecting, critical, or negligent, the patient will not feel cared about.

Encouraging Effective Communication

Negative beliefs about cancer alter communication patterns between the patient and many other people: physicians, nurses, family members, friends, and even casual contacts. These changes can be the most devastating part of cancer.[32] The patient may personally alter communication as a result of feelings of shame, unworthiness, guilt, fear, and movement into the passive, dependent role. Others may alter communication with the patient in an attempt to protect the patient or to avoid causing themselves emotional pain.

The nurse is in a strategic position at the crossroads of these communication patterns. Thus, the nurse may be able to intervene at many points to facilitate changes in communication patterns. Cancer patients may find that expressing their feelings is no longer acceptable to some persons. Disapproval is usually expressed nonverbally. The person may change the subject; facial expression, gestures, and body position may change; or the person may move slightly farther away from the patient. In some instances, the person may actually withdraw from the patient. This may sound like something that only an immature family member might do, but it commonly occurs with nurses and physicians. Patients become skilled in testing the people they talk to by first lightly expressing some nonthreatening feeling. If there is no reaction, the patient may test them with a stronger feeling. If the people show any sign of anxiety or withdrawal, the patient will make no further attempts to express feelings to them. Because of this, patients are often left with no one with whom they can express feelings. Nurses especially need to be very aware of their emotional reactions to the communications of cancer patients. It is foolish to believe that these personal reactions can be concealed.

Communication of permission to express feelings is often best done nonverbally. Openness can be suggested by keeping arms and legs in uncrossed positions and by leaning slightly toward the patient. When the patient expresses feelings, moving slightly toward the patient will encourage further communication of feelings. Touching can also be helpful with some patients. Other patients are very threatened by touch. Therefore, it is usually best to begin by reaching out toward patients and allowing them to reach out in response. Increased eye contact can also be useful in encouraging expression of feelings, but it can be overdone and become threatening.

Whenever possible, it is best to be on eye level with the patient for conversations. Sitting down is more effective than standing. Being near to the patient is also important. If the patient is in a hospital bed, standing in the doorway or at the foot of the bed is ineffective.

Listening is one of the most difficult parts of good communication. The good listener blocks out all other thoughts and is completely attentive to what the patient is saying. It is important to hear not only the words but their meanings. This requires noting nonverbal messages, tone of voice, and inflection as well as words. Nurses sometimes are so busy thinking of what they will say when the patient stops speaking that they do not really hear what the patient is saying.

Therapeutic communication by nurses requires that they be aware of their own personal feelings, body language, and expected effect of messages on the patient and at the same time be attentive to the patient's words, body language, and responses to their communication. This requires considerable energy expenditure by nurses and can be very tiring, especially to the inexperienced.

Sometimes nurses can be so strongly schooled in the idea that cancer patients should talk, express feelings, and cope that they will personally set goals, expecting that the patient will disclose private feelings and demonstrate effective coping within a given period of time. This type of approach can be as harmful as entirely avoiding communication. Not all patients have the same feelings; not all patients wish to express their feelings. The nurse should be available and communicate that accessibility to the patient. However, the patient should always remain in control of what, when, and how communication occurs.

Sometimes the most meaningful communication between patient and nurse takes place without the use of words. It may involve touching, eye contact, or mere physical presence. Usually this occurs only after an effective relationship has been established. It requires that the nurse have the inner strength to be still and silent — to be with the patients where they are, in an existential sense. This act requires practice and courage, but can be a very meaningful experience for both patient and nurse.[3]

Touching is also a valuable art that can be developed as a means of communication. Used in this way, touching can have very deep meaning for the patient. Necessary touching — to provide care — does not have the same effect. The nurse must be careful with this approach. Touching various parts of the body can have personal meanings to the patient that are not known to the nurse. Longer periods of touch can be more threatening than brief periods.

Cancer patients who have inadequate support systems or who have been socially isolated have an increased need for touch. Sometimes they will grab out for the nurse and hold on tightly. This can be very frightening to the nurse. If this occurs, it is important not to stiffen up but to remain calm and to move slightly toward the patient, not away. A soft, soothing voice can help. Attempts should then be made to determine the reasons for and extent of the patient's need. Plans should then be made to include increased touching in the patient's care.

Many of the communications that occur in our world are ritualistic. We ask a person "How are you?" The expected response is "Fine." We make a casual joke; the other person is expected to laugh. We feel angry and uncomfortable when people fail to respond in the expected way; then we may avoid them.

This pattern of communication is very common in health care situations. The nurse stands in the doorway and says "How's it going today?" Body language indicates that the nurse is in a hurry. The patient will ritualistically respond "OK." No meaningful communication has occurred. Although words have passed between two people, the patient may sudden-

ly feel more alone. This activity is so automatic that the nurse must be very conscious of this behavior to be aware of it when it is occurring.

Sometimes communication between the patient and significant others is ineffective. Both may avoid meaningful conversation and discuss only social trivia. Eventually, walls are built that separate them. The nurse can sometimes function as a guide to those wishing to improve effective communication.

Styles of communication vary from one person to another. There is no one right thing to say or way to say it. However, it is important to be genuine. An approach used very effectively by one nurse may be totally ineffective if used by another nurse.

Some counseling techniques may be helpful in developing an effective personal approach. In communicating, the nurse is using the self in a therapeutic way. In psychiatric nursing, this is a common and consciously developed practice. Unfortunately, in medical-surgical nursing, this art has not been as well developed.

Expression of feelings by the nurse can sometimes have a very therapeutic effect. Maintaining professional distance may protect the nurse, but it is not usually helpful to the patient. If the nurse is feeling sad or frustrated or uncertain about how to help the patient, it may be very appropriate to express these feelings. If genuinely felt, crying with the patient or family can be helpful.

Sometimes a nurse will dislike or feel very angry toward a patient. Although it may not be helpful to express them to the patient, these feelings need to be dealt with — perhaps by talking with other nurses — or they will be communicated to the patient in some form. Sometimes even these feelings are best conveyed to the patient. Saying "When you do _____, I feel very angry" will give the patient direct feedback on his or her behavior.

Nurses tend to expect gratitude from patients when they give "good" nursing care or do nice things. If expressions of gratitude do not occur, the nurse may withdraw and decrease efforts at nursing care.

Sometimes, cancer patients are not at a place, existentially, where they can feel gratitude or express it. Therefore, nurses working with cancer patients should be sufficiently inner-directed and mature to not depend on receiving gratitude from patients.

Evaluating the effectiveness of communication is difficult. Changes in communication patterns by patients or family can usually be observed. Evaluation of nursing interventions should not, however, be based on whether or not the patient chose to express feelings. The evaluation should instead be focused on the nurse's communication of receptivity. This is more difficult to measure. We sometimes see ourselves differently from how we are viewed by others. Therefore, it is helpful to get feedback from patients or their family members or from other nurses about our communication skills.

Promoting Effective Coping Mechanisms

The words defenses, adaptation, and coping are being used freely, sometimes interchangeably, in nursing today. They are not usually clearly defined and often their meaning changes when they are discussed. The meanings attached to these words vary greatly. The words, as used in this book, are defined below.

Defenses

Defenses are means of protection that all of us at times employ, at least temporarily, until we can find a way to manage a threatening situation more effectively. Some level of denial is found in all defenses.[69] Defenses commonly used by participants in the cancer situation are rationalization, affect reversal, suppression, displacement, passive acceptance, disengagement, projection, cooperative compliance, self-blame, impulsivity, minimization, and compartmentalization.[69]

Defenses are less effective when we recognize that we are using them as means of denial and avoidance. That recognition itself breaks through the denial. Therefore, people using defenses may not realize that a problem exists against which they are protecting themselves. Or they may feel generalized anxiety, but may not be able to define what the problem is. Problem solving is usually not possible as long as defenses are in place.

Some people automatically use defense strategies whenever a problem occurs. They are usually very rigid people who seek security above all other things. These people tend to resort to a few preferred defenses regardless of the problem. They are inclined to be dependent and pessimistic. Their anxiety level is often high. They may feel helpless, hopeless, and depressed and have a low morale. Their approach to life is often one of passivity and compliance. They tend to have a general feeling of victimization.

Adaptation

Many people use the words adaptation and coping interchangeably. There are some differences, however, that should be considered. Adaptation is an attempt to maintain sameness. From a physiologic point of view, out of which the idea of adaptation comes, this makes sense. From a psychosocial point of view, adaptation is often not the most effective or healthy strategy. Psychologically, it involves reacting to a situation by altering one's self to conform to environmental demands. It implies a passive, fatalistic acceptance of the situation as it is. From a systems perspective, the person alters himself or herself in order to maintain the present system. When this happens, the system becomes more important than the person. Watzlawick and colleagues[67a] call this first order change. Second order change, which changes the system, is more like coping. In coping, the person acts on a situation in order to change it in some significant way.

In the cancer situation, adaptation occurs when the cancer patient accepts the social isolation that often accompanies the stigma of diagnosis and adjusts his or her living pattern to fit within the framework of isolation. Adaptation occurs when the person accepts the role of passive, compliant patient that is imposed upon admission to the hospital. It occurs with the cancer patient in pain who, because of the system's rules, cannot get adequate pain relief and attempts to find some way to endure the pain.

In nursing we often reward adaptation. Patients who adapt may be seen as good patients. Copers may be seen as troublemakers. They are more likely to disrupt our comfortable way of doing things.

Coping

The goal of coping is problem resolution. Coping is a process that entails changes in both the situation and the person involved in the situation. It is based on the philosophy that change is possible. The individual is in control and can have an impact on the environment, nature, or the world. Coping involves a perception of the problem, action, evaluation of the effectiveness of the action, alteration of activity as necessary, and further action. This process requires directed, motivated behavior.[69] The resolution that occurs may not permanently solve the problem and the process will begin again. Coping persons use a wide variety of resources and may use both active and passive strategies, but confrontation is

always an integral part of their strategies. Weisman[69] lists 10 rules that people who cope well seem to follow:

1. Avoid avoidance; do not deny.
2. Confront realities and take appropriate action.
3. Focus on solutions or redefine a problem into solvable form.
4. Always consider alternatives.
5. Maintain open, mutual communication with significant others.
6. Seek and use constructive help, including decent medical care.
7. Accept support when offered; be assertive when necessary.
8. Keep up morale through self-reliance or resources that are available.
9. Believe that self-concept is as important as symptom relief.
10. View hope as self-pride, not self-deception.

People who cope well are usually oriented toward personal growth. They are independent, optimistic people who are autonomous and competent. They have a high morale and are resourceful and self-assertive. Although cancer is a serious problem in their lives, the disease seldom throws them into despair.

Most people use a combination of defenses, adaptation, and coping. Sometimes, a person may be coping with one problem while utilizing defenses with other problems.[69] However, people with a pattern of poor mental health practices throughout their life may primarily use defenses,

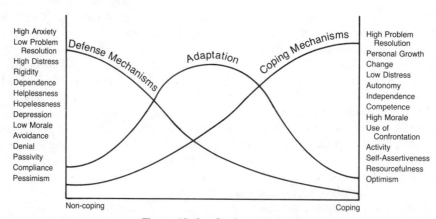

Figure 12–2. Coping patterns.

whereas some who have been oriented toward personal growth may primarily use coping. (See Fig. 12–2.)

Nursing Interventions

One of the assumptions of psychosocial nursing interventions is that people can sometimes be helped to cope better than they are presently doing. The goal of interventions, then, is to help the person achieve a higher level of successful coping. Included in this framework are actions to identify problems, reframe problems so that they can be solved, and increase self-esteem. Although the patient's chief problem may not be solvable, possible options or alternatives need to be identified and considered. Selection of appropriate interventions is dependent on an adequate psychosocial assessment. It is unrealistic to expect a person who has a history of multiple problems and who primarily uses defenses to be able to immediately move to a style of using mostly coping strategies. The intervention strategies used with these people should be different from those selected to assist people who cope more effectively. With any intervention designed to improve coping, the goal should be oriented toward accomplishing small steps, not great leaps.

Reaching this goal requires a trusting nurse-patient relationship and open communication. The nurse must be sensitive to the meanings of the patient's communication and know how to evaluate those meanings. Concerned, intuitive, and caring responses are important, but not sufficient, in assisting the patient. The nurse must be disciplined and knowledgeable enough to fit those intuitions into a framework in order to intervene effectively. Nurses are expected to have a comprehensive understanding of human physiology. It is just as necessary to have a thorough understanding of psychologic processes. Skills in psychosocial interventions are as important as technical nursing skills. Competence in only one of these areas does not constitute nursing practice.

Table 12–4.   Countercoping Strategies*

A. *Clarification and control*
1. Confront with salient problem and take appropriate action
2. Get or give more information
3. Redefine or reduce problems to manageable concerns
4. Consider alternative solutions

B. *Collaboration*
1. Mutuality/constructive sharing of concern
2. Submit problems to judgment of another
3. Prevent impulsive actions or ill-considered behavior
4. Be more directive and active in all alliance

C. *Directed Relief*
1. Elicit catharsis and unburdening
2. Temporary avoidance and suppression
3. Encourage diversions that worked in the past
4. Suggest new tactics that relieve

D. *Cooling off*
1. Modulate emotional extremes
2. Build morale through increased self-esteem
3. Rationalize and distract
4. Realistic resignation/be in silence

*From Weisman, A. D.: *Coping with Cancer.* New York: McGraw-Hill Book Co., 1979. Used by permission.

Weisman[69] lists interventions that are effective in cancer situations. He calls these interventions countercoping strategies. (See Table 12–4.) Freidenbergs and colleagues[25] have also provided a list of interventions. (See Table 12–5.)

Interventions that facilitate coping require the therapeutic use of self. Because of this, it is not possible to give step-by-step procedures for moving through the process. It truly combines art and science. The two unique personalities of the nurse and patient determine the approach and its effectiveness. However, it is helpful to have guidance, support, and feedback from another professional who has preparation in this area.

Some general suggestions may be helpful. Control should be left with the patient, not the nurse. Since the nurse is assessing a subjective experience of the patient, the nurse should not make definitive statements of what the patient is feeling. Any value judgments that are expressed should be offered by the nurse, not imposed on the patient. If the patient chooses not to accept

Table 12–5. Psychosocial Intervention Principles*

Educational

Clarifying/giving information about the medical system—e.g., explaining hospital procedures, teaching patients' rights, informing patients of existing outpatient services, etc.

Clarifying the patients' own medical condition—e.g., what types of cancer the patient has, the meaning of test results, etc.

Teaching about cancer and its side effects—e.g., the side effects to be expected from treatment, what the norms are regarding resumption of activities, etc.

Teaching what to do to relieve physical discomfort, emotional discomfort, etc., e.g., relaxation training, self-hypnosis, etc.

Reinforcing what *other* medical personnel have said, i.e., helping patients comply with prescribed medical regime—e.g., reinforcing the necessity of medical treatment, reinforcing M.D. statements about the medical condition or treatment, etc.

Teaching about the emotional reactions to cancer—e.g., what emotional responses can be expected by the patient himself/herself, what reactions can he/she expect from others, etc.

Counseling

Allowing or encouraging the patient to ventilate feelings.

Offering the patient reassurance or verbal support.

Helping the patient clarify own feelings and interpreting thoughts, feelings, and behavior in more psychodynamic terms to patient.

Encouraging the patient to act on his/her environment—e.g., urging patient to speak to medical personnel, to family; urging patient to ask questions.

Exploring the patient's past and/or current situation.

Offering indirect support, e.g., by listening to patient, chatting with patient about events unrelated to medical condition.

Environmental

Speaking with health care personnel about the patient.

Making a formal health service referral.

*Modified from Freidenbergs, I., Gordon, W., Ruckdeschel, M., and Diller, L.: Assessment and treatment of psychosocial problems of the cancer patient: a case study. *Cancer Nursing.* 3:111–119, 1980. Used by permission of Masson Publishing USA, Inc., New York. Copyright 1980.

the nurse's assistance at that point, the nurse should communicate willingness to assist later if the patient desires. Caution should be taken not to avoid or reject the patient in this situation.

Some examples of intervening in a nonthreatening way follow:

"You seem to be very distressed about ___. If you're willing to talk about it, perhaps I could help you consider some ways to deal with it."

"From my work with other patients, I believe it can be harmful to hold feelings inside the way you seem to be doing."

"If you want to talk about it later, let me know. Now, how about going for that walk we decided to take?"

Confrontation. Confrontation does not mean a direct attack. It means helping people face up to a situation or a problem and examining the alternative ways of handling it and the consequences of those alternatives. If confrontation is improperly

used, patients may react by increasing their defenses. Patients using denial will block the information. Properly used, confrontation can facilitate movement of patients toward problem resolution. Some examples of confrontation are:

I have noticed when observing you that you seem to be pulling away from your family. If you continue to do this, these are some of the things that may happen: ___. There are some other ways to handle the things that are happening within your family, which you might want to consider.

Are you aware that you are eating less of your food, that you have stopped doing your mouth care, and that you went outdoors yesterday without a coat? You don't seem to be taking very good care of yourself right now. What do you suppose is going on with you?

Teaching. Accurate and sufficient information is essential to promote effective coping. It is helpful to determine what the patient has been told, but even more important is to get the patient's interpretation of that information and the meaning attached to the information. Patients need to be informed about many things related to the cancer situation: their medical condition, the nature of the type of cancer they have, what to expect in the near future, interpretation of test results and physician statements, what to expect from their treatment, how to take care of themselves, ways to interact with the health care system, common emotional reactions to cancer, and ways to cope with these feelings.

Nurses sometimes have unreasonable expectations of patient behavior after information has been provided. They may expect the patient to immediately change behavior. The information is supposed to be valued above everything else already felt by the patient. The patient is presumed to have retained the information in the exact form it was given. Unfortunately, none of these expectations actually occurs.

Telling patients something does not mean that they will make that knowledge part of themselves. Even if they do, they may not choose to act upon it. Other things happening at that time may seem more important. They may distort the information and interpret it according to their present view of the situation. Information is very often value-laden and is given with the expectation that the patient will take on one value in favor of another. If the information is not in keeping with the patient's values, however, the information may be rejected.

Information should be provided in such a way that the patient is most likely to utilize it for effective coping. Information should be offered, not imposed. It should be understood that the patient is free to use the knowledge as desired and that the nurse is willing to assist if the patient wishes. Alternatives and consequences can be presented with the information.

The following are examples of this type of communication. "What did the doctor tell you? What did that mean to you? How did you feel when the doctor told you? How do you feel about that now?" "I can explain what that means, if you would like." "It

might be helpful for you to know more about the side effects of this treatment. Then you will be better able to take care of yourself."

If a change in behavior or lifestyle is sought in addition to the intake of information, this should be discussed. Alternative behaviors should be explored and the consequences of each behavior discussed. Consequences should be a direct result of the behavior, not punishment, disapproval, or rejection by the nurse or other health care givers. Punitive actions are not an effective way to achieve adherence with expected behavior and forces the patient into a passive, dependent role. Health care givers are not always the best judges of what behavior is "good" for a patient. "Good" must sometimes be considered from several perspectives.

Redefining. Redefining or reframing is commonly used as a psychosocial intervention. Redefining is a way of looking at the problem from a different, perhaps more positive perspective or a way of breaking it down into several components, some of which may be more solvable. Although medical-surgical nurses are not as familiar with the technique, it is frequently used in casual conversation. Patients often see a problem as overwhelming or impossible to solve. This may result in feelings of helplessness, hopelessness, and despair.

The problem can sometimes be seen as a situation that can be of benefit to the patient. It can be seen as an advantage or an opportunity, rather than a disadvantage. After all, it is not what happens to us in life, but what we do with it and how we respond to it that give meaning to life. If we can see ourselves as in some way controlling the experience of our existence or our death, we can endure and even transcend the unbearable.

Considering Alternatives. Proposing alternatives to the patient seems simple, but examining all the possible solutions requires some creativity. We are often inclined to think of two or three rather obvious solutions and then skip to examining the advantages and disadvantages of those choices without giving further thought to other alternatives. Performing this mental activity with the patient can be very stimulating to both nurse and patient.

Because each has dissimilar values, the patient and nurse may weigh alternatives differently. In presenting alternatives, it is easy for the nurse, by tone of voice and body language, to indicate "good" choices and "bad" choices. In order to be effective, the choice must be the patient's. The patient should not feel coerced into a decision. The patient, not the nurse, will experience the consequences.

Consideration of alternatives must always include the identification of the positive and negative consequences of each alternative. The evaluation of the consequence as positive or negative should be done by the patient, not the nurse. Again, care must be taken to consider all the likely consequences.

Being Directive. Every rule of counseling indicates that it is "bad" to give advice or tell someone what to do. However, in a crisis situation, the person is often incapable of making even simple decisions. In this event, it is appropriate to give simple directives or advice. The trick is to recognize when it is time to stop being directive. When the crisis is over, the patient can be supported in moving back into decision-making activities.

Expressing Concern. It is important for the nurse to express concern about the patient's situation. The mutual concern felt by both nurse and patient is very strengthening to the patient. It can be the beginning of problem solving. It can also give the patient the feeling of being truly cared for.

Providing Support. Patients can gain a great deal of strength and security from a trusting, supportive relationship in which feelings, successes, and failures are shared. Patients need the recognition by others of their strengths and assets. They need the warm, caring mutuality that has come to be associated with a nurse-patient relationship. Within a relationship such as this, a sense of optimism and positive self-esteem can be nurtured. The patient can truly feel understood.

Patients need to receive encouragement and praise for their efforts. Considerable energy output may be required to achieve even small gains. Sometimes only the nurse and the patient know the struggle involved in the achievement of a goal. The patient needs to know during the struggle and the achievement that someone else understands and cares. The effort and joy are much more satisfying when shared.

Caring for the Family

The cancer situation seriously disrupts the entire family. The consequences can be both severe and long-lasting. Family dynamics are altered, roles within the family change, communication patterns may be thrown into disarray, and social supports may fail. These changes can sometimes lead to the dissolution of the family. They may also impair the mental and physical health of family members, with effects lasting long after the cancer situation is over.

In spite of these alarming possibilities, family members are virtually ignored in most health care situations. They are often considered unimportant or in the way. Any interventions used are likely to be for the purpose of decreasing disruption to the health care system or to change a family member's behavior for the benefit of the cancer patient.

Thus, the family member is seen as an inconvenient appendage of the patient and must be tolerated and controlled. Time is not allotted for family care. Institutions are not reimbursed for family care and may, in fact, be dissuaded from conducting such activities. However, in spite of these discouraging circumstances, family members and the family as a group must be included in a very significant way in any nursing practice that focuses on the quality of life.

Crisis events within the cancer patient's situation disrupt the family and may throw it into disequilibrium. There are specific points at which this is most likely to occur: the time of diagnosis, the beginning of a new treatment, the end of a treatment, the discovery of a recurrence, the recognition of preterminality, dying, and death. The family system will adjust to the crisis in some way, healthy or not, within a month or two of its occurrence. During the period of disruption immediately after a crisis, the family is most susceptible and receptive to interventions that could improve its functioning. After equilibrium has been reestablished, interventions to improve functioning can be accomplished, but they require greater effort and time.[9]

Family members may exhibit problems during the course of the cancer situation that are a consequence of poor resolution of a family crisis. Helping a single family member to successfully manage a problem will in turn alter the family as a whole.

The Time of Diagnosis

When the diagnosis of cancer is learned, family members will react on the basis of their beliefs about cancer. Thus, the severity of the reaction is not always in keeping with the seriousness of the diagnosis or prognosis. The first reaction is one of shock and disbelief. Then gradually thoughts will turn to the effect that the disease will have on family functioning. Efforts will be taken to diminish those effects.

If the family learns the diagnosis before the patient does, attempts may be made by family members to keep the information from the patient. Their rationale is usually that the patient cannot deal with the diagnosis. They are really saying that the family cannot deal with it. They believe that keeping the diagnosis a secret will protect the family system from change. The more rigid and dysfunctional the family is, the more likely this is to occur. Dysfunctional families utilize avoidance and denial as defensive strategies against change. One way to avoid this situation is to tell the patient and family together. Functional families will also experience this as a crisis event and can use help in coping with it.

Families need as much privacy as possible in order to express feelings. Efforts to make contact with other family members and support systems should be facilitated. Expressions of fear and anger and negative beliefs about cancer should be allowed, with no attempt made at this point to dispel them. The presence of the nurse at this time can be helpful in many ways. The reaction is essentially one of grief over multiple losses. The presence of a caring, supportive nurse can be very comforting.

Concentration at this time is very poor. Anxiety is high and very little learning can occur. The patient and family will have trouble remembering what they were told by the physician. They may have even greater difficulty grasping the total significance of the information. This awareness will emerge gradually. The family members and the patient may need to ask the nurse on several occasions to repeat what the physician said. This should be done willingly and kindly.

The patient and family may need to be given simple directives from the nurse at this point. They may be incapable of making even the smallest decisions related to staying or going, eating, resting, whom to contact, or what to do next. The nursing care given at this time can help to facilitate coping during the resolution phase of the crisis.

As the family's awareness of the situation emerges, interventions can begin to promote coping and to maintain open channels of communication. The family at this point will be very receptive to learning and change. Family members will begin to seek answers to their questions. They need to understand the diagnosis, the treatment, and the side effects. They need to know how to take care of themselves and what things they can do to help the patient. They need to make plans for the future, usually in the face of uncertainty. They may need to reexamine their beliefs about cancer.

Nursing interventions designed to meet these needs should be based on an adequate assessment of the family. The interventions can take place with individual family members, the family as a group, or within support groups consisting of multiple families or families and patients combined. (See Chapter 16 for a fuller discussion.)

The family needs to understand the decisions it is making and think about the consequences of those decisions. Often decisions will be made about what communication patterns will be used and what role changes will occur. Based on these decisions, changes in behavior can occur even without anyone's recognizing that a decision has been made. If the behavior seems harmful or dysfunctional, the behavior and its consequences should be pointed out to the family by the nurse. Alternative choices can be discussed. The option, however, should remain with the family. It is easy, at this point, for the nurse to get caught up in family dynamics and begin to function with the family by its rules. If the nurse becomes enmeshed in family relationships, it will be less possible to use interventions that could change a dysfunctional system.

Beginning a New Treatment

When a new treatment is begun, family activities and the timing of activities change. Family roles may be altered. The family may be interacting with new groups of people, such as new physicians and nurses. Family members may have to learn the way around a different health care facility. The treatment may arouse hope, but at the same time may increase awareness of the existence of cancer. The side effects of the treatment will have to be managed. Family members may encounter patients with more advanced diseases and become increasingly anxious. New information and new ways of coping may be needed. The beginning of a new treatment may be seen as a turning point, a change, and thus a crisis.

Family needs and nursing interventions at this point are similar to those exhibited at the time of diagnosis. If the needed interventions were not provided at the time of diagnosis, problems may now be more severe. Continuity of care, ensuring that the family can continue working with

the same nurse, can greatly increase coping abilities. Unfortunately, the nurse may be encountering the patient and family for the first time, requiring a completely new assessment. In some cases, such as in some radiation centers, nurses may not be available to provide psychosocial care for families.

Since most treatment for cancer now occurs on an outpatient basis, patients and families often have few opportunities for nursing care during this time. Defenses and dysfunctional adaptation strategies may become fixed patterns that are incorporated into the family dynamics. The family may keep the patient in a dependent role, not allowing independent role behavior or decision making. They may tend to overprotect the patient and take on unnecessary responsibilities. Family goals may be abandoned unnecessarily and the family activity may revolve around the patient. Family members may drift apart from each other. When treatment is long and the chronicity of the disease seems apparent, the spouse may abandon the cancer patient. Sometimes an unexpected cure will also cause a severe family crisis or disintegration of the family.[12]

The End of a Treatment

Completion of a treatment seems more a time of relief than a time of crisis; however, it is still a change. Family activities and interactions have revolved around the treatment regimen. Relationships with health care givers may have been established. There was a feeling of hope because something positive was being done.

Suddenly, it is over. The family is on its own; so is the tumor. Will it begin to grow again? Will actions of the family make a difference in whether it begins to grow again? Is the patient still a patient? What do we do now? The future is uncertain. How do we live the rest of our lives in uncertainty? What family plans can be made?

Every symptom that the patient has may be interpreted as cancer. The family may be fearful of reinvesting in the patient when a recurrence is possible. Family members may feel that it is safer to maintain some distance.

Nursing contact in this family crisis is rare. Support groups or the family nurse practitioner can provide invaluable assistance in helping the family move back into the mainstream of life.

The Discovery of a Recurrence

The discovery of a recurrence is usually a greater crisis than the original diagnosis because it is very often the end of a hope for cure. This time the family knows more clearly what they are faced with. Grief reactions will predominate. The patient may be blamed, although this will not usually be openly expressed or even recognized by the family. Family members may feel that the patient has done it to them on purpose. Because this type of thinking is socially forbidden, the family may reverse the feeling and be syrupy sweet, act overly solicitous, and hover over the patient.

Again, the family dynamics must change. What will happen now? How long will it be? What symptoms can we expect? How do we handle it? How do we treat the patient? Do we have the courage to go through this? What does this mean to the family?

At this point, the family is again receptive to nursing interventions that can strengthen its functioning. The interventions discussed in the sections on coping and diagnosis will be effective. The family needs to consider placing the patient in the role of a person with a chronic, not a terminal, illness. (See Chapter 1.)

Recognition of Preterminality

When the patient begins to deteriorate physically and requires more assistance with the activities of daily living, the family dynamics will again change. Roles will be altered. The caretaker role will be implemented. (See Chapter 1 for a discussion of this role.) Family activities will often revolve completely around the patient. Demands in terms of time and energy may be exhausting.[31]

Society expects family members to devote themselves completely to the patient's needs. Meeting personal needs may be considered selfish. Family members may be working 8 hours a day and caring for the patient 16 hours a day. Sleep may be intermittent. Family members living outside the home may be called in for assistance; often these are young people with small children and responsibilities of their own. They may have mixed feelings about taking on additional responsibilities. Feelings are on edge. Quarrels may erupt easily. Divisions can occur that may never be resolved.

Family members may need permission from the nurse to take care of themselves. They need to know the consequences to their own physical and mental health of not taking care of themselves. Plans need to be made so that it is possible for family members to have time for themselves.

Family members will often begin to feel that the four walls of their home are closing in on and trapping them. There seems to be no way out. A type of panic is experienced with this feeling. Attending a support group at this time can be extremely helpful. The meeting provides a legitimate reason for family members to get away from the house. Other families can share their solutions to problems. It is a chance to ask questions and feel safe expressing negative feelings.

Family members need to get away on a regular basis — preferably to do something they enjoy doing. They need contact with the rest of the world. They need to be able to have fun and relax — even if it is for only a short time. But for it to be effective, they must do it without feeling guilty. One strategy is for the nurse to make a contract with the family member to do this for 1 hour and then share the experience with the nurse.

Dying and Death

The family crisis during dying will be discussed in detail in Chapter 14. During this time communication patterns need to change. Life review and the saying of good-bye need to occur. Family differences with the patient should be resolved. The family needs to begin looking beyond the death and prepare for and plan life without the patient. Imagining what life will be like should be encouraged. After death, the family will continue to need support and care. Only hospices currently provide nursing care during this period. It needs to be given by all institutions providing care to advanced cancer patients.

Facilitating Personal Growth

The cancer situation usually results in experiences that are allowed to be psychologically and socially destructive to the patient and family. These same experiences can, however, be used to facilitate growth. The patient or family member who is oriented toward personal growth can use the experiences in a positive way. The supportive care of a nurse who has experienced personal growth can facilitate this process. Sometimes a seemingly rigid patient will suddenly begin to change in a positive direction.

The confrontation with possible death seems to stimulate in some patients a reexamination of their values. Facets of life that have been taken for granted will suddenly be magnified. The person may learn to treasure the experience of the moment. The old adage of stopping to smell the roses may take on new meaning. Relationships with significant others may become more valued than money or business or other activities. Sometimes, family members (particularly spouses) and the patient will develop a much closer relationship than existed before the illness. The patient may seek ways to fulfill the spiritual part of being. The patient may become more introspective and philosophical. This behavior should not be confused with depression,

although the patient may be more quiet and interact less with others at times.

There seems to be nestled deep within all of us a small seed of yearning that guides us in the direction of reaching our potential. Becoming the best we can be, self-actualization, individuation — it is called by many names. We often keep this seed hidden and under control because we fear the changes that will come if it is released.

In crisis situations, the barriers seem to be lowered and personal growth may proceed rapidly and unimpeded. Two things seem to be needed for this to occur: a receptive person and an environment that is conducive to growth. The nurse can often be a catalyst to this beautiful blossoming of personality.

Strengthening Social Support Systems

The social support system is a rather ill-defined concept at this time. Support systems include a person's network of contacts or relationships with family members, friends, and community groups. The strength of the support comes from not only quantity but also intensity of the relationships and from interrelatedness of the various persons or groups. Although little research has been conducted on the impact of support groups on the cancer situation, it seems reasonable to assume that a network of support groups can give strength to the patient and family and help them cope. The absence of support groups, then, might be an indication of coping problems. The withdrawal of support groups could be detrimental to the ability of the patient and family to cope.

Cancer patients and families often find that immediately after diagnosis, family members, friends, neighbors, and religious groups are concerned and helpful, and visit frequently. As the disease progresses, however, these people make fewer and fewer contacts. If called by the patient or family, they usually make some excuse to avoid interacting. Although there probably are multiple reasons for this behavior, negative beliefs about cancer seem to be a major factor.

Actions that the nurse can take to maintain or restore support systems may improve the family's ability to cope. Two types of intervention may be helpful. The patient or family may be taught the importance of support groups and encouraged to maintain them, or the nurse can intervene directly with the support system. Working with the patient or family members to recognize early changes in communication may be helpful. Open channels of communication may make it safer for support persons to maintain contact. People in the community often do not know what to say to the person with cancer. They may want to help, but do not know how. They may feel depressed or afraid when they are reminded, by contact with the cancer patient, of their own mortality.

If the patient is hospitalized, the nurse can make contact with visitors and sometimes assist them in maintaining the relationship. The visitor can be allowed to express feelings. The nurse can encourage alternative ways for the visitor to cope. Concrete ways for the visitor to help can be suggested. The implications of this for the patient and family can be explored. Of course, this type of interaction cannot and should not occur with every visitor. And the well-being of the visitor as well as the patient and family must be considered.

Meeting with a group, such as a church or school organization, to discuss the cancer situation and its impact on the patient and family is also effective. Group members can be helped to examine their feelings about cancer and explore ways in which they could be helpful. In addition to helping the specific patient of concern, this type of action can stimulate changes in the community at large, in terms of its response to cancer.

SPECIFIC NURSING SITUATIONS

It is not possible to explore all of the intricacies involved in the psychosocial problems related to cancer. Some of the more common ones will be discussed and interventions will be suggested for each individual problem. Although problems will be explored separately, they will very rarely be seen clinically in isolation. Interventions for one problem must be combined in a workable manner with interventions designed for concurrent problems.

The nurse, it must be realized, is not a miracle worker. The causes for feelings cannot be magically removed. The patient usually has very valid reasons for the feelings being experienced. The nurse should not expect to be able to dispel all psychosocial problems. The goal of intervention should be to help the patient manage what is being experienced in the most constructive way possible.

Negative Beliefs About Cancer

Beliefs about cancer (as described in Chapter 1) can have very harmful effects on the patient. These beliefs are primitive and often have not been verbalized by the patient. Even the experience of recognizing and expressing the beliefs can be helpful. But intellectual understanding alone cannot alter beliefs. Having positive experiences while coping with cancer seems to alter some patients' attitudes. Observations of the way that other cancer patients are treated is also helpful. Gaining knowledge about the disease and its treatment may alter some beliefs. However, much research needs to be conducted to determine effective nursing interventions in this area.

Denial

Denial exists in varying degrees and in all kinds of disguised forms. We tend to place a negative value on it, but denial can sometimes be an effective coping strategy. Patients may deny that they have cancer, they may deny the seriousness of the diagnosis, or they may deny the impact of the diagnosis on their lives. If the patient denies having cancer, needed treatment may not be obtained. Denying or minimizing the seriousness of the diagnosis may prevent the patient from making necessary plans for the future. However, denying the impact of cancer on life may allow the patient to continue to function at a maximum capacity. Denial may be, in a sense, a role rejection. The patient may choose to function within the well role, rather than maintain the cancer patient role; this may facilitate coping.[58]

It is easy for the nurse to become caught up in the patient's inappropriate denial and to support it since, in the beginning, using denial prevents the patient from dealing with the disease's consequences. Nurse-patient interactions, however, should not generally support denial.[69] If the patient's denial is supported, movement will often be in the direction of further denial and avoidance.

The patient's denial will appear in nurse-patient conversations. If the patient's statements reflect inappropriate denial, the nurse can gently remind the patient of the facts. The patient may then swing to the opposite direction — that of despair. If this occurs, the nurse can point out the reality again and help the patient move in the direction of problem solving.

For some patients, denial may be the only present way of dealing with the situation. In this case, no attempt should be made to disrupt the denial. Patients will move out of the denial in their own time. For the most part, nurses need not be concerned about unintentionally dispelling patients' denial. Their denial is not fragile. Confronted directly with the facts, patients using denial will block out the communication; it will not be incorporated for cognitive processing.

Anger and Hostility

For the most part, assessing the existence of anger is not a difficult task. However, in some patients, it is kept carefully controlled and expressed only in very subtle ways. For example, the patient who is syrupy sweet and always praising the nurses may in fact be very angry. Patients are usually afraid of retaliation if they openly express their anger. Expressing anger from a helpless, dependent position is more risky than from a position of control. And yet, patients who openly express anger, are critical, and demand the kind of care that they think they should have seem better able to cope with their situation. Their response to their illness and treatment also seems better than more compliant patients.

Cancer patients feel anger at many things: the physician, God, their family, the world, their situation, and themselves. The anger they feel is frightening to them. Patients will often displace their anger and direct it at the nurses. This is difficult for nurses to handle. The patient may accuse the nurses of incompetence. Nurses may become afraid and defensive and withdraw from the patient. This increases the patient's anger and a vicious circle begins.

Providing quality nursing care to an angry patient is not an easy task. The patient is not likely to feel grateful or express gratitude for the care given. It is sometimes difficult to determine what care is needed. Planning care with the patient may be a problem if the patient is displacing anger onto the nurse.

Thus, the most logical first step is to confront the anger directly. Sometimes patients will deny that they are angry, while clenching their fists and gritting their teeth. It is helpful to describe their nonverbal behavior to them. Patients should be allowed and encouraged to express their anger. This will be safer if the nurse indicates a willingness to "be with" the patients while their anger is being expressed and not retaliate.

The causes for the anger can then be explored. Since the anger is a defense against deeper feelings of hurt and fear, this area must be approached gently and compassionately. Patient's displace their anger because it is more threatening to recognize its true source. Many patients are angry with God and terrified at what they imagine to be the consequence of this. It can be helpful to express the belief that God is big enough to accept our anger and understands. Explaining that the anger is a reasonable reaction to the patient's situation can also be helpful when the anger is expressed. The deeper feelings of hurt and fear may surface and must be dealt with eventually.

The patient needs to be encouraged to move beyond the anger to problem-solving strategies, in order to cope with the situation that caused the feelings. The nurse needs to realize that all of these actions will not magically eliminate the patient's feelings. Interventions can, however, alter what the patient does with the feelings. The patient will continue to need to express anger as it is experienced. Now, however, this can be done within a trusting nurse-patient relationship.

Some patients are so angry that trust is not possible. This usually occurs when the anger is not dealt with and a very unhealthy system of interaction develops. Some patients have had such negative experiences in other institutions or situations that trust develops very slowly, if at all. Great care must be taken, in this case, not to abandon the patient in any way. Although the nurse may have to plan the care without the active direct participation of the patient, the patient should be kept informed of the plan. The patient should be allowed as much control as possible and should not be treated like a disobedient child. The patient should continue to be perceived as a responsible problem-solving adult.

Many of these patients keep detailed notes of nursing care and medications. If the patient allows this, the notes can be compared with the nursing care plan. If the nurse needs additional information, the patient and the notes can be consulted. Some patients may hold on to the notes as a threat of retaliation to the nurse. These patients are extremely fearful of abandonment and will often interpret a slight delay or the absence of the nurse for illness or days off as a sign of abandonment.

This is a very difficult nursing situation, one in which the nurse will need the supportive concern of other nurses. The nurses should not yield to the temptation to assign the patient to a different nurse each day.

For the patient, this is another form of abandonment.

Depression and Grief

Depressed patients have turned their anger inward against themselves. The anger will not be recognized. Instead, feelings experienced will be those of deep sadness, despair, and hopelessness. These patients will move slowly, think slowly, and speak slowly. Motivation and energy will be very low. Depressed patients do not care what happens or what is done to them. Patients who are extremely depressed will have little desire or energy to communicate or express feelings. It may be extremely difficult for these patients to make decisions.

Other people tend to avoid the depressed person. Depression almost seems contagious — being around a deeply depressed person causes others to feel depressed. The depression is not always easy to "shake off." The desire is often to "cheer up" patients with happy, bubbly, enthusiastic talk. This does not usually work and may drive patients further within themselves. The most effective approach is to move slowly, speak slowly, and maintain a rather somber manner. Questions must be designed for brief replies. The nurse can verbally reflect the feelings that the patients' behavior expresses. The appropriateness of the sadness needs to be recognized. Patients can be encouraged to talk about their thoughts and feelings. Alternative ways of dealing with the situation can be described by the nurse. Consequences of continued depression need to be explored. The choice, however, remains the patients'. Remaining silently with patients for periods interspersed throughout the day can sometimes be helpful. Any reaction, positive or negative, from these patients should be reinforced. An expression of anger from a very depressed patient is like a breath of spring.

Some patients can feel very depressed and conceal the feeling behind a facade of "normal" or happy behavior. This type of depression is a serious drain on the patients' available energy. Signs of this depression will be much more subtle, but many of these patients will admit to feeling depressed if asked. Strategies should revolve around exploring the feelings, the problems that cause the feelings, and alternative methods of coping with them.

A feeling often accompanying depression is grief. Patients with a diagnosis of cancer must give up many things; they do not have to be dying to experience a sense of grief or loss. They are giving up the view of themselves as healthy, giving up usual roles, and sometimes giving up future plans, hopes, and fantasies. They may be giving up significant portions of their body. It requires work and sadness to give up these things. To go beyond resignation and accept a new type of existence requires even more effort and coping ability.

Anxiety

Anxiety is a generalized feeling. It is often accompanied by muscle tension. Patients with anxiety cannot usually identify what they are anxious about. Anxious patients have a much more narrow perceptual field. Their ability to learn is diminished. Patients may experience symptoms brought about by increased muscle tension. Anxiety also increases the pain level. Their ability to sleep restfully is diminished. Patients will tend to overreact to situations. Anxiety breeds upon itself; thus, the patient may be caught in an upward spiral of anxiety, tension, and emotional and physical pain.

Patients with high anxiety need a predictable environment. Unexpected happenings will increase their anxiety. Participating in the nurse's care planning is very important to them.

The nursing goal should be to lower the patient's anxiety level. The patient needs to understand the consequences of high anxiety. The anxiety and tension are a defense against things that, to the patient, are even more fearful. Giving up the anxiety will involve helping the patient move

in the direction of coping and problem solving. In a sense, the patient must "give up" the anxiety and "let go" of the tension. These defenses are, in a way, security blankets. The nurse must be very supportive during this effort.

The relaxation strategies described in Chapter 11 can be very helpful in lowering anxiety. Patients who have been anxious for a long period of time will have difficulty relaxing and must be encouraged. Repeated practice sessions may be required before any significant level of relaxation is achieved.

When the patient is relaxed, problem solving will be more possible. Teaching will be more effective and the patient will be better able to differentiate and express feelings. Anxiety reduction strategies will need to continue over the course of the cancer situation.

Fear

Patients with cancer are justifiably afraid of many things: pain, death, abandonment, dependency, recurrence. Some of the fears can be expressed, others cannot. Sometimes fears will be only indirectly expressed.

Some fears are based on inaccurate information and can be relieved by providing that information. Other fears, such as the anticipation of unrelieved pain, will require reassurance and a description of measures that will be taken to ensure the relief of pain.

Death is a real possibility for many patients and must be worked through philosophically. However, many patients are more afraid of the dying process than of death itself. They may have fantasies of the dying process that are unrealistic. Describing the actual process and the nursing measures that are used can be very reassuring.

Fear of abandonment is usually greater than the fear of death. The nurse cannot prevent others from abandoning the patient, but can give reassurances that the patient will not be abandoned by nurses.

The patient's behavior often encourages abandonment. Interaction patterns between the patient, family, and significant others can be explored and adjusted to decrease the possibility of abandonment.

Dependency and Passivity

One of the greatest fears of patients is taking on the passive, dependent role. This role requires the patient to regress to a more childlike state. It is now believed that this role may interfere with a positive response to treatment and a prolonged life. It prevents decision making and problem solving. The role encourages use of defenses, manipulative behavior, and withdrawal. It interferes with the possibility of personal growth. And yet, some degree of dependency must be present to allow necessary care that cannot be done by the patient. Most patients can tolerate this if they are sure that they will regain their independence as soon as possible.

Passive behavior is seldom a necessary accompaniment to dependency. Passivity is closely related to the loss of control and power. It is usually imposed and enforced by health care institutions and by nurses. Nurses in many settings have become addicted to having power and control of the patient. This behavior is not in the best interests of the patient and should be eliminated. Power and control should rightfully remain with the patient. Nurses have services to *offer,* not to *impose.*

Helplessness is another feeling related to dependency and passivity. The cancer situation can be viewed by some patients as a helpless one. If the passive, dependent role is imposed as well, the combination can be overwhelming, even to the well-adjusted individual.

Social Isolation

Social isolation can be a very subtle process involving decreases in verbal or nonverbal communication or both. This includes quality as well as quantity of communication. Feeling-level communication may not occur. The patient may be aware of decreases in eye contact and touching and of distancing. The patient may not be allowed to participate in family decisions and may not even be told of family activities. Numbers of visitors and frequency of visits may decrease. This is painful enough to endure, but when health care givers exhibit the same behavior, it is almost more than a person can bear.

These activities may occur because of the patient's behaviors, particularly those related to anger and depression. Once begun, the patient may perpetuate the process by reacting to the behavior of others. A state of resigned withdrawal may occur. The patient may lose interest in other people and the outside world. The longer this is allowed to continue, the more difficult it is to reverse.

Some patients will respond favorably to increased contact with other patients. Patients should not be placed at the end of the hall in a private room with the door kept closed. This is a tactic designed to socially isolate the patient, not — as nurses may explain — to provide quiet. Providing mechanisms for patients to be cared for at home when possible can help prevent the development of social isolation.

Social isolation also occurs with patients who have been treated and may be cured. It is a consequence of widespread negative beliefs about cancer. These people may experience distancing of family members or friends and difficulties getting a job. Religious and community groups may discourage attendance, as if this were in the best interest of the person with cancer. These activities can only be changed by community education designed to alter the negative beliefs about cancer.

Altered Body Image

Patients with cancer perceive their bodies as being eaten away by some unseen, uncontrollable, and unknowable thing. The disease alters not only their image of the structure of their body but also their idea of being able to have some control over body functioning. Treatments for cancer also alter the structure and function of the body in ways that are difficult for patients to accept.

The image of the body is very much associated with the image of the self. Patients may see changes in their body as not being acceptable. Ostomies may cause patients to feel unclean or "bad." Changes visible to the public may actually be repulsive to others and thus to the patient. This is particularly true of patients with head and neck cancers. Progressive weight loss and weakness also cause severe body image changes.

Patients with body image problems may feel safe in the hospital where they feel accepted by the nurses, but may be reluctant to leave that secure environment and return to the real world. The difficulties there are real. There is no point in trying to convince the patient that social reactions will not occur.

Contact with other patients experiencing similar problems is very valuable and can help facilitate coping strategies. Self-acceptance is a necessary prerequisite to acceptance by others. Making the most of present capacities is also important (this concept will be discussed further in Chapter 15).

Dysfunctional Sexuality

Sexuality involves several factors: being seen as a sexual being, being intimate, being able to perform sexually, and being able to sexually stimulate another.

The cancer situation affects sexuality in many ways. Sexual partners are sometimes reluctant to be intimate for fear of contagion. Others may be afraid of hurting the patient. For some partners, it is difficult to equate sickness and sexuality. Others may be "turned off" by changes in the patient's body. The disease process or treatment may alter the patient's ability to function sexually. Physical deterioration may also be an obstacle to sexual function-

ing. Psychologic problems related to cancer may result in a loss of sexual desire. A person who has a low self-esteem will often have difficulties with sexuality. Women who have had mastectomies often experience what could be called the "china doll syndrome," in which they are seen as fragile, delicate, and breakable. Their partners are afraid to embrace them for fear of hurting them.

A psychosocial assessment should include information about past and present sexual functioning as well as the state of the marital or sexual relationship. Both sexual desire and ability to perform sexually should be determined. It is also important to ask if the patient considers his or her present level of sexuality to be a problem.

Interventions will depend on the type of problem that is occurring. It is often helpful also to explore the problem with the partner. If the partner is helped to cope with personal problems related to the cancer situation, he or she will then be more able to reach out to the person with cancer.

Strategies designed to increase self-esteem are also helpful. Closer attention to grooming can be encouraged. Changes in position or approach to sexual activity can be suggested. Alternative means to achieving sexual satisfaction can be considered. If the patient is hospitalized, privacy can be provided for sexual activity.

Sometimes, partners are unable or unwilling to function sexually with a person with cancer. If this occurs, the patient will need additional help with self-esteem.

Role Changes and Loss of Self-Esteem

During the cancer situation, the patient may have to change roles many times. The first change involves taking on the sick role. (See Chapter 1.) Family dynamics may change and the patient's role within the family may be assumed by others. Employment status may change and with it the loss of a significant role. The patient's position within the community may be altered. Some of these role changes are necessary because of changes in the patient's health status and capacity to function. Others occur because of the expected behavior associated with the role of cancer patient. Still others are a result of negative beliefs about cancer.

Social roles are very closely related to the status and value of a person within society. A person's value depends on the contributions made to society. If society perceives that person as not contributing, roles will be withdrawn and the patient's social worth will diminish. Social worth is very important to our self-esteem. As social roles will be withdrawn and the patient's

The patient should be encouraged to maintain social roles, when possible. The family needs to understand the consequences of taking family roles away from the patient. With assistance, both patient and family can often find ways for the patient to function meaningfully within the family structure. Even if the patient is physically incapacitated, roles such as peacemaker, decision-maker, teacher, parent, and spouse can be maintained. It may be possible for the patient to take on roles previously held by another family member while that family member fills a role previously held by the patient.

Uncertain Future

One of the most difficult feelings that must be lived with in cancer is uncertainty. It is not always possible to determine who will live and who will die, who will have recurrence and who will not, whose treatment will be effective and whose will not. We tend to be very goal-oriented people. Our security comes from being able to anticipate what will happen tomorrow. The uncertainty of cancer leaves people feeling anxious, insecure, and out of control.

Patients who may have many years of life ahead of them need to recognize that only portions of their life are completely uncertain. Conversely, they also need to recognize that absolute certainty in life is always a delusion. In spite of uncertainty, life must be lived and decisions must be made.

Patients with a shorter projected future can be helped to function within a shorter time reference. Those who are able to do this find treasures in the experience of the moment that the rest of us fail to see. These patients need to be given as much information as is available to provide some predictability to their life. Treatment routines, nursing routines, and planning for tomorrow can all be helpful.

BIBLIOGRAPHY

1. Antonovsky, A.: *Health, Stress, and Coping.* Jossey-Bass Publishers, San Francisco, 1979.
2. Bahnson, C. B.: Psychologic and emotional issues in cancer: the psychotherapeutic care of the cancer patient. *Seminars in Oncology.* 2:293–309, 1975.
3. Benoliel, J. Q., R. McCorkle, and K. Young. Development of a social dependency scale. *Research in Nursing and Health.* 3:3–10, 1980.
4. Blumberg, B., M. Flaherty, and J. Lewis, ed.: *Coping with Cancer.* National Cancer Institute NIH Publication No. 80–2080, September, 1980.
5. Buchler, J. A.: What contributes to hope in the cancer patient? *American Journal of Nursing.* 75:1353–1356, 1975.
6. Burkhalter, P. K.: Counseling the oncology patient. In *The Dynamics of Oncology Nursing,* ed. by P. K. Burkhalter and D. L. Donley. McGraw-Hill Book Co., New York, 1978.
7. Burkhalter, P. K., and P. R. Russell: Sexuality and the oncology patient. In *The Dynamics of Oncology Nursing,* ed. by P. K. Burkhalter and D. L. Donley, McGraw-Hill Book Co., New York, 1978.
8. Cain, M., and C. Henke: Living with cancer. *Oncology Nursing Forum.* 5:4–5, 1978.
9. Caplan, G.: *Support Systems and Community Mental Health.* Behavioral Publications, New York, 1974.
10. Caplan, G., and M. Killilea: *Support Systems and Mutual Help.* Grune & Stratton, New York, 1976.
11. Cassileth, B. R., and J. N. Hamilton: The family with cancer. In *The Cancer Patient: Social and Medical Aspects of Cancer,* ed. by B. R. Cassileth. Lea & Febiger, Philadelphia, 1979.
12. Cassileth, B. R., and H. I. Lief: Cancer: a biopsychosocial model. In *The Cancer Patient: Social and Medical Aspects of Care,* ed. by B. R. Cassileth. Lea & Febiger, Philadelphia, 1979.

13. Cohen, M. M., and D. K. Wellish: Living in limbo: psychosocial intervention in families with a cancer patient. *American Journal of Psychotherapy.* 32:561–571, 1978.

14. Costello, A. M.: Supporting the patient with problems related to body image. In *Cancer: Pathophysiology, Etiology, and Management,* ed. by L. C. Kruse, J. L. Reese, and L. K. Hart. C. V. Mosby Co., St. Louis, 1979.

15. Creech, R. H.: The psychologic support of the cancer patient: a medical oncologist's viewpoint. *Seminars in Oncology.* 2:285–292. 1975.

16. Day, E.: The patient with cancer and the family. *New England Journal of Medicine.* 274:883–884, 1966.

17. Derogatis, L. R., M. D. Abeloff, and C. D. McBeth: Cancer patients and their physicians in the perception of psychological symptoms. *Psychosomatics.* 17:197–201, 1976.

18. Derogatis, L. R., and S. M. Kourlesis: An approach to evaluation of sexual problems in the cancer patient. *CA — A Cancer Journal for Clinicians.* 31:46–50, 1981.

19. Derogatis, L. R., M. D. Abeloff, and N. Melisaratos: Psychological coping mechanisms and survival time in metastatic breast cancer. *Journal of the American Medical Association.* 242:1504–1508, 1979.

20. Donovan, M. I., and S. G. Pierce. *Cancer Care Nursing.* Appleton-Century-Crofts, New York, 1976.

21. Duncan, S., and P. Rodney: Hope: a negative force? *The Canadian Nurse.* Mar. 1978, pp. 22–23.

22. Ehlke, G.: The psychological aspects of cancer. In *The Dynamics of Oncology Nursing,* ed. by P. K. Burkhalter and D. L. Donley. McGraw-Hill Book Co., New York, 1978.

23. Foley, V.: *An Introduction to Family Therapy.* Grune & Stratton, New York, 1974.

24. Francis, G. M., and B. A. Munjas: *Manual of Social Psychologic Assessment.* Appleton-Century-Crofts, New York, 1976.

25. Freidenbergs, I., W. Gordon, M. Ruckdeschel, and L. Diller: Assessment and treatment of psychosocial problems of the cancer patient: a case study. *Cancer Nursing.* 3:111–119, 1980.

26. Friedman, B. D.: Coping with cancer: a guide for health care professionals. *Cancer Nursing.* 3:105–109, 1980.

27. Froland, C., G. Brodsky, and L. Steward: Social support and social adjustment: implication for mental health professionals. *Community Mental Health Journal.* 15:82–93, 1979.

28. Garusi, G. F.: Psychological problems of the cancer patient. *Zeitschrift fur Krebsferchung und Klinische Onkologic.* 91:117–125, 1978.

29. Giacgunta, B.: Helping families face the crisis of cancer. *American Journal of Nursing.* 77:1585–1588, 1977.

30. Gigliotti, L. R.: Treatment environments and professional nursing: an interactive opportunity. In *The Cancer Patient: Social and Medical Aspects of Care,* ed. by B. R. Cassileth. Lea & Febiger, Philadelphia, 1979.

31. Goldstein, V., G. Regnery, and E. Wellin: Caretaker role fatigue. *Nursing Outlook.* 29:24–30, 1981.

32. Harker, B. L.: Cancer and communication problems. *Psychiatry in Medicine.* 3:163–171, 1972.

33. Holland, J. : Coping with cancer: a challenge to the behavioral sciences. In *Cancer: The Behavioral Dimensions,* ed. by J. W. Cullen, B. H. Fox, and R. N. Isom. Raven Press, New York, 1976.

34. Holland, J.: Understanding the cancer patient. *CA — A Cancer Journal for Clinicians.* 30:103–112, 1980.

35. Kaplan, D., A. Smith, R. Grabstein, and S. Fisherman: Family mediation of stress. *Social Work.* 18:60–69, 1973.

36. Konior, G. and A. S. Levine: The fear of dying: how patients and their doctors behave. *Seminars in Oncology.* 2:311–316, 1975.

37. Korner, I. N.: Hope as a method of coping. *Journal of Consulting and Counseling Psychology.* 34:134–139, 1970.

38. Krant, M., M. Beiser, G. Adler, and L. Johnston: The role of a hospital-based psychosocial unit in terminal cancer illness and bereavement. *Journal of Chronic Diseases.* 29:115–127, 1976.

39. Krant, M., and L. Johnston: Family members' perceptions of communications in late stage cancer. *International Journal of Psychiatry in Medicine.* 8:203–216, 1977–78.

40. Leiber, L., M. Plumb, M. Gustanzang, and J. Holland: The communication of affection between cancer patients and their spouses. *Psychosomatic Medicine.* 38:379–385, 1976.

41. Leonardson, G. R.: Relationship between self-concept and perceived physical fitness. *Perceptual and Motor Skills.* 44:62, 1977.

42. Letang, B. W.: Coordinated supportive services benefit the breast cancer patient. *Delaware Medical Journal.* 49:623–624, 1979.

43. Lewis, F. M., and J. R. Bloom: Psychosocial adjustment to breast cancer: a review of selected literature. *International Journal of Psychiatry in Medicine.* 9:1–17. 1978–79.

44. McCorkle, R.: The advanced cancer patient: how he will live — and die. *Nursing 1976.* 6:47–49, 1976.

45. McCorkle, R., and K. Young. Development of a symptom distress scale. *Cancer Nursing.* 1:373–378, 1978.

46. MacVickar, M. G., and P. Archbold: A framework for family assessment in chronic illness. *Nursing Forum.* 15:180–194, 1976.

47. Martin, P. J., M. H. Friedmeyer, and J. E. Moore: Pretty patient — healthy patient? A study of physical attractiveness and psychopathology. *Journal of Clinical Psychology.* 33:990–994, 1977.

48. Mastrorito, R. G.: Cancer: awareness and denial. *Clinical Bulletin.* 4:142–146, 1974.

49. Miller, C. L., P. R. Denner, and V. E. Richardson: Assessing the psychosocial problems of cancer patients: a review of current research. *International Journal of Nursing Studies.* 13:161–166, 1976.

50. Miller, M. W., and C. Nygren: Living with cancer-coping behaviors. *Cancer Nursing.* 1:297–302, 1978.

51. Minuchin, S.: Families and family therapy. Harvard University Press, Cambridge, 1974.

52. Morrow, G. R., R. J. Chiarello, and L. R. Derogatis: A new scale for assessing patients' psychosocial adjustment to medical illness. *Psychological Medicine.* 8:605–610, 1978.

53. Muranski, B. J., D. Penman, and M. Schmitt: Social support in health and illness: the concept and its measurement. *Cancer Nursing.* 1:365–371, 1978.

54. Parkes, M. C.: The emotional impact of cancer on patients and their families. *Journal of Laryngology and Otology.* 89:1271–9. 1975.

55. Robinson, L.: *Psychological Aspects of the Care of Hospitalized Patients.* F. A. Davis Co., Philadelphia, 1976.

56. Ryan, M. E., and B. Nevenshwander. Team approach of patients with neoplastic disease. *Radiologic Technology.* 49:285–289, 1977.

57. Sachtlebeu, C.: The role of belief systems in cancer therapy. *Delaware Medical Journal.* 50:71–72, 1978.

58. Sanders, J. B., and C. G. Kardinal: Adaptive coping mechanisms in adult acute leukemia patients in remission. *Journal of the American Medical Association.* 238:952–954, 1977.

59. Sheldon, A., C. Ryser, and M. Krant: An integrated family oriented cancer care program: the report of a pilot project in the socio-emotional management of chronic disease. *Journal of Chronic Diseases.* 22:743–744, 1970.

60. Silberfarb, P. M.: Psychiatric themes in the rehabilitation of mastectomy patients. *International Journal of Psychiatry in Medicine.* 8:159–167, 1977–78.

61. Skynner, A.: *Systems of Family and Marital Psychotherapy.* Brunner/Mazel, Inc., New York, 1976.

62. Smith, E. A.: *Psychosocial Aspects of Cancer Patient Care: A Self-Instructional Text.* McGraw-Hill Book Co., New York, 1976.

63. Sweeney, D. R., and D. C. Tinling: Differentiation of the "Giving-Up" Affects — Helplessness and Hopelessness." *Archives of General Psychiatry.* 23:378–382, 1970.

64. Thomas, S. G.: Breast cancer: the psychosocial issues. *Cancer Nursing.* 1:53–60, 1978.

65. Vachon, M., K. Freedman, A. Formo, F. Rogers, W. Lyall, and J. Freeman: The final illness in cancer: the widow's perspective. *CMA Journal.* 117:1151–1154, 1977.

66. Veffese, J. M.: Problems of the patient confronting the diagnosis of cancer. In *Cancer: The Behavioral Dimensions,* ed. by J. W. Cullen, B. H. Fox, and R. N. Isom. Raven Press, New York, 1976.

67. Warby, C. M., and R. Babineau: The family interview: helping patient and family cope with metastatic disease. *Geriatrics.* 29:83–94, 1974.

67a. Watzlawick, P., J. Weakland, and R. Fisch: *Change: Principles of Problem Formation and Problem Resolution.* W. W. Norton, New York, 1974.

68. Wegmann, J., and M. Ogrine: Oncology nursing conflict: a case presentation of holistic care and the family in crisis. *Cancer Nursing.* 4:43–48, 1981.

69. Weisman, A. D.: *Coping with Cancer.* McGraw-Hill Book Co., New York, 1979.

70. Weisman, A. D., and H. J. Sabel: Coping with cancer through self-instruction: a hypothesis. *Journal of Human Stress.* 5:3–7, 1979.

71. Weisman, A. D., and J. W. Worden: The existential plight in cancer: significance of the first 100 days. *International Journal of Psychiatry in Medicine.* 7:1–15, 1976–77.

72. Welch, D.: Assessing psychosocial needs involved in cancer patient care during treatment. *Oncology Nursing Forum.* 6:12–18, 1979.

73. Wellish, D., M. Mosher, and C. Van Scoy: Management of family emotional stress: family group therapy in a private oncology practice. *International Journal of Group Psychotherapy.* 28:225–231, 1978.

74. Wieder, S., J. Schwarzfeld, J. Fromewick, and J. C. Holland: Psychosocial support program for patients with breast cancer at Montefiore Hospital. *Quality Review Bulletin.* 4:10–13, 1978.

75. Winick, L., and G. F. Robbins: Physical and Psychological readjustment after mastectomy. *Cancer.* 39:478–486, 1979.

13

The Child with Cancer

THE FIELD OF PEDIATRIC ONCOLOGY

Cancer is the leading cause of death due to disease among children. The only factor causing a greater number of deaths is accidents.[60] The incidence of the various types of cancer in children is shown on Table 13–1.

During the last 10 years, great strides have been made in the treatment and cure of childhood cancers. The prognosis has improved significantly for leukemia, lymphoma, Wilms' tumor, rhabdomyosarcoma, and osteosarcoma.[51] Van Eys states that the cure rate for children with cancer under care at the M. D. Anderson Hospital and Tumor Institute Department of Pediatrics is 50 per cent.[57] Approximately 90 per cent of children with Wilms' tumor are still alive 2 years after optimum treatment.[57] At least 60 to 75 per cent of children with acute lymphocytic leukemia will survive 5 years or longer.[60]

The successes in this field are in part a result of centralization of care for children

Table 13–1. **Major Sites of Malignant Disease in Children under 15 Years of Age***

Site	Incidence for All Tumors in Childhood (%)
Leukemia and lymphomas	43.8
Central nervous system	18.6
Sympathetic nervous system	7.7
Soft tissue sarcoma	6.5
Kidney tumors	6.1
Bone tumors	4.6
Eye tumor — retinoblastoma	2.6
Other	10.1
	100.0

*Adapted from Silverberg, E.: Cancer Statistics, 1979. *CA–A Cancer Journal for Clinician.* 29:13, 1979.

(Source: SEER Program, National Cancer Institute, 1973–1976.)

in large cancer research centers and cooperation between pediatric oncology researchers in centers throughout the United States. This coordination has increased the probability that children with cancer will receive optimum care. It has also facilitated research on current and new approaches to therapy.

The philosophy of care that pervades pediatric oncology is like a breath of fresh air. It has been suggested that pediatric oncology is 10 years ahead of the rest of the field in patient management.[52] Pediatric oncologists, as a group, do not seem to have the ego need to adhere to the "captain of the ship" doctrine that is so evident in some fields of medical practice. The contributions of all who work within the team are recognized and highly valued. Roles are somewhat blurred. The need for mutual support is recognized and provided.[33, 51, 61] Psychosocial concerns and a family approach to therapy are emphasized. Researchers in pediatric oncology have been able to demonstrate that this approach makes a difference not only in quality of life, but also in length of survival.[51]

MEDICAL MANAGEMENT OF COMMON CHILDHOOD MALIGNANCIES

Leukemia

About 80 per cent of leukemias in children are acute lymphocytic leukemia (ALL). Other types are acute myelocytic leukemia (AML) and chronic myelogenous leukemia (CML). At the time of diagnosis, children will usually exhibit infection, bleeding, or pallor. Symptoms of low-grade fever, malaise, or anorexia may have been present for several months. Some children will complain of bone or joint pain.[16, 60] Bone marrow examination is required to confirm the diagnosis. Factors that appear to be related to survival include age, initial white count, organomegaly, and platelet count.

The greatest dangers to the child at the time of diagnosis are hemorrhage, anemia, infection, and uric acid nephropathy. Therefore, immediate steps must be taken to control these complications. If fever is present, cultures should be taken and antibiotic therapy initiated. Transfusions of packed red blood cells or platelet concentrates may be necessary. Uric acid nephropathy is a consequence of the rapid breakdown of leukemic blood cells. To prevent this complication, fluid intake may be increased to 3000 ml per square meter and the child may be started on allopurinol. Bicarbonate or citrate may be given to alkalize the urine.[59, 60]

Chemotherapy for leukemia occurs in two stages: remission induction and maintenance therapy. The drugs most commonly used for remission induction are vincristine and prednisone in combination. If these drugs are ineffective, L-asparaginase may be added. If this fails, Adriamycin will be used. Although these drugs are effective in inducing a remission, they are not useful in maintaining a remission. For this purpose, other drugs are used, including 6-mercaptopurine, methotrexate, or cyclophosphamide (Cytoxan).[59, 60]

Because none of these drugs crosses the blood-brain barrier, the central nervous system can serve as a reservoir for leukemic cells. Therefore, action must be taken to destroy cells in this area. Cranial radiation or intrathecal methotrexate may be used either alone or in combination. Treatment is continued for at least 3 years.

Recurrence of the disease (relapse) is a serious possibility that greatly diminishes the likelihood of cure. After a recurrence, steps will again be taken to induce a remission; however, each remission achieved after this point will usually be more brief.[59, 60]

Recently, bone marrow transplantation has been used as a therapeutic strategy for patients who have relapsed. In order to do this, a person — usually a family member — must be found who has a human leukocyte antigen (HLA) system identical to the child's. The procedure appears to be most effective when it is performed while the child is in remission. Drugs are first used to induce remission. Then, in preparation for the transplantation, the child is placed in reverse isolation. A laminar air flow system sometimes is used.

Cyclophosphamide is administered intravenously and intrathecal methotrexate may also be given. Because all of the child's white blood cells, normal as well as abnormal, will be destroyed by this process, there is a great risk of uric acid nephropathy. To prevent this complication, forced alkaline diuresis with furosemide is given intravenously. Then 1000 rads of total body irradiation is administered. While the radiotherapy is being given, the bone marrow donor is taken to surgery and multiple bone marrow aspirations are performed. Immediately following the irradiation, the bone marrow is administered intravenously to the child.[59, 60]

Several very dangerous complications may arise after bone marrow transplantation: graft-versus-host disease, infection, and failure of the engraftment. Intravenous methotrexate in low doses is administered to help prevent graft-versus-host disease, as are steroids and antihuman thymocyte globulin (ATG). Infections are the most common cause of death and are often due to organisms normally present in the body. The patient is treated with broad-spectrum antibiotics and sometimes with infusions of donor compatible granulocytes. Bleeding is also a risk and platelet and red blood cell infusions may be necessary.

There is a 25 per cent survival rate of at least 1 year for those given transplants while in relapse and a 50 per cent survival rate for those given transplants while in remission. In some patients who survive the graft, the leukemic process is found in the newly transplanted blood cells.[5, 49, 59]

Brain Tumors

The presenting symptoms of brain tumors are the result of increased intracranial pressure. They include headaches, impaired vision, cranial enlargement, convulsions, mental disturbances, and focal effects. Symptoms vary, depending on the exact location of the tumor. Diagnosis is made by radiologic studies and cerebrospinal fluid examination. Surgery is the treatment of choice, but cures are rare. Radiotherapy is being used, though only in a limited capacity because of the brain's low tolerance of radiation. As a group, brain tumors are quite sensitive to chemotherapy, yet neurosurgeons have been very reluctant to refer patients for this treatment.[58] Many chemotherapy drugs do not cross the blood-brain barrier; however, the brain tumor is often not protected by the blood-brain barrier. (Late in the disease process, when chemotherapy may finally be initiated, the center of the brain tumor is usually necrotic and the growth fraction is small, decreasing the possibility of effective drug therapy.) Intrathecal administration is not effective unless there is meningeal spread. Adjuvant chemotherapy has not yet been tried with brain tumors.[58]

Therefore, after initial treatment most therapy for brain tumors is palliative. Steroids are used to control cerebral edema. Shunts are sometimes performed to manage excess fluid formation. Anticonvulsant therapy is usually necessary. Many childhood tumors are slow growing and survival may be prolonged. Careful attention to the rehabilitative aspects of care can improve the patient's quality of life.[58]

Lymphoma

Hodgkin's Disease. The treatment of Hodgkin's disease in children is similar to that in adults, except that total nodal radiation is seldom used. Localized radiation is given, as is chemotherapy with nitrogen mustard, vincristine, prednisone, and procarbazine. Survival rates are similar to those of adults and are dependent on the stage of the disease.[60]

Burkitt's Lymphoma. Burkitt's lymphoma in an African child has a high cure rate if treated early with cyclophosphamide or methotrexate. Unfortunately, a child in the United States with this disease, even in an early stage, has a much more guarded prognosis. American children with this malignancy are now treated in a manner similar to children with leukemia, which is improving survival rates.[60]

Histiocytic Lymphoma. Histiocyte lymphoma has a very poor prognosis whether it occurs in adults or children. Satisfactory treatment has not yet been developed. Death usually occurs rapidly after the onset of illness.[60]

Neuroblastoma

These tumors usually develop from the sympathetic ganglia and adrenal medulla. Most originate in the abdomen and one-third start in the adrenal gland. Some of these tumors will undergo spontaneous maturation into benign ganglioneuromas. Children with a very advanced disease will sometimes have total resolution of their tumor and never experience recurrence. About half of these tumors occur before the age of 2 years and are sometimes present at birth. The most common presenting sign is a mass.[60]

Prognostic factors are stage of disease, age of patient, location of the tumor, and evidence of maturation of tumor cells. Overall survival is about 40 per cent. The survival rate for stage I disease is 90 per cent, then the survival rate rapidly drops for later stages.

Optimum treatment has not been established. Complete surgical resection is seldom possible; however, even partial resection can result in cure. The tumor is radiosensitive and sensitive to chemotherapy. The combination of vincristine and cyclophosphamide has resulted in cures. Clinical trials to determine optimum treatment are being conducted.[60]

Rhabdomyosarcoma

Rhabdomyosarcoma is a very aggressive malignancy that metastasizes early. The tumor is thought to develop from primitive skeletal muscle cells. Local recurrence after surgical resection and radiotherapy is common. Metastatic disease is present in 20 to 30 per cent of patients at the time of diagnosis. Common metastatic sites are lungs, lymph nodes, liver, and bones. Sixty-four per cent of primary tumors occur in the head and neck area; one-third of these are in the orbital area. There are two peak ages of incidence: from 2 to 5 years and from 15 to 19 years.[60]

If children with stage I or II disease are treated with surgery, radiotherapy, and chemotherapy, the cure rate is about 80 per cent. Children with stage III or IV disease have a poorer outlook, but 2 year survivals are now occurring more frequently.

The treatment for rhabdomyosarcoma has recently undergone a dramatic change. Multimodal therapy with surgery, radiotherapy, and chemotherapy is used. Radical surgical procedures such as orbital or pelvic exenteration are avoided. Radiation in the range of 5000 to 6000 rads is given over a 3 to 4 week period.[60] Chemotherapy includes vincristine, cyclophosphamide, and actinomycin-D and is continued for a minimum of 2 years. Experimental regimens to improve survival rates are under way.[60]

Wilms' Tumor

Wilms' tumor usually arises from the renal cortex. Use of surgery, radiotherapy, and chemotherapy in combination has increased the survival rate of children with localized disease to over 80 per cent.

The tumor is often found accidentally by parents or medical examiners who discover a hard mass in the abdomen. Hematuria may be present, and about 25 per cent of the children have hypertension. Fifty per cent of the children are anemic. Even for children with advanced disease, the survival rate is 50 per cent if optimum treatment is provided.[60]

Therapy involves surgical excision, during which time five biopsy specimens are taken of suspicious lesions on the other kidney and the liver. Periaortic chains are examined and suspicious nodes removed. Postoperative radiation is given to the tumor bed if staging is beyond stage I. A combination of vincristine and actinomycin-D is given as soon as possible after surgery.[60]

Bone Tumors

Bone tumors are diagnosed by a biopsy, preferably performed in an institution designed to provide multimodal therapy after diagnosis of this disease. Some clinicians recommend radiation with 1000 rads the day before and the day after the biopsy. This procedure will destroy 90 per cent of the tumor cells that could be disseminated by the blood stream as a result of the biopsy.[50]

Ewing's Sarcoma. This type of tumor occurs mostly in children, adolescents, and young adults. The primary tumor is usually in trunk bones or bones of the extremities. The most frequent sites are femur, innominate, rib, tibia, humerus, vertebra, fibula, and scapula. It occurs more frequently in males. Metastases will be apparent at the time of diagnosis in 14 to 28 per cent of patients. In the rest of the patients, rapid dissemination develops within a year.

Present treatment consists of radical radiation therapy combined with intensive and prolonged chemotherapy. Treatment is designed to destroy the primary tumor while preserving the function of the bone and to destroy metastatic sites. Chemotherapy consists of vincristine and cyclophosphamide.[50] This approach to treatment will eradicate the primary tumor; however, the long-term survival is still relatively poor, with only 25 per cent of patients surviving 42 months. More intensive chemotherapy with vincristine, actinomycin-D, cyclophosphamide, and doxorubicin increases survival rates so that 75 per cent of patients are disease free at 40 months.[50]

Osteosarcoma. The peak period of occurrence of osteosarcoma is from 10 to 25 years of age, with a higher incidence in males. It commonly involves bones in the extremities, particularly the legs. Treatment includes amputation, with removal of the entire involved bone. A hemipelvectomy is required if the ilium is involved. A forequarter amputation is often required for tumors in the proximal humerus and the head of the humerus.[50]

Osteosarcoma has in the past been resistant to chemotherapy but now high-dose methotrexate with leucovorin rescue has been shown to be very effective. Doxorubicin is also effective and some multidrug programs are being used.

Before the implementation of multidrug therapy, the overall survival rate was 10 to 20 per cent. The overall survival rate with multidrugs is 51 per cent. The survival rate for patients undergoing amputation, intensive multiple drug therapy, and high-dose methotrexate with leucovorin rescue is 79 per cent at 18 months. This is a dramatic change from previous results.[50]

Retinoblastoma

Retinoblastoma arises in the retina of one or both eyes and may occur in more than one site on the retina. It usually develops in children before the age of 2 years. In two-thirds of the patients only one eye is affected. In approximately 40 per cent of the patients, the disease has been transmitted genetically.[52]

Early signs and symptoms are not obvious. Eye abnormalities will be the first noticeable signs and may include strabismus and a whitish appearance of the pupil. A red eye, pain, and limited vision are late signs. When the disease is limited to one eye, enucleation is the treatment of choice. If the tumor is very small, radiotherapy

may be used rather than enucleation. If the malignancy involves both eyes, attempts will be made to preserve at least one eye. Chemotherapy is used only for patients with advanced disease and includes cyclophosphamide, vincristine, and doxorubicin. The mortality rate for this malignancy is 18 per cent and is a result of intracranial disease, distant metastases, or the development of second primary sites.[52]

NURSING CARE IN CHILDHOOD CANCER

Physical Care

Comprehensive supportive care is essential to the successful treatment of childhood malignancies. This care requires careful coordination of medical and nursing care. Medical care may involve such strategies as antibiotic therapy, total parenteral nutrition, blood component therapy, and utilization of well-equipped laboratory and radiology facilities to maintain surveillance of the child's physiologic status. High quality nursing care is essential to facilitate the most healthy response the child can make, physically and emotionally, in the face of assaults from disease, treatment, and sometimes environment. All of the physiologic problems of adult cancer patients are equally common in pediatric oncology. Interventions may need to be adjusted to suit the age of the child.

Infection. Infection is the leading cause of death from childhood malignancies. The disease process interferes with normal immune responses. Intensive antibiotic therapy may result in superinfections. Breaks in the continuity of skin and mucous membranes serve as portals of entry for infectious agents. As discussed in Chapter 11, the nurse must take extreme precautions not to transmit these agents to the patient.[12]

In addition to those infectious agents common to adults with cancer, other agents can cause serious or fatal infections in the child with cancer. The child with cancer can tolerate most respiratory and gastrointestinal viruses with little complication. However, the herpes virus group (including the chickenpox virus, herpes simplex, herpes zoster, and cytomegaloviruses) is extremely dangerous to the child with cancer. Measles virus can be fatal, as can infections following the administration of live virus vaccines, such as those for polio, smallpox, and measles.[12]

The most effective strategy to take for these viruses is prevention. If the child attends school, officials need to be alert to prevent the child from being exposed to viruses in the classroom. Siblings with these infections should be isolated from the patient. Passive immunization can be used with plasma or globulin after exposure has occurred. Measles immune serum and zoster immune serum are available from the Center for Disease Control.

Protozoal infections such as *Toxoplasma gondii* and *Pneumocystis carinii* both occur, particularly in patients with hematopoietic malignancies. Both of these infections require very complex medical management. *Pneumocystis carinii* causes a severe pneumonia that demands intensive nursing care. Oxygen therapy usually must be administered for prolonged periods of time and the levels must be closely monitored to prevent toxicity. Pentamidine or trimethoprim–sulfamethoxazole (Bacterim) is used to treat this infection. Both have very dangerous side effects.[62]

Nutrition. Maintaining adequate nutrition is extremely important for the child with cancer. In addition to the need for increased intake due to the disease and its treatment, the child has increased nutritional needs for growth. The nurse and parents may need to work closely together to devise creative ways to encourage eating. Total parenteral nutrition (TPN) may in some cases actually be life saving.[10, 12]

Pain. Children with leukemia frequently experience joint or bone pain. Acetaminophen and acetaminophen with codeine are usually effective analgesics for this symptom. Support of the extremity with firm pillows and proper body positioning can be helpful. Elevation of the extrem-

ity may also increase comfort. Application of heat to painful joints may decrease pain. Gentle passive range of motion exercises should be performed by the nurse or parent every 8 hours.[37] Some of the strategies described in Chapter 11, adjusted to the age of the child, may be very useful in pain relief.

Psychosocial Care

The Child

Many of the psychosocial interventions discussed in Chapter 12 are very appropriate for children. And yet, in each developmental stage children have problems and needs that are unique. Within the limits of their comprehension, children — even preschoolers — should be active participants in planning and implementing their care. This is much more possible than is generally thought.

For children, expression of feelings and working out ways of coping with their present situation are done through play. This process can be facilitated by providing the appropriate play equipment. This equipment should include items used in the children's treatments, such as unbreakable syringes, and small dolls or puppets that can represent family members and health care professionals. Drawing pictures is also a very significant way to communicate with children.[13] Taylor and Williams have suggested that the nurse working with children in hospitals, clinics, offices, or home care should become skilled in interpreting the communication that occurs in child's play and in using strategies for intervening through the medium of play.[34]

Children are very perceptive to the attitudes and feelings of adults. As Pearse notes, attempts to conceal the seriousness of the illness from the child are not usually successful.

Adults and children alike, given partial information, will fill in the rest with fantasy which may be more frightening than reality. Silence also creates distance and distrust, while honest answers to questions given with support and realistic hope, dispel unnecessary fears and promote closeness. Few people are comfortable with deceit, and it is rarely in anyone's best interest to conceal such a serious matter.[43]

Explanations must be given according to the child's developmental level. Young children will not understand the threat of death because death is not within their comprehension. They are, however, afraid of pain and abandonment. They need as much control over pain as possible and repeated assurances that they will not be abandoned.[57]

Children are much more focused on the present than the future. Their energies go into accomplishing the developmental tasks with which they are struggling. The most healthy nursing interventions include strategies that facilitate the child's achievement of these tasks in spite of the restraints of illness. This means interacting with the child in ways that promote increased independence, responsibility, and accountability and expectations of learning and personal growth. Strategies that allow the illness situation to interfere with accomplishment of these tasks can have long-lasting and even permanent detrimental effects.

The Family

The family of a child with cancer needs to be cared for as carefully as the child. There are several very serious problems that can occur in these families. Relationship problems between parents often develop. At the time of diagnosis, the parents may feel that they are in some way responsible for the child's illness. This can disintegrate into mutual blaming. Because of treatment needs, the mother is often thrust into constant close contact with the ill child and isolated from the rest of the family, while the father is isolated from the illness situation and expected to continue job-related and family-related activities. Siblings may be ignored and expected to function on their own. The entire family system is disrupted. The disruption can have consequences that last long after the illness situation is over.

The mother can become so close to the sick child that a symbiotic relationship is established. The child is overprotected and may refuse to communicate with anyone but the mother. The child regresses to a more infantile level and the mother loses interest in everyone but the ill child. The consequences can last a lifetime.[17, 34]

Both parents experience depression, anxiety, and decreased ability to function in social roles.[55] Marital problems often develop.[34] Emotional and physical illnesses are more frequent in all family members. Siblings may develop problems with school performance and behavior.[21, 28]

Interventions for these problems should be initiated at the time of diagnosis. Most families develop some mechanism for managing the situation within the first few months. If the mechanism is an unhealthy one, it is much more difficult to alter the pattern once it is well established.[2]

At the time of diagnosis, families should be alerted to possible unhealthy responses. Strategies for effective coping should be explored. Support groups for parents have been very effective in helping family members manage this very difficult situation.[20, 31, 32, 67] Throughout the course of the illness, nursing interventions should include the entire family. Continuous assessment should be used to determine how the family is managing.[19, 44, 47]

Treatment for pediatric cancer frequently occurs in a treatment center that may be at a great distance from the family's home. This may be very disruptive to the family unit and may increase social and financial problems. Some centers are developing living quarters near the hospital for families. This greatly eases the burden and presents opportunities for sharing concerns with other family members.

Home Care

Treatment for childhood cancer is now extended over a period of several years.

During most of this time, the child will be home, not in a hospital. The family and the community will need help to manage the situation in a healthy way. During this time, the family is in a state of uncertainty. No one knows whether the child will be cured or will die.

Parental behavior also tells children about their future. Under normal circumstances, parents discipline their children, place limitations on them and thus prepare them for adulthood. In many ways, they are telling their child: "I believe in your future enough to disappoint you in the present." If they stop doing this, if they never say no, if they overwhelm their child with presents long after he or she is home from the hospital and feeling better, they are saying, "You have no future," and the child hears this.[47]

If the child is treated as if death were expected, actions will be taken that do not facilitate development of the child. Van Eys proposes an approach to the "truly cured child."[57] In this approach, it is assumed that the child will be cured. Energies are focused on ensuring that the child is allowed to grow up and master needed skills. The child is treated as a normal child who has cancer. The cancer is not ignored; neither is it the overwhelming focus of life.[56, 57]

If the cancer were ignored by well-meaning people, the child's reality would be distorted, and he would not be accepted as the person he is. On the other hand, when the cancer is made the overwhelming concern, the "normal" in the child that wants to be recognized is ignored. Either produces despair.[57]

In order to accomplish this goal, neighbors and other support group members must be helped to manage the situation. Visits by health care professionals to school teachers, principals, and even classmates can be very helpful. The concept needs to be explained and ways to accomplish it discussed. Mechanisms for school officials to contact health care professionals when needed should be discussed. The school nurse should be included as a valuable team member.[27, 40]

Parents need to be taught to provide both physical and emotional care for the child to a greater extent. To implement this, nurses can function as teachers and resources. Physical care now done chiefly by nurses can be performed very effectively by many parents.[3, 23]

During the times that the child's illness is in remission, or when the child is doing well, the family may forget about the illness. The family system will return to a state of equilibrium. Visits to the physician may be resented. Complaints about side effects of drugs may increase. It may seem hard to believe that the illness was real. This denial is healthy and should be supported. If a relapse occurs, a new family crisis will develop.[48]

The Dying Child

The death of a child is one of the greatest social losses we experience. The anguish of the parents is great. The consequences of the death for the family can be far-reaching.

To help ease the trauma, families are now more often electing to care for the dying child at home. In order to accomplish this, the parents need to be assured of continued links with physicians and nurses. The family can remain functioning as a family and provide mutual support. Siblings are less likely to be shut off from needed relationships.

The child is frequently placed in the center of family activities, such as the family room, rather than in a bedroom. All family members assist in the child's care. Parents often do procedures commonly done by nurses. Community health nurses, home health care nurses, or hospice nurses are contacted to assist the family as needed. The nursing interventions discussed in Chapter 14 are helpful in providing care in this situation.

BIBLIOGRAPHY

1. Adams, M. A.: Helping the parents of children with malignancy. *Medical Progress*. 93:734–738, 1978.

2. Atkins, M. D.: Counseling Families. *Nursing Mirror.* 144:62–64, 1977.

3. Bloomquist, L. M., and M. J. Lewis-Hunstiger: To care for the child at home: discharge planning for the child with leukemia. *Cancer Nursing.* 1:303–308, 1978.

4. Brown, A., and J. Bjelic: Coping strategies of two adolescents with malignancy. *Maternal–Child Nursing Journal.* 6:77–85, 1977.

5. Cahan, M. P., and N. R. Lyddane: Bone marrow transplantation at UCLA. *Cancer Nursing.* 1:47–51, 1978.

6. Carns, N. V., G. M. Clark, S. D. Smith, and S. B. Lansky: Adaptation of siblings to childhood malignancy. *Journal of Pediatrics.* 95:484–487, 1979.

7. Churven, P.: A group approach to the emotional needs of parents of leukaemic children. *Australian Paediatric Journal.* 13:290–294, 1977.

8. Clapp, M. J.: Psychosocial reactions of children with cancer. *Nursing Clinics of North America.* 11:73–82, 1976.

9. Clausen, J. P.: Cancer diagnoses in children: cultural factors influencing patient/child reactions. *Cancer Nursing.* 1:395–401, 1978.

10. Cohen, I. T., A. M. Coulston, M. Ferrero, S. E. Siegel, and D. M. Hayes: The role of the nutritional team in the management of the child with cancer. *Journal of Pediatric Surgery.* 13:287–291, 1978.

11. Cotter, J. M., and A. D. Schwartz: Psychological and social support of the family. In *Malignant Diseases of Infancy, Childhood and Adolescence,* ed. by A. J. Altman and A. D. Schwartz. Philadelphia, W. B. Saunders Co., 1978.

12. Culbert, S. J., and J. Van Eys: Principles of total care — physiologic support. In *Clinical Pediatric Oncology,* ed. by W. W. Sutow, T. J. Vietti, and D. J. Fernbach. C. V. Mosby Co., St. Louis, 1977.

13. de Christopher, J.: Children with cancer: their perceptions of the health care experience. *Topics in Clinical Nursing.* 2:9–20, 1981.

14. Embleton, L.: Children, cancer and death: a discussion of a supportive care system. *Canada's Mental Health.* 27:12–15, 1979.

15. Fergusson, J. H.: Cognitive late effects of treatment for acute lymphocytic leukemia in childhood. *Topics in Clinical Nursing.* 2:21–30, 1981.

16. Fernbach, D. J.: Natural history of acute leukemia. In *Clinical Pediatric Oncology,* ed. by W. W. Sutow, T. J. Vietti, and D. J. Fernbach. C. V. Mosby Co., St. Louis, 1977.

17. Fife, B. L.: Reducing parental overprotection of the leukemic child. *Social Science and Medicine.* 12:117–122, 1978.

18. Fochtman, D.: How adolescents live with leukemia. *Cancer Nursing.* 2:27–31, 1979.

19. Fond, I.: Dealing with death and dying through family-centered care. *Nursing Clinics of North America.* 7:53–65, 1972.

20. Gilder, R., P. K. Buschman, A. L. Sitarz, and J. A. Wolff: Group therapy with parents of children with leukemia. *American Journal of Psychotherapy.* 30:276–287, 1976.

21. Gogan, J., G. P. Koocher, D. J. Foster, and J. E. O'Malley. Impact of childhood cancer on siblings. *Health and Social Work.* 1:42–69, 1977.

22. Goldfogel, L.: Working with the parents of a dying child. *American Journal of Nursing.* 70:1675–1679, 1970.

23. Goodell, A.: Perceptions of nurses toward parent participation on pediatric oncology units. *Cancer Nursing.* 2:38–46, 1979.

24. Iles, P. J.: Children with cancer: healthy siblings' perceptions during the illness experience. *Cancer Nursing.* 2:371–377, 1979.

25. Issner, N.: The family of the hospitalized child. *Nursing Clinics of North America.* 7:5–13, 1972.

26. Johnson-Soderberg, S.: The development of a child's concept of death. *Oncology Nursing Forum.* 8:23–26, 1981.

27. Kagen-Goodheart, L.: Re-entry: living with childhood cancer. *American Journal of Orthopsychiatry.* 47:651–658, 1977.

28. Kaplan, D. M., R. Grobstein, and A. Smith: Predicting the impact of severe illness in families. *Health and Social Work.* 1:71–82, 1976.

29. Keyser, M.: At home with death: a natural childdeath. *Journal of Pediatrics.* 90:486–487, 1977.

30. Klopovich, P., D. Suenram, and N. Cairns: A common sense approach to caring for children with cancer: the community health nurse. *Cancer Nursing.* 3:201–208, 1980.

31. Knapp, V. S., and H. Hansen: Helping the parents of children with leukemia. *Social Work.* 18:70–76, 1973.

32. Koch, C. R., J. Hermann, and M. H. Donaldson: Supportive care of the child with cancer and his family. *Seminars in Oncology.* 1:81–86, 1974.

33. Lane, D. M.: Principles of total care — psychologic support. In *Clinical Pediatric Oncology,* ed. by W. W. Sutow, T. J. Vietti, and D. J. Fernbach. C. V. Mosby Co., St. Louis, 1977.

34. Lansky, S., and M. Gendel: Symbiotic regressive behavior patterns in childhood malignancy. *Clinical Pediatrics.* 17:133–138, 1978.

35. Lansky, S. B., N. J. Cairns, R. Hassanein, J. Wehr, and J. T. Lowman: Childhood cancer: parental discord and divorce. *Pediatrics.* 62:184–188, 1978.

36. McCollum, A. T., and H. Schwarts: Social work and the mourning parent. *Social Work.* 17:25, 1972.

37. Manchester, B. P.: The adolescent with cancer: concerns for care. *Clinical Nursing.* 2:31–37, 1981.

38. Manchester, B. P., C. Ferrero, and M. M. Myers: The child with cancer — a plan of care. *Pediatric Nursing.* 4:72–76, 1978.

39. Martinson, I. M., G. D. Armstrong, D. P. Geis, M. A. Anglim, E. C. Gronseth, H. MacInnis, M. E. Nesbit, and J. H. Kersey: Facilitating home care for children dying of cancer. *Cancer Nursing.* 1:41–45, 1978.

40. Moore, I. M., and J. L. Triplett: Students with cancer: a school nursing perspective. *Cancer Nursing.* 3:265–270, 1980.

41. Parodi, B. A.: Psychological aspects in care of the leukemic child. *Haematologica.* 62:75–87, 1977.

42. Patton, J. H., E. J. Wimberly, and J. D. Feddis: Ministering to parents' groups. *American Journal of Nursing.* 68:1290–1291, 1968.

43. Pearse, M.: The child with cancer: impact on the family. *Journal of School Health.* 47:174–179, 1977.

44. Peck, B.: Effects of childhood cancer on long-term survivors and their families. *British Medical Journal.* 1:1327–1329, 1979.

45. Pochedly, C.: Guinea pigs get the best treatment: cooperative children's cancer therapy research. *Pediatric Nursing.* 4:64–67, 1978.

46. Pryor, A. S.: Cancer chemotherapy in children. *Issues in Comprehensive Pediatric Nursing.* 3:45–59, 1978.

47. Ross, J. W.: Social work intervention with families of children with cancer. *Social Work in Health Care.* 3:257–271, 1978.

48. Ross, J. W.: Childhood cancer: the parents, the patients, the professionals. *Issues in Comprehensive Pediatric Nursing.* 4:7–16, 1980.

49. Stream, P., E. Harrington, and M. Clark: Bone marrow transplantation: an option for children with acute leukemia. *Cancer Nursing.* 3:195–199, 1980.

50. Suit, H. D., Sutow, W. W., and R. G. Martin: Primary malignant tumors of the bone. In *Clinical Pediatric Oncology,* ed. by W. W. Sutow, T. J. Vietti, and D. J. Fernbach. C. V. Mosby Co., St. Louis, 1977.

51. Sutow, W. W.: General aspects of childhood cancer. In *Clinical Pediatric Oncology,* ed. by W. W. Sutow, T. J. Vietti, and D. J. Fernbach. C. V. Mosby Co., St. Louis, 1977.

51a. Sutow, W. W., T. J. Vietti, and D. J. Fernbach: *Clinical Pediatric Oncology.* C. V. Mosby Co., St. Louis, 1977.

52. Tapley. N.: Retinoblastoma. In *Clinical Pediatric Oncology,* ed. by W. W. Sutow, T. J. Vietti, and D. J. Fernbach. C. V. Mosby Co., St. Louis, 1977.

53. Taylor, C. I., M. DeAntonio, N. C. Draffin, and S. K. Morgan: A group experience for parents of children with malignancy. *Journal of the South Carolina Medical Association.* 44:290–292, 1978.

54. Taylor, M. M., and H. A. Williams: Use of therapeutic play in the ambulatory pediatric hematology clinic. *Cancer Nursing.* 3:433–437, 1980.

55. Tiller, J. W. G., H. Ekert, and W. D. Richards: Family reactions in childhood acute lymphoblastic leukemia in remission. *Australian Paediatric Journal.* 13:176–181, 1977.

56. Tisza, V. B.: Management of the parents of the chronically ill child. *American Journal of Orthopsychiatry.* 32:53–59, 1962.

57. Van Eys, J.: The outlook for the child with cancer. *Journal of School Health.* 47:165–169, 1977.

58. Van Eys, J.: Malignant tumors of the central nervous system. In *Clinical Pediatric Oncology,* ed. by W. W. Sutow, T. J. Vietti, and D. J. Fernbach. C. V. Mosby Co., St. Louis, 1977.

59. Vietti, T. J., V. J. Land, and A. H. Rajab: Management of acute leukemia. In *Clinical Pediatric Oncology,* ed. by W. W. Sutow, T. J. Vietti, and D. J. Fernbach. C. V. Mosby Co., St. Louis, 1977.

60. Vietti, T. J., and A. H. Ragab: Pediatric malignancies. In *Clinical Oncology,* ed. by J. Horton and G. J. Hill, II. W. B. Saunders Co., Philadelphia, 1977.

61. Villanueva, R., and C. P. Ajmani: Principles of total care — rehabilitation. In *Clinical Pediatric Oncology,* ed. by W. W. Sutow, T. J. Vietti, and D. J. Fernbach. C. V. Mosby Co., St. Louis, 1977.

62. Voors, B. B.: Pneumocystis Carinii in the immunosuppressed child. *Cancer Nursing.* 2:14–18, 1979.

63. Wallace, E., and B. D. Townes: The dual role of comforter and bereaved. *Mental Hygiene.* 53:327–332, 1969.

64. Wolf, W. J., and B. Bancroft: Early detection of childhood malignancies. *Pediatric Nursing.* 5:43–44, 1980.

14

Care of the Dying Patient

INTRODUCTION

For all patients with advanced cancer, the time will come when they are designated as actively dying. Although there are no clearly definable criteria by which the process of active dying can be differentiated from earlier disease states, usually there is more rapid tumor growth, failure to respond to treatment, and increased physical deterioration. Awareness of the implications of dying is usually gradual for patient and family and perhaps also for the involved health care professionals. Physiologic processes, functional status, and the psychosocial situation all change, requiring alterations in the provision of care.

Until recent years, the literature contained scant information about care of the dying. Discussion might emphasize the importance of switching from cure care to comfort care, but the process of providing comfort care was never described in detail. In recent years, the thanatology movement (the study of death and dying) has greatly expanded our knowledge of psychosocial care. The hospice movement has increased our understanding of symptom control. We can now unite the art of care for the dying to what is beginning to be the science of comfort care. It is hoped that the emerging humanistic approach to care of the dying will expand to encompass all of cancer care and eventually all of health care.

Death may be the result of a disease process, but that does not necessarily mean that death is the extreme negative end of a health–illness continuum. In some cases, dying may be the most healthy thing that can occur. The process of dying can progress in a very healthy way or an unhealthy way. How healthy the dying process is depends on previous health behaviors and the willingness of patients to be actively involved in the manner of their dying.

Given our interest, support, and guidance, the dying person may turn to use his available capacities to deal with the several distinct part-processes of dying. He can face death as unknown with the realization that he cannot know, and instead consider the process of dying that he can know and deal with. He can learn to endure the inevitable degrees of separation that begin to occur if he is not actually deprived of human contact. He can face the loss of relatives, friends, and activities and actively mourn their loss and become reconciled to it if this grief is defined and accepted. He can tolerate the loss of self-control if it is not perceived by himself and others as a shameful experience, and if he can gain control of himself to the degree that he is able. He can retain dignity and self-respect in the face of the completion of his life cycle, gradually relinquish the unattainable and respect himself for what he has been. Then one can place one's life in a perspective of both reunion and continuity with one's personal history and human tradition. If this is accomplished, then one can move toward an acceptable regression where the self gradually returns to a state of non-self.[71]

THEORY OF DYING

In the last two decades, research and theory development in the field of death and dying have burgeoned. The once untouchable subject of death and dying has come to the forefront of scholarly and public attention. So great has been the volume of written work on the subject that attempting to sort out an organized theoretic framework is not an easy task.

One of the seminal studies conducted in this area was a sociologic research project of several years duration performed by Glaser and Strauss. This study resulted in many publications, two of which — *Awareness of Dying* and *Time for Dying* — presented theory related to the dying situation.[29, 30] Kubler-Ross's well-known book *On Death and Dying* was published several years later and has had a profound effect on society's attitudes about the dying person. The following discussion incorporates these and other theorists' findings.

Levels of Awareness

Glaser and Strauss's first book, *Awareness of Dying*,[29] describes four levels of the awareness of death. The level of awareness may be used to describe the awareness of the patient, family members, and sometimes the nurse, although each may be at a different level. At the "closed awareness" level, patients are completely unaware that they are dying. This situation usually is associated with the conservative approach to care discussed in Chapter 1. According to Glaser and Strauss, physicians sometimes avoid telling nurses that a patient is dying, believing that the patient will get better nursing care if nurses do not know.[29]

At the "suspicion awareness" level, patients suspect that dying may occur, but are unable to get sufficient information to verify their feeling. Patients are almost totally dependent on health care professionals for accurate information with which to make realistic judgments. It is extremely difficult for patients to accurately evaluate the significance of symptoms that they are experiencing. However, the nonverbal behavior of those around the patients may give sufficient clues to arouse suspicion. The consequences of suspicion awareness are similar to those of closed awareness. However, the psychologic strain on family members and nurses is probably greater. A "collective mood of tenseness" develops, which tends to generate avoidance of the patients.[29]

The "mutual pretense awareness" level is perhaps more complex than any of the other awareness levels. In this situation everyone concerned knows that the patient is dying, but it is never discussed. A ritual pretense is enacted in which each participant pretends that the patient will recover. If one party slips up slightly, the others ignore the "slip." Conversation about the patient's death or future is avoided and centers instead around "safe" topics. Sometimes the patient may openly discuss death with one or two individuals and maintain mutual pretense with everyone else.[29]

A patient at the mutual pretense level can have some degree of dignity and privacy but may be deprived of close relationships. The feeling of isolation that comes with the inability to express feelings and talk openly can be very painful. This situation also eliminates any possibility of the nurse's helping the patient cope with impending death or move toward personal growth.

At the "open awareness" level, the patient, family, and staff know that the patient is dying and demonstrate this awareness in their actions. However, the patient's awareness may be qualified by lack of knowledge about other aspects of the death, such as length of time remaining, type of physical deterioration expected, or expected mode of death.[29]

The consequences of the open awareness situation are both positive and negative. As discussed in Chapter 1, when patients are aware of dying, they become responsible for acting in the role of the dying person. Aware patients may attempt to negotiate for more control over matters related to dying, such as routines or activities, nurses' time, location of the death, and presence of family. Patients may press for further information about time and mode of death. These activities may be viewed negatively by some health care professionals.[29]

Patients in open awareness have the opportunity to achieve closure on their life both in terms of personal growth and family interactions. However, not all patients are able to use this opportunity. There is less tension among nurses in an open awareness situation, but many nurses find frank discussions with patients about their dying difficult to deal with.[29] Nurses who have acquired counseling skills as well as a knowledge of oncology will be more effective in this field of practice.

Dying Trajectories

In *Time For Dying*,[30] Glaser and Strauss describe nursing care patterns, death expectations, and the dying process. The nursing work associated with dying varies as the pattern of dying changes. Although the Glaser and Strauss study describes a hospital situation, this is true regardless of the location of the dying. This work has features that are performed at a particular time, such as feeding, bathing, turning, administering drugs, monitoring condition, and providing treatments. The pattern of work alters as the patient progresses toward death.

Each hospital unit has a unique dying trajectory (the expected pattern of dying). The patterns of dying in an emergency room, a cardiac intensive care unit, a medical-surgical unit, and an oncology unit are all uniquely different. A dying patient being cared for on a particular unit is expected to die over a specific period of time in a predictable way. Glaser and Strauss identify four types of death expectations:

1. Certain death at a known time
2. Certain death at an unknown time
3. Uncertain death, but a known time when certainty will be established
4. Uncertain death and an unknown time when the question will be resolved

When possible, nurses must correctly assess when the patient will die and plan their work in accordance with those expectations. However, this assessment has not been clearly defined and at this time must be acquired through clinical experience. The patient's dying may be classed five different ways compared with the expected dying trajectory of a particular nursing unit:

1. Leading to too sudden a death
2. Having a vacillating pattern
3. Certain to die on time
4. Having a short-term reprieve
5. Lingering

Glaser and Strauss emphasize the importance of forecasting the dying trajectory:

When the staff's expectations closely approximate a dying patient's trajectory, their work with other patients, as well as with the dying patient, is made easier. For instance, critical junctures during his dying can be planned for so that manpower will not be withdrawn suddenly from other patients nor will the scheduling of tasks with them be disrupted. Miscalculations in forecasting or in perceiving trajectories can play havoc with the organization of work — as when one or more patients unexpectedly and swiftly begin to die. Each service usually has routine procedures for managing occasional expectable emergencies, but this organization machinery may not be sufficient to cope with crises stemming from gross miscalculations of trajectory. As we shall see, when such crises occur, the staff attempts to regain control over the disrupted organization of work as quickly as possible. Since a revised notion of the patient's condition may necessitate new procedures or additional time spent at his bedside, a considerable reordering of work — even changes in the division of labor — may be involved.[30]

The cancer patient is most likely to fit into the lingering category. Dying is slow and the period of time is unpredictable. Sometimes vacillation will occur, with brief periods of improvement interspersed with physical decline. Following a period in which death seemed imminent, the patient will sometimes achieve a short-term reprieve with marked improvement. The difficulty in predicting the trajectory is due in part to the present lack of understanding of the physiologic changes that occur in late stage cancer. Psychosocial responses to cancer and dying also have a great impact on the dying trajectory.

The Order of Nursing Care

Last Weeks. Glaser and Strauss divide the dying trajectory into last weeks, last days, and last hours. Nurses generally spend the last weeks juggling care activities and situations related to the patient's family and relationships. Managing space and dealing with the family are major problems. Space problems include increased equipment and supplies at a patient's bedside and an increased number of family members standing in the room and hallways. The patient is involved in leave-taking, examining the meaning of death, and tying up loose ends. Social isolation of the patient may increase. Otherwise forbidden behavior by the patient may be licensed.[30]

Last Days. During last days, family, health care providers, and sometimes the patient are confronted with decisions regarding whether or not to prolong life (or prolong dying). Nurses tend to resist extending the dying process. Physicians tend to resist "giving up." Family members often put pressure on the physician to end their ordeal. Or, if they have not accepted the death, they may push for intensive measures to prolong life. Choices must also be made about where the dying will occur: home, hospital, or nursing home.[30]

Last Hours. Three stages occur during the last hours: the death watch, the death scene, and the death itself.

The Death Watch. During the death watch, little is happening to the patient. Nurses must monitor the patient's condition closely. This watch is designed to maintain the order of nursing care and prevent an unpleasant death. Negligence is guarded against. Care focuses upon physical management of the patient, by control of his or her sleep, pain, or restlessness, for instance. It is considered important for the patient not to die alone. In some hospitals, a staff member will be assigned to stay with the patient if family members are not present. Nurses may encourage the family to eat or get some rest, assuring them that they will be called when death is imminent.

If nurses miscalculate the dying trajectory, the patient may die too soon, disrupting the order of nursing care and leaving no time to alert the family. The patient may also live longer than expected, resulting in a false watch, with the family requesting to be called again when the condition gets worse.[30]

The Death Scene. The death scene is brief and ends at the actual death. Many nurses prefer not to be present at this time and avoid it. Family members are allowed to witness the death scene if the patient is dying comfortably and in an acceptable way. Families who have demonstrated their ability to control themselves are more likely to be allowed to stay.[30]

The Death. The death is the brief period in which the patient dies and is officially recognized as dead. The official pronouncement is generally made by a physician.

After Death. After the death, there is still hospital work to be completed. The hospital "must dispose of the body; it must wind up its relationship with the family; it must write a conclusion to the patient's story."[30]

The Announcement. Unless the family has been present at the death scene, it is necessary for someone to inform the family of the death. Preferably, the announcement is made in a private place, allowing the family to express grief without disrupting the sentimental (emotional) order of the unit. However, with an illness like cancer, which has a lingering trajectory, the family is expected to accept the news of the patient's death with some degree of composure. Although announcement of death is usually the physician's role, in a lingering dying trajectory this task may be delegated to the nurse.

The Last Look. Often the family is encouraged to look at the patient before the body is taken to the funeral home. Nurses usually tidy up the body, the bed, and the room before inviting in the family. There is generally an unspoken agreement that the family will not make a scene.

The Last Touch. Family members often need to touch the body in an attempt to close the gap between life and death. The touch may trigger strong emotional feelings:

Happily, many last touches are gentle and moving, bringing to both the relative and the usher a modicum of composure — and perhaps closure. The relative may kiss the body, stroke the cheek, caress the hands, run hands through the hair, touch all the face areas. These touches seem to be a matter of assuring oneself that "everything is in place" and thus they help close the mystic gap. Such a final, formal farewell is made even more real by touching a body that is still warm. The relative realizes he is saying goodbye at the point of genuine departure. The staff member watches and waits for the right moment, when the disbelief in death disappears, then gently ushers the relative out and takes him back to the family group.[30]

The Usher. A hospital representative, often a nurse, serves as an usher to escort family members to see the body. This individual provides support during the last look and the last touch and is responsible for preserving the sentimental order of the unit. It is no easy task and many nurses either avoid it or refuse to allow the family to see the body.

Body Disposal. Body disposal is usually well organized by the hospital. Attempts are made to conceal knowledge of the death and the body from other patients and visitors. These attempts are usually unsuccessful. Doors to other patients' rooms are closed when the body is removed. When the body is being transported, attempts are made to prevent the appearance that a body is being moved. Usually an elevator is held open and the body is moved hurriedly down the hall and into the elevator, out of sight.

The Last Details. After the last look, the family must gather the patient's belongings and attend to the hospital details. Autopsy permits may have to be signed. Arrangements must be made with a funeral home. Many hospitals have private areas that families can use at this time. Support may be provided for the grieving family by the nursing staff. In a lingering trajectory, intense immediate grieving may be minimal. The intensity of support given the family will depend on how well the nurses know the family and how well the family members conduct themselves emotionally. The noisy, highly emotional family will often be quickly ushered out of the hospital. After the family has left, no further contact is usually made between nurses and family.

Disposition of the Patient's Story. The disposition of the patient's story is a psychosocial process that brings the situation to a close in the minds of the nurses. Those patients whose dying and trajectories were expected and typical are quickly forgotten. If the patient's death was sudden or unusual, a post-mortem story may be developed about the patient to explain what happened. If the patient's death was a significant social loss, if the patient was particularly obnoxious or wonderful, or if the family's characteristics made them outstanding, a post-mortem story may be generated. The story is brought to a close by repeated discussion by the nurses. Personal grieving and introspection by the nurses may accompany the story's close.

The post-mortem story is developed by talking. The scene is reconstructed and the nurses may review the situation for signs that were missed, discuss things that went wrong, reflect on what the patient seemed to be thinking, and evaluate the possibility of negligence. Most of this discussion subsides in a few days or weeks, but in some few cases the situation is still remembered on the unit years later.[30]

Stages of Dying

The Theory

Almost all discussion of death and dying is dated as before or after Kubler-Ross, who has had a significant impact upon society's attitudes about dying. Kubler-Ross's book *On Death and Dying* examines multiple case studies that graphically demonstrate meaningful interaction with the dying person. The impact of social isolation on the dying patient is clearly demonstrated.

Kubler-Ross describes five emotional stages that the dying person goes through: denial, anger, bargaining, depression, and acceptance. She discusses strategies that can help the patient move through the stages to the goal of acceptance. Kubler-Ross's definition of acceptance is one in which the person is not necessarily happy, but accepts the reality of dying and gradually withdraws from meaningful relationships. This orientation toward the dying has been so publicized that the dying person is now expected to move in sequence through these stages. Nurses gauge how effective they are by whether and how fast their patients move through these stages to acceptance. In a sense, the stages are being used as a check list, although Kubler-Ross never intended them to be employed in this way.

Criticism of the Theory

Unfortunately, Kubler-Ross did not use any research strategy to identify the stages; she used the case method. Although thanatologists recognize the significance of her contribution to care of the dying, the theory of stages is now being seriously questioned. Schultz believes that:

It is important to note that Kubler-Ross's *stages theory* is based on the impressions of one individual. No attempt was made to control or systematize the interview process or to check the reliability of the observations. Given these limitations, her conclusions are perhaps best viewed as hypotheses rather than as guides for policy formation. More sophisticated investigations are necessary to adequately evaluate speculations such as these.[82]

Kastenbaum[45] examines both the strengths and weaknesses of stage theory.

Weaknesses

1. The existence of the stages as such has not been demonstrated.
2. No evidence is presented that people do move from stage 1 through stage 5.
3. The limits of the method have not been recognized.
4. There is insufficient distinction between description (how particular individuals have died) and prescription (how one *should* die).
5. There is a questionable balance between emphasis on the response to the dying situation and the totality of the individual's life.
6. It is not acknowledged that the resources, pressures, and characteristics of the immediate environment can make a tremendous difference.
7. The available evidence, although not definitive, fails to provide support for a stage theory of dying.[45]

Strengths

1. The value of Kubler-Ross's work in improving sensitivity to the needs of the dying person has not been called into question.
2. It is not necessary that the stage theory be accepted or rejected in all of its particulars.
3. Some of the practical problems that have arisen in the wake of Kubler-Ross's presentations can be attributed to hasty and uncritical application rather than to problems with her observations and ideas.
4. The idea that there might be adaptive stages in the terminal process is worth attention.[45]

Kastenbaum also states that, in general:

The stage theory of dying requires careful evaluation. It was accepted quickly by some people as though it was a definitive and comprehensive account. Soon after the first Kubler-Ross book was published and its message repeated in hundreds of lectures, there was a social phenomenon worthy of analysis in its own right. Many readers and listeners behaved as though memorizing the five stages is equivalent to knowing what the dying process was all about and, therefore, what should and should not be done. The conceptualization exerted so much appeal that attempts at objective evaluation were decidedly unwelcome. Even subsequent efforts by Kubler-Ross to discourage rigid adherence to stage theory could not catch up to this phenomenon. Like any other attempt to understand human experience, the stage theory of dying must be examined with all the thoroughness and sensitivity that can be brought to the enterprise. The fact that it is concerned with life-and-death matters cannot be taken as a reason for lowering standards of evidence; if anything this intensifies our obligation to evaluate the theory with great care.[45]

Theories of the Response to Dying

Theorists differ in their analyses of how the patient responds to the dying process. The disengagement theory originated in the field of gerontology and proposes that the aged or dying person voluntarily gives up roles in life, loses interest in happenings in the world, and withdraws from even close family relationships. The person in this state is not happy and feels few emotions, but is peaceful. This is the state that Kubler-Ross calls acceptance. Role theorists suggest that the dying person is a more passive victim and that society takes away roles and isolates the dying person, leaving him or her without the social supports needed for growth.

The developmental theorists focus on change and personal growth, and place value on the process of self-actualization or individuation. This requires active energy expenditure on the part of the dying person. Emphasis is on introspéction, life review, and conscious reappraisal of the self. Individuation involves a search for meaning and development of the self; thus, preparation for death is very important. Theorists who hold this position include Jung and Erikson.[65]

People tend to manage the dying situation in the same way that they handle other problems in life. (See Chapter 12.) Thus, if patients tended to use defenses and denial in past situations, disengagement and avoidance might characterize their response. If patients tended to passively adapt to external forces, they may be more likely to accept and adapt to the taking away of roles and the social isolation. If patients were oriented toward personal growth, they ideally would cope with the experience of dying in such a way that further individuation would occur.

Responses to dying can be gradated on a scale:

Defenses	Adaptation	Coping
Disengagement	Social Role Removal	Personal Growth

The nurse whose response to death is at a point on the continuum to the left of the patient's response will not be able to help the patient move toward coping and personal growth. If the nurse and patient are at similar locations on the scale, each will reinforce the other's behavior and neither is likely to change. If the nurse is at a lower point on the continuum than the patient, the patient will sometimes expend energy to guide the nurse to a higher position on the continuum. Nurses who primarily use defenses and denial may tend to avoid caring for the dying patient. If providing care is unavoidable, minimal physical care

will be given and the patient will be socially isolated by the nurse. The nurse who has achieved some degree of individuation or personal growth can provide support and guidance to the patient or family member who chooses to move in this direction. The nurse, in turn, may experience further personal growth.

THE MEANING OF DEATH

The meaning of death has been examined by many philosophers, psychologists, and religious thinkers. Freud believed that the ego was incapable of comprehending the possibility of annihilation. Death anxiety and denial were strong, and yet there was a death instinct.[26] Jung, who strongly disagreed with Freud's views of death, believed that an important part of the process of individuation (or personal growth) was to recognize one's own mortality (in middle age) and then accept the responsibility or task of preparing for one's death.[42]

In 1973, Becker wrote a highly acclaimed book, *The Denial of Death,*[2] that extensively examined the theories of psychology, philosophy, and religion on death. Published at about the same time, Weisman's book, *On Dying and Denying,*[90] separated death denial into three degrees. First order denial involves repudiation of clinical facts, such as symptoms or diagnoses. Second order denial is negation of the consequences or implications of the symptoms or diagnosis. Third order denial means the denial of extinction, the inability to imagine personal death. Weisman proposes also the idea of middle knowledge. In middle knowledge, the person tends to vacillate between denial and acceptance.

Feifel proposes that individuals simultaneously experience both acceptance and avoidance of death. Consciously, there is limited fear; at the fantasy level, ambivalence, and at the unconscious level, outright aversion. Feifel believes this pattern serves an adaptational purpose, allowing us to maintain communal associations and at the same time prepare ourselves for death.[25]

Pattison has another view of the acceptance of death:

A very different death-accepting attitude might be termed *death integrating*. Existential thought has placed death at the center stage of life. Death is not physiological termination; it is our frail mortality. It is not the threat of body stoppage; it is the threat of one's own nonbeing. If we do not face and come to terms with the existential fraility of our existence — the fact that we plan life trajectories that will lead us to old age when, in reality, our life may be snuffed out at any moment — if we deny this fragile life, we become vulnerable to all the neurotic processes of denial.[71]

Our society tends to deny the existence of death. Increasingly, the dying person is placed in an institution to die. According to Schultz, 50 per cent of deaths occurred in hospitals in 1949. By 1958, institutional deaths had increased to 61 per cent.[82] This trend has continued to the present, with an estimated 70 to 80 per cent of deaths occurring in institutions.[17] We have turned over to experts many activities that were formerly done by the family. This tends to make death less real and less visible; it also has less of an impact on our daily lives. We see death as something that happens to old people whom we do not know. And it is deemed acceptable for the elderly to die because they have had the chance to live their life. As Corr notes:

A curious kind of widespread, but rarely acknowledged, socialization process mirrors these attitudes. It began with natural human death becoming less and less frequently a part of our lives. We were comforted by that fading presence and we encouraged the process whenever we could. Partly because we wanted to, we began to believe that death was not really a legitimate part of life and somehow should not break in on us. Death came to be regarded as unfortunate, undesirable, and even improper. When it had to be recognized, we treated it as something that ought to apply only to the elderly, a group to which none of us happened to belong. By such methods, we proceeded not only to reduce the frequency of death, but also — since it would continue to insist on striking some of those among us — to put it out of our sight wherever possible. In other words, we have coupled increasing distance with decreasing frequency. This is undoubtedly reflected in social practices that deal with death through *specialization* and *functionalization*. For example, in the recent past we have transferred a very large portion of the responsibility of caring for the elderly, the dying, and the dead to a select set of institutions and professional functionaries.[17]

Counteracting that approach to death is what Lofland calls the "happy death movement."[63] Lofland defines a change that is currently taking place. Since it is in progress, she describes general views, all of which are not held by all of the proponents of the movement. Lofland states that:

... the individuals, organizations, and activities which are the movement are concerned with promoting a change in American society with regard to its beliefs about death and dying, its emotional responses to death and dying, and its legal and normative practices relative to death and dying. They are attempting, that is, to "establish a new order of life" relative to death.... Participants — organizationally affiliated or otherwise — seem, to the degree this can be judged, generally to be white, relatively affluent, both "straight" and counterculture in style and, unsurprisingly, heavily representative of such occupations as physician, nurse, clergyman, social worker, psychiatrist, psychologist, and counselor.[63]

The beliefs of this group are that death has been a taboo subject in the United States and that this taboo is unhealthy. The movement has supported talk about death, both educationally and therapeutically. Another strategy of this group is to rearrange the bureaucratized structure of care for the dying. A new ideology of the meaning of death is in the process of emerging from the happy death movement. Lofland has identified three components of this ideology: immortality, positivity, and expressivity. Immortality is associated with belief in an afterlife. Although the exact character of this afterlife is undetermined, it is believed to be pleasant.[63]

Positivity is a break away from Western secularism and materialism and has a link with mysticism:

As a component of the ideology of the movement, positivity involves three interrelated assertions: (1) that the dying process may be the occasion for self-improvement and personality "growth" for the dying person; (2) that the dying process and subsequent grieving may be the occasion for self-improvement and personality "growth" for the family and friends of the dying/dead person; and (3) that death itself (the moment of death and what follows) may be blissful, serene, pleasurable, intensely contenting — perhaps even orgastic . . . the positive character of dying and death is not simply given in the nature of things. Quite the contrary; the growth and self-improvement that may emerge out of the dying process — one's own or others — and the ecstasy of death itself are largely to be *achieved*.[63]

One of the ways of achieving these experiences is through expressivity. This movement specifies that emotions about dying should be expressed and that suppressing emotions prevents the potential for growth. This expression specifically consists of talking about feelings; intellectualizing is discouraged.

In evaluating the effects of the happy death movement, Lofland states:

. . . it is fair to say that in at least *some* of the construction of new actions and beliefs relative to death and dying, something of great consequence is occurring. . . . Individually and collectively, modern humans seem to be "solving" the problems raised by the situation of modern death.

But solutions seem frequently — given the peculiarities of the human condition — to be double-edged swords. An accepted solution resolves a problem but it also reduces the availability of alternate solutions. When groups solve their problems they seem also to bondage themselves to their own creations, to hedge themselves in with those creations.[63]

The problems that Lofland foresees include dealing with the person who wants to prolong life at all costs and the person who does not wish to express feelings. These people will be considered odd and under pressure to change. The person who fails to use death and dying for self-improvement may be considered an underachiever and face still another failure.

Paul Ramsey, a philosopher and Christian ethicist, wrote an article entitled "The Indignity of 'Death with Dignity' " to protest the idea that dying was dignified. His contention is that although there is great nobility in caring for the dying, there is no dignity in dying. Dying persons must give up everything, every relationship. They must suffer the indignity of deterioration, dependence, and hopelessness.

Ramsey, however, sees acceptance of death and the indignities of dying as a task that has the potential for personal development:

One can, indeed, ponder that verse about the source of all evil in the apprehended evil of death together with another verse in Ecclesiastes which reads: "Teach us so to number our days that we may apply our hearts unto wisdom." The first says that death is an evil evil: it is experienced as a threatening limit that begets evil. The second says that death is a good evil; that experience also begets good. Without death, and death perceived as a threat, we would also have no reason to "number our days" so as to ransom the time allotted us, to receive life as a precious gift, to drink the wine of gladness in toast to every successive present moment. Instead, life would be an endless boredom and boring because endless; there would be no reason to probe its depths while there is still time. Some there are who number their days so as to apply their hearts unto eating, drinking and being merry — for tomorrow we die. Some there are who number their days so as to apply their hearts unto wisdom — for tomorrow we die.[75]

Weisman expresses caution about our new-found freedom from the denial of death. He believes that the fear of death is the root of most people's problems and "is woven into the solutions we propose."[91] To him, the increased interest in death is nothing but a resurgence of earlier attempts to understand (and thus control) death. Nonetheless, death is still death.

Destiny cannot be cheated. It is beyond quibble, quarrel, entreaty, and deception. Nevertheless, while we dread dying, we fear old age. Death is both sacred and sinister, embodying elements of evil or assurances of relief and release from suffering and injustice.

According to the now-popular opinion, we have stripped away the denial surrounding death. It is purported no longer to be a taboo topic because we talk more openly about death, implying that because of a new found candor we confront our own dying with equanimity. I am not convinced that resurgent interest in death-related topics is without its own anxiety. . . .

I do not deplore openness, but like other professionals I am concerned about death becoming a chic subject. The hidden factors of death and dying as a central human experience may be in danger of again being obscured by counterfeit enthusiasm. It is a little like a dreamer who wants to talk about an intriguing dream, but is reluctant to analyze the elements that go into the dream. People seem to want answers, but prefer oversimplified diagrams to the arduous task of asking researchable questions.

We are not so empirical that we do not dress up older ideas, as if they were innovations.

Truth is only what we believe today, fortified by a faith that it will be true tomorrow. In short, every action has an equal potential for abuse of action. There is no idea so sublime, certain, or self-evident that it cannot be distorted and even become a form of insanity. Preoccupation with "management of dying" is a noble and necessary quality of life, but it can also be a subtle tactic for exploitation of anxieties.[91]

What thoughts then can be organized from this vast array of ideas about dying? It would seem that we will never be able to eliminate death, nor will we ever be able to completely comprehend it. Both we and those we care for will experience both denial and acceptance of death, varying in intensity and expression over time. Some of those we care for and perhaps we ourselves will be able to respond to our fear of death in a creative, growth-promoting way. We must recognize and use the strengths of the new philosophy of caring for the dying and yet maintain enough distance to keep some objectivity about its limits. It is easy to romanticize an ideal that can blind us to the realities we must see in order to meet the often neglected needs of the dying person.

THE PHYSIOLOGY OF DYING

Defining the point at which dying begins in the cancer patient is difficult. The patient has usually been in a gradual physical decline over a period of months or years. However, a point often occurs when more rapid physical deterioration becomes apparent. The significance of this change may not be immediately comprehended by any of those involved. But as the deterioration continues, nearness to death is more easily recognized.

Very little is available in the literature that describes, either clinically or pathophysiologically, the physiologic changes that occur during the dying process. The science of pathophysiology is within the medical model and focuses on the understanding of a disordered function in order to cure or prevent or alter its natural processes. To understand these changes in order to provide support or comfort during an inevitable process may seem illogical

within the reasoning of the medical model and thus not worth the effort. However, from a nursing point of view, these changes are important to understand. Many interventions used with the dying are ineffective or unnecessarily discomforting to the patient and may meet more of the needs of the family and health care professionals. A nurse who can recognize the changes occurring and anticipate future changes likely in a particular patient's dying process is in a better position to effectively implement the nursing process.

Because of the lack of available literature, much of the information in this chapter will be based on clinical observation. Although this empirical knowledge is important and a point of departure for research in this area, the need is great for increased scientific knowledge on which to base a reasoned practice.

The onset of more rapid physical deterioration may take many forms. Patients may begin to experience more fatigue, greater weakness, and decreased functional status. Appetite may decrease, and mental acuity may fluctuate. The tumor may seem to grow more rapidly, interfering with the functioning of vital organs and using a greater amount of body nutrients. Additional tumors may appear suddenly, bony metastases may cause more fractures, and the level of pain may increase. The patient may become less and less able to perform even simple activities, such as turning or eating, without assistance.

At this point, the malignant process affects functioning at all levels of body physiology. Metabolism has been altered, depriving normal cells of nutrients needed for even minimal functioning. Protein is extracted from muscle tissue for use by the tumor. Fat is depleted, depriving normal cells of fat needed for essential structures within the cell. Hormone and enzyme levels that control body system interactions are altered and many abnormal substances produced by the tumor may influence chemical communications. Tumor growth obstructs the normal flow of fluids through the body, causing lymphedema in some tissues and anoxia in others.

These changes eventually reach the degree at which continuation of life is not possible. Multi-organ failure begins to occur and with this a cascade of events that leads to the death of the individual. This is the point at which active dying begins. Dying is not, as some nurses may suppose, a process that always happens quickly. As the end stage in a chronic disease, dying takes place over a span of several days. During this period, patients will often have generalized weakness to the extent that some patients are unable to talk and eventually are too weak to swallow. Patients usually have no desire for food, although they may experience extreme thirst. Severe nausea and vomiting can sometimes occur.

A shock syndrome, with a completely decompensated state of all body functions, occurs. This results in a cascade of events, many happening simultaneously, so that a step-by-step process is impossible to describe. Physiologic changes include "hypotension, decreased myocardial performance, high CVP (central venous pressure), increased transit time, low peripheral resistance and reduced oxygen consumption."[83] Multiple organ failure occurs, including cardiac, respiratory, hepatic, and renal failure; central nervous system depression with an altered state of consciousness; and nutritional failure with metabolic acidosis and coagulopathies. There is increased cellular metabolism occurring with inadequate oxygenation, which profoundly affects peripheral circulation. All available oxygen is extracted from the blood by the cells, peripheral vessels dilate, circulation is slower, and pooling of blood occurs. This results in hypovolemia, decreased cardiac output, pulmonary edema, increased oxygen demands, and decreased oxygen transport.[83] Cell death begins, ultimately leading to cardiorespiratory failure and death.

The patient will have more rapid respiration, using mouth breathing and abdominal breathing. Cheyne-Stokes respiration may occur. Urinary output will be decreased. The patient may have urinary incontinence or retention and fecal incontinence. The level of consciousness may vacillate. Some patients slip into a coma, whereas others may remain quite alert until death. Restlessness, with twitching and jerking, may occur as a consequence of air hunger and hypoxia or central nervous system malfunction. Some unconscious patients will moan rhythmically. The extremities will become cooler and sometimes will turn dusky in color. Some patients will emit an unpleasant odor, perhaps as a result of increasing numbers of necrotic tumor cells, uncontrolled expelling of flatus and feces, gastrointestinal bleeding, and alterations in intestinal bacterial flora. The skin may feel clammy. Petechiae and skin pigmentation changes may appear. Ascites and lymphedema may become more pronounced. Tumor masses will become more taut and rigid, sometimes bulging tightly against a shiny skin surface.

Dying seems to require an intense amount of the patient's energy. The patient's attention appears to be focused inward. Attempts at communication or care that distracts the patient may be met with indications of irritation or pulling away. The sense of touch seems to lessen in the extremities so that the patient may not feel a hand being held. Sensitivity to touch about the face and neck seems to persist. The sense of hearing remains acute, even if the patient is comatose. Vision may blur and the eyes appear glassy or cloudy.

Any romanticized ideas of dying are difficult to maintain when one is confronted with the realities that assault the senses while caring for the dying. Dying is repulsive. It smells and feels awful; it looks and sounds awful. It strikes at all of those qualities that we value about life.

Watching the dying person, it is easy to get caught up in the effort, the struggle, and the tremendous output of energy required of the patient. It is somewhat similar to the experience of watching an athletic event, straining with the athletes to make the extreme effort, and then feeling exhausted afterward. Providing care for the dying truly requires nurses who are willing to invest themselves in the process and who have enough mental stability and personal strength not to become submerged in the process.

NURSING CARE OF THE DYING

Goals

Before discussing the actual care of the dying, the goals of intervention must be considered. It is very easy in such an emotion-laden situation to respond instinctively, without thinking through our actions. These goals of care should be met:

1. The patient must be cared for as a person, not as an object.
2. The care should facilitate the highest quality of life possible for that patient at that time.
3. The care should be health promoting for both patient and family.
4. The patient should experience a sense of security and protection.
5. The care should facilitate the achievement of an appropriate death.

Physical Care

The major problem in care of the dying in hospitals is inadequate physical care. This was the chief complaint of both patients and family members, as reported in an extensive study by Castles and Murray,[14] and of cancer widows, as recorded by Vachon.[88] There are several barriers to the provision of adequate physical care:

1. The limitations of the institutions in which dying occurs.
2. The fact that nursing literature has not yet clearly delineated adequate physical care of the dying.
3. The ethical consideration of appropriate use of the nurse as a scarce resource.
4. The low value placed by our society on the elderly and the dying.
5. The reluctance of nurses to provide care for the dying.

Adequate physical care is essential before psychosocial care can be meaningful. The patient must feel cared for and safe before a sufficient level of trust can develop and before the patient can focus attention and energy on the psychosocial aspects of life. Castles and Murray's study indicated that patients and family did not necessari-

ly see psychosocial interventions as the duty of the nurse.[14] They perceived the primary duty of the nurse to be the provision of adequate physical care. This does not necessarily indicate that nurses should not attempt psychosocial care, but rather that until good physical care is achieved, patients and families will not be able to see beyond that to the potential that nurses have for much broader aspects of care. The core of nursing is, and must be, quality physical care.

Most of the physical care activities discussed in Chapters 6 and 11 are also appropriate in the care of the dying patient. As the patient becomes weaker, increasing amounts of personal care will need to be furnished. The nurses' manner of providing this care is also very important. Nurses can indicate in many ways their feelings about giving personal care. Is it done hastily and impersonally or gently and carefully? Does the nurse pay attention to details or skim the surface of what needs to be done? Can the patient and family participate in planning and providing care? Are they allowed some control over what, when, and how care is done?

Personal Care Aspects

Hair. Hair should be kept clean and not allowed to become oily, dirty, and matted. Clean and groomed hair is of great significance to the patients' self-image and self-esteem as well as their comfort. Adequate equipment is available for bed shampoos or dry shampoos to make this a realistic possibility. Alcohol sponges can also be used to remove some of the oil from the scalp and hair. The patient should be allowed to dictate hair style whenever possible.

Nose. Mucous crusts often collect on the nares of the dying patient and can be uncomfortable. Nasal cannulas used to provide oxygen may increase irritation to the nose. Mucous crusts should be gently removed with tissues or gauze moistened with normal saline. Nares should be kept moistened with water-soluble jelly.

Eyes. Eyes can become matted or

crusts may collect on the eyelids or corners of the eyes. These areas can be cleaned with cotton balls moistened with normal saline. During active dying, the blinking reflex may not occur and the eyes may stay open, causing dryness and sometimes corneal ulceration, which is very painful. Castles and Murray suggest instilling cottonseed oil in the conjunctival sac to prevent friction.[14] Because the patients' vision fails as they approach death, the room should be kept well lighted.

Mouth. The mouth requires much more intense care than that detailed in Chapter 11. The tongue becomes thickly coated, teeth are coated with mucus that hardens and dries as mouth breathing occurs, and lips become dry, crusted, and cracked. The mouth is dry and saliva is greatly decreased. Some patients complain constantly of thirst, but are too weak to swallow liquids.

Mouth care should be given hourly with a 1:1 solution of hydrogen peroxide and water. Lips should be kept moist with petroleum jelly. Castles and Murray suggest using a water-soaked gauze for the patient to suck on or chips of ice wrapped in gauze and placed back between the cheek and gums. If regurgitation is causing excess fluid in the mouth, gauze wicking placed between the cheek and gums and extending out between the teeth prevents choking. The patient should be carefully positioned to prevent the edematous tongue from blocking the airway. Positioning should allow gravity drainage of the mouth.[14] Suctioning may be necessary but should be kept to a minimum.

Skin. Early in the dying process, the skin becomes very dry, perhaps due to utilization of fats by the tumor. Care should be taken to avoid overuse of soap and to rinse the skin thoroughly. At this point many patients are receiving bed baths and soap is easily left on the skin. Cleansing preparations are available that can be used in the place of soap for dry skin. The skin should be kept as supple as possible with lotion. However, avoid using too much lotion, which may be sealed in by powders and gels, causing enzymes to become trapped on the skin and leading to excoriation. Backrubs reinforce skin integrity and are very soothing to the patient as well. Areas of skin pressure should be kept dry. Reddened areas and breaks in the skin should be promptly attended to. Decubitus care, as described in Chapter 11, should be meticulously performed.

As the patient nears death, diaphoresis occurs as the body temperature lowers. Incontinence may further increase problems with wet skin. Linens should be changed frequently to maintain clean, dry skin. The pubic and perianal area should be kept clean and dry, with ointment applied to irritated areas.

Elimination. Patients tend to lose bowel and bladder control as death nears. They may have urinary incontinence or problems with retention. It is often necessary to insert a catheter. Because of the patient's greatly decreased immune response and decreased urine output, urinary tract infections often develop and must be treated with antibiotics. Catheter irrigations may be necessary because of thick drainage.

Patients may have diarrhea and must also be watched closely for impactions, in spite of greatly decreased intake. This is often one of the greatest degradations for patients because of the social values placed on bowel functions. More than any other action, the manner in which nurses care for the bowel incontinent patient can communicate either gentle protective care or anger and rejection. Because of time demands and the unpleasantness of the task, it is one of the most difficult activities for nurses to perform gracefully.

A good preventive bowel regimen is very important, especially if the patient is receiving narcotics.

Positioning. Dying patients are too weak to hold themselves in any position other than recumbent and must be carefully positioned with pillows. Their position should be changed frequently and their bed linens straightened. Sometimes patients will assume positions that appear awkward to us but that, because of tumor masses or ascites, provide them with maximum comfort. They should be supported in these positions, making sure that the head is not bent forward enough to partially obstruct the airway. These positions should also be adjusted regularly.

Nutrition and Hydration. During the early stage of dying, patients should be allowed to have whatever they desire to eat, whenever possible. Small, frequent offerings of food are more likely to be accepted. The patient should be closely observed for choking, which can occur because of weakness. Patients should not be forced to eat if they do not wish food.

During active dying, the patient will usually be unable to eat, except perhaps for small amounts of liquids. Because of society's strong association of eating with life, family members may become very anxious about the patient's abstinence and attempt to press the patient to eat. This can cause discomfort for the patient. Food that is consumed most likely will not be digested and absorbed because the digestive tract has ceased functioning.

If the patient is hospitalized, intravenous fluids may be administered to maintain hydration. This may relieve the patient's thirst to some extent and may prolong the dying process. The site of administration may be another source of discomfort to the patient. As the circulatory system fails, intravenous fluids will be more difficult to maintain.

Pain. Patients may continue to experience severe pain during the dying process, even if their level of consciousness decreases. If they have been receiving large doses of narcotics before stupor occurs, this is not the time to abruptly stop pain relief. That might cause the patient to undergo withdrawal in addition to the discomfort of dying. It is very possible for the patient to experience pain and not be able to express it. Some patients experience a marked decrease in pain 1 to 2 days before death, requiring changes in titration of narcotics. Control of chronic pain is discussed in much greater detail in Chapter 11.

Restlessness. Restlessness may be due to air hunger, central nervous system (CNS) involvement, or psychological factors. The cause of the restlessness should be assessed before interventions are made. Air hunger may not be relieved by oxygen administration because of poor perfusion. If the restlessness is extreme and results in the patient's thrashing around in bed and using extreme amounts of energy, Thorazine, Haldol, and sometimes intravenous morphine may be given.

Dyspnea. Dyspnea is most likely to occur in patients who have malignancies of the lung. Patients may have more difficulty breathing while in a completely recumbent position. Elevating the head may decrease dyspnea. Oxygen may also be administered. Anxiety increases with dyspnea and hypoxia, even if the patient is semicomatose. The presence of a calm, familiar person can sometimes reduce the patient's anxiety. Tranquilizers may also be useful.

Physical care of the dying is very demanding, both in terms of time and mental energy. Dying patients are physically as dependent and helpless as newborn infants. Their care requires planning and coordination among nurses and shifts. If terminal care is being provided at home, it will usually require coordination by family members and perhaps the home health care team. But high quality comfort care certainly *can* be provided much more effectively than it presently *is* being provided in most of our health care institutions.

Psychosocial Care

There are several psychosocial needs that patients have during the dying process: to be kept informed about what is happening to them, to maintain some control over what is happening to them, to have some assurance of safe conduct through the dying process, to have their remaining life be meaningful, and to achieve an appropriate death. All of these are areas within which the nurse can make a major difference.

These factors can be examined in light of the fears of the dying person. Such fears occur as a result of the vulnerability inherent in the dying process. Dying people fear helplessness, hopelessness, loss of self-esteem, abandonment, suffering, dying alone, and a bad death.

The hopes and fears of the dying patient must be kept in mind while providing psychosocial care. Psychosocial care is not so much a set of distinct activities or interventions as it is a fluid, ongoing process that ebbs and flows and constantly changes character and direction in response to the patient's situation. Although interventions will be discussed as separate entities, in practice they are bound together along with other ongoing interventions in a dynamic process. The philosophy, theory, and goals that generate that process must be well defined and consistent.

Informing

One of the greatest complaints of both patients and families is the withholding of information. The withholding of information by health professionals is a very effective way of controlling a situation, affectively and behaviorally. Keeping people informed allows them to function as responsible adults, make more reasoned decisions, and use more effective coping strategies and fewer defenses.

Although physicians have the responsibility of informing the patient about diagnosis and the state of the disease process and treatment, nurses are involved much more in informing the patient about day-to-day activities. In addition, the nurse often must function as interpreter of the physician's explanations. Nurses can also be helpful by explaining the meaning of events and symptoms experienced by the patient. Defining institutional rules and social expectations can also greatly assist the patient and family.

Controlling the Situation (Autonomy)

The dying person is often placed in an unnecessarily dependent position. This position is the socially expected role of the dying person (described in Chapter 1). The patient may simply comply with the role expectation, not recognizing that there are options. Certainly, at this stage of the disease process, the patient *is* terminally ill and will need to become more dependent when that is necessary; for example, the patient must let personal care be provided by others.

There must, however, be a balance maintained between letting go and remaining involved. Involvement requires some degree of power and control. If this is taken away, the patient has no choice but to disengage and become dependent. This is one major difference between approaching care of the dying from a health perspective or an illness perspective.

There is a great difference between physical dependency and psychologic dependency. Patients can be totally dependent on others for physical care and yet maintain their own autonomy. This means that the patient has a voice in decisions and can influence, to some degree, the timing of activities, what communication occurs, and the immediate environment (i.e., where objects are placed in the room and who comes into the room). It means that nurses do not walk into the room and administer a medication or perform a treatment without the patient's understanding and consent. It means that the patient can say no. Control allows the patient to be involved in planning care and making reasoned choices after being provided with sufficient information to understand the consequences of each alternative. It means informed consent.

The patient who is often considered to exercise the extreme of autonomy — the dying person who seems to wield tremendous power, dictating and controlling the family and health care givers — is actually a very dependent person. This is not autonomy. This type of person is very afraid, lonely, and terrified of being abandoned. If this behavior reflects a long held pattern of family interaction, it is unlikely to change. However, if it is a change from previous behavior, the nurses can sometimes help the patient adopt more effective coping strategies, by demonstrating acceptance, setting reasonable limits, establishing trust by being reliable about providing care, and helping family members to manage the situation.

Family members may need assistance from the nurse to understand the need of the patient for control, how family dynamics might remove that control, and ways of leaving control with the dying person while maintaining family integrity. Families of dying patients are in a difficult dilemma: they must begin letting go of the patient and still continue to maintain involvement with the patient. Balancing these two acts requires effective coping strategies.

The nurse can often help family members manage this difficult situation. The nurse can serve as a role model of interacting with the dying person as an autonomous being. In dealing with the family or family members as clients, the nurse can facilitate interactions that utilize effective coping strategies and help families move toward a higher level of mental health. Strategies for accomplishing this are included in Chapter 12.

Safe Conduct

According to Weisman, safe conduct means "to behave cautiously and prudently, and to guide another through peril and the unknown."[92] Assurance of safe conduct requires a promise not to abandon the patient. It also precludes the initiation of social isolation, which is a form of desertion.

More positively, safe conduct means that the nurse will provide the needed physical care and maintain a supportive relationship with patients. As a guide, the nurse will have to existentially "be with" patients in the "peril and the unknown" while they move through the dying process. And yet the nurse must maintain enough distance to remain the guide, not the traveler.

As a guide, the nurse can help patients explore feelings and move through the experience of their dying in a meaningful way. Problems encountered along the way can be confronted together and managed together. The nurse can support the patients' most healthy use of coping strategies and can facilitate personal growth.

A Meaningful Life

Life for dying cancer patients can be grim. They may feel that their existence is purposeless, filled with lonely, meaningless pain and seemingly endless days. Relief of distressing symptoms is essential to the patients' increased awareness of self, others, and the environment. The patients can then be helped to use their remaining time in a meaningful way.

Communicating and Exploring Feelings. During the dying process, it is important for patients to have at least one significant other (sometimes a nurse) with whom meaningful communication can occur. This communication needs to be genuine, open, and include feeling-level conversation. New feelings may emerge, which need to be expressed and explored. Patients who have not previously had the opportunity may have a great need for this type of interaction; sometimes the nurse must become the significant other. The interventions suggested in Chapter 12 may be helpful to the nurse providing care during this period.

Dying patients often do not use the reserve and restraint usually present in conversation. They tend much more to be frank and direct, which can be both disconcerting and refreshing. This type of conversation, described very effectively in an article entitled "Terminal candor and the coda syndrome: a tandem view of fatal illness,"[40] is most often seen in patients who cope at a high level and have achieved some degree of resolution of their dying situation.

Conversing with a dying person should include more listening than talking; sometimes mutual silence is the most appropriate form of communication. The patient should be in control of both the timing and the topic of discussion. While the nurse is listening, an assessment can be made of feelings the patient is experiencing and where the patient is located on the coping continuum.[49]

The feelings of denial, anger, bargaining, depression, and acceptance described by Kubler-Ross[43] are common in dying patients, but rather than occurring in a sequence, they seem to be five threads that are always present, with one emerging to predominate at a given moment. The presence of all five can often be detected in a single conversation, or feelings may vacillate from one nursing contact to the next. In addition to these feelings, some level of anxiety is often present.

The nurse cannot "take away" the patients' dying. The feelings experienced by patients are their unique reaction to their situation and should be accepted. Feelings are neither good nor bad. They just are. The nursing interventions involve guiding patients to consider what will be done with the feelings. Feelings can be expressed and give temporary relief from the anguish. Feelings can be stuffed inside and kept secret. This is usually destructive because the patients' negative feelings, rather than being directed outward at the situation, are directed inward toward the self. Feelings that are denied are also expressed in some way in patients' behavior. In addition, containing these feelings requires a tremendous expenditure of energy, which could be directed to more positive uses.

Exploring the reasons behind feelings can be very useful. To say that the feeling is occurring because the person is dying is too general. There are usually specific problems related to certain feelings that can be explored and perhaps solved. Feelings usually come in layers: dealing with one will often allow others that are more deeply submerged to surface. The energy released by this process can then be directed toward personal growth.

Maintaining Connectedness. People tend to define their existence by the relationships they have. This is their connectedness with the world. According to Cassell, elements of illness include loss of connectedness and the patient's recognition of personal mortality.[13]

Castles and Murray see one of the nurse's functions as helping maintain the patient's connectedness. "If one accepts Cassell's notion that illness and disease are not synonymous, curing and healing may be different functions. The dying patient is ill and cannot be *cured;* he may be *healed* to the extent that he is helped to maintain his connectedness to the world."[14]

In order to accomplish this function, the nurse will need to help the patient maintain existing relationships with family and friends and, in some cases, help the patient find new ways to relate. This may involve exploring relationship problems, rehearsing interactions, participating as a third party in interactions in order to provide support or assist in new ways of interacting, and explaining new ways of interacting or working with family and friends to strengthen their connection with the patient. When these mechanisms fail, the nurses may have to become the connecting link between the patient and the world. This requires a more involved relationship with the patient.

Life Review. People who are dying tend to recall previous life experiences and evaluate them in terms of their present situation. This is, in essence, an attempt to make sense of their life as it nears its end. The life review may be entirely an internal process or it may be shared with a significant other. The review helps the person maintain a sense of continuity of the self over time. It is the result of a concern for identity and for reintegration of the self. Patients, when reviewing their life:

. . . see the chapters of their life unfolding, and the heightened awareness of finitude . . . brings them into the last chapter. As their autobiography draws to its ending in death, they want their story to be a "good" one, not necessarily a story of success, happiness, fame, and the like, but a story that "makes sense," that is meaningful.[65]

The person reflecting on the past may seem withdrawn and quiet or may want to talk a lot. The same stories may be repeated frequently. Previous successes and failures need to be explored and related to life as a whole. The nurse can facilitate this process by being willing to listen and by helping the patient explore the meaning of past events.

Closure of Unresolved Relationship Problems. Patients sometimes have friends or family members who have been estranged, perhaps for years. In some instances, contact with these persons can be made and the conflict resolved. With some significant others, estrangement has not occurred, but past conflicts may never have been resolved, placing a strain on the quality of the relationship. Open discussion of the past conflict between the patient and the significant other can often satisfactorily close the matter.

Resolution of this situation can have a major impact on both the patient and the significant other. The patient can use the released emotional energy in other more positive ways. The significant other will be relieved of a burden of guilt that might surface after the death of the patient, slowing down the grieving process and damaging mental health.

Resolution of Unmet Goals. Few patients have met all of their goals at the time they discover they are dying. These unmet goals can be a strong source of frustration and anguish. The nurse can often be of assistance in helping the patient identify these goals, some of which may never have been explicitly defined by the patient. The nurse can participate by examining alternative approaches to dealing with the goal.

Sometimes activity needs to be directed toward achieving the goal. In other cases, the responsibility for achieving the goal needs to be handed over to someone else. The other person's indication of willingness to accept the goal as his or her own can be very gratifying to the patient. In some instances, goals need to be given up either because of the patient's lack of time or in favor of currently more pressing goals. For example, the patient may be in the process of writing a book, but instead may choose to spend the remaining time with the spouse.

Goals that are delegated or given up will be mourned, along with all of the other losses experienced by the dying person. The nurse who is aware of this process occurring with the patient can be more supportive.

Introspective Search for Meaning. During the dying process, many patients begin to consider the meaning of life and the meaning of death. They may examine their life in terms of a greater whole. This is another process that may occur internally or be explored with another. If it is occurring introspectively, it may be interpreted by others as withdrawal.

The search for meaning takes many forms. For some it is religious or spiritual in nature, for others it is more philosophic. The search may result in a reaffirmation of beliefs previously established. However, some patients examine old beliefs, attitudes, and values and make drastic alterations in them. This is particularly true of the relative values of achievements and relationships. Family members often are seen as much more important. Money and world events become less important. Time perspectives change. The patient begins to appreciate the experience of the moment. The meaning of the phrase "stop and smell the roses" becomes clearer.

In order for the nurse to be helpful in this process, previous personal experience in the search for meaning must have occurred. It is not necessary to wait until dying to participate in this experience. But recognition of personal mortality and a previous examination of the meaning of life are necessary. It is a step toward transcendence of the self that can be shared. The self then becomes both a distinct entity and a meaningful part of a whole. It is then possible for the world view and the self to merge into a greater whole. And dying can become meaningful.

Living in the Here and Now. The values and goals of our society are future-oriented. The dying person, however, has very little future. To maintain the same orientation would cause existence to have little meaning. Some patients are able to become more present-oriented, with a greatly increased awareness of present sensual and perceptual experiences. This has been termed "living in the here and now."

The phrase can be illustrated by imagining a person riding on a train and looking out the window, and a person standing in a lovely summer meadow nearby as the train zooms past. The person on the train pays scant attention to the view out the window. The passenger's thoughts are on the future — activities occurring at a time and destination not yet reached. The person standing on the ground has a very different experience. The sound and smell and vision of the passing train are distinct. There are also pleasant sounds of bird songs and a trickling brook. A soft wind caresses the face, the sweet smell of wildflowers and grass is in the air, and the grass waves gently in the warm summer sun.

Although none of us can live all of our life enjoying a warm summer meadow, we tend to scurry by those "simple and unimportant" moments in life on our way to bigger and better things. The change in perception often comes with the personal awareness of mortality, whether or not this is accompanied by immediately impending death. If we, as nurses, have had this experience, we can guide the patient into the joys of it. Learning the process can be difficult for those who are almost completely future-oriented, but the effort is well worth it.

Good-by Saying. One of the advantages of dying of a chronic illness rather than having a sudden, unexpected death is the opportunity to say good-by to significant others. In some ways this is a painful experience, but it can also be a meaningful and liberating one. The significance of relationships can be validated by saying, for example, "I'm glad we were married. You mean a lot to me. We have accomplished many things in the years we have had together."

Saying good-by is a way of letting go and giving permission to let go. This can have a very positive effect on the mental health of the survivors. Saying good-by means it is a shared experience — a shared acceptance of the inevitable and a shared sorrow — but an involved participation in the movement of life and death.

The nurse can have a major role in the eventuality of this scene. The open communications that are a prerequisite must be facilitated. Relationships must be supported. The possibility of the situation's taking place may have to be suggested. Good-by-saying may occur over a period of time. Even so, family members often want to say a last good-by. However, sometimes families wait until too late, when the patient can no longer respond (although some patients remain alert throughout the dying process). The nurse, knowing more about the physiologic changes that are occurring, may have to identify the appropriate timing and alert those who wish to participate. The nurse also may wish the opportunity to say good-by to the patient.

One family in particular, with which the author was involved, comes to mind. The husband, in his early fifties, was dying of lung cancer. He and his wife were devoted to each other and had arranged for him to die at home. Their only son, who was away at college, had come home for a brief visit, knowing this would probably be the last time he would see his father. The husband kept insisting that his wife and son had to let him go. They agreed to do this but insisted that he also had to let them go. There was a tearful interlude with much hugging and touching. Feelings of endearment were expressed. The son promised to finish college — a major goal of the father. The wife promised to go on with her life and not to give up. They each solemnly said good-by and the son returned to college. Only a few days later the father died. The son and wife were grieved but also felt a sense of participation and successful closure. They were both able to move fairly quickly back into the mainstream of life.

Planning for the Future. Although the dying patient has very little future, actions may need to be taken concerning the future of family members and significant others. This may involve making a will, planning the funeral, arranging for burial, or making secure financial arrangements. It may be necessary for the patient to give family members permission to go on with their lives, to remarry, and to change and grow. The patient must at the same time both control the future and let go of it.

These activities need to occur while the patient still has the mental and physical energy to participate in them. The nurse can be instrumental in assisting in this process, often by referring the family to available community resources. These are difficult subjects to broach, and the nurse should do so carefully. Reluctance by the nurse to discuss these subjects, however, can have serious consequences for the family. In addition to these specific arrangements, family plans for the period after the patient's death may need to be discussed.

An Appropriate Death

Appropriate death is a term that was coined by Weisman and Hackett.[92] Their criteria for an appropriate death included:
1. Reduced conflict
2. Preservation or restoration of important relationships
3. Compatibility with the ego ideal
4. Consummation of basic instincts and wishes

An appropriate death is not one that seems foreign to the life of a patient, but is integrated into the style, meaning, and sequence of the person's past life. Therefore, an appropriate death is different for each person.

Pattison suggests that the following patterns of assistance help to promote an appropriate death:
1. Sharing the responsibility for the crisis of dying with the patient so that he has help in dealing with the first impact of anxiety and bewilderment.
2. Clarifying and defining the realities of the day-to-day existence which can be dealt with by the patient. These are the realities of his life.
3. Making continued human contact available and rewarding.
4. Assisting in the separation from and grief over the realistic losses of family, body image, and self-control, while retaining communica-

tion and meaningful relationships with those who will be lost.
5. Assuming necessary body and ego functions for the person without incurring shame or depreciation, maintaining respect for the person, and helping him maintain his self-respect.
6. Encouraging the person to work out an acceptance of his life situation with dignity and integrity so that gradual regression may occur without conflict or guilt.[70]

Weisman also gives his definition of appropriate death:

Just what is an appropriate death? It means an absence of suffering, preservation of important relationships, an interval for anticipatory grief, relief of remaining conflicts, belief in timeliness, exercise of feasible options and activities, and consistency with physical limitations, all within the scope of one's ego ideal. Resolution of qualms and equivocations about the inexorability of death ensures that a dying person, through the final version of an informed consent, will die with dignity, perhaps with greater self-esteem than was possible during life. The dying person can realize extinction without false promises, but with safe conduct, renouncing autonomy without feeling helpless. Appropriate death is not a visionary consummation, but one in which the reward is to confront our mortality as if we had created it.[91]

The activities discussed in the last few pages, facilitated by a caring family and/or a caring group of health care professionals, can lead to an appropriate death.

FAMILY CARE

Family members usually have more difficulty dealing with the dying process than the patient. Denial is more prevalent and access to health care professionals is usually infrequent. This is a serious problem because inadequate management of the dying situation and poor resolution of the grief process seem to lead to decreased levels of mental and physical health. This appears to be even more serious in the cancer situation than in death from other causes.[41, 64]

Anticipatory grief begins when the family knows for certain that the patient will die. Moving through the grief process is difficult work. It does not just automatically happen over time. Some family members never resolve their grief, but live with it the rest of their lives.

Nursing interventions for family members are discussed in Chapter 12. However, interventions specific to the dying process will be discussed here. When the family first realizes that the patient will die, there is a severe disruption of the family system. The family usually seeks help and is receptive to support and suggestions. Within 2 to 3 months, the system has reorganized and utilization of help may decrease.[32]

Family members need access to health care professionals who can give information, listen, and provide support. The person with the broadest skills in this area is the nurse. In order for an effective nurse-client relationship to develop, the family should have access to the same nurse over time. The nurse understands both physical and psychosocial components of the dying situation. A social worker may be helpful in participating in the psychosocial area but should be working in coordination with the nurse. A social worker may also be helpful in referring the family to community resources.

The family needs some idea of what to expect. The unknown is very frightening. Plans need to be made for managing situations that are likely to occur. Family members may need to learn new skills that may be required in order to provide care to the dying person.

The family needs to recognize changes that occur in family roles and communication patterns and the consequences of these changes. Alternative approaches to managing the changes can be suggested. Families can be encouraged to allow the patient to continue to function in important family roles, even if these are new roles.

The primary caregiver role is described in Chapter 1. A family member functioning in this role needs additional support. Family members often do not take care of their own health and need to be urged to do so.

The family needs a safe place to express feelings that may not be socially accept-able. Family members often feel angry with the dying person. They may resent the demands being placed on them by the situation or they may be angry that the patient is leaving them. At the same time, they may be angry with themselves for having these "selfish" feelings. They may have begun to fantasize what life will be like without the dying person and to set goals that reach beyond the death. Often, family members equate these behaviors with the wish that the person would die. Family members may also be secretly relieved that it is the patient who is dying and not themselves.

Although all of these feelings are normal and to be expected, they cannot openly be expressed because of social expectations. Considerable energy may be spent in suppressing them. To be able to voice some of these statements to the nurse and still be accepted is a great relief. On the other hand, it is not helpful for the nurse to confront the family member with feelings that have not been consciously recognized unless that nurse has considerable advanced training in counseling.

One strategy that is sometimes useful is to describe in general terms other situations that the nurse has encountered in which family members have experienced these feelings. The nurse can then express personal values related to these feelings. This strategy must be used cautiously, since the nurse is guessing what the family member is feeling. If the intuitive guess is wrong, it could alienate the family member and interfere with the possibilities of later, more effective interventions. The importance of the family member's envisioning life after the death of the patient can be stressed and the family member can be encouraged to do this. Planning for goals after the patient's death can sometimes be done within the nurse-client interaction.

The strategies described earlier in the chapter to promote personal growth of the patient can be explained to the family. If family members are aware of this process, the entire family can participate in it. Family members can then use the experience for their personal growth.

Whether or not this is possible will depend on the family members' state of mental health and their positions on the coping continuum when the dying process begins. Family members who have fragile mental health and cope poorly are very unlikely to suddenly move into rapid personal growth. This does not mean that the nurse should not assist the family. It means that the type of assistance given must be based on a thorough assessment of the family and designed for that unique situation.

INSTITUTIONAL CARE

At present, most dying occurs within an institution, although patients are spending more time at home prior to death. Institutions, for the most part, are geared to cure-oriented care. The emphasis is on management of life-threatening symptoms and monitoring of current physiologic conditions by laboratory and x-ray examinations. Psychosocial care and comfort care are not highly valued and time and personnel needed for them are usually not provided. In terms of physical structure, organizational structure, and institutional policies and values, as well as personnel qualifications, institutions are not well equipped to provide total care for the dying and their families.

Some research centers are now designing mechanisms for improving the institutional care of the dying cancer patient. These programs may be directed by a psychiatrist, psychologist, or clinical nurse specialist and usually use a team approach, with nurses, chaplains, and social workers participating. Group therapy for family members and patients may be provided. Institutions such as these may place a higher value on psychosocial interventions by the nurse.

HOME CARE

More patients and families are electing to go through the dying process at home. This has been made more possible by the provision of outpatient clinics, home health care agencies, and community health nurses. There are advantages and disadvantages to this choice.

The physician is usually less accessible. Access to nursing care is decreased. Family members will have to spend much more of their time providing care and may have to learn new treatment procedures, such as giving injections, changing dressings, and irrigating a colostomy. Personal care such as bathing, assisting with bowel evacuation, giving enemas, feeding, and turning is physically and emotionally difficult for some family members to do. However, after the patient's death, family members will often talk of the personal care they provided for the patient. These activities may have a great value in terms of the future mental and physical health of family members.

In our present society, most family members either work or go to school. This means that either someone quits a job or the patient is left alone during the day. Arrangements often leave the patient alone for several hours at a time, with easy access to food, liquids, medication, and the telephone. However, this often means that family members are working 8 hours and caring for the patient 16 hours. Sleep is often interrupted several times a night. Activities such as buying groceries or going to the bank become major undertakings. The services of a home health aide through a home health care agency can be extremely helpful. Volunteers from various organizations are often willing to assist in these types of activities if they are aware of the need. Nurses should maintain connections with these organizations. Churches can also be of great assistance. Often church groups do not know what to do to help and need guidance from the nurse.

Family members may begin to feel that the four walls of the house are closing in on them. There often seems no way to get away from the situation. If they do leave, they feel guilty. Previous support groups, by this point, have often pulled away, and the family is often left with few caring persons who can fill in for a respite. The physical health of family members may begin to fail. Depression and exhaustion may become more evident.

In spite of this unhappy picture, there are some advantages to home care that makes the effort worthwhile for some families. Some families are willing to go through this process to share in the experience of dying. Costs for care are greatly decreased. The patient is usually happier, retaining more control of activities and having access to home-cooked food, significant others, and familiar, treasured surroundings. Although it is exhausting, grief afterwards may be shorter and there seems to be less guilt. It allows for a smoother transition to life without the dying person. This is particularly true if there are small children in the family. Children can accept the dying as more natural and comprehend it better than when it is distant and unreal and they are confronted with it abruptly.

Families are more likely to be successful in this endeavor if support systems such as home health care or hospice care are available outside the family and if effective coping stragegies are used. A supportive physician and the availability of nurses seem essential to this undertaking. The availability of respite care may also determine the ability of the family to continue to provide home care.

HOSPICE CARE

Hospice care is an approach designed to provide more effective care of the dying and their families than has formerly been available. The concept originated in England with Dr. Cecily Saunders who established St. Christopher's Hospice in London. Hospice care requires an interdisciplinary team whose focus is on symptom control, comfort, and a caring, supportive, nurturing environment. Attempts are made to leave as much control in the hands of the dying patient as possible and to facilitate and reaffirm life. The focus of care is on the patient and family. This care may be provided in an inpatient facility or by hospice team members who make home visits.

Volunteers provide many types of services in addition to those provided by health care professionals. Counseling services are also considered an essential part of the care. Respite care focuses on giving some relief to family members, who are encouraged to get away, relax, and rest. Care continues after the death for several months as the family is supported in their bereavement.

The philosophy of hospice care is now being adopted by some existing institutions, which are beginning to examine the deficiencies in the care they provide for the dying. The concept holds promise for greatly improved care for the dying in the future.

The Process of Providing Hospice Care

Patients are generally admitted to a hospice when curative care is no longer considered appropriate and their life expectancy is 6 months or less. Patients are usually admitted because of problems in management of physical symptoms, usually pain, but may also be admitted because of the availability of psychosocial support. Most hospices in the United States provide care in the home. Nursing personnel are on call and available 24 hours a day, 7 days a week.

A home visit is initially made to assess the patient's physical problems and the psychosocial situation. Most hospices require that the patient have some degree of awareness of dying. However, having an awareness of death does not mean that the patient accepts it. A primary caregiver must be available. However, in some hospices, a patient without a primary caregiver may be admitted to settle affairs prior to placement in a nursing home or hospital. During this visit the hospice philosophy of care is explained and available services are described. The nurse, patient, and family spend some time getting acquainted. It is not unusual for the patient to express feelings about dying during the first visit, although patients are often in denial at this point. The family and patient will often describe some of their previous experiences with institutional care, and their expectations of hospice care are discussed. It is not unusual for this first visit to last 3 hours.

A planned approach to pain management is discussed, and the family is taught to keep records of the patient's experiences of pain and doses of medication administered. Family teaching of physical care management is initiated. Families may be taught to give injections, enemas, catheter care, and treatments. Strategies of personal care such as turning, bed baths, ambulation, and transfer from bed to chair will be taught as needed.

After the visit, a hospice team conference is held and a plan of care developed. At the second home visit, the nurse presents the plan of care for acceptance or revision by the patient and family. A home health aide may come to the home two or three times a week to give a bed bath and other physical care if needed. Social workers will make home visits to assist in counseling, coordinate family use of community services, and advise in financial and legal concerns.

The nurse visits whenever needed but minimum contact is usually once a week. Nursing activities involve providing physical care, psychosocial interventions, teaching, and coordination and collaboration with other health professionals. Telephone communications are an important part of contact with patient and family. Initially, patient and family may test the hospice personnel to determine if they really will respond to calls for help. Many problems can be managed by phone and do not require a visit. The primary caregiver often needs only some additional information and assurance to continue with the care.

The primary caregiver actually functions as a member of the health care team and is treated as such. Conversations between nurse and primary caregiver are like those of one professional consulting another for needed expertise. In many instances, the primary caregiver may be considered the expert.

When the patient's condition changes, the primary caregiver reports to the hospice staff. A visit is made to assess the change and adjust the care. The physiology behind the change is explained to the patient and family. The patient and family are usually kept informed about expected patterns of deterioration and how to manage them.

Continuing interactions in the management of symptoms occur between patient, primary caregiver, nurse, and physician. Physicians are usually enthusiastic about and supportive of the care being given. They are kept well informed and are encouraged to maintain contact with the family.

Psychosocial situations in the family are considered as important as physical problems and strategies are planned to intervene when needed. Counseling is ongoing and designed to meet the unique family situation. Counseling may focus on immediate situational problems, movement through the grieving process, or problems concerning family relationships. Many hospices have a chaplain available who can assist with spiritual care.

Volunteers have a major role in hospice care and may provide many varied services. They may do such things as deliver medication to the patient or carry a specimen to the physician for analysis. They may do light housekeeping, mow the grass, or provide respite care. Sometimes they buy groceries for the family or take the patient to the doctor. In some hospices, specific volunteers are assigned to particular patients so that an ongoing relationship can develop. In others, volunteers are assigned specific types of tasks or provide whatever services are needed within a given time frame. Some volunteers specialize in bereavement care.

If the patient is admitted to an institution, hospice personnel continue to visit, consulting with the institutional staff about patient care. Some hospices have arrangements with a hospital to admit their patients to a particular unit so that the same philosophy of care can be provided. This unit is sometimes referred to as a palliative care unit. In a very few instances, the hospice has its own inpatient care facility to which patients can be admitted.

When the patient enters the stage of active dying, hospice care increases. Physical care problems are more serious and time demands on family members are greater. Families may rethink whether or not they can deal with the dying patient at home. They are supported in whatever decision they make.

If death is to occur at home, the family is instructed in care during the process. They are informed of the physical changes likely to occur and how to manage them. The activities that must take place after the death are discussed. More frequent home visits are made. If possible, a nurse is present at the time of death. If not, the family calls at the time of death and the nurse comes to the home to assist in necessary procedures and to provide support to the family. In some hospices, a representative from the hospice attends the funeral.

The family continues to be followed by the hospice after the death as part of a bereavement care program. The length and intensity of the program vary greatly from one hospice to another and from family to family, based on need. The purpose of the program is to support family members during their grief and to facilitate their movement back into the mainstream of social activities.[10]

Problems in Hospice Care

The hospice program seems to work well to provide the care it was designed to give to its clients. At present, the clients cared for seem to be primarily drawn from the white middle class. However, studies currently in progress may show changes in this pattern. The select population from which hospice patients are drawn seems to be due, at least in part, to a difference in values about care of the dying among cultures and among socioeconomic levels of American society. The expectation that the patient will know of impending death and that the event will be openly discussed may not be well accepted by all segments of society. Most hospices have a philosophy of accepting clients regardless of their ability to pay, so cost does not appear to be the primary problem. Hospice care is generally available only to those with an available primary caregiver. With the trend in our society of families in which everyone either works or goes to school, many will not be eligible for these services.

Another problem encountered in hospice care is financial. Hospices are not presently reimbursed for many hospice services. Most of them are reimbursed for the same services provided by home health care agencies through Medicare, Medicaid, and some private insurance. None of these programs will reimburse for psychosocial care, so that an important facet of care is not covered by insurance. Presently, many hospices are being partially supported by private donations. Although the cost of hospice care is lower than hospital care, it is still expensive. Some experts are concerned about how long hospices can survive without a more financially stable base. The Health Care Financing Administration is currently funding research related to the effects of reimbursement of hospice care. In this project 26 hospices are being reimbursed for the Medicare and Medicaid patients receiving hospice care. Policy decisions resulting from this study may well determine reimbursement patterns by private insurers.

The people who are involved in the hospice movement have an almost evangelical fervor in their determination to institute this type of care. Hospice care is high quality care because of the firm commitment of these caregivers. But will there be enough committed people to staff the numerous hospices now opening across the United States? What will happen if people who are less emotionally bound to the hospice idea begin providing care? Will the commitment to the hospice cause last, or is it a fad that will become boring and fade away because of lost interest? If a firmer financial base is provided, will a different management group emerge? Will there be provision only of those services that are reimbursable? Will the same thing happen to hospice care that has happened to nursing home care, where people interested in profits but not in quality care took over management when reimbursement was provided? Is it possible that providing reimbursement could, in effect, destroy the movement? Is it possible to expand the services to include a broader span of cultures and socioeconomic levels? Does the hospice compete with existing institutions, taking patients away from them, or does it complement their care? What effect will hospice care have on institutional care and on nursing in particular? These are the questions being asked by concerned, reasoned people, but at present the answers are not known.

Research on Hospices

The first hospice was established in the United States in 1974. Since then the number of hospices has increased rapidly. Presently, little research has been conducted to examine this field. Differences between hospice and hospital care need to be identified and differences in costs examined. The care provided in a hospice must be described more carefully. Some of the major research that has been conducted in this area is discussed in a recent publication, *Hospice: The Living Idea*.[78] The Health Care Financing Administration is currently funding a three-year study of hospices prior to establishing criteria for reimbursement. The author is also presently conducting nursing research in the area of hospice care.[10]

THE PSYCHOLOGICAL AUTOPSY

The psychological autopsy originally developed as a strategy to identify the intentions of a person who died in uncertain circumstances. It was designed to determine if the death was possibly an accident, a suicide, or a homicide. The method was later modified by Weisman and Kasten-baum to study people who died in the hospital situation.[93] It is now being used for clinical teaching and research purposes.

The psychological autopsy takes place during an intensive case conference attended by as many people who cared for the patient as possible. The patient's life and health during hospital care are reconstructed in as much detail as possible, moving backward from the time of death.

In addition to gathering accurate facts about the events leading to the patient's death, people can share their feelings and perceptions about the patient and death. It allows the group members to learn from each other. At times it also serves a therapeutic function.[45]

This strategy would seem to be an effective mechanism for evaluating nursing care of the dying and in turn developing more effective techniques of care. It would be possible to examine the extent to which care plan goals were achieved. In what ways was the nursing care effective? In what ways did the nurses feel unsuccessful? Were these a failure of nursing strategies or an unexpected consequence of disease processes? Psychosocial interventions, which are not as concrete as physical care, could be more closely examined. The nurses' reactions to the situation could be explored. Possible alternative strategies could be considered for use with other patients. Nursing research studies could be developed using this strategy to systematically identify the nursing care that is actually being given and that which needs to be given. Problems not previously recognized could be identified and possible nursing care measures devised.

NURSES WHO CARE FOR THE DYING

Role Expectations

Nurses who care for the dying are expected to function in a specific manner. In Castles and Murray's study of institutions, nurses were expected by patients to always be cheerful, available, and informative.[14]

They were expected to be kind and friendly, gentle and pleasant. Patients hoped that the nurses would really care about them. Nurses were to be courteous to, respectful of, and interested in the patient. Patients placed great meaning on the provision of personal, individual attention. But nurses were expected to provide good care only if the patient cooperated. If the nurses' behavior did not meet these criteria, the patients usually justified the behavior. Patients believed that nurses did all they could do; expected that sicker patients were to be cared for first; and thought that nurses were often limited by institutional constraints, inadequate staffing, too much work, and an inability to get instructions from the physician. Nurses were not seen as independently functioning beings; they were viewed as well-meaning, somewhat powerless, and always busy.[14]

Responses to Caring for the Dying

The work of caring for the dying is difficult and demanding. It is a highly stressful job. In order to provide effective care, the nurse must have emotional maturity. The nurse must recognize the reality of personal death and must have philosophically examined the meaning of death. Even if these processes have taken place, death will always be difficult to witness and the feelings surrounding it will be painful. Nurses cannot always meet the expectations of the role.

Pattison describes well some of the feelings involved in caring for the dying:

Our own attitudes toward the dying are a panoply of positives and negatives, as they also are for the dying person, his family, relatives, and friends, and all professional staff. It is unrealistic to only expect positive attitudes in ourselves or in others. Sometimes we will be angered and frustrated by the dying. The situation of dying does not suddenly make people nice! Dying people are all types of human beings, some likeable, some not. Some people are easy to relate to, others not. Some dying persons we will feel like helping, others not.

Some people who die will cause us sorrow, others who die will provide us with a sense of relief, or maybe even with vindictive feelings of satisfaction! It is our task to identify and assimilate all these feelings in ourselves and others; to establish a pattern of nondenial of all such feelings; to recognize that the range of emotions is part of the human experience; to integrate both positive and negative feelings; and, finally, not to act upon raw emotion, but to filter our feelings through our conscious self, and act in accord with responsible integrity to ourselves and the dying.[71]

Work Problems

Nurses working constantly with the dying are often in an institution with short staff, low morale, little time to provide psychosocial care, and a poor support system. Personnel turnover is usually rapid and the situation is destructive to the health of the nurse. However, nurses are not as powerless as it might seem. Morale and support can be boosted by the nurses on the unit. Cohesiveness among nurses can make for a stronger voice that is more likely to be heard by administrative personnel. Nurses on a unit can work together to make their unit a desirable one on which to work and provide teaching and assistance to nurses who elect to work with them.

Nursing behavior can also change over time when caring for the dying. Pattison identifies two attitudes that greatly interfere with the quality of care and the mental health of the health care professional. *Exaggerated detachment* is a way of achieving emotional distance from the dying. Dying is made an object of scientific study; it is a thing. It is no longer a threat because now there is therapy for it. It is as though using open awareness communication patterns and providing psychosocial interventions that help the person "move toward acceptance" cures the dying. Death becomes an external problem. People are expected to die in rigid and logical patterns such as the stages described by Kubler-Ross. *Exaggerated compassion* is the extreme opposite. In this situation there is psychologic fusion with the dying. The caregivers identify with the dying and seek through their work to undo previous guilts and shames. They wish to restore their own self-esteem through their work. They use their work to anticipate their own dying and its anxieties. "They live, die, and are reborn with each dying person. Such vicarious identification is also a defense. The dying person is me, but then the miraculous occurs, for when the dying is dead, I am still alive. I have beaten death after all."[70] People with exaggerated compassion become overinvolved in their work and tend to criticize any signs of distance they see in others. They feel that if you really have compassion you must be totally involved.

Health Strategies

The nurse who works with the dying should plan strategies to maintain a high level of mental and physical health. Realistic limitations should be recognized and planned for:

Another aspect of self-helping is to recognize the phenomenon of *death saturation*; that is, we can only work with dying persons for so long, and with so much personal investment, and with so much intensity, before we have reached the limits of our personal tolerance. Helping the dying is a personally demanding task. We each have limits to our intimate exposure to dying. We must be able to identify our personal limits of saturation. Then we need to back off, to gain distance, relief, and reconstitution of ourselves. We readily recognize that our bodies need sleep in order to be fit to face the next day. Yet we less readily acknowledge that our human spirits get exhausted too. It is unrealistic to demand of ourselves the ability to face dying all the time on an intense basis and expect to survive psychically. If we do not build into our work and life schedule appropriate spaces for reprieve and reconstitution, our psychic defenses will do it for us, but not in desirable ways, for then we see the emergence of denial, callousness, emotional withdrawal, disinterest, and so on that are the probable manifestations of psychic exhaustion.[70]

Burn-out is a great risk among those who care for the dying. To combat this, Maslach suggests the following:

1. Training in interpersonal coping skills
2. Recognition and analysis of personal feelings
3. The availability of a support system
4. The use of humor with patients and other professionals
5. Varying the amount and type of patient contact
6. Making a sharp distinction between job and personal life
7. Strategies to maintain physical health[66]

Successful coping requires careful planning. It is important for the nurse to recognize when personal limits have been reached and establish ways to withdraw before the saturation point in order to regain personal strength. The provision of "mental health days" by institutions would be helpful.

Nurses are often reluctant to completely separate their work from their personal lives. After all, a truly dedicated nurse is a nurse 24 hours a day. However, bringing work home and thinking about patient problems at home eventually take their toll, leaving the nurse unable to function effectively, even while at work. Sharing experiences and feelings with other team members at work can be an effective way to let go of problems before going home.

It is critical for the health care practitioner's psychologic and physical well-being that a significant portion of his or her life be reserved for activities that are not job related. That is, a person needs regular free time to spend with family or friends, engage in sports, read or pursue hobbies, or simply rest and relax. The more that work cuts into this private time, the greater the risk of burn-out. Because it is so easy for a professional person's work to take over more and more of his or her home life, it requires real effort to keep the two separate. Parts of one's private life succumb to the job every time one brings home work to do in the evening or on the weekends, brings home unresolved negative emotions that are taken out on the family, puts in overtime, is "on call" (and thus never able to really relax at home), spends little time with family or friends because of a need to be away from people, and so forth.[66]

Promoting physical well-being involves

paying attention to one's self. Nurses often feel they should disregard their needs and spend that time and energy ministering to the needs of others. This does not work. A better strategy would be for nurses to view themselves as very valuable people who must be carefully nurtured and taken care of in order to maximize their ability to continue to care for others.

Adequate sleep, proper nutrition, decreased consumption of caffeine, and moderate use of alcohol are important measures. Valuing one's self enough to spend time and money for such things as clothing, entertainment, and hobbies is important. Careful attention to one's physical state is a way of taking care of one's self. Regular vacations that allow complete rest and revitalization are essential. Relaxation techniques can be very helpful. The nurse needs to be aware of personal signals of stress and its effects.

A regular program of physical exercise has been found in studies to be the most significant factor in preventing burn-out. Exercise can be any activity that is physically exhausting: playing tennis, dancing, swimming, jogging, walking, or bicycling. The work of caring for the dying may seem to be physically tiring but it is not — not in the same way as physical exercise is. Nursing is more likely to be emotionally exhausting. Physical exercise itself improves sleep, eating patterns, and mood.

From this discussion it seems apparent that most of the strategies to prevent burn-out must be the responsibility of the individual nurse. They are not activities that somebody else (i.e., the institution) "ought to" do for the nurse. Nursing care of the dying is at the same time rewarding and demanding. It requires a nurse who has some emotional maturity and is willing to become personally involved. There is a risk of emotional pain as well as the potential for personal growth. The care is very rewarding but often not socially valued. Thus, the nurse must have a well-functioning internal reward system.

BIBLIOGRAPHY

1. Amado, A., B. A. Crank, and R. Mileo: Cost of terminal care: home hospice vs. hospital. *Nursing Outlook.* 27:522–526, 1979.
2. Becker, E.: *The Denial of Death.* The Free Press, New York, 1978.
3. Becker, B. A., N. Hannon, and N. Russell: *Death and Dying: Individuals and Institutions.* John Wiley & Sons, New York, 1982.
4. Bleeker, J. A. C.: Brief psychotherapy with lung cancer patients. *Psychotherapy and Psychosomatics.* 29:282–287, 1978.
5. Brady, E. M.: Telling the story: ethics and dying. *Hospital Progress.* March, 1979, p. 57.
6. Brooke, B. N.: The Styx. In *Cancer: Pathophysiology, Etiology and Management,* ed. by L. C. Kruse, J. L. Reese and L. K. Hart. C. V. Mosby Co., St. Louis, 1979.
7. Brown, N. K., M. A. Brown, and D. Thompson: Decision making for the terminally ill patient. *Cancer: The Behavioral Dimensions,* ed. by J. W. Cullen, B. H. Fox, and R. N. Isom. Raven Press, New York, 1976.
8. Burkhalter, P. K.: Living until death: caring for the dying cancer patient. In *Dynamics of Oncology Nursing,* ed. by P. K. Burkhalter and D. L. Donley. McGraw-Hill Book Co., New York, 1978.
9. Burns, N.: Evaluation of a supportive-expressive group for families of cancer patients. Unpublished Ph.D. dissertation, Texas Woman's University, 1981.
10. Burns, N. and M. K. Carney: Evaluation of the first year of operation of a hospice. Research in progress, University of Texas at Arlington, 1982.
11. Cantor, R. C.: *And A Time To Live.* Harper & Row Publishers, Inc., New York, 1978.
12. Carey, R. G. and E. J. Posavac: Holistic care in a cancer care center. *Nursing Research.* 28:213–216, 1979.
13. Cassell, E. J.: Illness and disease. *Hastings Center Reports.* 6:27, 1976.
14. Castles, M. R. and R. B. Murray: *Dying in an Institution: Nurse/Patient Perspectives.* Appleton-Century-Crofts, New York, 1979.
15. Caughill, R. E.: *The Dying Patient: A Supportive Approach.* Little, Brown & Co., Boston, 1976.
16. Corbett, T. L. and D. M. Hai: Searching for euthanatos: the hospice alternative. *Hospital Progress.* March, 1979, p. 38.
17. Corr, C.: Living with the changing face of death. In *Dying: Facing the Facts,* ed. by J. Wass. Hemisphere Publishing Corp., Washington, D.C., 1979.
18. Corr, C.: Reconstructing the changing face of death. In *Dying: Facing the Facts,* ed. by J. Wass. Hemisphere Publishing Corp., Washington, D.C., 1979.
19. Cotter, Z. M.: Institutional care of the terminally ill. *Hospital Progress.* June, 1971, p. 43.
20. Craven, J. and F. S. Wald: Hospice care for dying

patients. *American Journal of Nursing.* 75:1816–1822, 1975.

21. Davidson, G. P.: Coming to terms with cancer. *New Zealand Nursing Journal.* 71:4–6, 1978.

22. Dobihal, S. V.: Hospice: enabling a patient to die at home. *American Journal of Nursing.* 80:1448–1451, 1980.

23. Donovan, M. I. and S. G. Pierce: *Cancer Care Nursing.* Appleton-Century-Crofts, New York, 1976.

24. Epstein, C.: *Nursing the Dying Patient.* Reston Publishing Company, Inc., Reston, Va., 1975.

25. Feifel, H., ed.: *New Meanings of Death.* McGraw-Hill Book Co., New York, 1977.

26. Freud, S.: Thoughts for the time on war and death. In *Collected Papers,* vol. 4, Hogerth, London, 1915.

27. Garfield, C. A.: *Psychosocial Care of the Dying Patient.* McGraw-Hill Book Co., New York, 1978.

28. Garrett, D. N.: The needs of the seriously ill and their families: the haven concept. *Aging Magazine,* Department of Health and Human Services, Washington, D.C., Nov. 1978, pp. 12–19.

29. Glaser, B. G. and A. L. Strauss: *Awareness of Dying.* Aldine Publishing Co., Chicago, 1965.

30. Glaser, B. G. and A. L. Strauss: *Time for Dying.* Aldine Publishing Co., Chicago, 1968.

31. Goleman, D.: We are breaking the silence about death. *Psychology Today.* 10:44–60, 1976.

32. Goluk, S. and M. Reznikoff: Attitudes toward death — a comparison of nursing students and graduate nurses. *Nursing Research.* 20:503, 1971.

33. Gottheil, E., W. C. McGurn, and O. Pollak. Truth and/or hope for the dying patient. *Nursing Digest.* 4:12–14, 1976.

34. Hamilton, M. and H. Reid: *A Hospice Handbook: A New Way to Care for the Dying.* W. B. Edermans Publishing Co., Grand Rapids, 1980.

35. Hardt, D. V.: *Death: The Final Frontier.* Prentice-Hall, Inc., Englewood Cliffs, N. J., 1979.

36. Hinton, J.: *Dying.* Penguin Books, New York, 1967.

37. Hinton, J.: Comparison of places and policies for terminal care. *The Lancet.* 1:29–32, 1979.

38. Holmes, F. F.: Terminal care needs. *Kansas Medical Society Journal.* 79:570–573, 1978.

39. The International Work Group in Death, Dying and Bereavement: Assumptions and principles underlying standards for terminal care. *American Journal of Nursing.* 79:296–297, 1979.

40. Jaffe, L. and A. Jaffe.: Terminal candor and the coda syndrome: a tandem view of fatal illness. In *New Meanings of Death,* ed. by H. Feifel. McGraw Hill Book Co., New York, 1977.

41. Janzen, E.: Relief of pain — prerequisite to the care and comfort of the dying. *Nursing Forum.* 13:48, 1974.

42. Jung, C. G.: *Modern Man in Search of a Soul.* Harcourt, Brace and World. New York, 1933.

43. Kaplan, D., A. Smith, R. Grabstein, and S. Fischman: Family Mediation of Stress. *Social Work.* 18:60–69, 1973.

44. Kassakian, M. G., L. R. Bailey, C. Stewart, and M. Rinker: A revival of an old custom: home care of the dying. *Cancer: Pathophysiology, Etiology, and Management,* ed. by L. C. Kruse, J. L. Reese, and L. K. Hart. C. V. Mosby Co., St. Louis, 1979.

45. Kastenbaum, R.: *Death, Society and Human Experience.* C. V. Mosby Co., St. Louis, 1981.

46. Kavenaugh, R. E.: Dealing naturally with death. *Nursing 76.* 6:22–31, 1976.

47. Keeling, B.: Giving and getting the courage to face death. 8:38–41, 1978.

48. Koff, T.: *Hospice: A Caring Community.* Winthrop Publishers, Inc., Cambridge, Mass., 1980.

49. Konier, G. S., and A. S. Levine: The fear of dying: how patients and their doctors behave. *Seminars in Oncology.* 2:311–316, 1975.

50. Krant, M.: Rights of the cancer patient. *Ca – A Cancer Journal for Clinicians.* 25:98–100, 1975.

51. Krant, M. J.: Sounding board. The hospice movement. *New England Journal of Medicine.* 299:546–549, 1978.

52. Krant, M. J., M. Theiser, G. Adler, and L. Johnston: The role of a hospital-based psychosocial unit in terminal cancer illness and bereavement. *Journal of Chronic Diseases.* 29:115–127, 1976.

53. Krant, M. J. and L. Johnston: Family members' perceptions of communications in late stage cancer. *International Journal of Psychiatry in Medicine.* 8:203–216, 1977–78.

54. Kubler-Ross, E.: *On Death and Dying.* The Macmillan Company, New York, 1969.

55. Kubler-Ross, E.: *Death, The Final Stage of Growth.* Prentice-Hall, Inc., Englewood Cliffs, N. J., 1975.

56. Lack, S., and R. W. Buckingham: *First American Hospice: Three Years of Home Care.* New Haven, Conn., The Connecticut Hospice, 1978.

57. Lack, S. A.: Hospice — a concept of care in the final stage of life. *Connecticut Medicine.* 43:367–372, 1979.

58. Lamerton, R. C.: Cancer patients dying at home. *The Practitioner: The Journal of Postgraduate Medicine.* 223:813–817, 1979.

59. Leiber, L., M. M. Plumb, M. L. Gerstenzang, and J. Holland: The communication of affection between cancer patients and their spouses. *Psychosomatic Medicine.* 38:379–389, 1976.

60. LeRoux, R. S.: Communicating with the dying person. *Nursing Forum.* 16:145–155, 1977.

61. Liaschenko, J. J.: Assessment of anxiety and depression in the dying patient. *Topics in Clinical Nursing.* 2:39–45, 1981.

62. Lofland, L. H.: *Toward a Sociology of Death and Dying.* Sage Publications, Beverly Hills, 1976.

63. Lofland, L. H.: *The Craft of Dying: The Modern*

Face of Death. Sage Publications, Beverly Hills, 1978.

64. Markel, W. M. and V. B. Sinon: The hospice concept. *Ca—A Cancer Journal for Clinicians.* 28:225–237, 1978.

65. Marshall, V. W.: *Last Chapters: A Sociology of Aging and Dying.* Brooks/Cole Publishing Co., Monterey, Ca., 1980.

66. Maslach, C.: The burn-out syndrome and patient care. In *Stress and Survival: The Emotional Realities of Life Threatening Illness,* ed. by C. Garfield, C. V. Mosby Company, St. Louis, 1979.

67. McCorkle, R.: Terminal illness: human attachments and intended goals. *Community Nursing Research,* 9:207–221, 1977.

68. McCorkle, R.: The advanced cancer patient: how he will live — and die. In *Cancer: Pathophysiology, Etiology, and Management,* ed. by L. C. Kruse, J. L. Reese, and L. K. Hart. C. V. Mosby Co., St. Louis, 1979.

69. McGrory, A.: *A Well Model Approach to Care of the Dying Client.* McGraw-Hill Book Co., New York, 1978.

70. Pattison, E. M.: The living–dying process. In *Psychosocial Care of the Dying Patient,* ed. by Charles A. Garfield. McGraw-Hill Book Co., New York, 1978.

71. Pattison, E. M.: Help in the dying process. In *Understanding Death and Dying,* ed. by S. G. Wilcox and M. Sutton. Alfred Publishing Co., Inc., Sherman Oaks, Ca., 1981.

72. Paulen, K.: Learning to discuss the unmentionable. *Cancer Nursing.* 1:197–199, 1978.

73. Pilsecker, C.: Terminal cancer: a challenge for social work. *Social Work in Health Care.* 4:369–379, 1979.

74. Pumphrey, J. B. and S. H. Eisman. Patient adaptation to terminal illness. In *The Cancer Patient: Social and Medical Aspects of Care,* ed. by B. R. Cassileth. Lea & Febiger, Philadelphia, 1979.

75. Ramsey, P.: The indignity of "death with dignity". In *Death Inside Out: The Hastings Center Report,* ed. by P. Steinfels and R. M. Vaetch. Harper & Row Publishers, Inc., New York, 1975.

76. Rovinski, C. A.: Hospice nursing: intensive caring. *Cancer Nursing.* 2:19, 1979.

77. Saunders, C. M.: *The Management of Terminal Disease.* Edward Arnold (Publishers) Ltd., London, 1978.

78. Saunders, C. M., D. H. Summers, and N. Teller: *Hospice: The Living Idea.* Edward Arnold (Publishers) Ltd., London, 1981. Distributed in the United States by the W. B. Saunders Co.

79. Schoenberg, B., et al.: *Loss and Grief: Psychological Management in Medical Practice.* Columbia University Press, New York, 1970.

80. Scott, M.: There are more answers than a deadly silence. *Health and Social Service Journal.* 88:1218–1219, 1978.

81. Schneidman, E. D.: *Death: Current Perspectives.* Mayfield Publishing Co., Palo Alto, 1976.

82. Schultz, R.: *The Psychology of Death, Dying, and Bereavement.* Addison-Wesley Publishing Co., Reading, Mass., 1978.

83. Shoemaker, W. C.: Pathobiology of death: structural and functional interactions in shock syndrome. In *Pathobiology Annual, 1976,* ed. by H. Ioachim. Appleton-Century-Crofts, New York, 1976.

84. Stoddard, S.: *The Hospice Movement: A Better Way of Caring for the Dying.* Stein & Day Publishers, New York, 1978.

85. Sudnow, D.: *Passing On: The Social Organization of Dying.* Englewood Cliffs, N. J., Prentice-Hall, Inc., 1967.

86. Swenson, E., J. Matsuura, and I. M. Martinson: Effects of resuscitation for patients with metastatic cancers and chronic heart disease. *Nursing Research.* 28:151–153, 1979.

87. Terrill, L. A.: The clinical specialist in oncology and the dying patient. *Journal of Neurosurgical Nursing.* 10:176–179, 1978.

88. Vachon, M. L. S.: The final illness in cancer: the widow's perspective. *Canadian Medical Association Journal.* 117:1151–1154, 1977.

89. Wegmann, J. A.: Avoidance behaviors of nurses as related to cancer diagnosis and/or terminality. *Oncology Nursing Forum.* 6:8–14, 1979.

90. Weisman, S. D.: *On Dying and Denying.* Behavioral Publications Inc., New York, 1972.

91. Weisman, A. D.: The psychiatrist and the inexorable. In *New Meanings of Death,* ed by H. Feifel. McGraw-Hill Book Co., New York, 1977.

92. Weisman, A. D. and T. D. Hackett: Predilection to death: death and dying as a psychiatric problem. *Psychosomatic Medicine.* 23:232–256, 1961.

93. Weisman, A. D, and R. Kastenbaum: *The Psychological Autopsy: A Study of the Terminal Phase of Life.* Behavioral Publications, Inc., New York, 1968.

94. Wellisch, D. M. Mosher and C. Van Scoy: "Management of family emotional stress: family group therapy in a private oncology practice. *International Journal of Group Psychotherapy.* 28:225–231, 1978.

95. Wentzel, K. B.: The dying are the living. *American Journal of Nursing.* 76:956–957, 1976.

96. Wilcox, S. G. and M. Sutton: *Understanding Death and Dying.* Alfred Publishing Co., Inc., Sherman Oaks, California, 1981.

97. Wiley, L., ed.: The other side of death: good memories and the strength to go on. *Nursing 78.* 8:40–45, 1978.

IV

Cancer Nursing Beyond the Hospital Walls

15

Rehabilitation and Cancer

THE PHILOSOPHY OF REHABILITATION

Rehabilitation was originally limited to treating a physical disability. Thus, the focus was on reparation of physical damage. As health care professionals became more knowledgeable about rehabilitation, they realized that repairing the physical damage did not necessarily restore patients to their maximum functioning potential. Rehabilitation has now been expanded to include psychosocial, vocational, and economic aspects and may involve not only the patient but the family and community.[9]

There are two different ethical viewpoints that are used to justify the time, effort, and money spent on rehabilitation. From the utilitarian point of view, rehabilitation is considered worthwhile because it is economically beneficial to society and allows people to fulfill social roles. A person who has been successfully rehabilitated is more likely to be a productive, contributing member of society. From the formalist point of view, rehabilitation helps restore to people their capacity, so that they can enjoy a higher quality of life, socially, emotionally, and psychologically.[9]

Because of the great advances in medical science in recent years, many people with congenital anomalies, diseases, and injuries who would otherwise have died can live. The importance of quality of life for these people has been brought to the forefront of public awareness. Our society has been willing to invest money and other resources in rehabilitation efforts. Thus, the number of rehabilitation specialists and the knowledge of the field of rehabilitation have expanded.[9]

Rehabilitation uses a team approach to therapy, recognizing the valuable contributions of those from many different professional fields. The care of the patient takes place over a long period of time and must include many facets of the person's life: family, community, culture, social roles, and emotions. All of these must be dealt with interdependently.[9]

Before an effective rehabilitation program can be developed, it is important to conduct a thorough examination of the patient and the situation. Along with a physical and psychosocial assessment, this should include an evaluation of the disability. Christopherson suggests evaluating four dimensions of disability: protensity, intensity, extensity, and autoviability.[9]

Protensity is the length of time from the onset of the disability to the present. The implications of a progressively deteriorating condition are different from those of a condition that is stabilized with no foreseeable recurrence. Factors that are affected by this dimension are medication, therapy, vocational goals, vocational pursuits, and relationships with others.[9]

Intensity is an estimate of the severity of the patient's disability in comparison to the severity of the same limitation in others. It is based on measures of endurance such as loss of motion, function, and mobility; active symptoms; medication; and disease-related residuals. Evaluating this dimension requires a high level of knowledge about the particular disorder. In a progressive disease, intensity will fluctuate. In a stabilized disease, intensity will "settle down" at a specific level.[9]

Extensity is a very complex dimension that describes the effect of the disability on the personality and behavior of the person. It measures the extent of adaptation or coping that has occurred or is likely to occur. Intensity is not an effective predictor of extensity. Low predictions of extensity by health care professionals can sometimes seriously limit the degree of rehabilitation achieved by the person.[9]

Autoviability means the ability of the individual to sustain life. Evaluating this dimension requires an assessment of the intrinsic and extrinsic resources of the person and how well the person uses them. Intrinsic resources include "intelligence, determination, strength, endurance and mobility."[9] Extrinsic resources include "the individual's economic means, his living accommodations, the quality of care available to him, his friends, equipment, education and occupational training."[9]

The aim of rehabilitation is to move people from a position of dependency and helplessness to one of dignity and self-respect. To do this requires some changes in the attitudes and behavior of those who work with the handicapped. Thoreson suggests that there is a tendency to believe that:

> The disabled serve as a reference group for gauging the dimensions of normality and in this way assist the "normal" in maintaining his sense of identity and personal integrity. We can expect some attempt at enforcement of this dichotomy by "normals" (such as employers) to "magically" ward off threat to their status.[32]

To the extent that health professionals who work with the disabled view their role as

> . . . helping the disabled person because he is disabled (and handicapped), the greater the potential danger of the counselor's promoting the dichotomy between the normal and disabled. (Help is defined here as a guilt-ridden reaction of a societal member toward a debased, piteous creature.)
> Conversely, the greater the tendency on the part of the rehabilitation counselor to view his role as helping the disabled person because he is another human being, the greater the potentialities for melting the rigid role barriers between the disabled and normal.[32]

The goal of rehabilitation is to help people to use all of their resources to function close to their maximum potential. Handicapped people can ill afford to make the halfhearted attempt at maximizing their potential that is made by most "normal" people. To help them reach their goal, the health care professional must never lose sight of the humanity of disabled individuals.

The field of medical rehabilitation repels a great many health personnel because, by necessity, it has the qualities of a mission. It is a phase of medical practice that requires a zeal for social benefit. It is deeply rooted in ethics and rests on a primary postulate of human value. Like every other movement dependent on zeal, there is the danger of emotion prevailing over judgment. At times, the problems of the severely handicapped are treated in a ritualistic fashion without deep understanding and without realization of the degree of adaptation and change required to shift the outlook of the disabled person from one of depression and despair to an attitude of hopefulness, accompanied by the desire and the energy to make a new start in life.

The goal of medical rehabilitation as a technique is the prevention or the reversal of those biologic tendencies that cause the ill, the disabled and the elderly to withdraw from life, to deteriorate and to become dependent. The goal of rehabilitation as a movement is more complex. Its objectives are more than the achievement of individual rehabilitation: they include the education of all of the professions involved in medical and supportive care in order to focus endeavors on human values rather than on mere technical success. They include the orientation of the public toward a fair deal for the handicapped in opportunities to work and to share the joys of living.[21]

USING REHABILITATION STRATEGIES IN THE CANCER SITUATION

Because of the dramatic advances in the medical treatment of cancer, more people with cancer are living many years with their disease and possibilities of cure increase each year. With this increase in the length of the cancer patient's life has come a greater interest in using rehabilitation strategies to improve the quality of that life. In a sense, the philosophy of rehabilitation is the philosophy of this book and can be found expressed throughout the chapters.

Rehabilitation ideally should begin at the time of diagnosis, continue during therapy, and follow the patient throughout the period of recovery or recurrence and decline. Unlike many disorders, cancer may not result in a physical disability; the residual handicap may be psychologic and social. Patients who have had mutilating surgery or damage from radiation will, in addition, have physical disabilities and body image problems.

Any person who has had cancer may be assigned by society to what Christopherson defines as the "cripple role." The individual's reference groups will change, expected behavior will change, and expected roles may change.

Interested and seemingly sympathetic persons will register shock, disbelief, and disapproval on receiving reports from a physically handicapped individual that he has been dancing, golfing, hunting, gotten married, or has otherwise violated the expectations that the well-bodied have of him.[9]

Employment opportunities may be altered by the cancer situation. People who maintain their job during their illness are fortunate. Employers are often reluctant to keep someone who has a history of cancer. They are concerned about absenteeism and other employees who may be reluctant to work with a "cancer victim." Group rates for insurance are increased if cancer patients who use the insurance for further medical treatment are included. Therefore, persons highly qualified in their field may have difficulty finding a job. Jobs taken may be on a lower status and pay scale than those previously held, in which case self-esteem is further damaged.

Economically, cancer is a devastating illness. Families often use all of their reserve resources during the illness. Afterward, job possibilities for the patient are diminished, large debts may have been incurred, and the family standard of living is lowered, perhaps for a lifetime.

Former cancer patients often are unable to obtain either medical or life insurance. The medical insurance that they previously held may have been job associated or may have been cancelled. If it is not cancelled, a rider may be placed on the policy, barring payment for future cancer-related treatment. This further increases the economic pressures placed on the family.

Two issues that are related arise in terms of cancer and rehabilitation. One involves when reconstructive surgery and rehabilitative efforts should be implemented. The other concerns whether scarce resources (money and health care professionals' time) should be used for a person who is dying of cancer.

Surgeons have often taken the position that reconstructive surgery should be withheld until the risk of local recurrence has decreased — usually a period of 2 or 3 years. Their rationale is that local recurrence is harder to detect and more difficult to treat if reconstructive surgery has been performed. This is particularly true of breast cancer.

The approach is unacceptable from a rehabilitative standpoint. In the span of 2 years, the person's body image and self-esteem have often been irreparably damaged. Social reaction to the person is firmly established. If a recurrence occurs in a patient who has undergone reconstructive surgery, it usually means that the person will eventually die of the disease. However, the quality of life has been improved by the rehabilitative strategies. Thus, the main issue seems to be the justification for expending scarce resources on a person who may die.

If only direct economic costs are considered, this may not be justifiable. However, the cost of a nonrehabilitated person to society is like a pebble causing ripples in a pool. The person's contributions to society are lessened. Family functioning is diminished over a long period of time. The psychologic and sociologic consequences of the failure to rehabilitate are subtle, but penetrate deeply into the fiber of society.

SPECIFIC REHABILITATION STRATEGIES

Amputation

Rehabilitation after an amputation is much more complex than might be imagined. Because of this, it is important for the nurse to be familiar with both the physiologic and psychosocial processes occurring after the amputation and the strategies that have been found to be effective in helping the person to overcome this sudden and dramatic disability.

We are inclined to think of the functional difficulties occurring after an amputation as being limited to the involved extremity. However, total body movement is dependent on a feedback type of communication that adjusts the body's activities to allow for coordinated movement. Therefore, an amputation will alter muscle function and the timing of movements throughout the body.

The term "unaffected side" sometimes used by professional persons to refer to the uninjured part is probably an unwarranted oversimplification. The high probability is that amputation results in an affected person, not a person with an affected and an unaffected side. The dependence of the dominant hand on the nondominant hand for feedback as to progress through stabilizing, holding, pushing, and so forth should provide a case in point. Another obvious example is the precision that is programmed into walking. Walking proceeds with the body weight being shifted from one foot to another, and with weight shifted from the heel of one foot to the toe of the same foot and to the heel of the other foot. The body's position in space, the relation of the center of gravity to the ground, the rate of speed, and other facts represent the feedback that provides for the purposeful and coordinated walking we take so much for granted. The loss of the mechanical function or the source of communication feedback necessitates a difficult period of relearning if walking is to be resumed.[10]

An amputee's perception of the extent of the disability has a greater impact on the success of rehabilitation than the actual physical limitations that occur. The personal meaning of the loss will greatly influence the person's self-concept. This perception is seldom accurate and contains many unrealistic and distorted beliefs. A major focus of rehabilitation is to change these distorted perceptions to a more accurate view of reality. At the same time, efforts are made to diminish the physical loss by means of medical strategies and to

train the person in the use of prosthetic devices.[15]

Fishman proposes that "specific psychologic, social and physiological human needs are thwarted" as a result of amputation.[15] It is necessary for the loss to be accepted and integrated by the person before rehabilitation can be successful. He identifies seven specific needs: physical function, cosmesis, comfort, energy costs, achievement, economic security, and respect and status.[15]

Physical activity and the use of one's physical resources are needs that can be seen even in an infant. The pleasure comes not from the physical activity itself, but from achievements that are a result of the activity. Cosmesis is related to the need to appear like others. It has two main facets, visual and auditory. Since people are often judged by their appearance, it is important for the prosthesis to provide the amputee with as normal an appearance as possible. Abnormal noises produced by a prosthesis are also problems. Air escaping from a socket, a prosthetic foot hitting the floor, an artificial joint locking in place are all evidence of difference, even though the sounds are of very low intensity and usually are not heard by people other than the wearer.[15]

Prostheses are not comfortable. They are heavy and often cause some level of pain or at least discomfort. Tissues exposed to the prosthesis become irritated, hot, and sweaty. Muscles must be used in unusual ways. The individual must simply learn to tolerate some level of discomfort.[15]

Physical tasks require more use of energy for the amputee than for the normal person. This energy must be diverted from energy that once went into other activities. Fatigue will be experienced more rapidly, and thus may cause frustration. Skilled use of a prothesis does not come automatically and requires conscious attention. This demands the intense concentration of the person and may divert attention from other concerns.[15]

Achievement and success are important values in our society. Because a prosthetic device is a machine, a reasonable amount of failure will occur. In learning to use it, the person may fall or drop things. The possibility of malfunction always exists. Such failures are embarrassing and are often generalized as a failure of the person, rather than of the prosthesis.[15]

White collar workers will probably not be hindered at their job by an amputation. Those in blue-collar or manual labor jobs, however, may be seriously impaired in their ability to be financially independent. Thus, vocational retraining may be a necessary part of rehabilitation.[15]

Respect and status are often altered after an amputation as a result of social reactions to amputation and the expectations of the "cripple role." This role is associated with inadequacy, charity, shame, punishment, and guilt. These attitudes lower self-esteem and the person may use defenses to protect his or her personal integrity.[15]

The limitations described above cannot be eliminated but can often be modified. One of the goals of rehabilitation is to assist the person to live within these limitations in such a way that there is minimum interference with other life activities.[15]

Nursing rehabilitative strategies should be started during the first nurse-patient contact. Before the surgical procedure, it is often helpful for the patient to have the opportunity to see a successfully rehabilitated amputee with a similar disability.

The nursing care after an amputation must, of course, include the usual interventions for a surgical situation. In addition, several factors must be carefully planned for. Proper stump care is essential to proper fitting of a prosthesis. Proper wound healing and prevention of contraction of skin and muscle away from the end of the bone are major concerns. Flexion contractures must also be prevented. The stump should not be elevated on pillows. The patient should be encouraged to lie on the abdomen as soon as possible, especially while sleeping.[22]

It is important to help the patient maintain as much independence as possible during surgical recovery. Patients should be encouraged to do as much as they can for themselves. Physical activity and mobility should be reinstituted soon after surgery. Sitting in a wheelchair seldom causes flexion contractures after leg amputations, if the patient is spending time lying on the abdomen. While lying in bed, the leg amputee should be carefully positioned and the stump aligned to prevent external rotation and abduction. Patients often experience phantom limb sensations that may last as long as a year. Pain from the surgical procedure should be controlled, but the patient should not be kept so heavily sedated that mobility and physical activities are compromised.

As soon as possible after surgery, training in the use of a prosthetic device should begin. The physical therapist and nurse will need to work closely together to facilitate good emotional and physical responses to prosthesis training. The patient will also need to be taught how to care for the stump. The skin over the stump is vulnerable to injury and infection. At home, skin care should be performed at night to allow drying before the prosthesis is reapplied. Soap should be carefully rinsed off. If the stump is wrapped, dressings should be washed daily and carefully reapplied.

Family members may feel sorry for the patient and attempt to wait on the patient excessively. The family should be an integral part of the rehabilitation team and be helped to understand and adopt the goals of the team.

Colostomy

The colostomy patient faces a situation in which feces are expelled in a less controlled way on the abdomen. This surgery may be associated by the patient with loss of control, uncleanliness, unacceptable odor, and shame. Even though the surgical procedure is explained beforehand, many patients do not experience the full impact of it until they see feces on their abdomen.

The patient will closely watch the facial expressions of the nurse as the dressings are changed. Immediately after surgery, the stoma is large, swollen, and bright red. Gradually, the patient will develop the courage to look at the stoma. This is a difficult experience and will require much care and support. The patient should be told that the stoma will decrease in size as the wound heals. After healing, the stoma will be much flatter against the abdomen.

Plastic colostomy bags are used to collect drainage. The drainage from the colostomy is irritating to the normal skin of the abdomen. The adhesive on the drainage bag may also irritate the skin. The drainage bag must be applied in such a way that skin irritation is avoided and drainage is not allowed to seep into the surgical incision.

The procedure suggested for applying collecting bags to draining wounds in Chapter 11 can also be used for colostomies. Bags should be emptied from the bottom rather than be changed several times a day. This will prevent much skin excoriation.

Some patients will require colostomy irrigations and others will not. Most patients can learn to perform this procedure alone in the bathroom. However, patients with advanced disease or other chronic disorders may need the assistance of a family member. In any case, it is wise for at least one family member to know this procedure before the patient leaves the hospital.

Some family members have great difficulty emotionally with this surgery; occasionally a spouse will abandon a patient. However, most of the time, with encouragement and emotional support, a family member can be taught to provide needed care. It is very helpful if an enterostomal therapist is available to help the patient and family manage this situation. There are many small "tricks" that can be used to make life much simpler and more pleasant. The enterostomal therapist should also be available when unanticipated problems occur after the patient has been discharged from the hospital.

Patients usually feel fairly safe in the hospital environment and at home, but may be reluctant to move into social situations outside their home. They are afraid of an "accident" or of odor. If proper rehabilitation strategies are not used, patients may withdraw and seldom venture outside the home. One patient cared for by the author had not gone outside her home into social situations for 20 years.

With proper teaching and care, most patients will no longer need to wear a colostomy bag for more than 6 months after surgery. A small flat dressing can be used. The stoma will be greatly reduced in size and normal clothing can be worn with no visible signs of the stoma. Although some patients may have to avoid specific foods, this varies from individual to individual and is seldom very limiting.

Patients can often be helped to reach this stage of rehabilitation by contact with another person who has a colostomy. The Ostomy Association affiliated with the American Cancer Society can be very helpful in guiding patients to complete rehabilitation. However, it is not wise for the patient to become so identified with other colostomy patients that movement back into the mainstream of society is impeded.

Ileal Conduit

An ileal conduit may need to be performed on a patient who has a large pelvic mass that is obstructing the ureters. In this case, no attempt is made to remove the tumor. The strategy is an attempt to divert the flow of urine above the tumor onto the abdominal wall. In other cases, the ileal conduit is performed in connection with a pelvic exenteration or for bladder cancer in which the bladder is removed. In these latter cases, the patient may have an extended life as a result of the surgery.

The surgery isolates a segment of ileum and attaches the ureters to it. An end-to-end anastomosis of the remaining ileum is performed. A cutaneous stoma is made into the isolated ileum, allowing urine to drain into an ileostomy appliance. Urine is extremely irritating to skin and great care must be taken to prevent skin contact. Urine dissolves karaya powder, which should not be used in the care of these stomas.[17]

Care must be taken to prevent urinary stasis, which can lead to reflux of urine through the ureters into the kidneys, hydronephrosis, and pyelonephrosis. Drainage should be checked each time the patient's position is changed, to ensure adequate flow of urine. Mucous plugs can sometimes obstruct the stoma and must be removed.

Home care of an ileal conduit is in some ways more difficult than that of a colostomy, but can be conducted by the patient and family, thus allowing increased quality of life and movement of the patient into social circles.

Some patients, particularly those who have had a pelvic exenteration, may have both a colostomy and an ileal conduit. This requires even more complex care to prevent contamination of the ileal conduit with feces. Emotional strength and the desire to live are important factors in determining the extent of rehabilitation that the patient achieves.

Mastectomy

Although rehabilitation for mastectomy should commence before surgery, the process only truly begins when the patient leaves the hospital. The rehabilitation process for mastectomy requires about 2 years. It is unfortunate that the small amount of rehabilitation that is attempted usually occurs while the patient is hospitalized. Teaching strategies may be used to help the patient recognize problems that may occur. If the patient is fortunate, a Reach to Recovery volunteer from the American Cancer Society may visit her. These volunteers are limited to one or two visits shortly after surgery and require the surgeon's permission before a visit can be made.

Most of the rehabilitation problems encountered by mastectomy patients occur after discharge from the hospital. Women often are not told where to purchase a prosthesis, what factors to consider in the selection, what a prosthesis looks like, how it should fit, or how much it will cost.[31] They are often given limited instructions for physical care and little psychosocial support. Women who have difficulties with rehabilitation may not be seen by health professionals for 2 or 3 years, during which time severely dysfunctional patterns of social behavior may develop. Those women who receive chemotherapy are fortunate, in a way, because of continued contact with supportive physicians and nurses over a period of a year or more.

An effective rehabilitation program for the mastectomy patient should provide access to familiar health care professionals for a period of 1 to 2 years. Potential problems that should be assessed and dealt with during this period include skin care, development of edema, proper prostheses, exercises, extent of range of motion, psychosexual adjustment, family functioning, and self-esteem and body image problems. Patients usually expect to feel better much sooner after surgery than they actually do. They often become depressed over their slow progress. For some patients, physical therapy may be very helpful. Husbands often need guidance in how to best help their spouse.

The risk of recurrence is an ever present shadow that clouds the future. This specter must be handled in such a way that life can be continued and enjoyed. Open family discussions of feelings and fears should be encouraged.

Successful treatment for mastectomy must include much more than a well-healed incision and a patient who can walk out of the hospital. The patient must be guided in effective ways to cope with the consequences of the disease and surgery.

Laryngectomy

The patient with a laryngectomy has two problems to live with: the presence of a tracheostomy and the inability to speak. Before going home from the hospital, the patient and family must learn the mechanics of caring for the tracheostomy. For most patients, this facet is not as difficult as the tragedy of losing the ability to speak. Rehabilitative strategies for learning to speak again are difficult to master and require months of intense effort. Mechanical voice boxes are being used, but for the most part are difficult to understand. Writing notes is slow and greatly diminishes nonverbal forms of communication that tell us so much of what a person is saying.

A large number of people who have laryngectomies are cured of the malignancy. It is very important that effective rehabilitative strategies be used to enhance the quality of life as much as possible. The American Cancer Society has an excellent program to assist in this area, and the Lost Cord Club can provide much needed support. A volunteer laryngectomee from the American Cancer Society or a speech pathologist can help the patient regain the ability to speak.

Baker and Cunningham[3] have developed an excellent assessment guide for the laryngectomy patient and discuss rehabilitation strategies in detail. Sexuality and employment problems may need to be considered. Some patients have difficulties with lifting. Patients should be cautioned against working in areas with high environmental pollution or extremes in temperatures.[3]

Changes in body image, self-esteem, and social roles are serious problems in this situation. Because of communication problems, these feelings may not be adequately expressed and explored. Family members may also need assistance to cope with the changes that occur as a consequence of this situation.

Face and Mouth Cancers

Face and mouth cancers cause difficult rehabilitation problems because the personality of the person is so associated with the face. The distortions caused by the malignancy and mutilating surgery cause strong negative reactions by others. Reconstructive surgery is usually performed over a 2 or 3 year period and facial prostheses are used to conceal facial abnormalities. It truly takes a courageous person to overcome all of the problems encountered during this period. Treatment should be conducted in a facility that has a well-prepared staff and the equipment to provide for the rehabilitative needs of these patients.

A patient with severe facial deformities even after reconstructive surgery may become a recluse if adequate assistance is not given. Assistance must be given in helping the patient to function and communicate as well as in ways of coping with an altered appearance. For these patients, regaining social approval can be a major breakthrough to successful rehabilitation.[12]

BIBLIOGRAPHY

1. Ahana, D. Y., and A. Takeuchi: Rehabilitation in cancer: concepts and application. In *Dynamics of Oncology Nursing,* ed. by P. K. Burkhalter and D. L. Donley. McGraw-Hill Book Company, New York, 1978.
2. Ainsworth, T. H.: The cost of cancer. *Cancer.* 36:283–284, 1975.
3. Baker, B. M., and C. A. Cunningham: Vocal rehabilitation of the patient with a laryngectomy. *Oncology Nursing Forum.* 7:23–36, 1980.
4. Blues, K.: A framework for nurses providing care to laryngectomy patients. *Cancer Nursing.* 1:441–445, 1978.
5. Blumberg, B., M. Flaherty, and J. Lewis: *Coping With Cancer.* U.S. Dept. of Health and Human Services, NIH Publication No. 80-2080, 1980.
6. Cain, M., and C. Henke: Living with cancer. *Oncology Nursing Forum.* 5:4–5, 1978.
7. Christopherson, V. A.: Role modifications of the disabled male. In *Rehabilitation Nursing: Perspectives and Applications,* ed. by V. A. Christopherson, P. P. Coulter, and M. O. Wolanin. McGraw-Hill Book Company, New York, 1974.
8. Christopherson, V. A.: The patient and the family. In *Rehabilitation Nursing: Perspectives and Applications,* ed. by V. A. Christopherson, P. P. Coulter, and M. O. Wolanin. McGraw-Hill Book Company, New York, 1974.
9. Christopherson, V. A.: Perspectives in rehabilitation. In *Rehabilitation Nursing: Perspectives and Applications,* ed. by V. A. Christopherson, P. P. Coulter, and M. O. Wolanin. McGraw-Hill Book Company, New York, 1974.
10. Christopherson, V. A., P. P. Coulter, and M. O.

Wolanin: *Rehabilitation Nursing: Perspectives and Applications.* McGraw-Hill Book Company, New York, 1974.

11. Dotson, T.: Only a ghost of a chance. *Texas Business.* August, 1977, pp. 18–23.

12. Dropkin, M. J.: Compliance in postoperative head and neck patients. *Cancer Nursing.* 2:379–384, 1979.

13. Entmacher, P. S.: Insurance for the cancer patient. *Cancer.* 36:287–289, 1975.

14. Fisher, S. G.: Psychosexual adjustment following total pelvic exenteration. *Cancer Nursing.* 2:219–225, 1979.

15. Fishman, S.: Amputee needs, frustrations and behavior. In *Rehabilitation Nursing: Perspectives and Applications,* ed. by V. A. Christopherson, P. P. Coulter, and M. O. Wolanin. McGraw-Hill Book Company, New York, 1974.

16. Frelick, R. W.: An overview of the cancer patient. *Occupational Health Nursing.* April, 1978, pp. 7–8.

17. Frenay, M. A. C.: A dynamic approach to the ileal conduit patient. In *Rehabilitation Nursing: Perspectives and Applications,* ed. by V. A. Christopherson, P. P. Coulter, and M. O. Wolanin. McGraw-Hill Book Company, New York, 1974.

18. Fried, D.: Rehabilitation of the cancer patient. *Cancer.* 36:277–278, 1975.

19. Grace, M., R. N. MacDonald, and F. Davis: Follow-up care of patients with cancer. *Canadian Journal of Public Health.* 68:403–406, 1977.

20. Harper, B. C.: Social aspects of cancer recovery. *Cancer.* 36:274–276, 1975.

21. Hirschberg, G. G., L. Lewis, and P. Vaughan: *Rehabilitation.* J. B. Lippincott Company, Philadelphia, 1976.

22. Kirkpatrick, S.: Battle casualty: amputee. In *Rehabilitation Nursing: Perspectives and Applications,* ed. by V. A. Christopherson, P. P. Coulter, and M. O. Wolanin. McGraw-Hill Book Company, New York, 1974.

23. Leopold, R. L., and E. L. Ramsden: Rehabilitation services. In *The Cancer Patient: Social and Medical Aspects of Care,* ed. by B. R. Cassileth. Lea & Febiger, Philadelphia, 1979.

24. Levy, S. W., and G. H. Barnes: Stump hygiene. In *Rehabilitation Nursing: Perspectives and Applications,* ed. by V. A. Christopherson, P. P. Coulter, and M. O. Wolanin. McGraw-Hill Book Company, New York, 1974.

25. O'Neill, M. P.: Psychological aspects of cancer recovery. *Cancer.* 36:271–273, 1975.

26. Paulen, A., and S. Sylvester: Caring for the patient who's "well." *RN.* April, 1978, pp. 56–58.

27. Rubin, R.: Body image and self-esteem. In *Rehabilitation Nursing: Perspectives and Applications,* ed. by V. A. Christopherson, P. P. Coulter, and M. A. Wolanin. McGraw-Hill Book Company, New York, 1974.

28. Rusk, H. A.: *Rehabilitation Medicine.* C. V. Mosby Co., St. Louis, 1977.

29. Smith, S.: The psychology of illness. In *Rehabilitation Nursing: Perspectives and Applications,* ed. by V. A. Christopherson, P. P. Coulter, and M. O. Wolanin. McGraw-Hill Book Company, New York, 1974.

30. Stone, R. W.: Employing the recovered cancer patient. *Cancer.* 36:285–286, 1975.

31. Thomas, S. G.: Breast cancer: the psychosocial issues. *Cancer Nursing.* 1:53–60, 1978.

32. Thoreson, R. W.: Disability viewed in its cultural context. In *Rehabilitation Nursing: Perspectives and Applications,* ed. by V. A. Christopherson, P. P. Coulter, and M. O. Wolanin. McGraw-Hill Book Company, New York, 1974.

33. Veronisi, U., and G. Martino: Can life be the same after cancer treatment? *Tumori,* 64:345–351, 1978.

34. Wilkes, E., A. G. Crowther, and C. W. Greaves: A different kind of day hosptial — for patients with preterminal cancer and chronic disease. *British Medical Journal.* 2:1053–1056, 1978.

16

Cancer Support Groups

INTRODUCTION

Cancer support groups are becoming a more frequent mechanism for helping those involved in the cancer situation to cope more effectively. Support groups are, in a sense, naturally occurring phenomena. They developed from health care professionals' observations of patients and families sharing experiences and feelings in waiting rooms and inpatient lobbies. The original groups met in cancer research facilities and were led by psychiatrists or psychologists. As the effectiveness of the groups became apparent, various strategies evolved to make them available to a larger number of people.

Because they are not designed to provide psychotherapy, the structure and dynamics of these groups differ from those designed for traditional group therapy. Change in personality is not the goal. Transference and resistance issues, developing a sense of belonging, and working through relationships with other group members are not primary concerns. The group leader's role is different from that of a psychotherapy group leader.[17] The group must be designed to meet the specific needs of the cancer situation.

THE THEORETICAL BASE FOR SUPPORT GROUPS

The first support group was organized in 1905 by Joseph Hershey Pratt, an internist in Boston who treated tuberculosis patients. Pratt was concerned about the poor, who were unable to enter a sanatorium for treatment. He developed a plan for home care, which included a tuberculosis class. Unable to get support from existing institutions, he was aided in his efforts by a Boston minister.[37]

Pratt was considered completely inexperienced in this field, since he had no knowledge of psychotherapy or group work. Group treatment for either mental or medical disorders was at this time unheard of. He was criticized by his peers for treating "nervous disorders" without the necessary expertise. As he conducted the classes, his understanding of the psychologic components of the illness increased, and the class changed gradually from one almost totally oriented toward physical care to one that included an emphasis on psychologic dynamics.[37]

Current cancer support groups merge strategies and theories that have been used in several fields of practice. This merger has resulted in a situation not unlike that of Pratt's in which practitioners are departing from tradition and implementing a new approach to care. These practitioners are often lacking in experience and knowledge and must learn as they go.

Psychiatrists, psychologists, and counselors may be skilled in group work with patients who have psychologic problems, but usually have little experience in dealing with "normal" people who need help to cope with a physical illness situation. Nurses, on the other hand, are skilled in working with "normal" people coping with a physical illness, but have little experience with group work. Social workers have skills in group work and may understand the illness situation, but have little experience with its physical and medical implications. Of these professionals, only nurses have a working knowledge of the physical, psychologic, and social implications of illness.

Nurses must not avoid implementing

support groups because they do not "know how," because very few people know enough to be considered experts at this point in time. It is a new and developing idea. Many nurses are interested in establishing these groups, but information on how to develop a group, the qualifications of facilitators, and the problems that may be encountered is difficult to find. Nurses must be committed to expanding knowledge and skills in this area by education, self-study, and supervised practice, in order to achieve optimum benefit from this intervention.

The theories that are used in support groups come from group therapy, group dynamics, family therapy, social work groups, and the support systems model. Each of these theories must be understood, but their strategies must be adapted for appropriate use in support groups. Adherents of each theory may insist that the traditional approaches must be used. It is easy to be intimidated by an "expert," rather than to think things out carefully on one's own. The practitioner must know the theory well enough to be able to apply its precepts in a new and different situation and alter it as necessary.

Group Therapy

Group therapy was developed primarily to treat people with mental disorders. It was an alternative to one-to-one psychotherapy. Therefore, the strategies were designed to facilitate the psychologic dynamics necessary for the treatment of disorder. Groups meet on a regular basis, usually weekly, for a predetermined number of sessions. They are "closed" groups, which means that no new participants can enter after a group has started. The process of the group is the focus of the sessions, and content is not preplanned. The leader is usually highly skilled in psychotherapy.

During the sessions, the interactions between group members are an important part of the therapy. Trust, cohesiveness, and transference are also important factors. The group moves through a process that involves identity with the group, possible group discord as transference develops, the working through of problems, and the termination of the group sessions. It is important to analyze the way group members interact with one another or to help group members change their interactions. The insight of group members is considered important.

The strategies of group therapy differ with each leader. Some may use confrontation, others may use role playing. Some may maintain rigid control of the group, whereas others may allow more democratic group functioning. Theorists who have been prominent in the group approach to therapy include Rogers, Berne, Burton, and Perls. Reading a book that introduces the various approaches to group therapy is helpful in understanding this field.[16, 24, 29, 33, 38, 41]

Group Dynamics

Group dynamics is another area of knowledge essential to the cancer support group. It is important to understand the normal interactions that occur in groups and how changes in group structure can alter the dynamics of the group. The definitive work on this topic is Cartwright and Zander's *Group Dynamics*.[9] Leadership style, arrangement of the room, timing, status of members, and many other factors can greatly influence the functioning of the group.

Family Therapy

Family therapy is a fairly new approach to the treatment of emotional problems. Theorists prominent in this field include Satir, Foley, Skynner, Minuchin, and Erickson.[12, 32, 39, 44] These theorists believe that the family functions as a unit and that problems that occur with an individual are actually problems of the entire family. In order to treat the individual who is identified as the "problem," the entire family must be involved. The family, as a group, sees the therapist. Communication styles, family rules, and family roles are explored. The focus is on changing the current family system.

Social Work Groups

Beginning in 1889 with Hull House, Jane Addams organized the first "settlement house," a neighborhood self-help group working for improved living conditions. The group was involved with providing community services and with changing adverse social conditions. This seems to have been the beginning of the social work group.[41] The focus of the social work group is on the interaction between human beings and society. The goal of the group may be recreation, socialization, or social service. The developing theoretical formulation of these groups draws heavily on theories of small groups, deviance, and systems. Two main theorists in this field are Vintner and Schwartz.[14]

Support Systems Model

In 1974, Gerald Caplan proposed a model of support systems, which evolved from his approach to crisis intervention.[7] Caplan defines support as the augmenting of a person's strengths to facilitate mastery of the environment. A support system is defined as an enduring pattern of continuous or intermittent support that plays a significant part in maintaining the psychologic and physical integrity of an individual over time. Caplan believes that during the course of a person's life, situations occur that disrupt the usual patterns of coping. During these periods, the person has an increased need for support and is more likely to respond to help offered by caretaking agents or informal caregivers. Caretaking agents are professionals whose roles give them the opportunity to influence the mental health of many individuals. Examples of caretaking agents are nurses, doctors, social workers, clergy, teachers, and police. Informal caregivers are individuals in the community who, because of personal experience or skills in relating to people, are sought out by people in the community in relation to mental health problems. Beauticians, barbers, bartenders, and former cancer patients are examples of people who may function in this role.[7]

Caplan considers the effectiveness of a person's support system to be a determining factor in the mastery of a crisis situation. This mastery is essential to future physical and mental health. He also believes that psychologic development, whether toward mental health or mental illness, is increased at times of crisis.[7]

Although family and friends can provide the needed support, they may also be in need of support during a crisis and temporarily unable to help. Caretaking agents or informal caregivers can provide effective assistance during a crisis. Even minimal interventions by caretaking agents at these times can lead to movement toward mental health.[7]

Caplan also proposes that sociocultural expectations affect people's beliefs, attitudes, and behavior and fix their place in the social structure. The strength of the individual's ego will also be a key factor in the outcome of a crisis. Ego strength is influenced by the quality of available support systems. However, the impact of sociocultural expectations on support systems and the outcome of crisis situations is not well defined.[7] Figure 16–1 shows a possible model of Caplan's formulations.

Research on Social Support

Caplan's presentation of a theoretic formulation of social support has led to increased research and theory development in that area. Gottlieb, in an excellent book entitled *Social Networks and Social Support*,[16a] has brought together some of the key theorists and researchers in this area. The questions raised by these authors are provocative. For example, it is not presently known what factors within a person's social

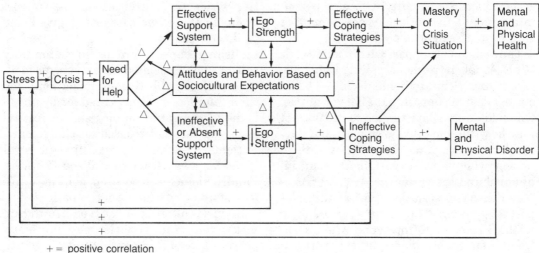

+ = positive correlation

− = negative correlation

△ = indefinite effect

Figure 16–1. Support systems theory.

network provide support. An inherent assumption has been that having a support system is good and not having one is bad. However, there can be disadvantages to a strong support system. Conformity with expected roles and behavior is often demanded by a strong support system and can sometimes be detrimental. If the support system does not believe that medical care is appropriate, treatment may not be utilized. The threat of social isolation or abandonment by the group is often enough to induce conformity with expected norms.

There is a question about what types of activities constitute support and who is best able to provide it. It has been fairly well documented that support improves coping abilities and functions in a preventive way to maintain physical and mental health. Several tools for measuring social supports are presented in Gottlieb's book and may be useful in assessing the support available to patients and families. Some of the researchers' findings are summarized here.

The provision of support seems to be situational rather than dependent upon its past availability. A patient who has had an effective support system for most developmental experiences in life may find that

no support is available in the catastrophic experience of cancer. In other cases, the patient's entire network of support may be involved in the crisis and may need outside assistance to continue functioning.

Support systems are examined in terms of density, range, and multiplexity. Density is a measure of how interrelated the members of the support system are. High-density systems such as extended families and small communities can be limited in ways of providing support and knowledge and in use of outside sources. A higher level of conformity is expected of the patient. Low-density systems involve contacts in a variety of settings who have differing value systems, more acceptance of nonconformity, and greater knowledge of outside sources of help. Low-density systems, then, provide a wider range of support. Multiplexity, meaning that multiple types of support come from the same person, is also an important factor in the effectiveness of support systems.

Many people tend to think of support as being completely separate from the sources of stress. Stressors are seen as coming from the environment external to the patient and the support system. This is not a clear picture of reality. Often, a person in a patient's network may be a source of both support and stress.

The division of support within a network is not equal, in terms of power, influence, or amount. Some individuals may obtain a great deal of support, but give very little. One individual who is linked to the patient may be willing to provide support, but may be influenced against doing so by a third person who has ties with both that individual and the patient.

In the cancer situation, the existing support system may fail or may need help itself. Strategies to intervene when a patient or family has inadequate support can occur at several levels. The patient and family can be helped to maintain or seek help from existing networks. An outside source of support specific to the cancer situation — volunteers or persons who have had cancer — can be sought.

The health professional can help to provide some of the complex types of support needed by cancer patients and their families. This latter approach is a strategy that has been used with greater frequency in recent years. With the increased awareness of the impact of support on the response to a health-related situation, it is a logical nursing intervention.

THE MECHANICS OF DEVELOPING A GROUP

Starting a group is usually best done by a planning committee. Advantages and disadvantages of various alternatives should be carefully considered. As the group is implemented, the effectiveness of various strategies can be evaluated and alterations made as needed.

Location

The most frequent location for a support group is within a facility providing cancer care, usually a hospital, outpatient clinic, or physician's office. This strategy effectively ties the activities of the support group to the other care being given and facilitates continuity of care. However, establishing support groups in community settings not associated with a specific facility can also be effective. Many patients and their families are being cared for by physicians who are not oncologists, in institutions that are not focused on cancer care. Patients and families may live in rural areas far away from specialized facilities. Family members who need help may live in a state or city far from the patient.

Rivalries often exist between health care institutions. Such rivalries may informally prevent people in the community from utilizing support groups within these institutions. Some groups are actually limited to those being cared for within the facility. Thus, people receiving high quality care are most likely to have access to support groups. Those receiving marginal cancer care, and who may therefore need greater support, are less likely to have access to this type of care.

Referral

Developing an effective referral system is essential to the success of the group. Referral processes are slow to develop. Health care professionals are justifiably cautious about a new group and will carefully observe its effectiveness and problems before being willing to refer patients to the group. It may be as long as a year after the group begins before confidence develops. Until this time, group attendance may be small — possibly just one or two persons — and sometimes no one will come. It is easy to become discouraged and stop the group before it has had a real chance to succeed.

Although a large number of referrals come from the supporting institutions, the greatest source of referral may be those who have attended the group or lay people who have heard about it. Nurses are the next most probable source of referral, followed by social workers. Physicians seem to be least likely to refer to the group, not because they disapprove, but because they are seldom oriented to the psychosocial aspects of the cancer situation.[6]

Facilitators

At least two facilitators (leaders) should be involved in conducting the group. One or two persons who can fill in when needed should also be available. The selection of facilitators is important to the effectiveness of the group. A facilitator should have a knowledge of the disease process, treatments and common problems, specific knowledge of physical care needs of the cancer patients, an understanding of psychologic and social processes and group dynamics, and skills in communicating and counseling. Because nurses have the broadest scope of knowledge and skills needed for this process, at least one nurse should be involved. Others who may be helpful are social workers, chaplains, physicians, psychologists, psychiatrists, and previous group members.

Nurses often do not have confidence in their ability to conduct this type of group, since they may not have had previous group experience. However, they may actually be more effective than others who are convinced of their expertise. There are many people who are anxious to get into counseling situations to meet their own personal needs. They believe they are excellent facilitators and are able to convince others that this is true. However, their performance belies their claims. Educational preparation in counseling is extremely important, but it is not a guarantee of effectiveness. Selection of a facilitator should be based on actual clinical performance and verbal evaluations from those who have worked with the person.

Open versus Closed Groups

Most cancer support groups are open groups. An open group allows members to enter the group at any time and attend for as many sessions as desired. Some may attend intermittently over a period of a year or more. Cancer is a situation within which multiple crises occur. If the group is oriented toward assisting with coping and personal growth, people must have access to the group at their time of need. If the group is primarily informational, it is usually a closed group with a great amount of structure.

Frequency of Meetings

Most groups reported in the literature met once a week for 1½ to 2 hours a session. It is possible, however, to have an effective group that meets twice a month. This may be more feasible, particularly if the facilitators are volunteers.

Structure

The amount of structure provided in the group is often based on the personal characteristics and needs of the facilitators. Those inexperienced in leading groups may feel more comfortable with a great deal of structure. The agenda may be carefully planned and each activity timed. This need for structure usually decreases as the facilitators gain more experience.

The goals of the group must be considered in planning the amount of structure. Some groups are primarily informational, with guest speakers invited and lecture topics planned. For example, nutrition may be discussed the first week, physical care the second week, and chemotherapy the third week. A brief time may be provided at the end of each session for discussion and expression of feelings. Some participants feel safer in this type of group. It is similar to the school system with which they are familiar and which allows for primarily passive participation. Little personal growth or behavioral change will occur in these groups, but many people are seeking information only and are not interested in the risk involved in exploring feelings and growing.

A process group is more concerned with providing emotional support, promoting expression of feelings, and facilitating coping and growth. These groups have less structure and tend to deal with the concerns and needs of the group members at the time of the meeting. The information sought by members is provided. Feelings are shared and ways of coping are explored. Participants are helped to examine alternatives in their unique situations. They are encouraged to move toward higher levels of mental and physical health. This type of group requires a more advanced level of counseling skills, but is certainly not beyond the realm of the nurse.

Participants

The criteria for selection of participants are an important consideration. Some groups include both patients and family members so that family communication is facilitated. Other groups are limited only to patients or to family members. Patients included may be restricted to those receiving chemotherapy or those who have had a specific type of surgery. The group may be limited to family members in order to allow expression of feelings that often cannot be exhibited with the patient present. The family members' needs may be different from those of the patient. Family members may definitely profit from a program geared specifically to their problems. (See Chapter 12 for a discussion of care for the family.) Family members can often benefit by sharing problems with other families and comparing their strategies. Another family member who has been through a similar experience can be very helpful.

The number of participants should also be carefully considered. A group that consistently has 15 or more people is too large to be effective and should be divided, if possible. A group with only one or two members is too small and focuses attention too closely on these participants, especially if there are several facilitators.

Conducting the Group

Conducting an informational group is usually formal and similar to a classroom situation. Chairs may be arranged in rows with the speaker in front of the group, perhaps with a table or podium. Audiovisual material may be used.

In a process group, the setting is more informal. Chairs are usually arranged in a circle, with room for some space between them. Too much closeness can cause people to feel uncomfortable. Group rules can be printed and given to each participant at the beginning of the session. These rules may include things such as the policies on confidentiality, turn taking, and smoking.

If it is an open group, the session can begin with introductions. Facilitators introduce themselves and then ask participants to introduce themselves and briefly express what they hope to achieve in the group. It is helpful if participants describe their cancer situation. This process is the beginning of the nursing assessment. Assessment should include physiologic, psychologic, and sociologic aspects of the situation, as well as family dynamics. The participants' description can be followed by questions to further assess the situation.

An explanation of what can happen within the group should follow. Participants need to understand that attendance at several sessions is necessary if help beyond the informational level is desired. The members should understand that active participation is necessary to achieve their goals.

The rest of the session will flow according to the response of the group. One participant may respond to a concern expressed by another. Much of the discussion may center on this type of interaction, with brief comments interjected by a facilitator. Interaction may occur between a facilitator and a specific participant. Other participants listen and usually gain much from these experiences. Opportunities should be provided for each member to participate. Occasionally, a participant may wish only to listen, particularly at the first session.

Facilitators can encounter several problems in conducting the group. Sometimes a participant will attempt to monopolize the session. This cannot be allowed to occur, since other members will not get the attention they need. A group member may attempt to take over leadership of the group. This, also, cannot be allowed to happen. Some group members may spend a great deal of time telling their sad story repeatedly in order to get sympathy, but show no desire to work to change their situation. Sometimes they can get all of the other group members working very hard to suggest solutions to their problem, none of which they will accept. They should not be allowed to control the direction of the group. These people can often drive away other members of the group, can exhaust facilitators who attempt to meet their desire for endless sympathy, help, and dependency, and can even destroy the group. It is sometimes necessary to speak with these people outside of the group and confront them with the observation that they do not seem to be willing to work with their problem or that they need a kind of help that cannot be provided in the group. Names of therapists willing to work with cancer patients or family members should be kept available for referral.

Social Maintenance

Time for refreshments and social interactions can be very helpful in providing additional caring and support for participants. This can be planned in the middle of the session or for a period after the session. Volunteer groups associated with the facility or religious or civic groups in the community may be willing to provide refreshments.

Record Keeping

Collecting data on participants can be very useful in terms of evaluating the group and adding to nursing assessments. Information such as addresses and phone numbers of participants should be available so that follow-up contacts can be made. Data collected can include such things as age, sex, occupation, income, type of cancer, and referring person. Additional assessment can be done by completing a questionnaire related to family members, social supports, physician, medical information, and other relevant data. It is also useful to keep a log of the activities of each participant in the group and their goals for further action.

Post-Group Meeting

A short meeting after the session is very helpful for facilitators. Discussion during the session can be reviewed, actions of facilitators can be explored, and feelings of facilitators can be expressed. In this way, facilitators can support each other and learn more effective strategies. Working in a group can be exhausting. The post-group meeting can provide a time to regain emotional strength before going on to another activity. The recording of group activities should also be done at the post-group meeting, while the important expressions and interactions are still fresh in the facilitators' minds.

Consultation

It is important for facilitators to have access to mental health professionals who can help them with problems that are beyond their capacities. Although psychologists or psychiatrists may not have time to conduct support groups, they are often willing to serve as consultants or members of an advisory committee. Without this help, facilitators can find themselves caught up in the unhealthy dynamics of a participant or may be unable to find effective strategies to help certain participants. This also allows a mechanism for maintaining the facilitators' mental health and providing the personal growth that is essential if other persons are to be helped.

Training

Many people are interested in attending a support group so that they can conduct a new group elsewhere. This is an important service to provide, but certain limitations should be established. The number of learners should be limited to one or two per session to prevent disruption of the group. Learners should begin by observing, not participating, and should not attempt to take over leadership of the group unless agreed upon by the facilitators. Learners should participate in the post-group meeting in order for maximum learning to occur.

Coordination with Other Care

To the extent possible, communication links should be developed with other health professionals providing care for each participant in the group. However, this communication should occur only with the knowledge and permission of the participant. The participant should feel confident that negative feelings and opinions expressed in the group will remain confidential. Health care professionals are usually more interested in the fact that the person is attending than in specific details. If a problem does occur, contact can then be made to discuss it.

TYPES OF GROUPS

Patient Groups

Patients have a natural tendency to gather into groups in hospital or outpatient settings. They compare treatments and give encouragement and sympathy to each other. They will often share strategies and tricks that have made life easier for them.

More formally arranged groups with a professional facilitator allow the same process to happen and go beyond it. Patients often do not understand their disease process or their treatment. It is often explained in terms that mean little to them. Patients are expected to comply, but are often not told the purpose of the expected behavior or the consequences of not complying. Interpreting the meaning of laboratory data can also be helpful.

The group also allows patients to express feelings, some of which are negative and socially unacceptable. Alternative coping strategies can be suggested and explored. Possibilities of personal growth can be considered. Patients are often far ahead of family members in dealing with their illness and need help in interacting with their families. Some have been socially isolated, or fear that possibility and need help in managing or avoiding it.

The group provides a caring community for people in a commonly stigmatized situation. It holds the possibility of helping patients to increase their ego strength in order to better manage their situation. Many patients experience the group as a safe haven in a sea of trouble. Sometimes, when the patient recognizes that others are experiencing similar problems, the struggle seems less lonely.

Family Groups

Family members are often left out of the mainstream of care in the cancer situation. And yet they are frequently confronted with multiple, complex problems with which they have had no previous experience. They may attend a group for information, support, or guidance in coping. Sometimes a very distressed family member will come to a group accompanied by one or two other members who are seeking help for the distressed member.

Family members of a dying patient may need to discuss such things as wills, funerals, and how to manage the dying. They may need to imagine what life will be like without the patient. Although some can discuss these things in the patient's presence, many cannot, at least not initially. After exploring these topics in the group and learning from the experiences of other families who have openly discussed them with the patient, they are more able to take the next step and develop more open communications with the patient.

Family groups can provide other types of help as well. For example, the patient is usually far ahead of other family members in dealing with the cancer situation. The family members need a chance to catch up before effective family communications can occur. In addition, family members may be functioning in the primary caretaker role (see Chapter 1) and may need guidance in functioning within this role. Often they also need help in knowing how to take care of themselves, mentally and physically.

Bereavement Groups

Family members continue to need support after the death of a cancer patient. Studies have indicated that families have more problems with both physical illnesses and emotional difficulties after a family member dies of cancer than those whose family member dies of other causes. The bereavement process seems to take longer. In some family support groups, family members continue to attend after the death and may attend sporadically for up to two years.

Many hospice programs offer a separate bereavement group to facilitate movement through the grief process. Parents of children who have died have organized support groups without professional facilitators to help in the long struggle to work through the loss of a child.

Self-Help Groups

Groups of patients with similar problems may organize to deal with the social implications of their situation. Some of these groups are Make Today Count, the Ostomy Association, and the Lost Cord Club. These groups can often help in a way that professionals cannot. However, the patient should not become so immersed in the group that movement back to normal society is slowed or diverted. (See Chapter 15.)

Nurse Support Groups

Working constantly in the cancer situation is very difficult and demanding, both emotionally and physically. Peer relation-

ship problems, lowered self-esteem, diminished job performance, and depression can occur if steps are not taken to maintain the physical and mental health of the nurse. Burn-out is the popular term currently being used to describe this situation.

A regular counseling group for a nurse who is already intensely involved in psychosocial interventions with others is only an added drain. Therefore, the support group must be different for the nurse. It should be a place for replenishing, nurturing, and facilitation of growth.

There are a number of activities that the nurse can take to prevent burn-out. These activities can be promoted and encouraged within a peer support group. Maslach, who has conducted much of the research on burn-out, suggests strategies that can reduce the destructiveness of burn-out.[31] These include increasing abilities in interpersonal skills, recognizing and constructive dealing with personal feelings, forming a support system, using humor, varying patient contact, separating work and home, and focusing on improving physical health.[31]

This last strategy is important because physical deterioration seems to accompany burn-out. The individual becomes exhausted, often is sick, experiences insomnia, and frequently has ulcers, headaches, and other more serious illnesses. There is often a habit of skipping meals, not getting enough sleep, or drinking too much coffee. There is a frequent pattern of use or abuse of tranquilizers, alcohol, or other drugs.[31]

Strategies that lead to good physical health should be encouraged. Maslach suggests developing support systems that encourage physical exercise such as running, tennis, swimming, bicycling, dancing, or other activities that physically tire the person. The nurse should avoid taking work home, either actually or mentally. Taking time-outs should be encouraged if stress becomes severe. This may involve having some days off or a change in job assignment. Nurses should always leave the unit for mealtimes and take coffee breaks away from the working area.[31]

If these behaviors are accepted as the group norm, the nurse is much more likely to adopt them. They should also be supported by nursing administration. These types of activities will increase the nurse's self-esteem and facilitate a higher level of professional functioning.

BIBLIOGRAPHY

1. Adams, J.: Mutual-help groups: enhancing the coping ability of oncology patients. *Cancer Nursing.* 2:95–98, 1979.
2. Bassett, S. D.: An oncology self help group. *American Protestant Hospital Association Bulletin,* 1977–1978, p. 794.
3. Berne, E.: *The Structure and Dynamics of Organizations and Groups.* Ballantine Books, New York, 1963.
4. Berne, E.: *Principles of Group Treatment.* Grove Press, Inc., New York, 1966.
5. Blumberg, B., M. Flaherty, and J. Lewis: *Coping with Cancer.* U.S. Dept. of Health and Human Services, NIH Publication No. 80-2080, 1980.
6. Burns, N.: *Evaluation of a Supportive-Expressive Group For Families of Cancer Patients.* Unpublished Ph.D. dissertation, Texas Woman's University, 1981.
7. Caplan, G.: *Support Systems and Mental Health.* Behavioral Publications, New York, 1974.
8. Caplan, G., and M. Killilea: *Support Systems and Mutual Help.* Grune & Stratton, New York, 1976.
9. Cartwright, D., and A. Zander: *Group Dynamics.* Harper & Row, Publishers, Inc., New York, 1968.
10. Cobb, S., and S. Erbe: Social support for the cancer patient. *Forum on Medicine.* 1:24–29, 1978.
11. Cohen, M., and D. Wellish: Living in limbo: psychosocial intervention in families with a cancer patient. *American Journal of Psychotherapy.* 32:561–571, 1978.
12. Foley, V.: *An Introduction to Family Therapy.* Grune & Stratton, New York, 1974.
13. Friel, M., and C. B. Tehan: Counteracting burn-out for the hospice care-giver. *Cancer Nursing.* 3:285–293, 1980.
14. Galinsky, M. J., and J. H. Schopler: The social work group. In *Models of Group Therapy and Sensitivity Training,* ed. by J. B. P. Schaffer and M. D. Galinsky. Prentice-Hall, Inc., Englewood Cliffs, N.J., 1974.
15. Gardner, K. G.: Supportive nursing: a critical review of the literature. *Journal of Psychiatric Nursing and Mental Health Services.* 17:10–16, 1979.
16. Gazda, G. M.: *Basic Approaches to Group Psychotherapy and Group Counseling.* Charles C Thomas, Publisher, Springfield, Illinois, 1975.
16a. Gottlieb, B. H.: *Social Networks and Social Support.* Sage Publications, Beverly Hills, Ca., 1981.
17. Gussow, Z., and G. S. Tracy: The role of self-help clubs in adaptation to chronic illness and disability. *Social Science and Medicine.* 10:407–414, 1976.
18. Haley, J.: *Uncommon Therapy: The Psychiatric Techniques of Milton Erickson, M.D.* W. W. Norton, New York, 1973.
19. Hare, A. P.: *Handbook of Small Group Research.* The Free Press, New York, 1976.
20. Herzoff, N. E.: A therapeutic group for cancer patients and their families. *Cancer Nursing.* 2:469–474, 1979.
21. Jersild, E. A.: Group therapy for patient's spouses. *American Journal of Nursing.* 67:544–549, 1967.
22. Johnson, J. L., and P. A. Nurby: WE CAN WEEKEND: a program for cancer families. *Cancer Nursing.* 4:23–28, 1981.
23. Kelly, P. P., and G. Coats-Ashby: Group approaches for cancer patients: establishing a group. *American Journal of Nursing.* 79:914–915, 1979.
24. Kemp, C. G.: *Perspectives on the Group Process.* Houghton Mifflin Co., Boston, 1970.
25. Kleiman, M. A., J. E. Mantell, and E. S. Alexander: RX for social death: the cancer patient as counselor. *Community Mental Health Journal.* 13:115–124, 1977.
26. Kopel, K., and L. A. Mock: The use of group sessions for the emotional support of families of terminal patients. *Death Education.* 1:409–422, 1978.
27. Krumm, S., P. Vannatta, and J. Sanders: Group approaches for cancer patients: a group for teaching chemotherapy. *American Journal of Nursing.* 79:916, 1979.
28. Lansky, R. G, and A. E. Dell Orto: *Group Counseling and Physical Disability: A Rehabilitation and Health Care Perspective.* Duxbury Press, North Scituate, Mass., 1979.
29. Levine, B.: *Group Psychotherapy: Practice and Development.* Prentice-Hall, Inc., Englewood Cliffs, N.J., 1979.
30. Lynch, J.: *The Broken Heart: The Medical Consequences of Loneliness.* Basic Books, Inc., New York, 1977.
31. Maslach, C.: The burn-out syndrome and patient care. In *Stress and Survival,* ed. by C. A. Garfield, C. V. Mosby Co., St. Louis, 1979.
32. Minuchin, S.: *Families and Family Therapy.* Harvard University Press, Cambridge, Mass., 1974.
33. Mullan, H., and M. Rosenbaum: *Group Psychotherapy: Theory and Practice.* The Free Press, New York, 1978.
34. Newlin, N. J., and D. K. Wellisch: The oncology nurse: life on an emotional roller coaster. *Cancer Nursing.* 1:447–449, 1978.
35. Okun, B. F., and L. J. Rappaport: *Working With Families: An Introduction to Family Therapy.* Duxbury Press, North Scituate, Mass., 1980.
36. Rogers, C. R.: *Carl Rogers on Encounter Groups.* Harper & Row, Publishers, Inc., New York, 1970.
37. Rosenbaum, M.: Group psychotherapy: heritage, history and the current scene. In *Group Psychotherapy: Theory and Practice,* ed. by H. Mullen and M. Rosenbaum. The Free Press, New York, 1978.

38. Rosenbaum, M., and A. Snadowsky: *The Intensive Group Experience*. The Free Press, New York, 1976.

39. Satir, V.: *Conjoint Family Therapy*. Science & Behavior Books, Palo Alto, 1967.

40. Satir, V.: *Peoplemaking*. Science & Behavior Books, Palo Alto, 1972.

41. Shaffer, J. B. P., and M. D. Galinsky: *Models of Group Therapy and Sensitivity Training*. Prentice-Hall, Inc., Englewood Cliffs, N.J., 1974.

42. Shubin, S.: RX for stress — your stress. *Nursing 79*. 9:52–55, 1979.

43. Silverman, P. R.: The widow-to-widow program, an experiment in preventive intervention. *Mental Hygiene*. 53:333–337, 1969.

44. Skynner, A.: *Systems of Family and Marital Psychotherapy*. Brunner/Mazel, Inc., New York, 1976.

45. Smith, D. W.: Survivors of serious illness. *American Journal of Nursing*. 79:441–446, 1979.

46. Spiegel, D., and I. D. Yalom: A support group for dying patients. *International Journal of Group Psychotherapy*. 28:233–245, 1978.

47. Wellish, D. K., M. B. Mosher, and C. van Scoy: Management of family emotion stress: family group therapy in a private oncology practice. *International Journal of Group Psychotherapy*. 28:225–231, 1978.

48. Whitman, H. H., J. P. Gustafson, and F. W. Coleman: Group approaches for cancer patients: leaders and members. *American Journal of Nursing*. 79:910–912, 1979.

49. Winder, A. E., and J. R. Elam: Therapist for the cancer patient's family: a new role for the nurse. *Journal of Psychiatric Nursing and Mental Health Services*. 16:22–27, 1978.

17

Home Care of the Cancer Patient

As cancer treatments have extended the life of cancer patients and the costs of hospitalization have increased, more of the care of cancer patients has shifted to the home. The family has been confronted with a greatly increased responsibility for caring for the patient, a responsibility for which some families are ill prepared in either knowledge, skills, or available caregivers. (See Chapter 1.)

The patient need not be dying to require some type of assistance with home care. The complex medical therapies now utilized, curing some and greatly prolonging the life of others, bring with them the need for longer and more complex nursing care in a variety of settings. Today there is also a stronger focus in health care on quality of life. The patient is more likely to be supported in efforts to stay at home whenever possible.

In spite of this trend, little is available in the literature regarding home care of the cancer patient. The concept and the nurses who provide it have remained, for the most part, unseen and unheard.

THE THEORETIC FRAMEWORK OF COMMUNITY HEALTH NURSING

Community health nursing operates within a prevention framework, with a focus on health promotion.[27] (See the Leavell and Clark model of prevention, Chapter 18.) Its theoretic base is the public health model, in which the client is the community.[25] The rationale for working with individuals or families must be that those actions will benefit the community as a whole.[27] Systems theory is heavily utilized to provide an orientation to the interrelatedness of individuals, families, and communities.[25, 27] Sociologic theories of family dynamics, group dynamics, and roles are also used. Nursing practice is divided into episodic and distributive modes, with hospital nursing considered episodic and community health nursing distributive. Of the two modes, distributive nursing is seen as having a much greater impact on health.

According to Helvie, the basic assumptions of community health nursing are:

(1) the essential dignity and worth of the individual, (2) the possession by individuals of potentialities and resources for managing their own lives, (3) the importance of freedom to express one's individuality, (4) the great capacity for growth within all social beings, (5) the right of the individual to basic necessities (food, shelter, medical care) without which fulfillment of life is often blocked, (6) the need for individuals to struggle and strive to improve their life and environment, and (7) the right of the individual to help in times of need and crisis.[27]

Helvie sees community health nursing as having four major goals. These are:

(1) helping individuals, families, groups and the community (systems) reach the highest level of health compatible with human potential and desire, (2) providing comprehensive care to these systems, (3) preserving the autonomy of the system, and (4) improving nursing and public health practice.[27]

Helvie believes that the outcome of public health nursing is "a client who is more independent or interdependent in relation to health."[27]

It is considered important for the community health nurse to understand and

352

accept various cultures and lifestyles and to work within the patient's cultural framework when providing care. There is a strong belief that the nurse's values should not be imposed on the client. This is an interesting notion, in light of the fact that health is a value and community health nurses treat as clients even those who do not request (or even desire) nursing care.[24] Rather than claim to be value-free, it would seem more reasonable for the nurses to recognize those values that they hold to be important. It would then be possible to share these owned values with clients, who are left free to adopt or reject them.

The role of the community health nurse has involved assessment, teaching, referral, identification of community needs, participation in policy making, and manipulation of the environment to promote community health. For the past few decades it has involved a minimum of hands-on personal care of individuals. Because of funding priorities, most of the care has been given to the poor, except in the area of communicable diseases.

Many community health nurses work for community health agencies. School nurses, industrial nurses, and nurse practitioners are generally viewed as functioning within this framework of practice. For many years, the requirement for entry into the practice of community health nursing has been a baccalaureate degree, which allowed for educational exposure to the field's theoretic framework.

How Does Community Health Nursing Fit into Nursing as a Whole?

When the community health nursing theory is compared with other theories of nursing, many commonalities can be found. The focus of most nursing theories is on health, with an emphasis on promotion and prevention. Nursing theories emphasize the importance of family. The key difference is that although most nursing theories speak to the care of individuals, families, and communities, most are oriented primarily to individuals and families. The ethical position of community health nursing — that in order for the nursing activity to be justified it must be of benefit to the community — is not espoused.

It does seem possible to merge these two orientations. Nursing theories must expand to more carefully explore the nursing care of the community. Although it can be argued that any activity that benefits an individual in turn must benefit the community, the consequences of taking this ethical position should be examined in more depth.

Certainly the community health nurse's focus on prevention and promotion is important and must continue. But the sick will always be with us, no matter how effective our prevention strategies are, and they also must have nursing care. Yet, with the current increase in chronic illnesses such as cancer, providing that nursing care only episodically is no longer sufficient.

HOME HEALTH CARE — THEN AND NOW

The concept of the home health care nurse originated with Florence Nightingale and William Rathbone. Rathbone, wealthy and able to provide good care for his wife, who died after a long illness, was concerned for the many others who did not have this advantage.[8, 53] Florence Nightingale provided guidance for him to organize a training school for nurses, which opened in 1862. Together they developed the idea of district nurses, who originally were visiting nurses for the sick poor in Liverpool. These nurses primarily provided bedside care but also did health teaching. Family members were taught personal hygiene, healthy living patterns, and how to care for the sick.[53]

In the United States, the first visiting nurses provided care through the New York City Mission, beginning in 1877.[53] The Visiting Nurse Society of Philadelphia originated in 1886. These nurses provided care for the sick poor and also for the sick who were able to pay. Chicago followed suit in 1889 and the Henry Street Settlement, founded by Lillian Wald, was established in 1893.[8] These programs and the others that followed expanded their services to include case finding, control of environmental conditions, health teaching, and many of the present day concerns of community health nursing.

With the passage of time, home care of the sick diminished as other concerns took priority. Now, in community health agencies, home care of the sick is somewhat of a stepchild. A low value is placed on it in terms of funding, personnel, and importance.

Third-party reimbursement for home health care by Medicare and Medicaid has stimulated a revival of these services. But along with the funding has come red tape, regulations, and limitations on the care that is reimbursable. The poor and the elderly qualify for care. Because of governmental control, however, many community health agencies have opted not to provide the service. Home health care agencies emerged in response to this situation. The agencies vary in structure. Some are community nonprofit, some private nonprofit, and some proprietary (or for profit). The competition for clients has increased as more agencies have opened. The quality of nursing care provided by these agencies varies greatly. In some agencies, the achievement of discrete tasks is the goal. The use of the nursing process is not encouraged. An increased volume of visits is important. Time for psychosocial interventions is not allowed. Nurses do not have assigned patients to follow over time but see different patients each day, which prevents the establishment of meaningful nurse-patient relationships. Other agencies place great emphasis on quality nursing care. They have developed useful assessment guides. Each nurse is assigned a case load of patients. Psychosocial interventions are valued and time for care is more flexible than it is when within the constraints imposed by reimbursement.

Hospital-based home health care agencies are now being developed. Thus the hospital can continue to provide care to the patient after discharge. Health maintenance organizations (HMOs) also may provide home health care as part of their services. It is difficult to anticipate all of the changes in the health care system that may occur as a result of these new approaches.

The focus of home health care is not the community but the patient and family. As in most nursing theories, the ethical value that the care must benefit the community in order to justify its provision is not held. Value is placed on improving the patient's and family's quality of life.

This process of treating more patients at home may very well be the beginning of a major change in the health care system and in nursing practice. It may result in the merging of episodic and distributive modes of nursing, of the theory of community health nursing with a more positive value placed on care of the individual and family. As hospital costs rise, it seems conceivable that only patients requiring intensive nursing will be admitted to hospitals, that funding for third-party reimbursement by private insurance of home health care will increase, and that the majority of nurses will work in outpatient clinics and home care programs rather than in hospitals.

The Role of the Home Health Care Nurse

The nurse providing care within a home health care agency may not have a baccalaureate education or a knowledge base that includes the theoretic framework of community health nursing. These nurses have often entered this area of practice as part of the mass exodus from employment in hospitals. They do not see themselves as hospital (or episodic care) nurses, but they also may not see themselves as community health nurses. Presently, many of them seem to have no identity with a particular field of practice. This is most likely one of the primary reasons for the dearth of literature in the field.

Baird has identified five functions of the home health care nurse: "coordinator of services, deliverer of skilled care, teacher of patients and families, counselor and supporter, and facilitator for the utilization of community resources."[5] Many cancer patients are being cared for by more than one physician, sometimes through two or more health care facilities. Multiple agencies may be providing services. Many times none of the health care givers knows what the others are doing. The home health care nurse is in an ideal position to coordinate this care. These nurses must also be very familiar with community resources and how to get through the red tape required to obtain services.[5] Providing care, teaching, and counseling are activities common to nursing practice in many other settings. Although providing skilled physical care in the home may differ in some significant ways, it is just as important at home as in the hospital. Patient and family teaching may be more effective at home because of increased motivation to learn and the increased ability of the nurse to assess the learning needs and evaluate the effectiveness of teaching. In the home there is greater opportunity to function as counselor and supporter. Knowledge of the home situation and the more relaxed atmosphere often make the counseling more effective.

HOME HEALTH CARE DURING THE CANCER SITUATION

Home nursing care for the cancer patient is underutilized, with only 5 per cent of cancer patients receiving these services.[42] Many physicians and nurses are unaware of the extent of services available. When home health care is provided, the patient is usually in an advanced stage of illness and is dying. The family has often been providing care with no outside assistance for months or even years. As a result, the quality of life for both patient and family has sometimes been needlessly lowered. The patient may be unnecessarily dependent and have a lower level of health than

should occur. Important family functions may have been abandoned in favor of caring for the patient. The family support systems may have been lost.

If contact were made earlier in the disease process, family members could be helped to arrange the environment for more efficient care. Measures could be started to teach the family how to care for the patient and ways of providing emotional support and guidance. The patient could be assisted in maintaining independence and important family roles. Networks of support could be maintained. The family could continue to function in more diverse ways.

The entire structure of health care is based on reimbursement patterns, which greatly influence what care is provided and to whom. Services not reimbursable are often not available, even to those able to pay. Although this arrangement may not be ideal, it is real. Nurses must demonstrate the cost-effectiveness as well as the care-effectiveness of services before they will be included in the reimbursement system.

Referral

Nurses and physicians alike are uncertain of the types of problems that warrant referral for home health care. They are often limited in their knowledge of the patient and family because of an inadequate assessment and a lack of awareness of the patient's home environment.

In order for patients to qualify for home care under Medicare or Medicaid, they must be homebound. This means that they are unable to come to an office or an outpatient clinic for care. Private insurers vary in their requirements, but many seem to follow Medicare guidelines.

The need for skilled nursing care must be documented in order to justify home health care. Care includes activities such as patient and family teaching and nursing procedures such as dressing changes or catheter care. Evaluation of physical status is also considered skilled nursing care. Although the patient may **need physi-**

cal therapy, social service counseling, or a visit by a dietitian, these services cannot be provided unless skilled nursing care is also required.

Referral to a home health care program should be a part of the discharge planning process implemented shortly after the patient's admission to the hospital. It should be discussed with the patient and family. As adequate an assessment as possible should be made of the family's living environment and social supports. A hospital visit by the home health care nurse would be helpful in allaying some of the apprehension commonly experienced when leaving the security of the hospital.

Although referral requires a doctor's order for reimbursement purposes, it may be up to the nurse to suggest referral. Patients and family members, made aware of this alternative, may also approach the physician for an order. Physicians often have a very limited understanding of nursing practice. The referral and the medical orders for care requested often reflect this fact. Many physicians still do not see the nurse in the role of assessing, evaluating, or making judgments about care. Therefore, the order may be only for a discrete nursing task. The physician may provide very little information about patients or their medical diagnosis, believing that it is not needed in order for the nurse to accomplish the task. The nurse must take the initiative to approach the physician to obtain the needed information. The physician should be kept informed about the comprehensiveness of the care being provided and the evaluation of that care. Demonstrated competence in quality nursing care and exposing the physician to the science of nursing practice by sharing the dynamics of the nursing process will often increase both the number and type of referrals being made.

PROVIDING HOME NURSING

Although the few articles available in the literature extoll the virtues of home health care, little information is available to give direction to the nurse who is entering this field of practice. Much of this knowledge is available only by establishing an apprentice-type relationship with a nurse skilled in providing home health care.

In some ways, home nursing is very similar to nursing in the hospital, but there are some striking differences. The nurse is entering the family's territory rather than the reverse. Space, rules, patterns of activity, timing, and placing of objects are all under the control of the family, not the nurse. The patient and family are in a stronger position to make decisions regarding care and may opt not to follow the instructions of the nurse. Family members will retain the final judgment about what is best for them rather than seeing the nurse as the expert, as is often the case in the hospital. Although the interaction between nurse and patient is different, nursing practice remains essentially the same. The processes of care provided, although performed in a less familiar environment for the nurse, are the same. The nurse is able to function in a far more autonomous manner than is possible in a hospital setting. It is more possible to provide care based on a professional nursing practice model than is usually possible in more traditional settings. Because the care given is more visible, the nurse is more accountable for nursing actions — to the client, the family, the agency, and the referring physician.

The Initial Visit

When the home visit is made, one of the nurse's first actions will be to demonstrate to the family that she or he is providing a needed service and is an expert. It is very possible to be an expert in an area but not to be perceived as such. The nurse's bearing, clothing, manner of speaking, and body language are all important factors in communicating expertise. At the same time, it is essential to communicate recognition that the patient and family are in control and that the nurse will function as a helper, advisor, or consultant. These two major activities will begin within minutes of the initial contact with the family in either a planned or an unplanned fashion.

Making a Contract

In home care, in contrast to a hospital setting, there is a much clearer contract made between nurse and client and between the client and the agency through which the nurse practices. A discussion of the services to be provided, the timing of services, the cost, and the length of time for which services will be provided are openly discussed by the nurse, client, and family. Thus, the nurse makes clear what types of nursing care can be offered and the clients may elect to avail themselves of these services.[7, 19, 25, 50]

Spradley presents a good discussion of the concept of contracting.[53] Contracting demands active participation. The contract is a working agreement between involved parties in which there is shared understanding and consent to the terms and purposes of the transaction. The four characteristics of contracting identified by Spradley are partnership, commitment, format, and negotiation. Spradley believes that all contracting involves shared participation and agreement (partnership). The decision to enter the contract binds all parties to fulfill the purpose of the contract (commitment). The contract defines the terms (or format) of the relationship. The contract always involves negotiation. During negotiation ideas are discussed, compromises made, and conclusions reached. Agreed upon terms often need modification during the period of the contract and renegotiation then occurs. This allows for built-in flexibility and gives contracting a dynamic quality.[53]

Spradley summarizes the advantages of contracting as follows:

1. It involves clients in their own care.
2. It motivates clients to perform necessary tasks.
3. It individualizes care by focusing on a client's unique needs, whether the client is an individual or a group.
4. It increases the possibility of achieving health goals identified by both client and nurse.
5. It develops problem-solving skills of both nurse and client.
6. It fosters client participation in the decision-making process.
7. It promotes clients' autonomy and self-esteem as they learn self-care.
8. It makes nursing service more efficient and cost effective.[53]

Contracting occurs in stages and is a complex process. Spradley states:

Consider the fact that this working agreement depends on knowing what the client wants, agreeing on goals, identifying methods to achieve these goals, knowing the resources that the nurse and client bring to the relationship, utilizing appropriate outside resources, setting limits, deciding on responsibilities, and providing for periodic reviews. Each of these tasks requires discussion between, and decision making by, nurse and client.[50]

Sloan and Schommer provide a sequence of phases in the process of contracting that can be helpful:

1. *Exploration of needs.* Assessment of client's health, problems, and needs by client and nurse.
2. *Establishment of goals.* Discussion and agreement between client and nurse on goals and objectives.
3. *Exploration of resources.* Defining what client and nurse each have to offer to and expect from each other; identifying appropriate resources such as significant others, agencies, and other professionals.
4. *Development of a plan.* Identifying methods and activities for achieving the goals.
5. *Division of responsibilities.* Negotiating the activities for which client and nurse will each be responsible.
6. *Agreement on time frame.* Setting limits for the contract in terms of length of time or number of visits.
7. *Evaluation.* Periodic and final assessment of progress toward goals occurring at agreed-upon intervals.
8. *Renegotiation or termination.* Agreement to modify, renegotiate, or terminate the contract.[53]

Assessment

As in any field of nursing practice, care begins with a thorough assessment. If possible, at least a 2-hour period should be reserved for the first visit. In home care, it is usually possible to do a more thorough assessment than could occur in a hospital setting, since the nurse can assess the family dynamics in the home environment and can get a better picture of the social support network. .Of course, assessment will continue with each visit, but the initial assessment is crucial for quality care.

Most home care agencies have developed forms to use for the history and physical examination. In addition, it is important to assess the psychological and social situation of both patient and family.

Factors that should be identified include:

1. All people living in the home, their age, relationship to the patient, educational level, and level of health.
2. All family members living outside the home who are directly involved in care activities, their age, relationship to the patient, educational level, and level of health.
3. The person who is functioning as primary caregiver, his or her age, relationship to the patient, educational level, and level of health.
4. The care responsibilities of primary caregiver, feelings, needs, problems, and extent to which personal life is disrupted.
5. The care responsibilities of other family members.
6. The roles of various family members.
7. The relationships between family members.
8. The daily routine of the family.
9. The family's coping patterns.
10. The social support network (Norbeck has recently developed an easy-to-use tool for assessing the social support system.[40])
11. The response of patient and family to the present health situation.

It is important to determine the patient's diagnosis, stage of cancer, and current treatment. The patient should be carefully questioned and examined for side effects of treatments. Careful questioning should be conducted to determine medications being taken and medications previously ordered but no longer being taken. Patients do not always take medications as ordered; therefore, it is important to determine how each drug is being utilized. More accurate information will be obtained if the nurse is not perceived as being judgmental or critical. It is important to communicate acceptance of the type of care being provided by the family.

Since much of the funding for these services is available through Medicare, a large number of patients currently being treated by home health care agencies are elderly. Because of age-related impairments, these patients and their families often have trouble remembering dates and times and instructions given verbally. They may require very careful questioning to determine what is actually being done in the home. A tolerant, kind approach is essential. The elderly person is very sensitive to impatient, rude questioning, becomes anxious and more confused, and is then less likely to be able to provide accurate information.

Nutrition, sleep patterns, pain, and pain management are important factors to assess in the cancer patient. The Karnofsky scale is a useful tool for determining level of activity (see Chapter 9). The patient and family should also be asked to identify problems that concern them. Such problems may seem minor to the nurse and are often easily remedied but can be major concerns to the patient.

With the current focus of nursing on the identification of problems, it is easy to overlook the family's strengths. Strengths may consist of previous successful experiences in dealing with a serious health situation, effective coping strategies, a strong support system, good ego strength, knowledge and education sufficient to facilitate effective problem-solving strategies, sufficient finances to manage needs, a cohesive and committed family, a religion or philosophy that provides stability, and a preventive health orientation.[4] These strengths should be assessed as carefully as the problems. It is necessary to identify them in order to determine the family's potential for movement toward a higher level of health. It is also important to identify the family's values related to health and personal growth.

Planning

Much of the information that is obtained from assessment can be expressed to the patient and family and planning can then be conducted together. Alternative approaches to care can be discussed. Because the family and the patient will have active roles in implementing the plan of care, it is important that it be understood and accepted by them. It is often important for the patient and the family to be aware of the consequences of the alternatives being considered while planning care.

The plan may include utilization of other personnel such as dietitians, physical therapists, social workers, occupational therapists, nurse's aides, and homemakers. Some of these services are reimbursable by Medicare and Medicaid but only if the need for skilled nursing care can be documented.

Edstrom and Miller have listed topics identified by family members as needed in order to care for a cancer patient at home.[18] (See Tables 17–1 and 17–2.) Much information about these topics is simply not currently available to families. Family members are left to struggle on their own as best they can. Their needs become more visible to the nurse during a home visit, when the family members usually feel freer to express their concerns. The family and patient need more than the teaching of "how to's" in order to maintain an optimum level of functioning. They also need emotional support, and this requires access to continuity of care. Home care for the cancer patient may be more complex and more intense than that provided to the typical

Table 17–1. Topics Identified by All (**N** = 8) Family Members Participating in the Needs Assessment Questionnaire as Desired for Inclusion in the Home Care Course*

(1) Skin care, how to prevent and treat skin breakdown.
(2) Administration of medications, including injections.
(3) Methods of pain control, including comfort measures and medications.
(4) Information on maintaining activity and dealing with activity limitations.
(5) Dealing with family changes and problems when living with a member who has a chronic illness.

*From Edstrom, S., and Miller, M. W.: Preparing the family to care for the cancer patient at home: a home care course. *Cancer Nursing.* 4:49–52, 1981. Masson Publishing USA, Inc., New York, copyright 1981. Used by permission.

Table 17–2. Topics Identified by a Minimum of Four Family Members Participating in the Needs Assessment Questionnaire as Desired for Inclusion in the Home Care Course*

(1) How to give a bed bath.
(2) How to use a bed pan and urinal.
(3) How to change an occupied bed.
(4) How to transfer the patient from bed to chair.
(5) Information regarding observations to make in assessing the ill person's condition.
(6) Information on nutrition and feeding.
(7) Dealing with nausea and loss of appetite.
(8) Dealing with constipation.
(9) How to use oxygen at home.
(10) Information regarding resources and services available in your community.
(11) Information on costs of home care.
(12) How to cope with economic changes within the family.
(13) How to utilize support systems.
(14) How to deal with children's questions and involving them in care.

*From Edstrom, S., and Miller, M. W.: Preparing the family to care for the cancer patient at home: a home care course. *Cancer Nursing.* 4:49–52, 1981. Masson Publishing USA, Inc., New York, copyright 1981. Used by permission.

home health care patient (see Chapters 11 and 12). Services need to be available 24 hours a day, 7 days a week. Although this increases the cost of home care, it is still considerably below that of hospitalization.

Intervention

Availability of a nurse's aide 2 or 3 days a week to bathe the patient, change bed linens, wash the hair, shave the patient, and provide other personal care can be extremely helpful to family members. Homemakers can sometimes come to the home to assist with housekeeping activities.

Some home health care agencies provide a type of primary nursing care in which the professional nurse carries a case load of patients. This is certainly more effective than randomly assigning a nurse to visit different patients each day. The latter strategy perpetuates the task-oriented focus of the hospital, which is such a serious impediment to the ability to practice professional nursing. Since the goal of cancer nursing is to help the patient cope as effectively as possible with the situation, the nurse must know the patient's status as well as possible in order to effectively intervene. This is not possible if a different nurse sees the patient each visit.

Activities such as colostomy irrigation, dressing changes, wound irrigation, and catheter changes are common procedures performed by professional nurses in the home. Blood samples may be drawn for laboratory study. Family members may be taught to give enemas or injections or how to ambulate the patient. Teaching will often include an emphasis on nutrition and pain management.

Psychosocial interventions, such as those discussed in Chapter 12, form an essential part of nursing care. These interventions must be conducted in conjunction with physical care, since third-party reimbursement will not pay for psychosocial nursing interventions alone.

Recently, more complex nursing care has begun to be provided in the home to decrease costs and improve the quality of life for cancer patients and their families. Some community health nurses are providing home administration of total parenteral nutrition (TPN) and chemotherapy.[30] This avoids costly, painful, and sometimes impossible trips to the hospital, clinic, or physician's office. These strategies should be provided by nurses skilled in the field of oncology nursing. At present, these approaches are experimental and usually provided in conjunction with a medical research center. One research hospital has developed a program in which a well-equipped van is available to transport physicians, oncology nurses, psychologists, psychiatrists, and other specialists to the patient's home to provide highly skilled care, which would otherwise require hospitalization.[57] Patients and family members have been enthusiastic about the service and the opportunity to be treated at home.

Evaluation

Nurses are just beginning to conduct studies to determine the effectiveness of home care. Even though the nurse may feel that the home visits have positively affected the lives of the patient and family,

finding measurable ways to demonstrate this change is difficult. However, it will be necessary to show this difference in measurable ways in order to justify use of scarce health care dollars for this purpose. Although patient and family satisfaction can be measured as a demonstration of their improved quality of life, this approach to evaluation will not be sufficient to justify the care unless it can also be demonstrated to be cost effective. With cancer patients, it is often not possible to show an improvement in physical condition, since the patient is deteriorating as an expected consequence of the disease process. Legge and Reilly have attempted to measure the outcomes of home care for cancer patients.[37] In this study, although patients' physical condition deteriorated, a large number were able to avoid rehospitalization because of the home care that was provided. Further studies in this area are needed.

Home health care seems to hold great promise for the future. One great question is the extent to which nurses will have a voice in shaping this future — or will choose to use that voice to participate in the policy making and planning that will be occurring over the next decade. The concept has the potential for catalyzing some of the second-order changes so badly needed in the current health care system.

BIBLIOGRAPHY

1. Allen, D. V., P. L. Kuhns, H. H. Werley, and S. R. Peabody: Agencies' perceptions of factors affecting home care referral. *Medical Care.* 12:828–844, 1974.
2. Amado, A. J., and B. A. Cronk: Home health care and the terminally ill. Treating the terminally ill at home: opportunities of change. *Home Health Review.* 2:38–44, 1979.
3. Anderson, J. L., and M. L. Brown: The cancer patient in the community: a nursing challenge. *Nursing Clinics of North America.* 15:373–388, 1980.
4. Antonovsky, A.: *Health, Stress and Coping.* Jossey-Bass, Washington, D.C., 1979.
5. Baird, B.: Nursing roles in continuing care: home care and hospice. *Seminars in Oncology.* 7:28–38, 1980.
6. Barnes, S. Y.: Your safety first. *Nursing 79.* 9:87–90, 1979.
7. Baulch, E. M.: *Home Care: A Practical Alternative*

to *Extended Hospitalization.* Celestial Arts, Millbrae, Ca., 1980.

8. Benson, E. R., and J. O. McDevitt: *Community Health and Nursing Practice.* Prentice-Hall, Inc., Englewood Cliffs, 1980.

9. Berry, N. J.: Measuring and projecting demand for home health care. *Home Health Review.* 3:24–27, 1980.

10. Bohnet, N.: Total nursing assessment of the home care patient. *Home Health Review.* 3:13–15, 1980.

11. Brickner, P. W.: Health care services for homebound aged maintain independence, limit costs. *Hospital Progress.* 61:56–59, 1980.

12. Brofman, J. L.: An evening home visiting program. *Nursing Outlook.* 27:657–661, 1979.

13. Cowper-Smith, F.: Changes in health visiting, part 1. *Nursing Times.* 75:615–618, 1979.

14. Cowper-Smith, F.: Changes in health visiting, part 2. *Nursing Times.* 75:660–663, 1979.

15. Coyle, E. H.: Homemaker-home health aide services. *Journal of Gerontological Nursing.* 2:37–41, 1976.

16. Davis, A. J.: Disability, home care and the caretaking role in family life. *Journal of Advanced Nursing.* 4:49–52, 1981.

17. Dawson, N., and M. Stern: Perception of priorities for home nursing care. *Nursing Research.* 22:145–148, 1973.

18. Edstrom, S., and M. W. Miller: Preparing the family to care for the cancer patient at home: a home care course. *Cancer Nursing.* 4:49–52, 1981.

19. Ford, M.: Bridging the gap between hospital and home. *The Canadian Nurse.* 77:44–47, 1981.

20. Freeman, R. B., and J. Heinrich: *Community Health Nursing Practice.* W. B. Saunders Co., Philadelphia, 1981.

21. Fromer, M. J.: *Community Health Care and the Nursing Process.* C. V. Mosby Co., St. Louis, 1979.

22. Good news about home health care. *Life and Health.* 95:19, 1980.

23. Greany, L.: The visiting nurse service. *The Australian Nurses' Journal.* 8:32–34, 1979.

24. Hall, J. E.: Distributive health care and nursing practice. In *Distributive Nursing Practice: A Systems Approach to Community Health,* ed. by J. E. Hall and B. R. Weaver. J. B. Lippincott Co., Philadelphia, 1977.

25. Hall, J. E., and B. R. Weaver: *Distributive Nursing Practice: A Systems Approach to Community Health.* J. B. Lippincott Co., Philadelphia, 1977.

26. Harris, M. D.: Evaluating home care? Compare viewpoints. *Nursing and Health Care.* 2:297–309, 1981.

27. Helvie, C. O.: *Community Health Nursing: Theory and Process.* Harper and Row Publishers, Inc., New York, 1981.

28. Hennessey, M. J., and B. Gorenberg: The significance and impact of the home care of an older adult. *Nursing Clinics of North America.* 15:349–360, 1980.

29. Hickmore, R.: Family support and friendly visiting. *The Canadian Nurse.* 77:50–54, 1981.

30. Hunter, G., and S. H. Johnson: Physical support systems for the homebound oncology pa-

tients. *Oncology Nursing Forum.* 7:21–23, 1980.

31. Inue, T. S., K. M. Stevenson, D. Plorde, and I. Murphy: Needs assessment for hospital-based home care services. *Research in Nursing and Health.* 3:101–106, 1980.

32. Jackson, P. A.: Developing an ostomy specialty role in a home care agency. *Journal of Enterostomal Therapy.* 7:9–14, 1980.

33. Karafiath, D. D.: Home care makes sense today. *Journal of Nursing Administration.* 76:31–34, 1976.

34. Lash, M. E.: Community health nursing in a minority setting. *Nursing Clinics of North America.* 15:339–348, 1980.

35. Laver, P., S. P. Murphy, and M. J. Powers: Learning needs of cancer patients: a comparison of nurse and patient perceptions. *Nursing Research.* 31:11–16, 1982.

36. Legge, J. S., and B. J. Reilly: Assessing the outcomes of a home nursing programme: previously hospitalized versus non-hospitalized patients. *Journal of Advanced Nursing.* 5:561–572, 1980.

37. Legge, J. S., and B. J. Reilly: Assessing the outcomes of cancer patients in a home nursing program. *Cancer Nursing.* 3:357–363, 1980.

38. Littlejohn, C. E.: What new staff learned and didn't learn. *Nursing Outlook.* 28:32–35, 1980.

39. Moulthrop, H. E., and J. Roxborough: Network support for the aged: the viable alternative to institutionalization. *Journal of Gerontological Nursing.* 4:64–66, 1978.

40. Norbeck, J., and N. Sheimer: Single-parent functioning. *Research in Nursing and Health.* 5:3–12, 1982.

41. Novak, B.: Home nursing program on an Indian reservation. *Public Health Reports.* 89:545–550, 1974.

42. Oleske, D., and E. Jeide: Planning for regional home care for cancer patients. *Oncology Nursing Forum.* 6:4–6, 1979.

43. Physical dependence of home patients. *The Australian Nurses' Journal.* 8:45–47, 1978.

44. Pieper, C. J., and M. A. Grundy: Respite care program. *Journal of Gerontological Nursing.* 3:49, 1977.

45. Prichard, E. R., J. Collard, J. Starr, J. A. Lockwood, A. H. Kutscher, and I. B. Seeland: *Home Care: Living With Dying.* Columbia University Press, New York, 1979.

46. Pritchard, M. A.: A concept of continuing care. *Nursing Times.* 76:169–172, 1980.

47. Reeves, R.: Nurse, what are you all about? *American Journal of Nursing.* 79:2145–2147, 1979.

48. Reines, M. O.: A visiting nurse in a problem-oriented group practice. *American Journal of Nursing.* 79:1224–1226, 1979.

49. Richardson, I. M.: General practitioners and district nurses: a study of referral patterns in the city of Aberdeen. *British Journal of Preventive and Social Medicine.* 28:187–190, 1974.

50. Rosenbaum, E., and I. Rosenbaum: Principles of home care for the patient with advanced

cancer. *Journal of the American Medical Association.* 244:1484–1487, 1980.

51. Ryan, S. J., and C. Wassenberg: A hospital-based home care program. *Nursing Clinics of North America.* 15:323–338, 1980.

52. Smith, J. A., J. Buckalew, and S. M. Rosales: Making the right moves in discharge planning: coordinating a workable system. *American Journal of Nursing.* 79:1439–1440, 1979.

53. Spradley, B. W.: *Community Health Nursing: Concepts and Practice.* Little, Brown and Co., Boston, 1981.

54. Stein, R. E. K.: Pediatric home care: an ambulatory "special care unit." *The Journal of Pediatrics.* 92:495–499, 1978.

55. Ventura, C. A.: Levels of knowledge about aging among homemaker/home health aides. *Home Health Review.* 3:16–23, 1980.

56. Vinciquerra, V., T. Degnan, J. Dicner, D. Budman, P. Schulman, J. McCartney, M. O'Connell, and M. Vargas: Home oncology medical extension: a new home treatment program. *CA — A Cancer Journal for Clinicians.* 30:182–185, 1980.

57. Williams, G. O.: The elderly in family practice. *Journal of Family Practice.* 5:369–373, 1977.

58. Ziegler, J. C.: Physical reconditioning–Rx for the convalescent patient. *Nursing 80.* 10:67–69, 1980.

18

The Nursing Impact: Cancer and the Social and Political Systems

THE PHILOSOPHY OF PREVENTION

Leavell and Clark's Model

The most familar concept of prevention was proposed by Leavell and Clark in 1958.[17] They defined prevention as "the science and art of preventing disease, prolonging life, and promoting physical and mental health and efficiency."[17] Leavell and Clark viewed health and illness as a continuum. The position of human beings on the continuum is not stationary: humans engage in a constant battle against biologic, physical, mental, and social forces that tend to disturb their health equilibrium.

In the struggle for health maintenance, people use internal and external defense mechanisms, great margins of safety and tissue reserves, and physiologic processes of repair. Leavell and Clark view disease as a process rather than a static entity, a process that begins before the body is actually affected. Each disease occurrence has multiple causes, many of which are in the environment. Prevention involves taking measures to intercept or counteract these causes. It requires knowledge of the causes of a disease and knowledge of how the causes may be intercepted or counteracted. Success, then, depends on the completeness of knowledge about a disease process, the opportunities to use the knowledge, and the actual application of the knowledge.[17]

Leavell and Clark classify prevention into three phases: primary, secondary, and tertiary. Primary prevention is oriented toward promoting optimum general health or protection against specific disease agents. Secondary prevention is directed toward early diagnosis and prompt and adequate treatment. The aim of tertiary prevention is rehabilitation.[17] Leavell and Clark developed a model to further clarify the concept. (See Fig. 18–1.)

Antonovsky's Model

In 1979, Antonovsky proposed a new conceptualization of health and prevention that goes beyond that of previous theorists.[3] Antonovsky suggested moving from searching for the causes of illness to attempting to determine how some few people manage to stay healthy. He proposed a new word, salutogenesis, which means the origins of health. He criticized the typical approach of medicine as having too narrow a focus on disease states rather than illness, and on illness to an almost total exclusion of interest in health. Instead, Antonovsky sees health as a separate continuum from illness. He uses several concepts to explain the factors present at a given location on the health continuum, which he calls the health ease/dis-ease continuum.[3] (See Fig. 18–2.)

The Sense of Coherence. The central concept of Antonovsky's model is the sense of coherence. He defines the sense of coherence as:

. . . a global orientation that expresses the extent to which one has a pervasive, enduring though dynamic feeling of confidence that one's inter-

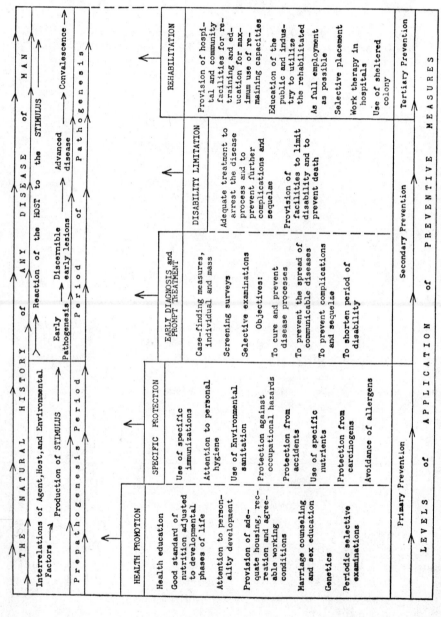

Figure 18–1. Levels of application of preventive measures in the natural history of disease. (From Leavell, H. R., and Clark, E. G.: *Preventive Medicine for the Doctor in His Community.* Copyright 1965 by McGraw-Hill, Inc. Used by permission of McGraw-Hill Book Company.)

nal and external environments are predictable and that there is a high probability that things will work out as well as can reasonably be expected.[3]

The sense of coherence is a way of perceiving the world and one's self within the world. It is not specific to any area of life, any situation, any time, or any specific stressor. It is "a crucial element in the basic personality structure of an individual . . . ," developing as a result of early childhood experiences and "shaped and tested, reinforced and modified . . . throughout one's life."[3]

The sense of coherence is a continuum. Those people with a strong sense of coherence view the internal and external environment as predictable and comprehensible. They have a clear perception of reality and an attitude of autonomy and competence. They feel a sense of confidence, of faith, of lawfulness. Events are predictable. There is a feeling that, for the most part, things will work out well.[3]

People with a weak sense of coherence tend to expect things to go wrong. The world makes no sense and is not predictable. These people do not expect their needs to be fulfilled. A sense of hopelessness and helplessness pervades their thinking; thus, they give up easily. Powerlessness, arbitrariness, and bewilderment are associated with a weak sense of coherence.[3]

An individual's position on this continuum is not permanent, but tends to change only slightly in one direction or the other with usual life events. However, dynamic changes that have more lasting effects can occur. These include events such as marriage, moving, or change of occupation.

Two types of situations can cause significant transformations in a person's sense of coherence. One is a cataclysmic stressor, which transforms life experiences rapidly. The person has had no choice, no experience, and no preparation for the situation. The experience invariably results in a significant weakening of the sense of coherence. A diagnosis of cancer is often a cataclysmic stressor.

The second type of occurrence is never sudden, almost always has an element of choice. (either conscious or unconscious), and can result in either weakening or strengthening the sense of coherence. "Movement toward the strong end of the continuum always requires hard work."[3] An example of a change toward strength would be the process of psychotherapy.

Generalized Resistance Resources. Generalized Resistance Resources are factors that greatly influence the strength of an individual's sense of coherence. These factors provide a person with sets of meaningful, coherent life experiences. The major Generalized Resistance Resources are financial resources, knowledge and intelligence, coping strategies, social supports, commitment, cultural stability, a philosophy that provides a stable set of answers, and a preventive health orientation.[3]

Stressors, Tension Management, and Stress. Everyone is continuously exposed to stressors — physical, mental, or emotional stimuli. The stressors commonly experienced have been discussed in depth in the literature. Illness has often been believed to be caused by such stimuli. Antonovsky, however, believes it is necessary to distinguish between stressors, stress, and tension. A person responds to a stressor with tension. The consequences of tension can be either negative, neutral, or salutogenic, depending on the effectiveness of tension management. Successful tension management is dependent upon the availability of Generalized Resistance Resources and a strong sense of coherence. If tension management is successful, stress does not occur. Unsuccessful tension management leads to a state of stress. Stress may contribute to the development of illness. Thus, successful tension management is important to the prevention of illness and the promotion of health.[3]

Breakdown. Movement toward the dis-ease end of the continuum is described by Antonovsky as breakdown. Unsuccessful tension management can lead to a state of stress that interacts with pathogens and weak links to move a person toward breakdown. The stress, however, does not determine the breakdown's particular nature.[3]

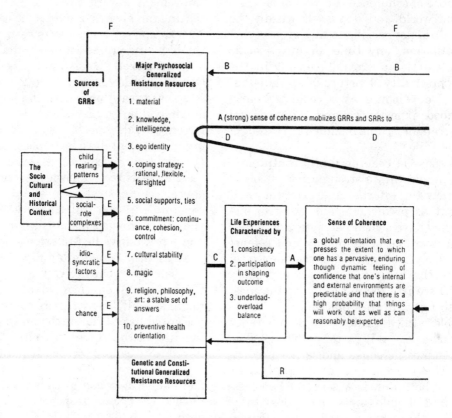

Key to Figure 1

Arrow A: **Life experiences shape the sense of coherence.**
Arrow B: Stressors affect the generalized resistance resources at one's disposal.
Line C: **By definition, a GRR provides one with sets of meaningful, coherent life experiences.**
Arrow D: **A strong sense of coherence mobilizes the GRRs and SRRs at one's disposal.**
Arrows E: **Childrearing patterns, social role complexes,** idiosyncratic factors, and chance **build up GRRs.**
Arrow F: The sources of GRRs also create stressors.
Arrow G: Traumatic physical and biochemical stressors affect health status directly; health status affects extent of exposure to psychosocial stressors.
Arrow H: Physical and biochemical stressors interact with endogenic pathogens and "weak links" and with stress to affect health status.
Arrow I: Public and private health measures avoid or neutralize stressors.
Line J: A strong sense of coherence, mobilizing GRRs and SRRs, avoids stressors.

Figure 18–2. The salutogenic model. (From Antonovsky, A.: *Health, Stress, and Coping.* Washington, D.C.: Jossey-Bass Publishers, 1979. Used by permission.)

Illustration continued on opposite page

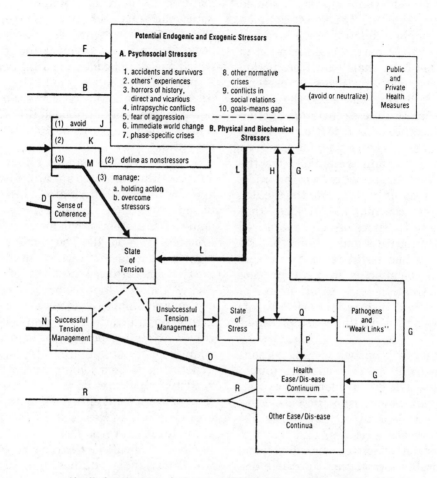

Line K: A strong sense of coherence, mobilizing GRRs and SRRs, defines stimuli as nonstressors.

Arrow L: **Ubiquitous stressors create a state of tension.**

Arrow M: **The mobilized GRRs (and SRRs) interact with the state of tension and manage a holding action and the overcoming of stressors.**

Arrow N: **Successful tension management strengthens the sense of coherence.**

Arrow O: **Successful tension management maintains one's place on the health ease/dis-ease continuum.**

Arrow P: Interaction between the state of stress and pathogens and "weak links" negatively affects health status.

Arrow Q: Stress is a general precursor that interacts with the existing potential endogenic and exogenic pathogens and "weak links."

Arrow R: Good health status facilitates the acquisition of other GRRs.

Note: The statements in bold type represent the core of the salutogenic model.

Figure 18–2 *Continued*

PRIMARY PREVENTION

General Preventive Measures

General preventive measures are aimed at promoting health. The most common way to accomplish this is by health education. For the most part, the assumption in the past has been that health promotion could only occur if illness was not present. When the individual moved to the illness end of the health-illness continuum, action moved to secondary and tertiary prevention. Antonovsky's description of health as a separate continuum accommodates the idea that health promotion can be effectively used at any point on the health ease/dis-ease continuum. Actions that strengthen or facilitate use of Generalized Resistance Resources and actions that result in more successful tension management should be effective in health promotion. Elimination or diminution of stressors should also promote health, as should strengthening the sense of coherence.

If Antonovsky's model works, persons high on the health ease/dis-ease continuum should have a lower incidence of cancer. Persons with cancer who increase their utilization of Generalized Resistance Resources, decrease stressors, and learn to manage tension effectively should respond more favorably to treatment of their disease. If the disease is progressive, they should react to the situation with more ease and less distress.

If Antonovsky's model is valid, it would seem advisable to develop effective tools for measuring the extent of Generalized Resistance Resources and the effectiveness of tension management. Nursing strategies should be created to facilitate development and strengthening of Generalized Resistance Resources, promote effective tension management, and identify and control stressors that are influencing the cancer situation. The Generalized Resistance Resources that seem to be most amenable to nursing interventions are ego identity, coping strategies, social supports, commitment, and a preventive health orientation.

One strategy to strengthen ego identity is by promotion of the active patient role. Ways of improving coping strategies and social supports are discussed in Chapter 12. Commitment is strongly associated with continuity, cohesion, and control of care, all of which are discussed in this book. Commitment involves the extent to which one is embedded in social networks. A preventive health orientation can be promoted during the cancer situation by helping people take responsibility for maximizing their physical and mental health potential.

Stressors in the cancer situation are often within the nurse's realm to identify and diminish or eliminate. These might include nutritional inadequacies, pain, and many of the other problems identified in Chapters 11 and 12. The nurse's role in tension management also takes on a greater importance, in light of Antonovsky's concept. Relaxation, guided imagery, and problem solving may have a much greater significance than previously perceived. Helping people to identify and change primitive, inaccurate, and fear-generating beliefs about cancer to more realistic beliefs may do much to strengthen their sense of coherence and mobilize available Generalized Resistance Resources.

All health care professionals should be involved in health education directed toward individuals, families, and community groups, with the goal of improving Generalized Resistance Resources and increasing tension management. Efforts should be made to alter the negative beliefs and social stigmas that have long been associated with the cancer situation.

Specific Preventive Measures

The aim of specific preventive measures should be twofold. First, biologic stressors such as environmental carcinogens should be identified and eliminated wherever possible. Second, persons at high risk should be identified and given information and support to minimize their risk factors.

The Political Arena

Identifying environmental carcinogens is a difficult task, one requiring close interdisciplinary work. (Environmental factors related to cancer are discussed in Chapter 3.) Merely identifying them, however, seems like child's play compared with the effort needed to minimize or eliminate them from the environment. This difficult task, which is also an interdisciplinary one, requires actions in areas that nurses have traditionally avoided; specifically, politics and economics.

Health is not the only important consideration in our society; nor is it the most vital concern of many people. Frequently, health and economic issues are at odds. Many of the actions that need to be taken to decrease the incidence of cancer are extremely costly to industry and government. The cost to society as a whole is also great, since these actions would require changes in our lifestyle.

Many pragmatists say that we cannot have a risk-free world. One of the prices that we pay for an industrial society is human lives. The question then becomes, how many human lives is the use of a specific carcinogen worth? And who is to make that decision?

Nursing, as the chief promoter of health in our society, must go beyond the simplicity of individual nurse-client relationships to do battle in the complex world of politics, economics, and industry. In a sense, the client must become society, with the nurse facilitating actions that promote society's greater health. Society must be confronted with the consequences of a disregard for health. Increasing the awareness of society as a whole will diminish the power of the few to make decisions affecting the health of many. At the same time, we must not be so narrow-minded that we cannot see the other values that must be weighed along with health in making choices. In other words, society, not nursing, must ultimately make its own choices about health and accept responsibility for the consequences.

The problem at the present time is that nursing is not being heard. The arguments

in favor of preventive health measures are weak and ineffective. In order to become effective in this arena, nurses must gain greater knowledge in the fields of politics, economics, and industry. Moving into this arena will require large doses of courage and determination. However, the greatest impact on the prevention of cancer will come from these activities.

High Risk Groups

Attempting primary prevention of a disease by altering some of the causative factors in a high risk group assumes that "most if not all health problems are theoretically preventable at some stage in their development."[10] In order to identify high risk groups, at least some of the causative factors of the health problem must be known. It then must be possible to intervene to alter the natural course of events caused by that factor.

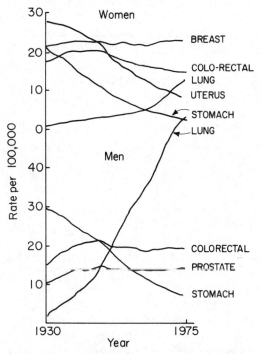

Figure 18–3. Trends in death rates from cancer in the U.S. population. From American Cancer Society Statistics, 1978. (From Negendank, W.: Cancer detection and screening. In *The Cancer Patient: Social and Medical Aspects of Care,* edited by Cassileth, B. R. Philadelphia: Lea & Febiger, 1979. Used by permission.)

Given the rapid increase in lung cancer, the single factor that could have the greatest impact on the development of cancer is smoking. (See Fig. 18–3.) The economic realities, politics, and lifestyles related to smoking make it a complex issue. Nurses, who should be functioning as role models of health promotion, are in the one health profession whose incidence of smoking has increased.

Other high risk factors that can be identified prior to the development of cancer are premalignant lesions, genetic predisposition, excessive exposure to sun, exposure to environmental carcinogens, and improper diet. Since the goal is prevention of the occurrence of cancer, not early detection, interventions should be directed toward decreasing the causative factor.

SECONDARY PREVENTION

Early Diagnostic Screening

In secondary prevention, the goal is to detect the health problem early. The assumption is that early detection will alter the natural course of the problem so that a greater level of health is maintained. Early detection, then, should result in prolongation of life, higher quality of life, or increased numbers of cures. Lewy has listed the following criteria that should be met to justify the worth of early screening.

1. The problem must be important; i.e., it must be of significance to the individual and detrimental to health if left untreated.
2. Effective treatment must be available. There is no need to identify a disease for which no treatment exists.

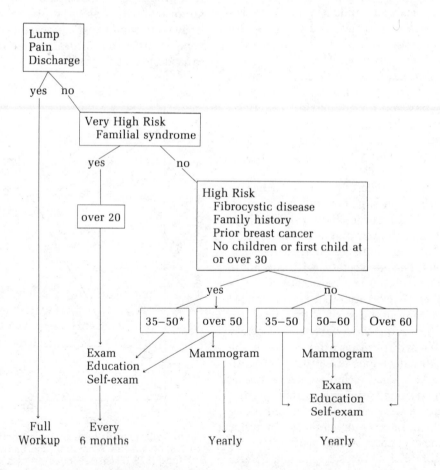

*Or whenever risk factor is noted.

Figure 18–4. Breast cancer screening. Prevalence in adults 2.5/1000. (From Negendank, W.: Cancer detection and screening. In *The Cancer Patient: Social and Medical Aspects of Care,* edited by Cassileth, B. R. Philadelphia: Lea & Febiger, 1979. Used by permission.) There is currently controversy over the use of mammograms in women at high risk of cancer (see Chapter 4). Self-exam is monthly.

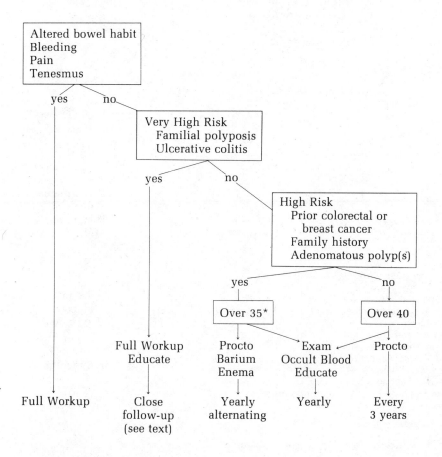

*Or whenever risk is noted.

Figure 18–5. Colorectal cancer screening. Prevalence in adults 1/1000. (From Negendank, W.: Cancer detection and screening. In *The Cancer Patient: Social and Medical Aspects of Care,* edited by Cassileth, B. R. Philadelphia: Lea & Febiger, 1979. Used by permission.)

3. Treatment should be accessible. Persons found in need of treatment should have treatment facilities available.

4. The test and treatment must be acceptable to the patient. Screening tests should be easy and quick to perform and present minimal discomfort to the patient. The patient should also be willing to undergo the treatment for the disease.

5. Early detection should be advantageous. Early diagnosis should lead to more efficient treatment and a better prognosis.

6. The course and natural history of the disease should be understood. There should exist a latent and early symptomatic phase that could warrant detection during this period.

7. The condition should either have some prevalence in the community or be especially serious.

8. Tests should be sufficiently sensitive and specific. There should be few false negative and false positive results.

9. Disease identification should be cost-effective. The cost of detecting a case must be reasonable in relation to the individual and the community.[18]

The screening physical examination for the individual has been described in Chapter 4. Screening large numbers of presumably unsymptomatic people in order to detect early cancer sometimes requires different patterns of decision making. Negendank has developed decision matrices for the most commonly occurring cancers and those with clearly identified risk factors.[23] These are also helpful to use in addition to the individual screening physical examination. (See Figs. 18–4 to 18–10.)

In 1980 the American Cancer Society changed its recommendations for the screening of high risk populations. These changes have been very controversial and are based on the cost-effectiveness of screening and on the effect of each discovery on treatment and cure. For example, early discovery of lung cancer seems to make little difference in the trajectory

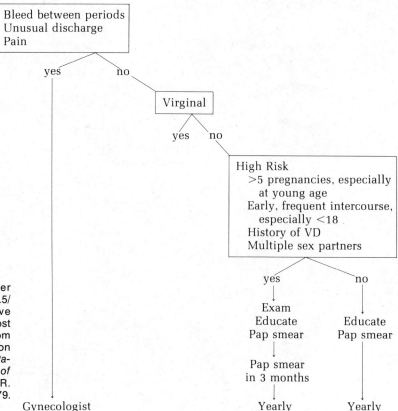

Figure 18-6. Cervical cancer screening. Prevalence about 2.5/1000. Prevalence of positive Papanicolaou (Pap) smears (most in situ) about 4/1000 smears. (From Negendank, W.: Cancer detection and screening. In *The Cancer Patient: Social and Medical Aspects of Care,* edited by Cassileth, B. R. Philadelphia: Lea & Febiger, 1979. Used by permission.)

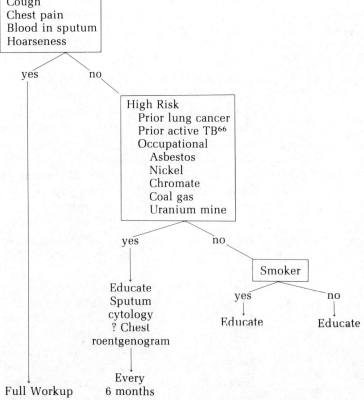

Figure 18-7. Lung cancer screening. Prevalence in adults 1/1000. (From Negendank, W.: Cancer detection and screening. In *The Cancer Patient: Social and Medical Aspects of Care,* edited by Cassileth, B. R. Philadelphia: Lea & Febiger, 1979. Used by permission.)

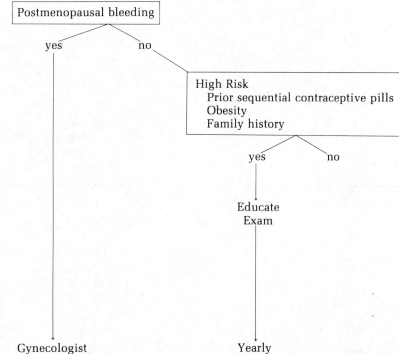

Figure 18–8. Uterine cancer screening. (From Negendank, W.: Cancer detection and screening. In *The Cancer Patient: Social and Medical Aspects of Care,* edited by Cassileth, B. R. Philadelphia: Lea & Febiger, 1979. Used by permission.)

of the disease. Cure is no more likely and treatments for lung cancer, for the most part, are ineffective. What, then, is accomplished by each detection? If mammo-grams increase the risk of breast cancer, their use cannot be justified. If a patient has had two negative Papanicolaou (Pap) smears, some clinicians believe further

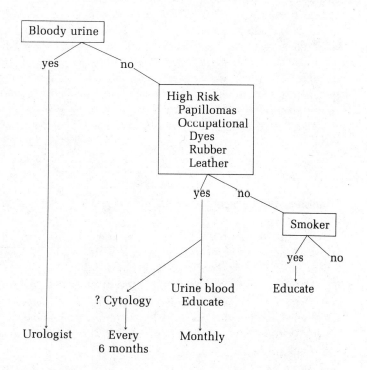

Figure 18–9. Bladder cancer screening. (From Negendank, W.: Cancer detection and screening. In *The Cancer Patient: Social and Medical Aspects of Care,* edited by Cassileth, B. R. Philadelphia: Lea & Febiger, 1979. Used by permission.)

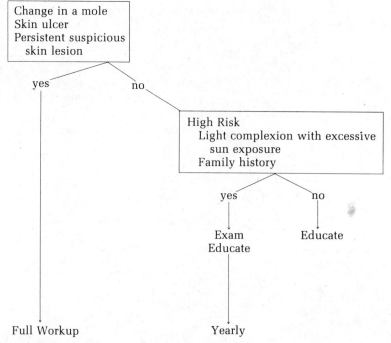

Figure 18–10.   Skin cancer and melanoma screening. (From Negendank, W.: Cancer detection and screening. In *The Cancer Patient: Social and Medical Aspects of Care,* edited by Cassileth, B. R. Philadelphia: Lea & Febiger, 1979. Used by permission.)

yearly Pap smears cannot be justified. Other clinicians strongly protest these changes, believing that without extensive screening some patients will be missed who could be cured or more effectively treated. This goes back to the ethical utilitarian view of the greatest good for the greatest number. If third-party reimbursement is based on these recommendations, it means that patients who desire more frequent or extensive screening must pay out of pocket for it.

Disability Limitation

After the health problem has been identified, actions are directed toward diminishing its impact. Medical treatment at this point is aimed at cure or treatment of the disease. Nursing care is directed toward promoting the most healthy response to the disability.

Quackery

One of the major problems encountered after the diagnosis of cancer is quackery. Because the cure rate for cancer is still low and medical treatment is unpleasant, many people are vulnerable to promises of a quick cure, a sure cure, or a secret cure. One of the greatest harms that occur with unproven methods of cancer treatment is delay in effective treatment, thus allowing the malignancy to grow, perhaps past the point of cure or control. It is important for the nurse to be familiar with current unproven methods of treatment and sources of those treatments in the community. (See Table 18–1.) The nurse should know the "logical" arguments used to persuade and the fallacies of those arguments.

Another serious danger of quack treatments is the change that occurs in the physician-patient and the nurse-patient relationships. Physicians and nurses often reject patients who have sought or accepted

Text continued on page 379

Table 18–1.   Summary of Some Unproven Methods of Cancer Therapy or Management*

Name	Advocates	Year	Description	Method of Administration
Anticancergen Z50 and Zuccala lytic test	G. S. Zuccala, Sc.D.	1960	An extract of pooled cancer tissue, the autogenous material from the patient's own oxalated blood or morning urine.	I.M.
Antineol	H. K. Wachtel, M.D.	1948	An extract of the posterior lobe of the pituitary glands of cattle. It is said to be a cancer-checking lipide (CCL).	Not known P.O.?
Bamfolin ("S. N. K.")	M. Oshima, Ph.D. H. Yokoyama, Ph.D. others	1959	An extract from the leaf of Yakusasa, a species of bamboo grass.	P.O.
H. H. Beard methods	H. H. Beard, Ph.D.	1902	Pancreatic enzymes, chymotrypsin; Laetrile with diet; chymotrypsin, Laetrile, Pangometin (CLP).	I.M., I.M. & I.T., etc.
Biomedical detoxification therapy	M. C. Zamora, R.N. M. Cates, R.N. M. E. Mathison, D.O. J. H. Friend, D.O.	1967	Gerson-like diet with Hoxsey method and Koch antitoxins.	P.O., I.M.
Bonifacio anticancer goat serum	L. Bonifacio, D.V.M. several others	1950	Extracts prepared from the intestinal villi of goats.	I.M.
Cancer lipid concentrate and the malignancy index	R. R. Citron, M.D.	1945	Equine anticancer antibody. Involves the injection of a variety of cancers into a variety of animals that are said to develop "antibodies" to cancer.	I.M.
Carcin, neocarcin	(Dr.) J. Pawlotzky, physician and chemist (Dr.) J. Issels S. A. Lugano	1902 1953	Glands and plant extracts, corrective substances, mesothorium and thorium X; also a serum from selectively bred white mice.	P.O., I.M.
Carzodelan	S. M. Gaschler (Dr.) W. Zabel	1955	Parenteral enzyme therapy, a proteolytic enzyme of the character of trypsin claimed to be capable of dissolving tumor protein.	I.M.
CH-23	P. Christoff C. Christoff (Dr.) J. Issels (Dr.) E. Berger (Dr.) F. Westrick	1959	An alkaloid medicine obtained from plants, which is said to destroy cancerous tissue without damaging normal tissue.	I.V.
Chaparral tea	H. H. Hogle, M.D.	1969	An Indian (U.S.) tea from a desert shrub.	P.O.
Chase dietary method	(Dr.) A. Chase	1965	A diet that soaks out undesirable wastes.	P.O.
C.N.T. (compleso attivo sulla omeostasi cellulare)	E. Spina (Dr.) A. Alecce	1967	Ovarian and testicular dried products plus other substances.	P.O.
Coley's mixed toxins, mixed bacterial toxins (MBT)	W. B. Coley, M.D. H. C. Nauts	1893 1960	Strains of *Bacillus prodigiosus, Streptococcus erysipelatis,* and other bacteria.	I.M., I.T.
Collodaurum and bichloracetic acid Kahlenberg; also KelZvme	H. H. Kahlenberg, Ph.D.		Metallic gold in pure water.	P.O., I.M.
Compound X	Vipont Chemical Co.	1973	Galangal, bloodroot and zinc chloride (an escharotic).	Topical

Table continued on following page

Table 18–1. **Summary of Some Unproven Methods of Cancer Therapy or Management** * *– Continued*

Name	Advocates	Year	Description	Method of Administration
Contreras methods	E. C. Rodriguez, M.D.	1966	Laetrile plus other methods; Beard therapy.	I.M., I.T., P.O.
Crofton immunization method; also Glover serum	W. M. Crofton, M.D.	1958 and earlier	Killed bacterial antigen.	I.M.?
Diamond carbon compound	Antubhai Vaidya, D.Sc.	1945	Powder of the cortical crystals of pure diamonds mixed with lime water.	?
Dimethyl sulfoxide (DMSO) with hematoxylin	Tucker, E. J., M.D.	1971	Promotes absorption and aids transport across cell walls.	Topical
Ferguson plant products	W. Ferguson	1931	Head shrinking compound from Ecuador; 30 separate plant compounds.	I.V.
Fresh cell therapy (CT)	P. Niehans, M.D.	1936	Injection of fresh embryonic cells from organs of animals similar to the organ or tissue that is dysfunctioning.	I.M.?
Frost method	I. N. Frost, M.D.	1961	Organic food diet plus vaccines, Krebiozen, Koch antitoxins, and Mucorhicin.	P.O., I.M.?
Gerson method of treatment for cancer	M. Gerson, M.D.	1942 (U.S.)	Diet of uncanned fresh fruits, vegetables and oatmeal, specially cooked and supplemented with vitamins.	P.O.
Gibson methods	F. Gibson, M.D.	1960	A group of unproven methods, including Carzodelan, Krebiozen, Laetrile, and Mucorhicin in various combinations; also Antineol.	P.O., I.M.
Glover serum	T. J. Glover, M.B. J. E. White, M.D.	1920	Serum of horses injected with a virus(?)	I.M.?
H-11	J. H. Thompson, B.Sc. G. J. W. Ollerenshaw, M.A., B.M., B.Ch.	1969	Normal human male urine extract.	I.M., topical, P.O.
Hadley vaccine and blood and skin tests	H. G. Hadley, M.D.	1960	Vaccine of *Bacillus cereus* plus two tests.	I.M.?
Heat therapy or hyperthermia	M. Von Ardenne, physicist and mathematician	1965	Bath with head relatively cool, 40° C, and body hot, 44° C.	—
Hemacytology index (HCL)	T. E. Arthur, M.D.	1963	A cytologic test for the diagnosis of cancer by leukocyte morphology.	Test
Hendricks natural immunity therapy	W. G. Hendricks, M.D.	1954	Lincoln bacteriophage lysates, Koch oxidation catalysts, and a newly developed antigen derived from patient's blood, urine, sputum, or feces.	I.M.
Hett "cancer serum" and Gruner blood smear test	J. E. Hett, M.D. O. C. Gruner, M.D. N. C. Hamilton, M.D.	1931	A serum of unknown derivation. Contained both *Escherichia coli* and *Streptococcus fecalis* on examination.	I.V.
Hoxsey method or Hoxsey chemotherapy	H. M. Hoxsey H. A. Galbraith, D.O. H. Stegman, D.O.	1920's	Internal medicine, external compounds, supportive therapy. Multiple benign drugs.	P.O.
Iscador	(Dr.) R. Steiner (Dr.) Anna Koffler (Dr.) Wegman	1958	Mistletoe extract (Viscum album).	?

Table 18–1. Summary of Some Unproven Methods of Cancer Therapy or Management*–_Continued_

Name	Advocates	Year	Description	Method of Administration
Issels combination therapy	(Dr.) J. Issels (Dr.) F. Gerlach	1971	Consists of a number of unproven products and possibly a specific immunobiologic substance.	?
Kanfer neuromuscular handwriting test	A. Kanfer (Dr.) D. F. Casten	1935 1965	A specific type of handwriting said to be diagnostic of cancer.	Test
KC-555	K. Sarkisian	1962	A botanical extract from a variety of plants with Chianti wine added.	P.O.
Kelley malignancy index and ecology therapy	W. D. Kelley, D.D.S.	1969	Five factors: nutrition, detoxification, well-balanced diet, neurologic stimulation, and spiritual attitude.	P.O.
Koch antitoxins	W. F. Koch, Ph.D., M.D.	1919	Glyoxylide plus partially oxidized inositol. Also two antitoxins.	I.M., P.O.
Krebiozen, Carcalon	S. Durovic, M.D. A. C. Ivy, Ph.D.	1950's	A natural process said to slow down the growth of cancer; a chalone.	I.M.?
Laetrile, vitamin B_{17}; also sold as Krebiozen amygdalin, Nitriloside, Aprikern, Bee 17	E. T. Krebs, M.D. E. T. Krebs, Jr. B. A. Krebs, D.O. (M.D.) H. H. Beard, Ph.D. E. L. McNaughton J. Beard	1920	Contains amygdalin, ineffective against cancer in humans and animals.	I.M.
Lewis methods	A. J. Lewis, B.A. J. E. Ayre, M.D.	1969	A coupled tumor protein antigen (CTPA) administered by injections into the thigh after a positive Lewis Test.	I.M.
Livingston vaccine	V. Wuerthele-Caspe, M.D. (nee Livingston) E. Alexander-Jackson, Ph.D.	1953	An organism in the blood and urine of patients with cancer and used as a vaccine.	I.M.
Makari intradermal cancer tests (ICT)	J. G. Makari, M.D. W. H. Schultz	1955	A skin test with presumed cancer antigens for the diagnosis of early cancer.	Subcutaneous; test
M-P virus	M. Molomut, Ph.D. M. Padnos, Ph.D.	1965	A lymphocytopenic virus used as a vaccine.	I.V., I.M.
Mucorhicin	P. L. Drosnes L. M. Lazenby J. W. Wilson, M.D. P. A. Murray, M.D.	1943	"An enzymatic product . . . biologically processed whole wheat grain. . . ."	P.O.
Multiple enzyme therapy	S. L. Shively, Sr., M.D.	1959	Trypsin, chymotrypsin, ribonuclease, desoxyribonuclease, pepsinogen.	I.V.
			Lipase, alpha and beta amylase.	P.O.
Naessens. Also called Anablast and G.N. 24.	G. Naessens	1950	"Chemotherapeutical medication." Anablast has been called a serologic medication; also, ". . . an element that provokes the proliferation of cancer cells."	I.M.
Nichols escharotic method	P. L. Nichols, M.D. J. A. Ottman, M.D. S. E. Simpson, M.D. L. R. Kerns, O.D. R. F. Sutter, O.D.	1914	Escharotic pastes of arsenical or zinc compounds.	Topical
Orgone energy devices; also COE.	W. Reich, M.D.	1936	"Orgone energy," "cosmic orgone energy," "COE." A "shooter" is used to concentrate "orgone energy" on certain sites.	Topical

Table continued on following page

Table 18–1. Summary of Some Unproven Methods of Cancer Therapy or Management* – *Continued*

Name	Advocates	Year	Description	Method of Administration
Polonine	J. W. Blaszczak, D.V.M.	1958	Compound of B vitamins; later called a "ribonucleoside." Said to have an antimetabolic effect.	P.O.
Rand-coupled fortified antigen (RCFA) and delayed double diffusion (3D) test.	H. J. Rand A. J. Lewis S. M. DeCarvalho, M.D.	1966	A vaccine said to benefit or cure cancer and a test for cancer, based on a presumed viral etiology of cancer.	I.M.
Revici cancer control	E. Revici, M.D.	1941	Adjusts the body's acid-alkaline level through diet and the use of lipids or lipisides. Also described as "biologically guided chemotherapy."	P.O.
Samuel's causal therapy; endogenous endo-crinopathy	J. Samuels, M.D.	1938	Diagnosis by a special test consisting of a spectrographic estimation of the reduction of the oxyhemoglobin in the skin. Treatment consists of short wave radiation of pituitary or gonads.	Radiation
SF I, SF II, SF III.	L. Burton, Ph.D. F. Friedman, Ph.D. D. D. Thaler, M.D.	1963	SF I is composed of serum of humans with neoplasia; SF II is serum from non-neoplastic donors; and SF III is composed of blood cells of neoplastic donors. Blood is taken from patients with cancer and processed at the Immunology Research Foundation (IRF). An extract of this is then probably injected into the patient.	Not known
Spears hygienic system	L. L. Spears, D.C. D. Spears, D.C. H. Spears, D. C.	1952	The segments of the spine are adjusted to correct vertebral distortions interfering with the nerve supply needed for function (chiropractic).	Physical
Staphylococcus phage lysates; also called Lincoln bacteriophage lysates	R. E. Lincoln, M.D. A. E. Mills, M.D.	1948	Bacteriophage human serum albumin (lincolnii) Beta was used initially in the treatment of cancer. HSA lincolnii Alpha was used first in the treatment of many other diseases and later given to cancer patients.	S.I. nasal spray
Ultraviolet blood irradiation intravenous treatment	R. C. Olney, M.D. and others in the American Blood Irradiation Society	1969	Blood is drawn from a patient with cancer, pasteurized with ultraviolet rays, and injected into the patient's circulation. Used in combination with many other unproven methods, including diets and trace elements.	I.V. plus others
Zen macrobiotic diet	G. Ohsaw	1960	A diet based on the opposing principles of yin (female, passive) and yang (male, active), ancient forces of Chinese cosmology. Macrobiotic diet No. 7 is currently the most popular.	P.P.

*From Olson, K. B.: Drugs, cancer and charlatans. In *Clinical Oncology,* edited by Horton, J., and Hill, G. J. II. Philadelphia: W. B. Saunders Co., 1977. Used by permission.

Many of these data are summarized from the American Cancer Society's monograph, *Unproven Methods of Cancer Management* (1966).

Names of these methods vary in different parts of the world; only those believed to be the best-known or prominent names are included here. Many of the therapies are combined with other unproven or (at times) proven methods of therapy by their proponents.

Dates are not precise but indicate the approximate time at which a treatment method became known or prominent.

The method of administration is not always clear. When in question, it is marked with a question mark. I.T. indicates therapy into the tumor, and Test indicates that it is a test for cancer and not a mode of therapy. Educational degrees are listed when known. (Dr.) indicates a title, but the kind of doctorate is not known.

a quack treatment. Even if this rejection does not occur, patients may expect it to and withdraw from the relationship, thus forfeiting further appropriate treatment. They may feel guilty and ashamed and feel that they deserve to be punished. Or they may feel angry and displace that anger onto the health care professionals. Sometimes they will espouse the quack treatment method with the fervor of a new convert to a religion or cause. They think that if they believe in it hard enough, the method will work. Behind this fervor may be the recognition that if they admit that the treatment was quackery, those patients will have to recognize what they have done to themselves. This is too difficult for many people to confront. It is easier to keep up a false front of belief.

Patients or family members will often reveal utilization of quack treatments to the nurse, but not the physician. It is important to avoid immediate condemnation. The nurse should listen and assess the situation. What factors about the treatment are dangerous? What effect will it have on current medical treatment? This information should then be conveyed to the patient or family member. It is important to remember that we offer nursing care, we do not impose it. The patient is a responsible decision maker. The nurse may not always agree with every decision made by the patient.

If the nurse simply rejects the patient, further opportunities to promote the patient's health may be lost. Therefore, it is more effective to indicate disagreement with the decision, but acceptance of the patient. This will leave the situation open for further discussion at a later time, particularly if problems arise.

TERTIARY PREVENTION

Tertiary prevention is oriented toward helping the patient move back to a higher level of health, which has been lowered as a result of a health problem. This orientation is the focus of rehabilitation, as discussed in Chapter 15.

NURSING RESEARCH NEEDS

Much of current nursing practice is not based on a solid foundation of scientific knowledge: it is based on intuition and tradition. It is imperative that nursing validate the care presently being given and develop strategies to improve it. This requires research based on a sound theoretical foundation of nursing practice. To simply seek out random bits and pieces of knowledge through scattered, unrelated research is neither helpful nor meaningful. Nursing research must be conducted so that it adds to an organized body of knowledge. It must give meaning to the whole of nursing practice.

If nursing is seen as the means of promoting the most healthy physical, emotional, and social responses to a health situation, and if Antonovsky's model of health is used, the following are important areas of research:

1. Methods of measuring ego identity
2. Methods of facilitating or strengthening ego identity
3. Methods of measuring coping strategies
4. Methods of strengthening effective coping strategies
5. Methods of measuring support systems
6. Methods of strengthening support systems
7. Methods of determining effective health teaching
8. Methods of improving the continuity of care
9. Alterations of current health care that allow the patient and family greater autonomy and control
10. Descriptions of economic factors related to nursing practice
11. Examination of cost containment strategies that maintain or improve current quality of care
12. Mechanisms of decreasing psychosocial stressors:
    a. Denial, anger, depression, anxiety, and fear
    b. Social isolation

c. Unrealistic beliefs related to the health situation
d. Communication barriers
e. Dependency
f. Altered body image
g. Dysfunctional sexuality
h. Role changes
i. Loss of self-esteem
j. Uncertain future
13. Mechanisms of decreasing physiologic stressors:
   a. Inadequate nutrition
   b. Nausea and vomiting
   c. Stomatitis
   d. Pain
   e. Infection
   f. Thrombophlebitis
   g. Pulmonary embolism
   h. Bleeding
   i. Constipation
   j. Diarrhea
   k. Incisions and lesions
   l. Lymphedema
   m. Fractures
   n. Impaired mobility
   o. Decubiti
14. Methods of measuring tension management
15. Methods of facilitating effective tension management
16. Methods of measuring the sense of coherence

THE FUTURE OF NURSING AND CANCER

Both nursing and the cancer situation are in a state of rapid change. Nursing is becoming a more autonomous profession supported by a more clearly defined body of scientific knowledge. Nursing is moving into the areas of community and home care, with more nurses providing care as family nurse practitioners, home care nurses, hospice care nurses, industrial nurses, and school nurses. Cancer care will move increasingly away from inpatient care and will be conducted more in comprehensive community cancer centers that promote continuity of care.

The future is hopeful, but permanent changes take time. Nurses must continue to promote change, look for small gains, and accept some failures and lost battles, but they must ultimately refuse to give up the fight. The apathy, frustration, and negative views of nursing as reflected by those nurses who are burned-out and have given up must not be allowed to stifle enthusiasm for the future. These nurses are victims of the present system and should be helped and cared for, not rejected. Strategies must be found to prevent the high level of casualties among nurses in nursing practice situations.

Cancer nursing care must improve, the theoretical basis for nursing practice must become more cohesive, and the nursing profession must be more socially valued. As these things happen, cancer nursing will become a much more satisfying field of care.

BIBLIOGRAPHY

1. American Cancer Society: *Unproven Methods of Cancer Management.* American Cancer Society, New York, 1971.
2. American Cancer Society: *Laetrile: Background Information.* American Cancer Society, New York, 1977.
3. Antonovsky, A.: *Health, Stress and Coping.* Jossey-Bass Inc., Publishers, San Francisco, 1979.
4. Antonovsky, A., and O. Anson: Factors related to preventive health behavior. In *Cancer: The Behavioral Dimensions,* ed. by J. W. Cullen, B. H. Fox, and R. N. Isom. Raven Press, New York, 1976.
5. Baird, S. B.: Economic realities in the treatment and care of the cancer patient. *Topics in Clinical Nursing.* 2:67–80, 1981.
6. Berg, J. W., R. Ross, and H. B. Latouretee: Economic status and survival of cancer patients. *Cancer.* 39:467–477, 1977.
7. Burkhalter, P. K.: Cancer quackery: what you need to know. In *Dynamics of Oncology Nursing,* ed. by P. K. Burkhalter and D. L. Donley. McGraw-Hill Book Co., New York, 1978.
8. Cahill, L. M.: Industrial cancer education service. *Cancer Nursing.* 1:391–394, 1978.
9. Carbone, A.: Laetrile, the continuing controversy. *Hospital Formulary.* August, 1978, pp. 589–590.
10. Clark, D. W., and B. MacMahon: *Preventive Medicine.* Little, Brown & Co., Boston, 1967.
11. Collins, N.: Cancer detection clinic serves community. *Occupational Health and Safety.* January/February, 1979, pp. 40–41.
12. DeWys, W.: Changing attitudes toward cancer. *Journal of Chronic Diseases.* 29:545–548, 1976.

13. Epstein, S. S.: *The Politics of Cancer.* Anchor Books, Garden City, 1978.
14. Fink, R.: Delay behavior in breast cancer screening. In *Cancer: The Behavioral Dimensions,* ed. by J. W. Cullen, B. H. Fox, and R. N. Isom. Raven Press, New York, 1976.
15. Green, L. W.: Site and symptom-related factors in secondary prevention of cancer. In *Cancer: The Behavioral Dimensions,* ed. by J. W. Cullen, B. H. Fox, and R. N. Isom. Raven Press, New York, 1976.
16. Janssen, W.: Cancer quackery: past and present. *Hospital Formulary.* August, 1978, pp. 592–593.
17. Leavell, H. R., and E. G. Clark: *Preventive Medicine for the Doctor in His Community.* McGraw-Hill Book Co., New York, 1965.
18. Lewy, R.: *Preventive Primary Medicine.* Little, Brown & Co., Boston, 1980.
19. Mattlin, C., V. McCoy, F. Nuchereno, and G. P. Murphy: The role and impact of the cancer education nurse in industrial health programs. *Oncology Nursing Forum.* 7:18–22, 1980.
20. Mechanic, D.: *Politics, Medicine and Social Science.* John Wiley and Sons, New York, 1974.
21. Mechanic, D.: *Medical Sociology.* The Free Press, New York, 1978.
22. Morgan, R. M.: Prospects for preventive medicine. *Canadian Journal of Radiography, Radiotherapy, Nuclear Medicine.* 9:169–173, 1978.
23. Negendank, W.: Cancer detection and screening. In *The Cancer Patient: Social and Medical Aspects of Care,* ed. by B. R. Cassileth. Lea & Febiger, Philadelphia, 1979.
24. Oberst, M. T.: Priorities in cancer nursing research. *Cancer Nursing.* 1:281–290, 1978.
25. Olson, K. B.: Drugs, Cancer and Charlatans. In *Clinical Oncology,* ed. by J. Horton and G. J. Hill, II. W. B. Saunders Co., Philadelphia, 1977.
26. Somers, A. R.: *Promoting Health:* Consumer Education and National Policy. Aspen Systems Corp. Germantown, Md., 1976.
27. Stillman, M. J.: Woman's health beliefs about breast cancer and breast self-examination. *Nursing Research.* 26:121–127, 1977.
28. Strauss, A. L.: *Where Medicine Fails.* Transaction Books, New Brunswick, N.J., 1973.
29. Stromborg, M. F., and S. Bourque-Nord: A cancer detection clinic: patient motivation and satisfaction. *Nurse Practitioner.* January/February 1979, pp. 10–11.
30. Trotta, P.: Breast self-examination: factors influencing compliance. *Oncology Nursing Forum.* 7:13–17, 1980.
31. Walter, C. A., B. B. Gallucci, D. M. Molbo, B. L. Pesznecker, and T. H. Holmes: The association of numerous life changes with cervical dysplasia and metaplasia. *Cancer Nursing.* 3:445–449, 1980.
32. White, L. N., J. L. Cornelius, A. F. Judkins, and J. E. Patterson: Screening of cancer by nurses. *Cancer Nursing.* 1:15–20, 1978.

INDEX

Page numbers in *italics* refer to illustrations; (t) denotes tabular material.

Abdomen, physical examination of, 71
Actinomycin D, 159
Adaptation, as coping strategy, 269–270
Adrenocorticosteroids, 165
Adriamycin, 158–159
Aflatoxins, as carcinogens, 56
Alcohol, carcinogens and, 49
Alkeran, 158
Alkylating agents, 157–158, 157(t)
Allopurinol, 163
Alopecia, chemotherapy and, 175, 188
Alpha-fetoprotein, 34
Alpha particles, 123
Alternatives, consideration of, 273–274
Amethopterin, 161–162
Amputation, 333–335
Androgens, 165
Anemia, 34–35
Anger and hostility, 280–281
Angiogenesis factor, 28
Angiosarcoma, of liver, 46
Animal research, 40–41
Antibiotics, 158–160, 159(t)
Antibodies, 27
Antiestrogens, 164–165
Antimetabolites, 161–163, 161(t)
Antineoplastic drugs. See *Chemotherapy.*
Antonovsky's model of prevention, 363, 365, *366–367*
Anus, physical examination of, 72
Anxiety, 282
1-β-D-Arabinofuranosylcytosine, 162–163
Arm muscle circumference, measurement of, 212, 212t
Asbestos, as carcinogen, 47
L-Asparaginase, 168
Aspirin, 233, 234(t), 235
Autopsy, psychological, 323
Awareness of Dying, 299
Axilla, physical examination of, 71
5-Azacytidine, 163

Bacillus Calmette-Guérin, 194
    complications of, 199
Backrub, 220, 231
Basal energy expenditure, 213
Basic care, 83–84
Bereavement groups, 349
Beliefs, negative, 279
Beta particles, 123
Betatron, 125

Biopsies, 74
Bladder, cancer screening of, *373*
    catheterization of, 239
Bleeding, 244–245
    increased risk of, chemotherapy and, 187
Bleomycin (Blenoxane), 159–160
Blood, clotting of, increased, 35
    flow, 30
    route, 32
    tests, 73
Blood-forming tissues, radiotherapy and, 134
Blocking factor, 28
Body image, altered, 283–284
Body metabolism, 35–37, 210
Body reaction, to radiotherapy, 125, 134
Bone, pathologic fractures of, 252–253
    radiotherapy and, 136
    tumors, in children, 291–292
Bone marrow, aspiration of, 74
    depression of, chemotherapy and, 172–173, 172–173(t)
    transplantation of, 289
Brain tumors, in children, 290
Breast, cancer of, 44
    risk factors in, 55(t)
    screening for, *370*
    examination of, 71
    radiotherapy and, 136
Burkitt's lymphoma, 290
Busulfan, 158

Cachexia, 209–216, 212t
Cancer, beliefs about, research in, 5
    categorization of, 74–76
    changing impact of, 7–8
    classification of, 76, 76t
    connotations of, 3
    effects of, on health care, 5–7
    expressions about, in literature, 4–5
    incidence of, 62, *63*
    negative beliefs about, 279
    registries, as research approach, 41
    social consequences of, 3–4
    theories of, 42–43
    therapy of, aggressive philosophy of, 8–9
        conservative philosophy of, 7
        unproven methods of, 374, 375–377(t), 379
Caplan, G., 342

Carbohydrate metabolism, 36
  following surgery, 110
Carcinoembryonic antigen, 33–34
Carcinogens, chemical, 44–50
  classification of, 45
Carmustine (BCNU), 158
Carotid blowout, 245
Cartilage, radiotherapy and, 136
Catheterization, bladder, 239
Cell(s), adoptive immunity of, 196
  cancer, biology of, 24–27
  cycle, 21, *21*
    chemotherapy and, 147
    in cancer, 25
  differentiated, 22
  doubling time of, 103, *104*
  hypoxic, 127
  kill, chemotherapy and, 148
  kinetics, 25
  proliferation of, 31
  radiation damage to, 126–127
  resting, 22
  stem, 29
  structure and function of, 19–21
Cell-mediated immunity, 23, *23*
Cell membrane, 19–20
  in cancer, 24–25
Cellular immunity, 27
Centrioles, 20
Cervical cancer screening, *372*
Cesium-137 teletherapy unit, 124
Chalones, 28–29
Chemicals, as carcinogens, 44–50
  in food, 56–58
Chemotherapy, 8, 146–190
  administration of drugs in, 179–184
  alkylating agents in, 157–158, 157(t)
  alopecia following, 175, 188
  antibiotics in, 158–160, 159(t)
  antimetabolites in, 161–163, 161(t)
  assessment of drug effect of, 184
  bone marrow depression in, 172–173,
    172–173(t)
  calculating doses of, 168, *169–171*
  development of drug resistance to, 155
  development of new drugs for, 148–150
  diarrhea following, 185–186
  fatigue following, 187–188
  for leukemia, 289
  gastrointestinal toxicity in, 173, 175
  hormones in, 163–166, 164(t)
  host variables in, 151–155, 152–153(t),
    154
  increased risk of bleeding with, 187
  increased risk of infection with, 186–187
  mechanisms of action of, 146–148,
    147–148
  mutagenicity, 175
  nausea and vomiting following, 184–185
  nursing assessment prior to, 176–178,
    178(t)
  nursing interventions prior to, 178–179
  pharmacology of, 155–156, *156*
  radiotherapy and, 129–130, 151
  stomatitis following, 185
  tumor variables in, 150–151
  vinca alkaloids in, 160–161, 167(t)
Chest, physical examination of, 71
Childhood cancer, 288–297

Chlorambucil (Leukeran), 158
Chromosome(s), 21
  Philadelphia, 44
Cisplatin, 168
Classification, of cancer, 76, 76(t)
Clinic, outpatient, 99
Clinical case studies, as research
  approach, 41
Clomiphene (Clomid), 165
Clone formation, 27–29
Cobalt-60 teletherapy unit, 124
Cocarcinogen, definition of, 45
Coherence, sense of, 363, 365
Coley's toxin, 193–194
Colon, cancer of, *57*
Colony stimulating factor, 24
Colorectal cancer screening, *371*
Colostomy, 107, 335–336
Communication, effective, 266–269
Community cancer center, 99
Community health nursing, 352–353
Complement, 24
Confrontation, 272
Constipation, 92, 245–248
Contract, for home health care, 357
Coping strategies, 263(t)
  promotion of effective, 268–274, *270,*
    271–272(t)
    adaptation, 269–270
    defenses, 269
  with pain, 223
Cortisol, 165
Cortisone, 165
Corynebacterium parvum, 194
  complications of, 199
Cosmegen, 159
Cutaneous stimulation, for pain, 231–232
Cyclophosphamide (Cytoxan), 157–158
Cytarabine, 162–163
Cytoplasm, 20

Dacarbazine (DTIC), 158
Dactinomycin, 159
Daunomycin, 158–159
o,p'DDD, 166
DDP, 168
Death rates, *63–65, 68, 369*
Decisions, quality of life and, 81–84
Decubiti, *254,* 255–256, *257,* 258
Dedifferentiation, of cells, 26
Defenses, as coping strategy, 269
Delalutin, 165
Denial, 279–280
Dependency and passivity, 283
Depression and grief, 281–282
Derepression, 42–43
Dexamethasone, 165
Diagnosis, 62–76, 106
  family and, 275–276
  stage of cancer at, *67*
Diagnostic screening, 370–371, *370–374,*
  373–374
Diarrhea, 92, 248–249
  following chemotherapy, 185–186
Diet, as carcinogen, 55–58
Diethylstilbestrol, 164
Distraction, for pain, 228

Dosimetry, 125–126, *126*
Doubling time, for cells, 29
  chemotherapy and, 147
Doxorubicin (Adriamycin), 158–159
Draining wounds, 249–250
Dressings, 240
Drugs. See also *Chemotherapy.*
  carcinogenic, 49–50, 50(t)
  for pain, 232–233, 233–234(t), 235, *236*
Dying, 298–328
  child and, 295
  family and, 278, 317–319
  home care of the, 319–320
  hospice care of the, 320–323
  institutional care of the, 319
  meaning of, 304–307
  nursing care of the, 309–317, 323–326
  physiology of, 307–308
  psychological autopsy of the, 323
  theory of, 298–304
Dysgeusia, 209
Dyspnea, in dying, 311

Ear, radiotherapy and, 135
Elimination, dying and, 310
Elspar (L-Asparaginase), 168
Embolism, pulmonary, 242–244, 243(t)
Emotional factors, 58
Emotional responses, to pain, 222
Endometrial cancer, risk factors in, 55
Endoplasmic reticulum, 20
  in cancer, 25
Endoscopic examinations, 73
Enemas, 237
Epidemiology, as research approach, 40
Epidermitis, 133
Estrogens, 164
Ethical decisions, 78–80
Etiology of cancer, 39–61
Ewing's sarcoma, 291
Expectations, social role, 9–15
  nursing and, 15–16
Extremities, physical examination of, 72
Eyes, dying and, 309–310
  physical examination of, 70
  radiotherapy and, 135

Face and mouth cancer, rehabilitation for, 338
Family(ies), 94
  caring for, 98, 274–278
  dying and, 317–319
  groups, 348
  in childhood cancer, 294
  nursing history of, 70
  support, during pain, 235–236
  therapy, 341
Fat, metabolism of, following surgery, 110–111
  stores, muscle mass and, 212(t)
Fatigue, following chemotherapy, 187–188
  following surgery, 112
Fear, 282

Feelings, communicating and exploring, 313–314
  impact on diagnosis, 62
Feifel, H., 304
Fever, high, 240
Financial factors, chemotherapy and, 154
Fistulas, 249–250
5-Fluorouracil, 162
Fluoxymestrone (Halotestin), 165
Food, chemicals in, 56–58
  intake, altered, 35
Formalism, as ethical theory, 79
Fractures, pathologic, 252–253
Fragmentation of care, 94–95

Gamma rays, 124
Gastrointestinal toxicity, chemotherapy and, 173, 175
Generalized Resistance Resources, 365, 368
Genetic factors, 42–44, 43(t)
Genitalia, physical examination of, 71–72
Goals, development of, 97
Golgi complex, 20
Gompertzian growth curve, 147–148, *147*
Gonads, radiotherapy and, 135
Grading, of cancer cells, 75
Grief, depression and, 281–282
Group dynamics, 341
Group therapy, 341
Guided imagery, for pain, 230

Hair, care of, in the dying, 309
  loss, 175, 188
Halotestin, 165
Head, physical examination of, 70
Head and neck surgery, 108
Health care, effects of cancer on, 5–7
Heart, radiotherapy and, 135
Hemorrhage, 244–245
Heredity, cancer and, 44
Herpesviruses, cancer and, 52–53
Hexamethylmelamine, 167
High fever, 240
High risk groups, 369–370
Histiocytic lymphoma, 290
Hodgkin's disease, 8
  in children, 290
Homans' sign, 241
Home care, 99, 352–361
  for dying, 319–320
  in childhood cancer, 294–295
Hormones, 29, 54–55, 163–166, 164(t)
  thymic, 198
Hospice care, 320–323
Hospital care, 89–101
Hostility, anger and, 280–281
Humoral immunity, 22
Hydration, for dying, 311
Hydromorphone (Dilaudid), 233(t)
Hydroxyprogesterone caproate, 165
Hydroxyurea (Hydrea), 166
Hyperthermia, 132

Hypnosis, for pain, 229
Hypogeusesthesia, 209
Hypoxic cells, 127

Ileal conduit, 336–337
Imagery, for pain, 230
Immune responses, alteration of, 104
Immune ribonucleic acid, 196
Immune system, 22–24, *23,* 27–28
  failure of, 54
Immunity, decreased, following surgery,
  112
Immunocompetence, decreased, 35
Immunologic factors, chemotherapy and,
  153–154
Immunotherapy, 191–206
  active nonspecific, 193–195
  active specific, 195, 199
  adoptive immunity, 196–197
  combination, 199
  complications of, 199–200
  effectiveness of, 200, 201(t)
  immunorestorative, 197–198
  local, 198–199
  passive, 195–196, 200
  process of, 200–205, *203*
Impaired mobility, 253–255
Industrial carcinogens, 46–47
Infection, 237–241, 237(t)
  increased risk of, chemotherapy and,
    186–187
  with childhood cancer, 292–293
Institution, cancer beliefs and, 7
Institutional care, for dying, 319
Intensive care unit, 99
Interferon, 24, 197
Interstitial fluid, in tumor, 30
Intravenous sites, 239
Ionizing rays, types of, 122–124
Isolation, 283

Justice, as ethical theory, 79

Kidney, radiotherapy and, 135
Kubler-Ross, E., 302–303

Laryngectomy, 337–338
Laxatives, use of, 247
Leavell and Clark's model of prevention,
  363, *364*
Legislative rights, health care and, 80
Leukemia, acute lymphatic, 8
  chronic myelocytic, 44
  in children, 288–290
Leukeran, 158
Levamisole, 198
  complications of, 199
Levorphanol, 233(t)
Life review, 314
Linear accelerators, 124
Linear energy transfer radiation, 131
Lipid metabolism, 36

Liver, angiosarcoma of, 46
  radiotherapy and, 135
Lofland, L. H., 305–306
Lomustine (CCNU), 158
Lung(s), cancer of, 44
    hemorrhage with, 245
    screening for, *372*
  embolism of, 242–244, 243(t)
  radiotherapy and, 135
Lymph node permeability factor, 24
Lymph route, 32
Lymphatics and lymph nodes, role of, 105
Lymphedema, 250–252
Lymphokines, 23–24, 27, 197–198
Lymphoma, in children, 290
Lymphotoxin, 24
Lysodren, 166
Lysosomes, 20

Macrophages, 27
Malnutrition. See *Nutrition.*
Massage, 231
Mastectomy, 107, 337
  lymphedema with, 251–252
McGill-Melzack Pain Assessment
  Questionnaire, *224–225*
Meaning, search for, 315
Mechlorethamine hydrochloride, 157
Megestrol acetate (Megace), 165
Melphalan, 158
Meperidine, 232, 233(t)
6-Mercaptopurine, 163
Metabolic changes, 35–37
Metabolic rate, increased, 37
Metabolic response to surgery, *109,*
  110–113
Metabolism, 210
Metastasis, 31–33
  residual, effect of, 105
Methadone (Dolophine), 233(t)
Methotrexate, 161–162
Mid-arm muscle circumference, 212, 212t
Migration inhibitory factor, 23–24
Mithramycin (Mithracin), 160
Mitochondria, 20
  in cancer, 25
Mitomycin-C (Mutamycin), 160
Mitotane, 166
Mobility, degree of, chemotherapy and,
    177
  impaired, 253–255
Molecular biology research, 41
Morphine sulfate, 233(t)
Mouth, cancer of, 338
  care of, in the dying, 310
  chemotherapy and, 177
  physical examination of, 70–71
Mucous membranes, radiotherapy and, 132
Multicentric cancers, 105
Muscle mass, and fat stores, 212(t)
Mustargen, 157
Mutagenicity, chemotherapy and, 175

Nafoxidine, 165
Nausea, following chemotherapy, 184–185
  nutrition and, 213
  surgery, 108

Neck, physical examination of, 71
Necrotic centers, 30
Negative pi-mesons, 124
Nervous system, radiotherapy and, 135
Neuroblastoma, in children, 290
Neurologic examination, 72
Neutrons, 124
Nitrogen mustard, 157
Nitroso compounds, as carcinogen, 56
Nitrosoureas, 158
Nolvadex, 165
Nose, care of, in the dying, 309
NSC-13875, 167
NSC-85998, 166–167
NSC-102816, 163
Nucleoside analogues, 162
Nucleus, of cell, 20
    in cancer, 25
Nurse support groups, 349
Nursing care, cancer beliefs and, 6
    psychosocial aspects of, 261–287
    related to physiologic conditions,
        209–260, *210*
Nursing history, 69–70
Nursing research needs, 379–380
Nurturing, 266
Nutrition, 210–216
    chemotherapy and, 152–153, 176
    for the dying, 311
    in childhood cancer, 293

Odors, control of, in infections, 240
    in draining wounds, 250
Omega vulnerability rating scale, *264–265*
On Death and Dying, 302–303
Oncogene theory, 53
Oncology intensive care unit, 99
Oncology outpatient clinic, 99
Oncology unit, 96–99
Oncovin, 160–161
Operative care, 116–117
Option rights, health care and, 80
Organelles, 20–21
    in cancer, 25
Orthovoltage X-ray machine, 124, *125*
Osteosarcoma, 292
Outpatient clinic, 99
Ovary, cancer of, 55
Oxymorphone (Numorphan), 233(t)

Pain, 216–237
    assessment of, 218–223, *221,* 222(t),
        224–225
    dying and, 311
    factors influencing, 216–218, *218*
    family support during, 235–236
    in childhood cancer, 293
    interventions for, 227–235
    relief of, 81–83
        evaluation of, 236–237
        planning for, 223, 226–227
Palliation, 106
L-PAM, 158
Pap smears, 73, 75
Paraneoplastic syndromes, 34
Passivity, dependency and, 283

Pathologic fractures, 252–253
Patient, cancer beliefs and, 6
    groups, 348
    teaching, 72
Pediatric oncology, 288–297
Perineal care, 239
Personal care, 91–93, 98
Personal growth, 278
Pharmacology, of chemotherapeutic drugs,
    155–156, *156*
Phenylalanine mustard, 158
Philadelphia chromosome, 44
Philosophy of care, establishment of, 96–97
Physical examination, 70–72
Physician, cancer beliefs and, 6
Physiologic conditions, nursing care
    related to, 209–260, *210*
Plan of care, design of, 97–98
Platinum complexes, 168
Political arena, nursing and, 369
Polycyclic aromatic hydrocarbons, as
    carcinogen, 56–57
Positioning, for the dying, 310
Postoperative care, 117–120
Precarcinogen, definition of, 45
Prednisone, 165
Preoperative care, 113–116
Pressure, 34
Pressure sores, *254,* 255–256, *257,* 258
Preterminality, family and, 277
Prevention, philosophy of, 363, *364,* 365,
    366–367
    primary, 368–370
    secondary, 370–379
Primary tumor, removal of, 104
Procarbazine, 166
Progestins, 165
Proliferation inhibitory factor, 24
Prostaglandins, 24
Protein binding, 156
Protein metabolism, 35–36
    following surgery, 110
Psychological autopsy, 323
Psychosocial assessment, 261, 262–263(t),
    263, *264–265,* 266(t)
Psychosocial care, 93–94, 98, 261–287
    for dying, 311–317
    in childhood cancer, 293–295
    nursing interventions in, 271–274
Psychosocial factors, chemotherapy and,
    154, 177
Pulmonary embolism, 242–244, 243(t)
Purine analogues, 163
Purinethol, 163

Quackery, 374, 375–377(t), 379
Quality of life, 80–81

Radiation, 50–52, 51(t)
Radiodermatitis, 133
Radiographic examinations, 72–73
Radiosensitivity, 129
Radiotherapy, 122–145
    alteration of tumor kinetics in, 127–128,
        128
    cell biology and, 126–127

Radiotherapy (*Continued*)
  chemotherapy and, 129–130, 151
  complications of, 132–136, 133(t)
  dosimetry, 125–126, *126*
  effect on body tissue of, 125
  effect on immune response of, 128–129
  effectiveness of, 129–132, 130(t), *131*
  equipment for, 124, 125, *125*
  external, 136–138
    nursing care with, 140–142
  internal, 138–140, *139*
    after loading of, 139
    nursing care with, 142–144
  response to, 128
  skin-sparing effect of, 125
  terms used in, 123(t)
  types of ionizing rays, 122–123
Rapid tissue proliferation, 54
Recognition factor, 28
Reconstruction, 106
Recurrence, family and, 277
Rectum, physical examination of, 72
Redefining, 273
Registries, cancer, 41
Rehabilitation, 92, 331–339
Relationships, 314, 315
Relaxation, for pain, 229–230
Research approaches, 40–42
Research center, 100
Research needs, 379–380
Respiratory infections, 239
Restlessness, in dying, 311
Retinoblastoma, 42, 292
Rhabdomyosarcoma, in children, 291
Ribosomes, 20
  in cancer, 25
Rights and duties, 80
Role changes, 284–285
Role expectations, dying and, 323–324

Saccharin, as carcinogen, 57
Salivary glands, radiotherapy and, 135
L-Sarcolysin, 158
Sarcoma, Ewing's, 291
Screening, diagnostic, 370–371, *370–374,*
  373–374
Self-esteem, loss of, 284–285
Self-help groups, 349
Semustine (Methyl-CCNU), 158
Septic shock, 240
Sexuality, dysfunctional, 284
Skin, carcinogens and, 48
  care of, in the dying, 310
  chemotherapy and, 177
  physical examination of, 70
  radiotherapy and, 125, 133–134
  stimulation, for pain, 231–232
Smoking, 44, 48–49, 370
Social consequences, of cancer beliefs, 3–4
Social history, of patient, 70
Social isolation, 283
Social role expectations, 9–15
  nursing and, 15–16
Social support systems, strengthening of,
  278–279
Social work groups, 342
Sodium, tumor growth and, 36–37

Staffing problems, 90
Staging, of cancer cells, 75–76, 106
Starvation, following surgery, 112
Stem cells, 29
Stomatitis, following chemotherapy, 185
Streptozotocin, 166–167
Stress, 365, 368
Suffering, 223
Support, provision of, 274
Support groups, 340–351
Support systems model, 342, *343*
Surgery, 102–121
  chemotherapy and, 151
  history of, 102–103
  one-stage vs. two-stage procedures,
    105–106
  recovery from, 108, *109,* 110–113
  strategies of, 105–107
Surgical risk, determination of, 108
Survival rates, *66*
Symptoms, 69
  control of, 98
Systems review, 70

Talc, as carcinogen, 57
Tamoxifen, 165
Taste, 209
  change in, 35
Teaching, as coping strategy, 272–273
  patient, 72
Testolactone (Teslac), 165
Testosterone propionate, 165
Tests, diagnostic, 72–74
Therapeutic touch, for pain, 232
Therapy, family, 341
  group, 341
Thermal regulation, alteration of, 112
6-Thioguanine, 163
Thrombophlebitis, 241–242, *241–242*
Thymic hormones, 198
Thymus, 23, 27
Thyroid gland, radiotherapy and, 136
Tissues, blood-forming, radiotherapy and,
  134
  body, effect of radiation on, 125
Tobacco, as carcinogen, 48–49
Total parenteral nutrition, 215
Touching, 268
  for pain, 232
Trace elements, 58
  imbalance of, following surgery, 111
Transcutaneous electrical nerve
  stimulation, 232
Transfer factor, 24, 196–197
Transformation, of cells, 26–27
Transmission theories, 53
Treatment, aggressive philosophy of, 8–9
  conservative philosophy of, 7
  failures, 104
  family and, 276
Triceps skin-fold thickness, 212
Triethylenethiophosphoramide
  (Thio-TEPA), 158
Trust, establishment of, 69
Tumor(s), bone, in children, 291–292
  brain, in children, 290
  chemotherapy and, 150–151, 184

Tumor(s) (*Continued*)
  growth, factors affecting, 30
    systemic effects of, 34–37
  kinetics, alteration of, radiotherapy and,
    127–128, *128*
  products produced by, 33–34
  solid, structure of, 30–31
  Wilms', 291
Tumor promoter, definition of, 45
Tumor stemlines, 29–30

Ulcer(s), decubitus, *254*, 255–256, *257*, 258
Ulcerating metastatic lesions, 249–250
Uric acid nephropathy, 289
Uterine cancer screening, *373*
Utilitarianism, as ethical theory, 78–79

Values, 77–78
Vascular network, 30

Vinblastine (Velban), 160
Vinca alkaloids, 160–161, 167(t)
Vincristine (Oncovin), 160–161
Vinyl chloride, 46, 57
Viruses, as carcinogens, 52–54
Vitamins, 58
  metabolism of, following surgery, 111
Vomiting, following chemotherapy,
  184–185
Vulnerability, correlates of, 266(t)
  rating scale, *264–265*

Water, 36
  carcinogens in, 47–48
Weakness, following surgery, 112
Weight loss, following surgery, 112
Weisman, S. D., 304, 306
Welfare rights, health care and, 80
Wilms' tumor, 291
Wound(s), draining, 249–250
  healing of, following surgery, 113